CW00518830

Child Psychopathology

This textbook covers the classification, causes, treatment and prevention of psychological disorders in the infant through the adolescent years. Chapters balance the social and historical context of psychopathology with the physiological roots of abnormal behavior, leading students to a comprehensive understanding of child psychopathology. The book is totally up-to-date, including coverage of DSM-5 and criticisms of it. In four parts, this textbook describes the empirical bases of child psychopathology as well as the practice of child psychologists, outlining the classification and causes of disorders in addition to methods of assessment, intervention and treatment. Students will be able to evaluate the treatments used by professionals and debunk popular myths about atypical behavior and its treatment. Complementing the lively writing style, text boxes, clinical case studies and numerous examples from international cultures and countries add context to chapter material. Study questions, diagrams and glossaries offer further learning support.

Barry H. Schneider is Professor Emeritus of Psychology at the University of Ottawa, now teaching at Boston College.

Child Psychopathology

From Infancy to Adolescence

BARRY H. SCHNEIDER

with Paul Hastings, Amanda Guyer,
Mara Brendgen and Eli Cwinn

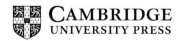

CAMBRIDGE
UNIVERSITY PRESS

CAMBRIDGE
UNIVERSITY PRESS

University Printing House, Cambridge CB2 8BS, United Kingdom

Published in the United States of America by Cambridge University Press, New York

Cambridge University Press is part of the University of Cambridge.

It furthers the University's mission by disseminating knowledge in the pursuit of education, learning and research at the highest international levels of excellence.

www.cambridge.org
Information on this title: www.cambridge.org/9780521152112

© Barry H. Schneider 2014

This publication is in copyright. Subject to statutory exception
and to the provisions of relevant collective licensing agreements,
no reproduction of any part may take place without the written
permission of Cambridge University Press.

First published 2014

Printed in the United Kingdom by TJ International Ltd. Padstow Cornwall

A catalogue record for this publication is available from the British Library

Library of Congress Cataloguing in Publication data

ISBN 978-0-521-19377-1 Hardback
ISBN 978-0-521-15211-2 Paperback

Additional resources for this publication at www.cambridge.org/barryhschneider

Cambridge University Press has no responsibility for the persistence or accuracy
of URLs for external or third-party internet websites referred to in this publication,
and does not guarantee that any content on such websites is, or will remain,
accurate or appropriate.

This book is dedicated to Dr. Sonja Poizner, the supervisor of my first clinical internship. Sonja could not complete her formal education during World War II because she had to flee her native country to escape persecution. She completed her doctorate many years later and then went on to inspire me and many other future psychologists to make judicious use of their knowledge of child psychopathology in the ethical and responsible practice of psychological assessment. She continues to inspire me long after her retirement.

CONTENTS

FIGURES

TABLES

BOXES

PREFACE

In the psychology department where I have taught for the past 32 years, I am regarded as one of the more research-oriented of the clinical-psychology professors and one of the most clinically oriented of the researchers. Although the commitment to bridge research and practice is strong in North America, tension between the two pillars of clinical psychology emerges all too often. Such tension is often much greater in the countries where I have collaborated and worked around the world. My need to resolve as much of this tension as possible for the students I teach and for my overseas colleagues was the primary impetus for this book. My course on child psychopathology has always been among my favorites. However, I have never found a textbook that bridges research and practice very well or one that my students enjoy reading. I have endeavored to provide such a resource by writing this volume. Let me mention some of its distinctive features.

Consistency of writing style. I want to tell the story from the beginning to the end in a coherent way. Therefore, I have been actively involved in writing all the chapters. Except for a few for which I needed the expertise of co-authors in areas that are outside my main fields of competence, I have written them all.

Just the right amount of information. Other books in this field provide either an entertaining but sketchy overview or too much encyclopedic detail.

Empirical basis. It is important to me to teach not only what is known but also how it is known and how well it is known. I have attempted to do this without excessive detail about individual studies or picky methodological objections.

A balanced perspective on the medical model. It is important for students to become familiar with the

DSM and ICD schemes, which are essential tools of the field, without accepting them uncritically.

Social and historical context. Theories and beliefs about child and adolescent psychopathology do not emerge entirely from advances in science. Students should be aware of the roots of new ideas and methods.

Physiology and genetics. Although many psychology students bring little background in these areas to their study of child and adolescent psychology, it is imperative that they familiarize themselves with the physiological bases as well as the social and familial bases of abnormal behavior. Together with colleagues, Paul Hastings, Mara Brendgen and Amanda Guyer, I have presented this material in language that should be accessible even to science-phobes.

A truly multicultural, international perspective. Most previous textbooks in this area mention culture only in passing. It is an undeniable fact that researchers in the United States have been the most active contributors to knowledge in this area. Without minimizing the importance of work done in the United States, this book is suitable for readers around the world. It is my firm belief that students in the United States benefit from an appreciation of the multicultural nature of that country and of the psychological functioning of people in other countries.

Readability. One of my foremost objectives has been to provide a book that is authoritative but also a volume that students will enjoy reading.

Critical but constructive stance. I believe it important for psychology students to neither accept blindly everything they read nor engage in picky, trivial criticism to the point of not appreciating the value of a very useful theory or research study.

Aids to learning

Although I have used non-technical language to the fullest extent possible, glossaries are provided with concise definitions of the terms that the student most needs to know.

Diagrams are provided to illustrate the more complex processes involved in child psychopathology, especially its physiological aspects.

Boxes present interesting material that is sometimes tangential to the main presentation of material but enriching.

Case studies of different lengths are included, first of all, as examples of the disorders and their treatment. Another purpose of these case studies is to portray the children and adolescents affected in a way that increases empathy and reduces stigma. Most of the case studies enable the reader to follow the child through a course of psychological treatment.

Chapter summaries and glossaries are provided to assist students in remembering the material and preparing for examinations.

Study questions are useful to the students in gauging their mastery of the content.

Structure of this book

The book is divided into four parts:

1. Basic concepts and processes. The first part begins with definitional issues pertaining to the delineation of normal and abnormal behavior within the context of normal child and adolescent development. This part includes chapters devoted to the possible causes, processes and correlates of psychological distress, including genetics, physiological roots, family factors, culture and peer relations. A capsule history of the field is included as well. The part concludes with an overview of the work of the psychologist in terms of prevention, assessment and intervention.

2. High-incidence disorders. This part is devoted to the psychological problems that are the most frequently referred to psychologists and about which there has been the most research.

3. Developmental disorders. This part presents a psychological perspective on these disorders, which typically originate during the childhood and adolescent years and that often (but not always) persist throughout the lifespan.

4. Less frequent and less clearly defined forms of psychopathology. This part is devoted to disorders that emerge less frequently than those in the previous parts and/or that are less clearly characterized as separate, well-defined mental health conditions. Some of these conditions are infrequent in childhood and more common in adolescence. These conditions are omitted in some textbooks, which is unfortunate. Less research has been devoted to these disorders than to those discussed in the earlier parts; consequently, these conditions are introduced only briefly. In the last chapter, on gender variance, the issue of what constitutes psychopathology is reprised together with information about the disorder.

Acknowledgements

I would like to thank, first of all, my colleagues and friends, Paul Hastings, Mara Brendgen, and Amanda Guyer, who agreed to collaborate with me on the chapters on genetics and psychophysiology, making those chapters much better than if I had written them myself. I would also like to acknowledge the dedicated assistance of the following gifted psychology students: Julian Caza, Eli Cwinn, Laura Galliana, Tanner McInnis, Kojo Mintah and Jesse Roberts.

Concluding note

The final thing that I would like readers to know is that writing this book has been an immense pleasure.

Part I | Basic concepts and processes

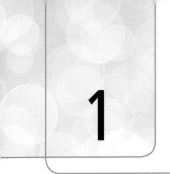

1

Normality and abnormality in the context of human development
Basic definitions

> The difference between a word and the right word is like the difference between lightning and a lightning bug.
>
> MARK TWAIN

> A word is not a crystal, transparent and unchanging; it is the skin of a living thought and may vary greatly in color and content according to the circumstances and time in which it is used.
>
> OLIVER WENDELL Holmes (Justice of the US Supreme Court)

Scholars of several disciplines use different terms to refer to children's psychological problems. The quest for a global descriptor that is accurate and that avoids stigma has so far been unsuccessful. In fact, there is probably not even a euphemism that enables its users to avoid debatable analogies and connotations that they would probably prefer not to evoke. This chapter is devoted to definitional issues, starting with the definitions of pathology and disease. Problems with all of the terms in common use to describe children's and adolescents' psychological problems are highlighted. Many of the issues raised in this chapter recur in subsequent chapters on the classification of mental illness and the physiological basis of child and adolescent psychopathology. Estimates of the total prevalence of psychopathology appear near the end of the chapter, followed by remarks about the notion of recovery in the context of mental illness.

Pathology; disease

Although the concepts of mental illness and disease have existed since ancient times, it is only in the past 200 years that coherent attempts have been made to differentiate transitory problems associated with the stressful experiences suffered by most

people from full-blown conditions that merit more enduring concern and professional care. The German psychiatrist, Karl Kahlbaum, renowned in his own time but almost unknown since, is credited with introducing, in 1863, the idea that the concept of mental illness should include the course of the illness, its effect on the individual's psychological well-being, the developmental stage at which it occurred and any accompanying conditions to which it might be secondary. Kahlbaum also applied these ideas to the study of children's mental disorders, especially early forms of psychosis (Kahlbaum and Berrios, 2007; Millon, Grossman and Meagher, 2004). His delineation of mental illness and health, with considerable refinement, has become an integral part of mainstream thinking about child psychopathology.

The word "pathology" is composed of two Greek words that refer to illness and to knowledge or understanding. This term is used to refer to the gathering of knowledge about the causes and effects of disease or diseases. Psychopathology is, thus, the science of the diseases that affect a person's psyche or mind. The *Oxford English Dictionary* (Simpson and Weiner, 1989) lists several alternative definitions of the noun "disease," all of which could arguably be considered descriptive of the major psychological problems of childhood:

absence of ease; uneasiness, discomfort; inconvenience, annoyance; disquiet, disturbance; trouble. (For long *Obs.* but revived in modern use with the spelling *dis-ease*.)

a cause of discomfort or distress; a trouble, an annoyance, a grievance. *Obs.*

a condition of the body, or of some part or organ of the body, in which its functions are disturbed or deranged; a morbid physical condition; "a departure from the state of health, especially when caused by structural change." Also applied to a disordered condition in plants.

an individual case or instance of such a condition; an illness, ailment, malady, disorder.

any one of the various kinds of such conditions; a species of disorder or ailment, exhibiting special symptoms or affecting a special organ.

fig. A deranged, depraved, or morbid condition (of mind or disposition, of the affairs of a community, etc.); an evil affection or tendency.

The term *disorder* is very closely related to the term *disease.* Although the original meaning of the word "disorder" is confusion or lack of order, that noun in the context of psychological problems signifies "an illness that disrupts normal physical or mental functions" (Simpson and Weiner, 1989).

Not all of these definitions inherently imply that a psychological illness has the exact characteristics of a physical illness, although the term psychopathology inevitably evokes that association. The *medical model* is often attributed to Freud, who was indeed a physician and who became interested in studying and treating the problem of hysteria among women in Vienna in the 1920s. He described the hysteria as a disease and described his "talking cure," which might involve, for example, allowing a sufferer to express grief over a traumatic event, as a treatment to be administered by a "doctor." This delighted many of his contemporaries who had previously believed that mental illness was biologically caused and incurable.

The *medical model* is the prevailing mode of thinking and communicating by and among many if not most professionals in the mental health field. It has become common in everyday conversation to refer to individuals suffering from psychological distress as "sick." Critic David Elkins has remarked that many psychologists use medical model language so readily that they do not realize that they are doing so, being no more capable of articulating the model than fish are capable of explaining what water is (Elkins, 2009).

However, there are fervent objections to the medical model, with the most vociferous articulated by proponents of the anti-psychiatry movement in North America and the Critical Psychiatry Network in the UK. The best-known opponents of the medical model are the late Scottish psychiatrist R. D. Laing (e.g., Laing, 1960) and late Hungarian-born American psychiatrist Thomas Szasz. Szasz, for example, objects to applying the concept of "disease" to difficulties of human thoughts, emotions and relationships. He would prefer that we referred to such psychological difficulties as *problems in living.* A disease, Szasz insists, is caused by a bodily lesion that a physician can identify and treat, as by medication or surgery. Problems in living do not work this way, he argues. He offers the analogy of a television program that is not of high quality. A technician or repairman could do nothing to improve it. Szasz argues that members of the health professions cannot improve the quality of human interactions by working on the "wiring." They propagate this myth, he insists, because their professional status is maintained and enhanced by this kind of thinking. Unfortunately, he continues, the medical model restricts the freedom of many individuals afflicted by problems in living and stigmatizes them unnecessarily (Bracken and Thomas, 2010; Szasz, 1974, 2007). Along similar lines, the late French philosopher and social critic Michel Foucault maintained that, over the past two centuries, society has been targeting the mentally ill as objects of abuse who can be isolated, repressed and punished, replacing the lepers who filled the roles of outcasts in earlier eras (Foucault, 2006). There has been similar criticism of the "medicalization" of child psychiatry. For example, Timimi (2002), a child and adolescent psychiatrist who works for the British National Health Service in Lincolnshire, compares "biomedical" child psychiatry to a religious cult, a cult that practices racism and sexism and imperialistically imposes Western values on non-Western peoples. Disputing the very existence of the disease entities that occupy the time of contemporary child psychiatrists and psychologists, Timimi advocates a diagnosis-free helping process in which therapists and their clients exchange, as equals, their personal narratives and the feelings they arouse. Needless to say, Szasz, Timimi and those who share their views reflect only the opinion of a vociferous minority, whose opinions are repudiated by most of their colleagues. More will be said in the next chapter about the historical evolution of the medical model and about ideas pertaining to the causation of psychological disorders during the childhood years.

Mental or psycho-

The adjective "mental" in "mental illness," "mental disorder," "mental health," and even "mental hygiene" has been the subject of almost as much controversy as the nouns that the adjective is used to describe. The prefix "psycho-" similarly implies that the location of psychological distress is in the mind or psyche. However, any such dichotomy of mind and body is incongruent with what has been known for a long time about the ways in which physiological processes affect thinking and behavior. The dynamic interplay of biological and mental processes has been known since ancient times. The rejection in modern medical science of any artificial distinction between the two is sometimes attributed to the influential psychiatrist Adolf Meyer (1866–1950), who taught that human beings are integral organisms. Their thoughts and emotions can affect biological function down to the cellular and biochemical level. Conversely, processes

at the lowest biological levels can affect thoughts and emotions (Cicchetti, 2006).

Georgaca (2013) observed that many people with mental illness find it comfortable to believe and assert that their problems are of physiological origin. They see doing so as legitimizing their problems and relieving themselves of responsibility for them. On the other hand, anything they might then say about their problems may be understood by other people as the result of the distorted thinking of a "sick" person.

Atypical or abnormal

The concept of normality and its opposite, abnormality, can be interpreted in a number of different ways, each conveying different metaphors and each having advantages and disadvantages. Abnormality can be understood, first of all, statistically: What is quantitatively unusual or atypical is considered abnormal. This does, of course, have the advantage of objectivity; all that is needed is information about the frequency in the population of the behavior in question. Invocation of the adjective "atypical," however, can also be construed as a glorification of the typical. Some infrequent behaviors can be innocuous, even positive. Creative genius, for example, is rare. It is surely inappropriate to consider a child who cultivates musical, artistic, literary or mathematical talents as abnormal, however few such children might be.

Furthermore, there may be nothing inherently wrong or dysfunctional with behaviors that characterize a minority. The classic example of this is homosexual behavior, which, after a generation-long battle within the mental health professions, is no longer considered abnormal per se. Hence, although many authors use the terms *atypical development* and *atypical behavior*, few do so wanting to reinforce the tyranny of the majority in any way. It is important to note that, as with much of the terminology discussed in this section, the adjective "abnormal" has acquired a negative connotation in common parlance that is not inherent in its dictionary definition.

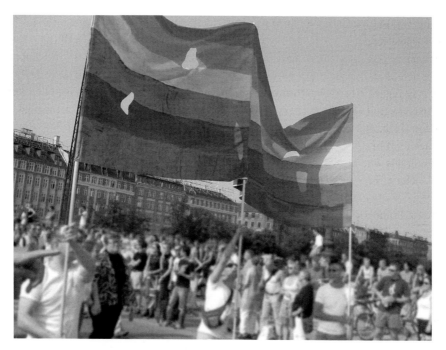

Figure 1.1 Homosexuality is no longer regarded as a mental disorder.

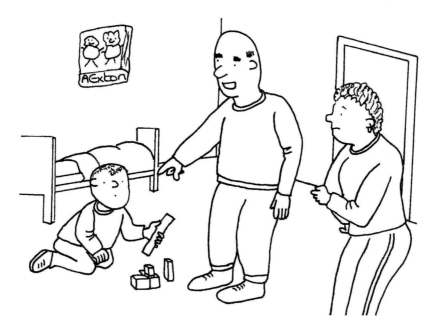

"You'll have to excuse George: he suffers from perfectly normal child disorder."

Figure 1.2 "Symptoms" must be understood against the backdrop of normal human development.

Discarding the notion of atypical or abnormal in the strict statistical sense in favor of a definition based on what society defines as abnormal does not constitute much of an improvement because many cultures may regard some behaviors or traits as deviant for reasons that are arbitrary or even wrong from a moral standpoint. Even though the behaviors need not interfere with either the lives of the individuals who display them or the functioning of society, the sanctions imposed by the culture may create maladjustment for the stigmatized group. Homosexuality is, again, the classic example.

Abnormal as maladaptive

Mealey (2005) proposes an evolutionary definition of normality/abnormality in which traits, behaviors or attributes that reduce an individual's chances of adaptation, survival and reproduction are considered abnormal. He extends this concept to traits, behaviors and attributes that may not necessarily affect the likelihood of survival, adaptation and reproduction of the people who exhibit them but which interfere with the potential of other people to survive, adapt and reproduce. As an example in child psychopathology, he cites conduct disorder, which violates the rights of other children and/or adults even though it may enable the child diagnosed with conduct disorder to achieve some misguided objective of their own.

This evolutionary definition is somewhat different from a medical definition of abnormality, which refers to some part of the human organism not working properly. Related to it is the notion that the dividing line between normal and abnormal should be drawn on the basis of danger to the person or to those around him or her (Comer, 2006). This concept is not invoked very frequently because many forms of child psychopathology, disabling as they may be, constitute no real danger to anyone but those who suffer. This is especially the case for anxiety and depression, which are very common.

Emphasizing the dysfunction in daily living that results from a disorder or condition has been widespread since Freud, who, in response to a question, stated that *lieben und arbeiten* (love and work) are the defining features of adaptation, happiness and mental health. In reflecting on how this idea might be applied to adjustment and maladjustment during childhood, eminent American child psychologist David Elkind suggested adding the element *spielen*, play, as the work of children (Elkind, 1988). Elkind is a fierce opponent of young children being pressured into precocious academic achievement and adult roles. However, it is certainly reasonable to consider schooling from the start of formal education as the major work of children. Given the importance of relations with other children for adjustment from that stage on, schooling and relationships might well be considered the childhood analogues of work and love in the adult psychoanalytic literature. Whatever disrupts success in those two domains might be considered pathological.

Development, not individuals, seen as abnormal, atypical or pathological

It is important to reflect upon exactly what is considered maladaptive, abnormal or atypical – children or their development. A basic precept of the emerging interdisciplinary field of developmental psychopathology is that the focus should be on development. Development can be considered abnormal, atypical or dysfunctional if it fails to achieve its purpose, which is to bring about adaptation to the environment and maturity (Cicchetti, 2006). The field of developmental psychopathology is based on the centrality of developmental processes in the conceptualization of mental illness and mental health. One of its core assumptions is that much can be learned about normal functioning by studying abnormal functioning and that, vice versa, studying abnormal developmental patterns can help elucidate the nature of normal developmental patterns (Cicchetti, 2006; Rutter and Stevenson, 2010).

Developmental psychopathology has been defined as "the study of the origins and course of individual patterns of behavioral maladaptation" (Sroufe and Rutter, 1984, p. 18). Developmental psychopathologists focus on the interplay between normal and abnormal development. Individuals can "cross the line" between normal and abnormal in either direction at many different points in life. The maladaptive symptoms evident at the moment at which they surface must be understood in broader perspective as elements of a process that has been going on for a long time and that will continue. The onset of a disorder is unlikely to be the one-to-one, linear result of some traumatic event, although a traumatic event may be its trigger (Perret and Faure, 2006). Therefore, it is important for researchers to study the development of individuals throughout the lifespan, focusing particularly on important transition points. Developmental psychopathologists are interested in comparing the *trajectories* of development for individuals who are and who are not experiencing psychological difficulties. They seek to learn why individuals who have experienced different background conditions and processes may end up in the same state (*equifinality*) and why individuals who start out at essentially the same point and seem initially to be developing in the same ways turn out differently at the end (*multifinality*). In illustrating the concept of a developmental trajectory, Sroufe (1997) offers the metaphor of a growing tree. Its various branches share a common trunk, representing the species-wide programming for development, which then subdivide and grow in their own directions. However, they might meet again, at some later stage. A developing child may follow a trajectory consisting only of successful adaptation to the successive crucial tasks that are encountered at different stages. Another individual's trajectory may start and continue with unsuccessful adaptation. Individuals following a trajectory that starts with successful adaptation at the early stages of development but continues into a failure to adapt

at later stages are likely to come to the attention of mental health professionals. However, the opposite trajectory – starting with a failure to adapt that is overcome at later stages – is highly informative, though often overlooked, as will be discussed shortly.

In the few decades since the emergence of developmental psychopathology as a movement and way of thinking, considerable progress has been made in tracing across time and developmental stages the course of many forms of adjustment and maladjustment. Still, much less is discussed about resistance to disease than about susceptibility to it. This is true of both physical and mental diseases throughout the lifespan. *Resilience* or *resiliency* refer to the capacity to achieve good adaptation despite being exposed to risk factors. The study of the processes associated with resilience is especially important in developmental psychopathology. Resilience has emerged as a distinct area of enquiry in the past 40 years, although as a research field it is minuscule in comparison to the largely opposite processes by which a child comes to display a mental health problem. Much of the initial impetus for studying the *protective factors* that may explain why some children who are exposed to many of the *risk factors* that often lead to mental illness came from the identification of some individuals who failed to develop adult schizophrenia despite clear signs that they are at risk because of genetic endowment or parental history of psychosis. The late American psychologist Norman Garmezy coined the term *invulnerable* to refer to this phenomenon (Garmezy, 1991). Hopefully, researchers will continue the legacy left by his pioneering work, equipped with the scientific knowledge and tools that have emerged in recent years in the areas of behavioral and molecular genetics (see Chapter 4).

Developmental psychopathologists emphasize the study of human development across the lifespan. They emphatically refute the contention that an individual's destiny is fully shaped in the early childhood years although they very definitely recognize the importance of those years. Instead, they argue that an individual is affected by experiences that occur at all points in life (Perret and Faure, 2006; Sroufe et al., 1999). Despite its emphasis on development across the lifespan, the developmental psychopathology movement has done much to facilitate a conceptualization of psychopathology that is suitable for children. It has disseminated a depiction of children not as junior adults but as organisms that are undergoing active growth and change and who are adjusting to a social environment that is itself undergoing change in most cases. It has been several centuries since childhood has been regarded by most of Western society as a distinct period characterized by its own challenges and miracles. We no longer think of children as adults-to-be needing a bit of care before they can assume their places at work in the fields beside their parents and older members of their communities. Instead, we now provide schools and other institutions to foster their development in a variety of ways. However, it unfortunately remains important to invoke quite frequently the fact that conceptual schemes designed to organize the mental health field in general may not fully fit the trials experienced by children and adolescents. Also overlooked all too frequently is the fact that the developing minds and bodies of children are not likely to react to treatments of all kinds in the same ways that adult bodies and minds do.

At the same time as it has raised awareness of the importance of developmental processes, the field of developmental psychopathology has raised the methodological standards of the research that is needed before ideas are accepted and rejected. It has done so by placing a premium on longitudinal research, especially longitudinal research that encompasses multiple causal factors, both genetic and environmental, as well as multiple outcomes. Influential longitudinal studies of child psychopathology have been conducted not only in large cities of the United States and the UK but also in such places as the Hawaiian island of Kauai (Werner, 1989), the Isle of Wight, off the southern coast of England (Rutter et al., 1970) and the island nation of Mauritius in the Indian Ocean (Raine et al., 2010).

Developmental psychopathologists might not object to the diagnosis of a disorder in a child at a particular moment in time. However, they have done much to remind us that the moment in time at which the diagnosis occurs is just that – a moment in time. That diagnosis might be just one part of the data that should be considered in studying the developmental trajectory of an individual in distress and in gathering the information needed to help bring that individual back onto a trajectory of adaptation to successive developmental tasks. Other data that might inform the demarcation of a developmental trajectory might consist of overt behaviors, information about interpersonal relationships and internal mental representations of the self and of the social environment (Perret and Faure, 2006; Sroufe et al., 2000).

Developmental psychopathologists revere the natural processes of human development but do not resist efforts at changing them to assist individuals or groups of individuals who are experiencing challenges in adapting to their environment. In fact, they regard intervention as a learning opportunity. By changing one element in a sequence of events, much can be learned about the effects of the phenomenon that has been modified. The eminent American developmental psychologist Uri Bronfenbrenner influenced the field by proposing that "if you want to understand something, try to change it" (Bronfenbrenner, 1979; Perret and Faure, 2006).

Although prediction in the field of child psychopathology remains a very imprecise endeavor, the longitudinal studies that have emerged in the past century have greatly enhanced understanding of the comings and goings of the psychological disorders that affect too many children and adolescents. Among the important first fruits of the developmental psychopathology movement are the findings that certain forms of disorder, such as disruptive behavior disorders (see Chapter 12) tend to be more or less debilitating and more or less stable depending on the ages at which they first appear. The challenge facing the next generations of theorists and practitioners is not only how to continue and refine this longitudinal research but also to discover how to use the findings to alter the course of psychopathology over the childhood and adolescent years.

How common is child psychopathology?

Prevalence refers to the number of people in a sample or population who are affected by a particular disorder. Incidence rates indicate the number of new cases that are diagnosed within a specified time frame, often 1 year. One of the reasons why it is difficult to estimate the population prevalence of child psychopathology is the divergence in the ways in which psychopathology can be defined, as discussed in the previous sections of this chapter. Another difficulty is the fact that many children suffer from psychological problems that never come to the attention of professionals. Therefore, although data on the use of professional time for the mental health problems of children and youth are interesting for other reasons, they do not provide the best estimates of the rate of psychopathology. Better answers come from studies in which large samples of the child population are screened for indicators of psychological problems. Population estimates can be derived, first of all, by tallying the numbers of children who can be diagnosed as suffering from a particular disorder. As will be discussed in Chapter 3, the result will depend on the diagnostic criteria used. For example, many children may be very sad but their sadness does not reach the level or the chronicity needed to formally diagnose them as having major depression. Therefore, there are advantages to estimating the prevalence of psychopathology according to the known prevalence of some of the behaviors that are linked to it, such as suicide or substance abuse.

The time span studied is an important variable in the interpretation of prevalence data. It is of some interest to find out how many children display signs of psychopathology at a particular moment in time. It is, however, probably more important to determine how many will experience mental health problems over their lifetime or significant parts of it. This is studied more rigorously by following the same children over a period of years in a longitudinal study, avoiding a number of possible pitfalls in a *cross-sectional* study – one in which children of different ages are studied at one specific moment. Furthermore, only a longitudinal research strategy can help distinguish between transitory difficulties that will usually disappear with maturity and stable problems that all too often persist over a lifetime.

Another issue to be considered is the age at which the study begins; relatively few longitudinal prevalence studies begin at birth or during the preschool years (Beyer and Furniss, 2007). This is one of the reasons why relatively little is known about the manifestation of several forms of disorder in very young children. Finally, it is important to remember that a study of the prevalence of child psychopathology, like any other study, can be no better than its measures and sampling procedures. The sample must be representative of the population. The measures, be they interviews or questionnaires, must be valid. Interviews are often more accurate because an interview can probe in detail the responses provided, revealing more subtle forms of psychological difficulty. Another important methodological feature is the scope of the problem behaviors being studied. As discussed in Chapter 3, there is considerable overlap among the various psychological disorders. The researcher must take this into account and not simply measure the individual disorders (Rutter and Stevenson, 2010). Because many of the influential longitudinal studies are by now over 50 years old, *era effects* must be considered in interpreting the statistics reported. The historical period when the study began may or may not have been one of particular political upheaval or stress. In many cultures, awareness of psychological problems has increased over time, which might increase the likelihood of respondents reporting them in a truthful manner. In general, child and adolescent mental disorders appear to have increased over the past 50 or 60 years. The reasons for this are not fully understood. New discoveries about the disorders and better training of professionals may account for much or most of the change. However, the increasing complexities and stresses of modern life may have some effect, as may some unknown change in the environment (Maughan, Iervolino and Collishaw, 2005).

The prevalence rates of specific disorders are discussed in the subsequent chapters devoted to them. However, it may be useful at this point to note that the prevalence rates for the disorders vary greatly. The more common forms of child psychopathology – anxiety, depression, attention deficit and disruptive behavior disorders – each affect at least one child in fifteen to twenty, whereas most other diagnosed disorders each affect less than 1 percent of the child population (e.g., Faravelli et al., 2009). For that reason, the chapters in this book are not of equal length: More in-depth treatment is provided to the more common disorders.

It is also useful at this point to provide some global estimate of the prevalence of child psychopathology. The influential Great Smoky Mountains Study in the United States conducted with children from 9 to 16 years, using a rigorous interview methodology, indicated that almost 37 percent of children suffer from some form of psychological disorder at some point during that 7-year period. Just over 13 percent could be diagnosed as having a disorder at a given 3-month time point within the range covered by the study (Costello, Compton et al., 2003). A similar prevalence rate of almost 13 percent was reported in the UK for children of 13–15 years old but the prevalence rates for younger children were somewhat lower (Ford, Goodman and Meltzer, 2003). Studies in many countries, including, for example, Brazil and Russia, indicate very similar prevalence rates (Ford, Goodman and Meltzer, 2003; Goodman, Slobodskaya and Knyazev, 2005). Importantly, in longitudinal studies that begin during childhood and continue into adulthood, such as the influential Dunedin longitudinal study conducted in New England, it has been found that most adult mental health disorders first occur during the childhood and adolescent years (Beyer and Furniss, 2007; Kim-Cohen et al., 2005). In brief, child psychopathology is far from rare.

Recovery and the "politics of hope"

If psychological problems can be seen as diseases, it is logical to speculate about the likelihood of recovery from them. Up until very recently, experts felt it important to distinguish between conditions that were likely to be lifelong and conditions that might be transitory. As will be detailed in the chapters that follow, longitudinal studies have often revealed that many of the disorders that affect children and adolescents are remarkably stable. Although experts are very wary of generating false hope and keenly aware of "miracle cures" that are quickly debunked, research in several areas has revealed what appear to be total cures for conditions once deemed incurable. The most outstanding example is a 2013 study by Fein (2013) about thirty-four individuals previously diagnosed with autism spectrum disorder who no longer show any symptoms of the disease. Small as this sample is, it lends credence to isolated case studies indicating recovery from autism that have appeared in the years since the disorder was first identified (see Chapter 17). This publication can be considered a landmark, leading many mental health experts to become less reluctant to use the "r" word (recovery; Ozonoff, 2013). Already, there is lively debate in the field about how to define recovery. It is unclear at this stage whether "recovery" implies the total absence of the original disorder, of any diagnosable mental disorder or even of the types of psychological problems that are quite common but that do not correspond to the criteria for any disorder. As more professionals recover from their anxieties about talking about recovery, some clarity about what recovery might mean will hopefully emerge.

Summary

- There is not yet a universally used term for children's psychological problems.
- Only in the last 200 years have efforts been made to differentiate between conditions requiring long-term care and transitory problems associated with stress. "Pathology" originates in Greek words for knowledge and illness, referring to the study of diseases. Thus "psychopathology" is the study of illness affecting the mind.
- The *Oxford English Dictionary* lists a number of relevant definitions of the word "disease," including "absence of ease," "a cause of discomfort or distress," "a condition of the body... in which its functions are disturbed or deranged," "an illness ailment malady, disorder," "a species of disorder or aliment, exhibiting special symptoms or affecting a special organ," "a deranged, depraved or morbid condition."
- The term "disorder" is related to "disease," and, in this context, refers to an illness that disrupts normal physical or mental functions.
- The medical model is often attributed to Freud, who used a "talking cure" to treat hysteria in Viennese women, who had been previously seen as untreatable.
- The medical model is now the primary mode of thinking in mental health, its language strongly ingrained among those in the field and in their language.
- Critics of the medical model include the anti-psychiatry movement in North America and the Critical Psychiatry Network in the UK as well as the late Scottish Laing and American Szasz. Szasz argues that psychological problems are not diseases, as they cannot be repaired simply by physically fixing a part of the body, and that the medical model restricts the freedoms of those with problems. He compares the treatment of the mentally ill to that of lepers. It has been argued that "biomedical" child psychiatry is sexist, racist and imposes Western values on non-Western people. These views represent only a loud minority.
- Terms used to describe psychological distress have a tendency to imply a mind–body dichotomy. However, mental and physical processes have dynamic interaction, affecting each other reciprocally.
- The terms "atypical" and "abnormal" and their derivatives must be used with care. While they describe behavior that is outside of statistical norms, this behavior is often benign, if not beneficial. The terms tend to "glorify" the typical. Mealey (2005) proposes viewing normality/abnormality in an evolutionary context, by effect on ability to survive, adapt and reproduce. The idea that normality and abnormality are defined by an individual's level of danger to those around is similar. The medical definition of abnormality refers to part of the organism functioning improperly.
- Freud considered love and work the key indices of mental wellness. Friendship and play or love and schoolwork have been suggested as equivalents for children.
- The emerging field of developmental psychopathology focuses on evaluating mental health in the context of children's development processes. Normal development is studied by comparing it to abnormal development.
- Developing individuals can change between normal and abnormal over their lives. Disorder is unlikely to be caused by one trauma, though it may be the trigger. Developmental psychopathologists study individuals' developmental trajectories, attempting to understand how they end up in their final states. Individuals adapting successfully in early stages but not in later ones are likely to come to the attention of mental health professionals.

- Much effort has been made to study susceptibility to disease, but not so much to resistance to disease or individual resilience, an area of study emerging in the last 40 years. Study of these protective factors was initially spurred much by the failure of some Children, called "invulnerable" by Norman Garmezy, to develop adult schizophrenia, despite clear risk factors.
- Developmental psychopathologists argue that an individual is shaped by experiences at all points of life. They have encouraged the view of children not as "junior adults," but developing organisms. Though children are generally no longer viewed as needy, small adults, the mental health field still has not perfectly adapted to their needs.
- Developmental psychopathology has raised the standards of research by placing a premium on longitudinal research, particularly with multiple causal factors and outcomes.
- Developmental psychopathology does not reject diagnosis of a disorder at a particular moment in time, but it holds that the diagnosis is one point of data in a developmental trajectory of adaptation.
- The natural process of development is revered.
- Prediction in child psychopathology remains imprecise, but, thanks to longitudinal studies, has improved, with greater understanding that certain disorders can be more or less debilitating at different ages.

- Varying definitions of psychopathology and children with problems not coming to the attention of professionals make data on use of professional time poor estimates of the incidence of child psychopathology. Estimates are best made with large-sample studies.
- The time span of a study is very important to its interpretation. Individual moments are interesting, but not as important as following the same children over years in longitudinal study, which distinguishes between transitory problems and stable problems.
- The age at which a study begins must be considered; few begin at birth or in preschool years. A study is only as valid as its measures and sampling methods. Interviews are often more accurate than questionnaires. The wide range of overlapping problem behaviors must be considered, as must the overlap of various psychological disorders.
- Due to the age of many major studies, era effects must be considered, such as political upheaval or increase in awareness of psychological problems. For reasons not fully understood, child and adolescent disorders have become more prevalent over the last 50 to 60 years.
- Prevalence of disorders varies greatly. The most common forms – anxiety, depression, attention deficit disorder and disruptive behavior disorder – affect at least one child in fifteen to twenty, whereas others affect much less than 1 percent of the population.

Study questions

1. To what extent is the analogy between mental and physical illness valid?
2. What is the major problem in using the adjective "mental" in the terms "mental health" and "mental illness"?
3. In your opinion, what is the best way of differentiating between normal and abnormal child or adolescent behavior? What are the advantages and disadvantages of the criterion or criteria you suggest?
4. What are the core principles of the developmental psychopathology movement?
5. What are some problems in estimating the overall prevalence of psychopathology?

History

From ancient wisdom to the behavioral and cognitive revolutions

2

This chapter provides a historical introduction to most of the major theories that have influenced and still influence both theory and practice. Like most historical accounts, this chapter is organized in roughly chronological order as far as possible. However, so much of the intellectual history in this area began in the late nineteenth and early twentieth centuries that many important developments occurred almost simultaneously at that time. One important insight to be gained from this historical journey is that ideas about children and their psychological difficulties do not develop in a vacuum. As will become apparent, theories of psychopathology are influenced by the intellectual, social and political climates of the eras in which they emerge.

Children's symptoms as an economic burden to their families

Most scholars who attempt to trace the historical roots of the study of child psychopathology are struck by what they see as the indifference of adults during most of the years of recorded history to children's psychological difficulties (e.g., Kanner, 1962). Indeed, there is relatively little reference in literature or folklore, medical or theological writings about the subject before the nineteenth century. This indifference is not really surprising given the fundamental differences between the implications of mental illness in childhood and adulthood. Regardless of the historical period, adult psychopathology is more likely to cause economic hardship than child psychopathology (Ries, 1971, cited by Gelfand and Peterson, 1985). That the economic burden of psychopathology would

be a prominent concern may be shocking to the contemporary reader, who is probably privileged to live in the relatively recent historical period in which children and their special needs are known and when child labor is no longer common in the Western countries though it unfortunately persists in some parts of the world.

Faint glimmers of interest by the ancients

As indicated in the writings of Hippocrates (c. B.C. 460–c. B.C. 370), the ancient Greeks believed that mental disorders were caused by imbalances in the basic body fluids or "*humors*" – blood, phlegm, yellow bile and black bile. They believed that such imbalances affected both mind and body. Disciples of Hippocrates also developed a rudimentary classification system for mental illness, differentiating epilepsy, paranoia, mania and melancholia (Alexander and Selesnick, 1966). Little is said about how this classification system might apply to children. Nevertheless, there is an isolated reference to melancholy in young children in the writings of the Greek physician Rufus of Ephesus, who practiced in the second century A.D. (Jackson, 1986; Rutten, 2008). Thus, in at least some Greek writings, there are traces of effort made to understand abnormal behavior. Understanding may often constitute the beginning of caring and helping, although that is hardly the picture that emerges from the ancient and medieval documents that have been recovered, as we shall see in the next few paragraphs (Jensen and Hoagwood, 1997).

Some sources portray the ancients as cruel in their handling of children whose thoughts or behavior were disorganized or unusual. Seen as an economic

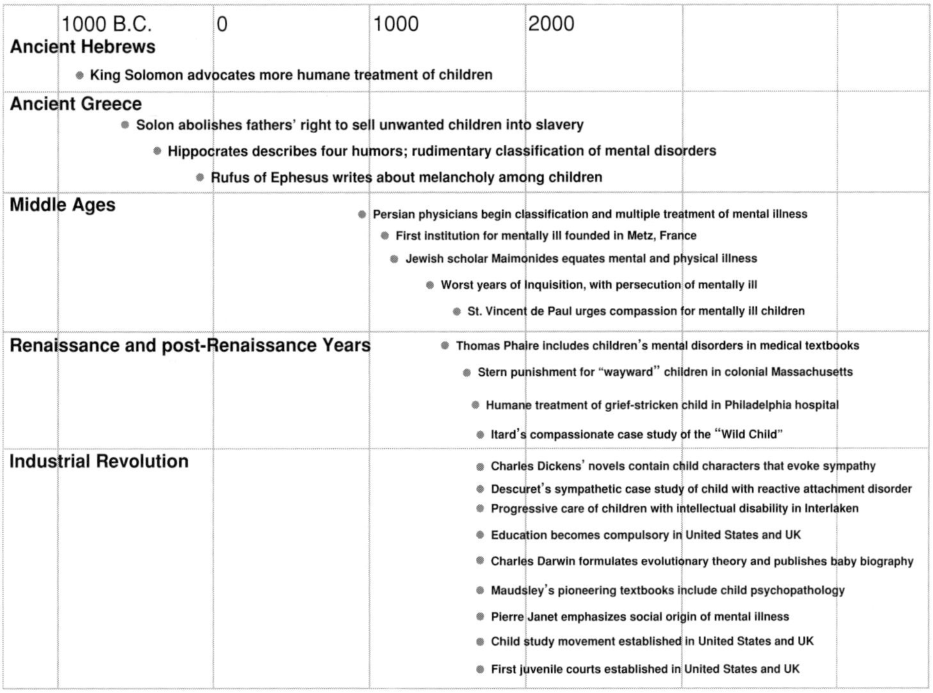

1000 B.C.	0	1000	2000		
Ancient Hebrews					
● King Solomon advocates more humane treatment of children					
Ancient Greece					
● Solon abolishes fathers' right to sell unwanted children into slavery					
● Hippocrates describes four humors; rudimentary classification of mental disorders					
● Rufus of Ephesus writes about melancholy among children					
Middle Ages					
		● Persian physicians begin classification and multiple treatment of mental illness			
		● First institution for mentally ill founded in Metz, France			
		● Jewish scholar Maimonides equates mental and physical illness			
		● Worst years of Inquisition, with persecution of mentally ill			
		● St. Vincent de Paul urges compassion for mentally ill children			
Renaissance and post-Renaissance Years					
		● Thomas Phaire includes children's mental disorders in medical textbooks			
		● Stern punishment for "wayward" children in colonial Massachusetts			
		● Humane treatment of grief-stricken child in Philadelphia hospital			
		● Itard's compassionate case study of the "Wild Child"			
Industrial Revolution					
		● Charles Dickens' novels contain child characters that evoke sympathy			
		● Descuret's sympathetic case study of child with reactive attachment disorder			
		● Progressive care of children with intellectual disability in Interlaken			
		● Education becomes compulsory in United States and UK			
		● Charles Darwin formulates evolutionary theory and publishes baby biography			
		● Maudsley's pioneering textbooks include child psychopathology			
		● Pierre Janet emphasizes social origin of mental illness			
		● Child study movement established in United States and UK			
		● First juvenile courts established in United States and UK			

Figure 2.1 Early history of child psychopathology.

burden and embarrassment to their families and communities, they could be abandoned and put to death (French, 1977). It is known that infanticide was a very common way of dealing with unwanted children in ancient Greece. Death would be the fate of children in Sparta who did not develop in ways that would make them fit for service to the state (Nathan and Harris, 1988, cited by Peterson and Burbach, 1988). The usual method of killing unwanted children in ancient Greece was to abandon them in the wild where they would not survive. Sometimes, however, they were asphyxiated by large ceramic vessels (Despert, 1965; Peterson and Burbach, 1988).

In the Old Testament, there is a passage in Deuteronomy (21:19–21) enjoining parents to bring unmanageable sons to the city elders, who would order the men of the city to stone the child (Peterson and Burbach, 1988). On the other hand, in the Old Testament book of Genesis, there is a fleeting reference to children being important and needing sympathetic treatment: "And he said unto him, My Lord knoweth that the children [are] tender, and the flocks and herds with young [are] with me: and if men should overdrive them one day, all the flock will die" (Genesis, 33:13). Furthermore, at one point in the book of Psalms, children are said to be "a gift from God" (Psalms 127:3; Peterson and Burbach, 1988).

Writings from the Roman Empire are similarly inconsistent in their depiction of children and their difficulties. As in Athens, fathers had the power to decide the fate of their children. Children who displayed physical or mental illness would be abandoned. However, Roman writings also contain some evidence of special, privileged (in fact, excessively privileged) status of children. Indulging children with too many sports and games, at the expense of their moral education, was sometimes cited as the cause of the defeat of the Roman Empire (Goodsell, 1934, cited by Peterson and Burbach, 1988).

The plight of the atypical child: part of the darkness of the Dark Ages?

Throughout the Middle Ages (A.D. 500–1300), the Catholic Church believed in the doctrine of original sin – that human beings are born evil. Children had to be educated in the ways of righteousness in order to overcome their inherent nature. If they displayed unusual behavior, they could be summoned by the Inquisition, the religious court system empowered by the kings. Very often, their family members would testify against them lest they also be considered evil and condemned to the same fate as the accused. Condemned children might be forced to serve the Church for their lives or might be burned at the stake as witches (Kroll, 1973; Neugebauer, 1979; Peterson and Burbach, 1988). Sometimes, "evil" symptoms were ascribed not to the inherent evil nature of children but to their being possessed by demons or evil spirits (Schendel and Kourany, 1980). Given the assumed connections between psychopathology and the forces of evil, people who embraced the professional work of caring for the insane were, not surprisingly, called "alienists," a now-obsolete term which shares the Latin root of the word "alien."

Despite this gloomy portrait, there were some important advances during the "Dark Ages." The first institution for the insane was established in Metz, France in the year A.D. 1100. According to Mora (2008), there is no reason to believe that treatment there was any less humane than in the psychiatric hospitals of the seventeenth to nineteenth centuries in England or Continental Europe. Mora (2008) also notes that while ecclesiastical courts were probably quite merciless, "monk-doctors" in monasteries were actually quite creative and benevolent in their treatments.

Recent scholarship casts doubt on the prevailing image of wanton cruelty to the mentally ill of medieval Europe. In many communities, local churches were in fact kind to mentally ill people, providing refuge for them against townspeople wanting to expel them or agents of royal families who had the right to take over the property of subjects who had been declared incompetent. Mora (2008) speculates that most mentally ill adults and children were cared for by their families. For much of the medieval era there were only two diagnoses of mental illness – idiocy, now known as intellectual disability or intellectual disability, or lunacy, now known as psychosis or schizophrenia. Differential diagnosis had important legal implications. Idiocy was deemed to be incurable; therefore an idiot's property would be confiscated and assigned to the State. Lunacy was considered curable; a lunatic's assets would be held for him/her pending recovery. English court records document many attempts by abusive relatives to have people declared idiots, giving the relatives access to their possessions; many such petitions were refused (Neugebauer, 1989). Neugebauer (1989) also cites records of mentally ill persons being cared for compassionately in the homes of medieval physicians. Mora (2008) documents Church writings allowing penalties for deviant behavior to be reduced when mitigating circumstances were in evidence as well as provisions for compassion in the writings of medieval Christian philosophers who followed the doctrines of Augustine. In the sixteenth century, St. Vincent de Paul voiced stringent objection to the vicious treatment of children who displayed atypical behavior, asserting that mental illness is not different from physical illness and that Christianity demands that those who are able must protect and cure its victims (Graziano, 1975). The epithet "Dark Ages" does not fit the historical period outside of Europe. Islam from its outset displayed a far more compassionate attitude toward mental illness than the medieval Catholic Church. Islamic writings declare unequivocally that the mentally ill are loved by God (Mora, 2008). In traditional Islamic society, families are enjoined to care for family members afflicted with mental illness (Youssef, Youssef and Dening, 1996).

Some Jewish writings emanating from the Middle East or Arab-controlled Mediterranean countries suggest that there was some understanding that

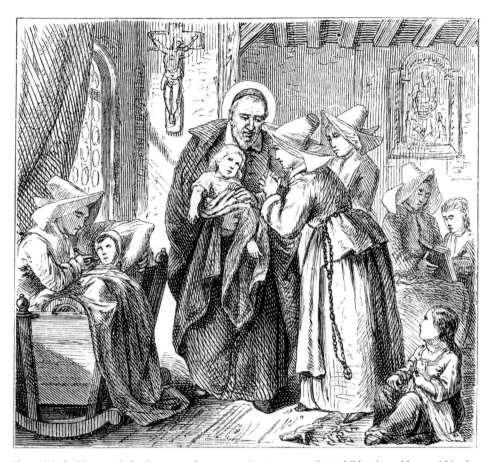

Figure 2.2 St. Vincent de Paul promoted a compassionate approach to children's problems within the Catholic Church.

children might differ in their basic dispositions and that some of these dispositions are more maladaptive than others. For instance, rabbis whose debates are contained in the Talmud, a sacred Jewish text of the Middle Ages that comprises commentaries on the Old Testament, introduced the metaphor of four sons to the Jewish Haggadah, which is read during the Passover holiday to this day. In the Haggadah, parents are instructed on how to explain things to four different types of sons – wise, wicked, simple and sons who do not even know how to ask questions. This medieval text thus foreshadows in a small way the contemporary "goodness of fit" approach that is the basis of recent writings about different types of

child temperament and the environments in which children of each type are likely to flourish (Seifer et al., 2000). Unlike the medieval Christian teaching that humans are born in a state of original sin, which might be manifest in psychopathology, traditional Jewish beliefs since the third century A.D. depicted a balance between *yetzer hara* (evil inclination) and *yetzer hatov* (good inclination). Children were thought to be born with *yetzer hara* but to naturally acquire the benevolent *yetzer hatov* afterwards (Luzzatto, 1997). Consistent with this balanced attitude and with his reverence for the intellectual faculties of the human species, the eminent Spanish-Jewish scholar Maimonides (1134–1201) commented that people

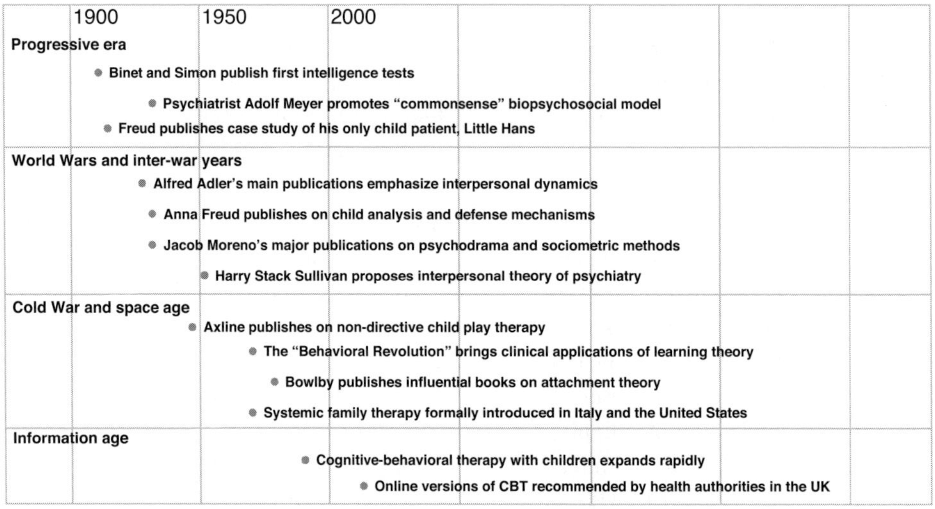

	1900	1950	2000				
Progressive era							
	• Binet and Simon publish first intelligence tests						
		• Psychiatrist Adolf Meyer promotes "commonsense" biopsychosocial model					
	• Freud publishes case study of his only child patient, Little Hans						
World Wars and inter-war years							
		• Alfred Adler's main publications emphasize interpersonal dynamics					
		• Anna Freud publishes on child analysis and defense mechanisms					
		• Jacob Moreno's major publications on psychodrama and sociometric methods					
		• Harry Stack Sullivan proposes interpersonal theory of psychiatry					
Cold War and space age							
	• Axline publishes on non-directive child play therapy						
		• The "Behavioral Revolution" brings clinical applications of learning theory					
		• Bowlby publishes influential books on attachment theory					
		• Systemic family therapy formally introduced in Italy and the United States					
Information age							
		• Cognitive-behavioral therapy with children expands rapidly					
		• Online versions of CBT recommended by health authorities in the UK					

Figure 2.3 Important events since 1900.

who run wild in the streets should not be considered insane, but that people whose thinking is confined to fixed ideas should, even if they appear perfectly normal (Maimonides, 1956; Barcia, 2005; Mora, 2008).

Vakili and Gorji (2006) maintain that medieval Persian practitioners can be considered the first psychologists or psychiatrists, long before those professions were formally constituted. Between the ninth and twelfth centuries A.D., Persian practitioners described and classified mental disorders, using such categories as melancholia, mania, paranoia and "passionate love disease," an obsessive condition. They developed a variety of therapies for treating these disorders, including an early form of psychotherapy that included advice and support. They also introduced diet therapy, music therapy, bloodletting and even electrical-shock therapy (Vakili and Gorji, 2006). The entire medieval Muslim world, known for its valuable spices and oils then as now, saw pioneers develop natural medicines for both physical and psychological ailments (Mora, 2008; Vakili and Gorji, 2006).

Enlightenment and unenlightenment in the Renaissance and post-Renaissance periods (1300–1800)

The Renaissance period brought profound progress to many fields of inquiry in the Western European countries. However, the period cannot be considered as bringing major innovations to theory or practice in the area of child psychopathology. As time went on, the Catholic Church condemned infanticide as a mortal sin. Nevertheless, the Church endorsed the abandonment of children who displayed atypical behavior to institutions, many of which it sponsored. Given the high death rate in the orphanages of the time, several historians commented that this institutionalization was almost tantamount to infanticide (de Mause, 1974; Peterson and Burbach, 1988).

In a conceptually important but apparently isolated contribution, the British physician Thomas Phaire (1510–1560) included some aspects of child psychopathology in what is considered the first textbook of pediatrics in the English language. Among the childhood psychological problems discussed by Phaire were nightmares and bedwetting (Still, 1931). Interest in more extreme cases of atypical child behavior emerged in the eighteenth and early nineteenth centuries from the ongoing philosophical quest to determine the fundamental nature of humans, evil or good, which did not end in the Middle Ages. One example is that of a 7-year-old girl who avoided contact with people by hiding in closets or running away. Because the local physician could do nothing more than speculate that she might be insane, she was placed in the care of the local minister. The minister tried in many ways to scare off the "baneful and infernal" power within her, including whipping, isolation and starvation. The girl died within a few months, leading to what is described as widespread relief (Hauch, 1946).

However, at least one important record belies the impression of wanton cruelty at the time. The most famous is the case study by the French physician Jean-Marc Gaspard Itard (1774–1838) of the "taming" of a "wild child" who had been raised in the woods (Itard, 1962[1806]). Itard's beneficent and highly humane treatment of the Wild Child has been portrayed as a precursor of the humanistic, child-centered psychotherapies that were to be introduced in the 1960s (Benzaquén, 2006). If Itard's "psychotherapy" had any philosophical underpinnings, it was to show that atypical children are not as evil as his contemporaries believed, in fact, not evil at all. Itard's case study of "the wild child" was the subject of a successful film released in the 1970s. Truffault's film *The Wild Child* is widely regarded as having influenced contemporary views about the fundamental nature of the child.

Although the colonization of North America may have brought freedom to some adults who had been persecuted in Europe because of their religious beliefs, it did not bring better treatment of children with psychological problems until well into the nineteenth century. Children and adolescents were more likely than others to be brought to trial as suspected witches, as in the famous witch hunts in Salem, Massachusetts in 1692. The colony of

Massachusetts passed a Stubborn Child Law in 1654, which prescribed penalties as strong as death for disobedient children. That law remained on the books of the State of Massachusetts until 1973. The death penalty appears not to have been applied very often because children's work was vitally needed in the colonies; however, severe corporal punishment of wayward children appears to have been very common (Katz, Schroeder and Sidman, 1973; Peterson and Burbach, 1988). In contrast to the general image of harsh treatment that is portrayed in most sources, there were other indications of the beginnings of compassionate treatment. For example, one of the first patients admitted to the Pennsylvania Hospital in 1765, 11 years before the American Revolution, was a 13-year-old girl seized by incessant and uncontrollable grief after the death of her mother. The girl was treated well there and considered cured (Duffy, 1976).

By the early nineteenth century, blatant cruelty to children displaying psychological problems seems to have abated somewhat. Because virtually nothing was known about the treatment of these difficulties, isolation and exile became the norm. Banished to asylums, forced to toil in workhouses or completely exiled from their native countries, troubled children could do no further harm to the communities they came from (Costello and Angold, 2000). The motives behind such ostracism, however, do not seem very cruel, as indicated in a quotation from Wade (1829, cited by Costello and Angold, 2000): "It appears to us that it would be real humanity toward these unfortunate creatures to subject them to compulsory and permanent exile from England" (p. 603). Although nothing was done to treat or rehabilitate them, their custodial treatment appears to have been tolerant and reasonably compassionate.

In 1841, the eminent Swiss physician Johann Guggenbuhl established the first institution for children and adults with various forms of intellectual deficiency near Interlaken, Switzerland. Importantly, Guggenbuhl prescribed a variety of measures that would go beyond confinement and custodial care.

There were memory-training exercises as well as various methods to care for the residents' bodies, such as massage and physical training. Although Guggenbuhl was discredited 20 years later for having made exaggerated claims about the efficacy of his treatment, the belief that institutionalization for proper care could be helpful for people with intellectual disabilities remained, unchallenged until the mainstreaming movement of the late twentieth century, which is discussed in Chapter 16.

In summary, the Renaissance and post-Renaissance periods, known for the rebirth of learning in many areas of inquiry, can be considered an era of only isolated progress in the understanding of child psychopathology.

Enlightened thinking about the downtrodden

The mid-nineteenth century is often regarded as a turning point in thinking about psychopathology in general. At that time, scientific methodology, scientific theories and social concern all advanced rapidly. The emerging science of child psychopathology benefited greatly from both the scientific and social progress of the times. The increased interest in the welfare of the downtrodden is often attributed to the French and American Revolutions, which transformed not only political systems but also general thinking about the rights and needs of persons. The lives of children and the challenges of growing up began to be captured by writers. By the late nineteenth century, novelists such as Charles Dickens (1812–70) sensitized the Western world to the plight of many downtrodden members of society, including children, especially orphans and child laborers. The results were widespread, including the introduction of child labor laws and universal compulsory education in many Western nations. By the beginning of the twentieth century, the child welfare movement in the United States began raising interest in children growing up in poverty (Brooks-Gunn and Johnson, 2006).

Leo Kanner (1962) offers a case example from the writings of Jean Baptiste Félix Descuret (1795–1871), a French physician, as an illustration of the transition to a more sympathetic stance and the decline in explanations based on theological or moralistic postulates (Descuret, 1841). It is the case history of a boy who was raised by a nurse while he was a baby. Brought to live with his parents at the age of 2, he became totally unresponsive and melancholy. The child was treated by having the nurse visit, initially for the full day. The nurse's presence was gradually faded out, first for a few hours, then for days, then weeks; the child became responsive and happy. This treatment indicates a rudimentary, probably intuitive awareness of some of the ideas embodied in contemporary attachment theory (see Chapter 6) and systematic desensitization, which is an important component of the treatment of phobias (see Chapter 15).

Juvenile delinquency seen as a manifestation of mental illness

In both North America and Britain adults became concerned that the urban environments that were increasingly common were not providing optimal conditions for the growth of well-adjusted children and adolescents. Writers and social reformers in the United States became concerned about what would happen to the masses of "idle" youth who gathered aimlessly on city street corners (Katz, 1976, cited by Silk et al., 2000). Separate juvenile courts were established, recognizing that criminal offense may relate to mental illness and that exposing young offenders to seasoned criminals might worsen them. The first juvenile courts in the United States were established in Denver and Chicago in 1899. The juvenile court in Chicago was founded at the instigation of the women's club members who volunteered their services to a local group home (borstal) for wayward young people in Chicago. These women were convinced that juvenile delinquency was caused by the lack of proper family upbringing, an idea that was quite novel in an era when family factors in psychopathology were not yet commonly known or accepted (Clapp, 1998).

Public campaigns for the more humane treatment of juveniles became particularly intensive in the 1890s and 1900s. These campaigns intensified as part of the general despair about the state of the recruits to the British army for the Boer Wars at the very beginning of the twentieth century. Concern that Britain was losing its position in the world was linked to the beliefs that children were not being raised properly. It was widely supposed that working-class parents were raising a generation of thugs rather than productive, fit workers and citizens (Bradley, 2008). The Children's Act of 1908 introduced the juvenile court to British legal systems, prescribed school meals, more humane conditions in reformatory schools and prohibitions against cruelty to children and their exposure to smoking and alcohol in pubs. The men and women alike who advocated for progressive juvenile justice seem to have been preoccupied with the proper socialization of boys. Young female offenders were rare, and appear to have been treated more harshly, especially for sexual offenses (Bright, Decker and Burch, 2007). Interestingly, some scholars maintain that young female offenders remain to this day mistreated and misunderstood by juvenile courts (Acoca, 1998; Logan, 2005).

Concern about the plight of children working in the factories that appeared during the Industrial Revolution led to expansion of laws prescribing free, compulsory education for all throughout the United States and the UK (Katz, 1976). With the advent of compulsory schooling, new tasks were added to those that might delineate normal, adaptive behavior and psychopathology: Children had to be attentive and obedient and were supposed to master the lessons they were taught.

Childhood recognized as a developmental stage

A by-product of new, enlightened thinking was the emergence of the concept of childhood as a distinct stage of development, replacing the earlier notion that children were simply adults-in-the-making who were to be introduced to productive adult work as soon as possible. The philosophical foundations for this transformation in thinking were put into place centuries earlier by John Locke (1632–1704) and Jean-Jacques Rousseau (1712–78) but not translated globally into concrete improvements in the lives of children at the time they were first disseminated. The ideas of these two philosophers were cornerstones of the new thinking that accompanied the American and, especially, the French Revolution. Locke argued against the idea that an individual's character is largely innate, emphasizing the role of environmental experiences in filling in the *tabula rasa* or empty slate. Rousseau emphasized the special and crucial nature of the childhood years, introducing a stage model to explain qualitative differences in the child's thinking at various stages. Unlike both Locke and the predominant European theological traditions of the previous centuries, Rousseau believed that children were born *inherently good*. He saw children as "noble savages" who would learn and adjust without much need for intervention if they were given the proper nurturing environment (Curren, 2007).

In the nineteenth century, adults became aware of the thoughts, feelings and worries of children. They began to represent children's mental space in their fiction writing. Charles Dickens, the British novelist, is the best-known author to introduce depictions of children in need and their emotional lives. The French author, Alphonse Daudet (1840–97), often accused of imitating him, provided French readers with stories written from a child's perspective.

Scientific observation of children's behavior

Scientific inquiry flourished in the eighteenth and nineteenth centuries, including interest in the observation of children's behavior, inspired by early evolutionary theory. Charles Darwin's (1809–82) research with children consisted largely of notes on the development of his own son that were compiled for 5 years. Although Darwin himself devoted relatively little time to the observation of children, his theory inspired members of the emerging discipline of child psychology to begin systematic observations of children's behavior and development (Charlesworth, 1992; Green, 2009). Several scientists published "baby biographies" documenting the sequence of development, often using their own daughters and sons. In doing so, they tried to document every detail of every aspect of their children's development, often without prior expectations or guiding theory. Darwin's biography of his son William is notable not only for the data about William's development but also for the speculations and reflections Darwin interspersed about the development of personality during the childhood years. Darwin's work betrays a man who complemented his scientific bent with intense love as a father. Darwin's emotional intensity is surely related to the premature deaths of three of his children. His very well-written baby biography was circulated widely and influenced thinking about child psychology so extensively that some historians regard this publication as a major turning point, clearing a path for future theories and research in child psychology (Fitzpatrick and Bringmann, 1995).

Dissatisfied with the imprecision of single-subject baby biographies, the pioneering American psychologist Stanley Hall (1844–1924) began a research program in the 1880s using questionnaires about child development. This marked the start of the child study movement, which made scientific study of children a legitimate scientific endeavor (Brooks-Gunn and Johnson, 2006). Hall is noted for reconciling the biological and social influences on children's development and adjustment, describing social interaction as a "catalyst for internal organization" (White, 1992). Hall is also noted for promoting the concept of adolescence as a discrete and important stage of development. Emphasizing the psychological consequences of puberty and adolescent cognitive development, he saw this distinct stage as needed to represent completely the

parallelism between biology and mental adjustment (or maladjustment) that scientists before him had established. He depicted adolescence as a time of "storm and stress" punctuated by more frequent experiencing of depressed mood than at any other stage of life. He attributed this unhappiness to adolescents' self-consciousness and insecurity regarding their own identities. He also described the compensatory mechanism of sensation-seeking during adolescence (Arnett, 2006; Cravens, 2006). Hall's work resulted in widespread recognition of puberty as a physiological cause of mental disorder. Prior to his time, adolescent disorders were regarded as essentially identical to adult mental disorders (Parry-Jones, 2001). Adults' awareness of the childhood stage resulted in increasing demands on parents to shape their children's development and character. Providing guidance to parents became a major focus of the emerging effort to *prevent* child psychopathology, as is discussed in Chapter 10.

A scientific approach to classification – and resistance to it

The leader identified with the major advances in the scientific study of child psychopathology at the beginning of the twentieth century is Alfred Binet (1857–1911). Binet was trained as a biologist but became interested in psychology after reading some early works in the field, including those of the German Wilhelm experimentalist Wundt (1832–1920). He was completely self-trained as a psychologist. Writings about Binet clearly establish him as a latter-day "Renaissance man" – an eclectic scientist with a keen commitment to the practical applications of psychological findings among many other interests. It is undoubtedly Binet's liberal political leanings that led him to an interest in applications of psychology to "abnormal children" (that was indeed the title of his first book, Binet and Simon, 1907). Binet is best known as the father of intelligence testing. Some infamous psychologists after him were to use intelligence testing to exclude rather than include (see Gould, 1981 for a very readable account of this sordid chapter in the history of psychology) individuals from schools, jobs, army ranks and countries. However, Binet's motives are almost surely beyond reproach despite the efforts of some French psychohistorians, described by Guillec (2000) as ideologically motivated, to discredit his work. Aptly capturing the tragic and very common misconceptions about Binet and his work, Siegler (1992) lamented that it is ironic that Binet's contribution is often summarized as "reducing intelligence to a single number" (p. 179) given the scope of his work and his fervent efforts at capturing the diversity of children's development and adjustment, providing great detail on not only general developmental processes but also individual differences. Binet's methods were far more varied than is often thought, including not only the memory and recognition tasks that formed part of intelligence tests but also measures of blood pressure and electrical activity, analysis of the biographies of creative individuals, case histories, inkblots and word associations, not to mention his intensive observations of his two daughters (Cairns and Cairns, 2006).

As part of the movement in France to make education free, compulsory and secular (as embodied into law in 1881 and 1882), Binet was concerned with extending education to children with atypical behaviors that he firmly believed required special educational techniques that could not be delivered in regular classrooms. It must be remembered that, at the time, the distinction between intellectual disability and other disorders was not fully established. In fact, one of Binet's objectives was to differentiate between the major subtypes of "abnormal children." However, Binet differed with some theorists of the time, such as the Italian criminologist Cesare Lombroso (1835–1909), who portrayed low intelligence, criminality and psychopathology as essentially the same condition and one that should be characterized as degenerate and frightful. It was Binet's intent that the special classes established for "abnormal children" be used

to provide them with the opportunity to engage in the "mental orthopedics" that would enable them to make the best use of their capacities (Foschi and Cicciola, 2006). At the same time, "experimenting" to see how successful these mental exercises might be would inform science about the nature of intellect and psychological adaptation.

Such attempts at classifying children's psychological problems met with considerable resistance because of the new recognition of childhood as a distinct stage of life, as mentioned earlier. This resulted in so great a reverence for the natural processes of development that there was strong objection to the idea that any abnormal pattern of childhood behavior should be considered pathological in the way that adult disorders were. This resistance reached a crescendo in the 1940s, as chronicled by Kanner (1962). The early child analyst Beata Rank (1866–1907), one of the many disciples of Freud who became disenchanted with his teachings and left his circle, introduced the concept of the "atypical child." She deliberately obliterated the lines of the diagnostic classifications that were emerging for adult disorders, as between neuroses and psychoses, as they were then called. Defending her stance, Rank (1949) maintained that all these conditions had a common origin, namely problems in the child–mother relationship. Those firmly opposed to the formal delineation and classification might have won the day had it not been finally decided that psychotic symptoms – such as mania and hallucinations – previously thought to occur only in adults, could occasionally occur in children. It was widely believed in the nineteenth century that insanity could not emerge before adolescence because children's minds were too unstable for harmful mental impressions to have any permanent effects. However, isolated accounts of suicide and melancholia, as well as psychosis, belied this contention (Parry-Jones, 1989). By the mid-nineteenth century, some medical textbooks, especially in psychiatry, contained reference to childhood "insanity"; these include Robert John Maudsley's influential 1867 treatise entitled *The Physiology and Pathology of the Mind* (Parry-Jones, 1989). Interestingly, Maudsley was criticized so scathingly for having dared to include child psychopathology in his writings that he was compelled to add an apologetic preface to the second edition (Kanner, 1973).

As early as 1900, a variety of case studies appeared documenting instances of psychotic behavior in children, which apparently astonished readers at the time (Kanner, 1962). This gradually brought closure to a debate that had raged for many decades about the possibility of psychotic disorder in children, although it was also concluded that mental illness was much less frequent in children than adults. This was aptly captured in a statement by Maudsley, the most prominent psychiatrist in England and prolific author of professional materials, "How soon can a child go mad? Obviously, not before it has some mind to go wrong, and then only in proportion to the quantity and quality of mind it has" (Maudsley, 1895, cited by Parry-Jones, 1989). Some of Maudsley's contemporaries, however, especially the eminent British psychiatrist James Chrichton-Brown (1860, cited by Parry-Jones, 2001; b. 1840–d. 1938), insisted that although children appear to be blissful and free of mental suffering, their apparent adjustment is only superficial, concealing a range of disorders including melancholia and hypochondriasis. The nineteenth-century German neurologist and psychiatrist Wilhelm Griesinger maintained that all forms of insanity occurred before puberty, although not very often (Parry-Jones, 2001). The pioneering work of Pierre Janet (1859–1947) at the Salpêtrière Hospital in Paris reinforced this idea to some extent. An important part of Janet's enduring contribution to the mental health field is his discovery of childhood trauma that can affect a person's psychological functioning throughout life (Van der Kolk and Van der Hart, 1989).

It is probably out of reverence for the variety and instability that the developmental process brings that it was only in the 1930s that the by then well-established disease models began to be commonly applied to children's mental health disorders. Even then, the focus was on the most visible and intrusive of disordered behaviors – childhood schizophrenia. Nevertheless, by that time, pediatricians had begun to recognize child psychopathology as a debilitating condition, although they had already considered for centuries several physical disorders that have psychological dimensions, such as enuresis (bedwetting), convulsions and insomnia (Phaire, 1546, cited by Parry-Jones, 1989) without conceptualizing these problems as mental disorders of children.

Disease models of child psychopathology debated

Early in the nineteenth century, Jean-Étienne Dominique Esquirol (1772–1840), an eminent French psychiatrist, distinguished intellectual deficiency from psychosis. The importance of this development is discussed in greater detail in Chapter 3, on the classification of childhood mental health disorders. Esquirol can also be credited for probably the first emphatic designation of physicians as authority figures in mental health institutions: "physicians with special training should be 'the vital principal of a lunatic hospital. It is he who should set everything in motion . . . The physician should be invested with an authority from which no one is exempt'" (Goldstein, 1987, p. 130–2).

The "medical model" became the predominant view among psychiatrists by the early twentieth century. The prevailing view was that a diseased brain was the primary cause of psychopathology. However, not all leading figures in the history of nineteenth- and twentieth-century mental health converged in attributing child psychopathology to physical causes exclusively or primarily. Among the dissenters was Pierre Janet, whose work was mentioned earlier in this chapter. Janet argued vociferously that both organic dysfunction and being reared in a pathogenic environment contributed to some childhood disorders. He emphasized the *sociogenesis*, or social origin, of all higher psychological processes, including thinking, volition and memory. He believed that these processes develop initially in interpersonal relationships before they become internalized by the individual child (Janet, 1929).

Janet's work is not widely known at this point. However, it has been argued that he rather than Freud should be considered the father of psychoanalysis and psychotherapy. Janet's ideas also remain alive to some extent by means of his influence on the Soviet psychologist Lev Vygotsky (1896–1934), whose work still attracts widespread interest. Inspired at least partly by Janet, Vygotsky's theory emphasized the role of culture and relationships in child development. Vygotsky went much further than Janet in explicating how the learning acquired in interpersonal relations becomes internalized by the growing child. Perhaps for that reason, contemporary educationalists around the world find his work, which was not available outside the Soviet Union for many years, highly insightful (Janet, 1929; Van der Veer and Valsiner, 1988; Wertsch, 1985).

Another important departure from the prevalent thinking of the mid-twentieth century was the *biopsychosocial theory* of Adolf Meyer, in which psychopathology is understood as the reaction of the entire organism to unfavorable environments and stressful experiences (Masten and Curtis, 2000; Menninger, Mayman and Pruyser, 1963). Meyer, a Swiss psychiatrist who immigrated to the United States and became perhaps the most influential American psychiatrist of the first half of the twentieth century, was a proponent of patient-centered treatment of all diseases, mental and physical. He resisted, first of all, the dominant movement at the time to classify mental illnesses within a disease model, which he criticized as biological reductionism. Instead of "single-word diagnoses," he favored a comprehensive assessment of the physical, social and cultural factors that impinge on an individual's mental health. At the same time, although he actually employed John B. Watson (1878–1958), father of the behavioral movement (discussed later in this chapter) to teach psychology to medical trainees at Johns Hopkins in Baltimore, he also dismissed the concept of behavior therapy as reflective of an "immature attitude" (Double, 2007). Meyer attempted to integrate the various causes of mental disease by developing a hierarchy of mental functions, with higher functions better explained by some causal agents than lower functions. Consequently, he proposed that "higher" and "lower" functions – and the disorders related to them – were differentially related to the competence of the various mental health disciplines (e.g., psychiatry, psychology, neurology, social work). Although Meyer's general idea of multiple causation, his fervent advocacy of eclecticism and the term *biopsychosocial* have all survived until the present, his attempt at integrating the multiple avenues of causation in a convincing theoretical model has been dismissed as "nothing more than an accumulation of the platitudes of the day" (Shorter, 2005, p. 10). Nevertheless, Meyer is to be remembered for making it scientifically respectable to draw on multiple theories about multiple causes in explaining child psychopathology.

Several other far-fetched theories about the origins of children's psychological disorders attracted little more enduring attention in the nineteenth century, when they were first proposed, than they would now. These included the contention that excessive masturbation leads to schizophrenia and that immoderate use of one's intellectual faculties leads to neurosis, especially in girls and women (Silk et al., 2000).

Psychoanalysis: psychopathology as the reacting organism in "shellshock"[1]

By the end of the nineteenth century, most "alienists" believed that psychopathology was caused by brain dysfunction. Soon afterwards, a complementary position emerged – that mental illness was triggered by the environment but that an important part of

[1] Expression introduced by Menninger et al. (1963).

the individual's reaction was biological. Menninger and his colleagues (1963) graphically described the reaction of the human psyche to early trauma as "shellshock."

Freud introduced a totally revolutionary perspective on psychodiagnosis and psychotherapy. Although he himself applied his theory mostly with adults, he emphasized the causal role of developmental stages of childhood, childhood sexuality and experiences during childhood. Trained as a medical doctor, Freud did not deny the biological origins of these processes, but presented a theory that radically altered thinking about how biology operates. His theory inspired widespread interest in the study of the childhood origins of psychopathology (Silk et al., 2000). His psychoanalytic theory garnered broad appeal among practitioners, cutting across the disciplinary divide that separates those with and without training in medicine or biology. To this day, many psychologists who do not use any Freudian technique or other form of psychoanalysis revert to Freud's insightful work as a framework for understanding some of the complex workings of the present day; that was even more common in the early and mid-twentieth century.

Despite the established belief by psychoanalysts at the time that many adult problems had their roots in traumatic experiences in childhood, the general climate in the analytic field at the time has been described as "child phobic" (Kahr, 1996). This is somewhat surprising given the very active research with children at the Vienna School of Developmental Psychology, led by Karl (1879–1963) and Charlotte Buhler (1893–1974), in the same city at the same time; it is well documented that there was little contact between the fledgling developmentalists and the fledgling psychoanalysts (Rollett, 1997). Freud himself never worked directly with a child patient. However, he was involved in a "supervisory" role in the analysis of a 5-year-old commonly called Little Hans and published a very famous case study about the child's problems, their origin and treatment. In his published report about the case, Freud remarked that he only took it on to validate his theories about children's unconscious inner motivations; he had no interest in establishing child psychoanalysis as a therapeutic technique (Anthony, 1986). In his case report, Freud concluded that he had "learned nothing new," meaning that he believed his theories of infant sexuality to be confirmed by the analysis of Little Hans (Anthony, 1986).

The case study emerged as a landmark work in the analytic field, one that is still read and even reanalyzed today. Aside from the insight it contains, the case study is valued for "the pioneer spirit, the novelty, the naiveté and freshness of this first direct exploration of a child's thoughts, feelings and fantasies" (Blum, 2007, p. 750). Prior to this case study, Freud had derived many of his conclusions about the psychic life of children from the notes he directed his followers to gather on the development of their own children. One of his most loyal followers was Hans' father, Max Graf. Freud agreed to devise a treatment for Little Hans' fear of horses and to supervise Graf's administration of the treatment at home to his own son. Of course, such role conflict – being both the patient's father and therapist – would not be acceptable in contemporary professional circles. In fact, he believed at the time that parents might actually be the best therapists for their children, which is unthinkable in modern psychoanalytic circles (Fordham, 1989). Nevertheless, as noted by Blum (2007), this arrangement is consistent with the theme still present in some psychoanalytic thinking that the therapist must assume, in essence, a paternal role. Little Hans was not a totally passive participant. He knew about his father's connection to Freud and helped compose his father's notes to the professor. At one point Hans even asked his father if Freud communicated with God. Little Hans' therapy lasted 4 months, far shorter than the course of traditional psychoanalytic treatment but no longer than some short-term dynamic therapies. Among the conflicts discovered was the classical Oedipal conflict, with Little Hans seen as covertly wanting to replace his father as his mother's lover. Freud directed Graf to share this insight with little Hans. Freud believed

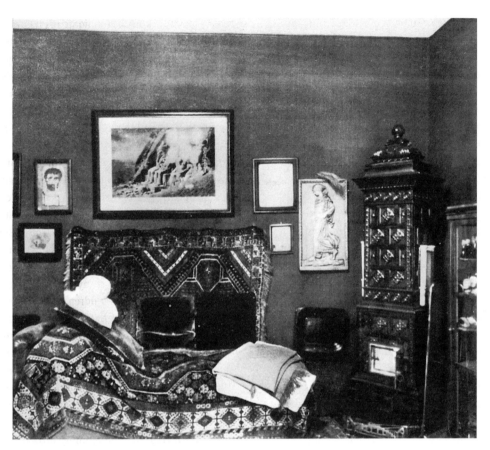

Figure 2.4 The couch in Sigmund Freud's consulting room.

that this conflict was the most potent determinant of Hans' psychopathology. Over the course of treatment, Hans' fear of horses abated (Blum, 2007). Freud was later surprised that Little Hans as an adolescent and young adult had little recollection of his earlier psychoanalysis. Little Hans, whose real name was Herbert Graf, was interested in music. He later became stage manager at the Metropolitan Opera in New York, part of a very successful career as a musician. He sought psychoanalysis as an adult because of an unhappy marriage (Quinodoz and Alcorn, 2005). Contemporary analysts looking back at the case history have commented on Freud's apparent inattention to several traumatic elements in the family life of the Grafs. Little Hans' parents fought with each other constantly, finally ending in divorce.

The young Hans also witnessed the physical beating of his sister while she was still a toddler (Blum, 2007). At the time of the analysis of Little Hans, Freud was not very attuned to the implications of mothering for child development, in spite of the fact – or maybe because – he himself was treating Little Hans' mother in psychotherapy (Anthony, 1986). Freud was subsequently criticized for that weak link in his theory, which he tried to correct in subsequent years, leading to important psychoanalytic work on mothering by Freud's daughter Anna, especially during her work at Hampstead Hospital in London in the 1940s (Young-Bruehl, 2004).

Freud's lack of interest in developing child psychoanalysis as a therapeutic method was not matched by many of his associates, who saw great promise in the idea. Methods of conducting child psychoanalysis were among the many areas of disagreement. However, the ex-disciples did disagree with "Papa Freud" on many important matters of basic theory and technique. The disputes between Freud and many of his associates are often discussed in terms of personality clashes. As they diverged further away from Freud's initial goal of discovering in analysis the roots of psychopathology in infant sexuality, some of the "revisionists" were accused of "wild analysis." Ironically, it is not Freud's daughter Anna who remained closest to her father's teachings or developed a child psychotherapy that can be considered a "junior version" of Sigmund Freud's psychoanalysis – child psychoanalyst Melanie Klein (1881–1960) was a far more faithful heiress to Freud's traditions as they might be applied to children (Nuffield, 1988). Anna Freud was accused by Klein of diluting the experience of therapy for children by devoting too much attention to building rapport with the child, failing to interpret negative aspects of the child–therapist relationship and dwelling too extensively on the child's relationships with his or her parents (Anthony, 1986). Despite their differences, Anna Freud, Melanie Klein and their contemporaries succeeded in establishing the tradition of child psychoanalysis, which has survived to the present day, although it is far more widely practiced in some places than others.

There were – and still are – some efforts at using the same classic psychoanalytic techniques with children as with adults. However, with time, this became relatively rare. First of all, few children can be brought to an analyst's office for as many therapeutic sessions as are usually required for classical psychoanalysis, that is, several times a week for a number of years. Anna Freud considered children poor candidates for this type of analysis, because their "weak ego structures" changed as part of the natural course of development. For these reasons, psychodynamic therapies for children evolved on a course separate from that of adult psychoanalysis, with the goals of "loosening . . . fixations and increasing the child's capacity for

reality testing (Brody 1964, cited by Peterson and Burbach, 1988). Through the use of dramatic play and art therapy, unconscious conflicts can be brought into the child's awareness (Bornstein, 1988, cited by Peterson and Burbach, 1988; Nuffield, 1988). In fact, the medium of play has become the core of the method of *play therapy*, which is often conducted outside psychoanalytic circles with the objective of using the safe, therapeutic environment and, especially, the relationship between the child and the therapist, to help the child achieve self-acceptance. Axline (1964) developed play therapy as a way of adapting the theories of Carl Rogers (1902–70), the father of client-centered psychotherapy (see Chapters 8 and 10), to children. Like Rogers' therapy with adults, Axline's play therapy is non-directive; the therapist helps the client by providing unconditional positive regard and by reflecting the child's feelings back to him/her. There is no attempt to uncover unconscious motives in the child's psyche or to make the child aware of them (Axline, 1964; Nuffield, 1988).

Attachment theory: a psychoanalytically inspired focus on child–parent bonds

Among the many prominent scholars who have reanalyzed the Little Hans material (see above) is John Bowlby (1907–90), the developer of attachment theory. Bowlby observed that Freud had ignored a number of possible alternative explanations of the case material about Little Hans' relationship with his parents. In explaining Little Hans' phobia, Freud did not take into account the fact that Hans' mother had threatened him with being sent away if he misbehaved. Importantly, Freud disregarded the fact that the phobia emerged soon after the birth of his younger sister a year earlier and the fact that Hans was in fact separated from his mother for a period of time after his sister arrived (Bowlby, 1973; Wakefield, 2007).

Given Bowlby's personal life, it is unsurprising that he could not gloss over the importance of child–parent bonding as easily as Freud did. Bowlby's father was a renowned surgeon but a shy, aloof man who lost his father at age 5; his father was brutally tortured to death during the Anglo-Chinese Opium War. John Bowlby was largely raised by a nanny in "traditional English fashion" (Coates, 2004, p. 573); his mother typically saw her children for only 1 hour a day, when she read to them. His beloved nanny left the home when Bowlby was 4 years old. His father went off to war soon after Bowlby was sent to boarding school, an experience, he later remarked, that should not be inflicted even on a dog. After his medical studies at Cambridge, at which he excelled, he decided to train as an analyst at the Maudsley Hospital in London. Among his supervisors during his psychoanalytic training was Melanie Klein, whose influence on him was paradoxical. While working with an anxious, agitated 3-year-old, Bowlby noticed the anxiety and distress in the boy's mother. Klein forbade Bowlby to even speak to the mother! Bowlby was horrified at her lack of interest. However, Bowlby was more influenced by the Hungarian school of psychoanalysis, which had always emphasized the child–mother bond (Coates, 2004).

In Bowlby's attachment theory, the child is seen as forming an *internal working model*, or mental representation, of how close interpersonal relationships work. The model depends on the security of bonds with early caregivers, especially the mother. From the "secure base" provided by the caregiver, the child explores other close relationships, including friendships and romantic relationships in later life (Bowlby, 1973; Schneider, Atkinson and Tardif, 2001).

The early interpersonalists vs. advocates of diagnostic typologies

As noted earlier, Freud's career was punctuated by bitter disputes with associates and disciples, many of whom could not accept psychoanalytic doctrine as it unfolded. Probably the most important difference of opinion of the time was between Freud and Alfred Adler (1870–1937), another medical doctor who chose to specialize in psychoanalysis and develop psychoanalytic thinking. Adler's career was already well established before he began his 9 years of collaboration with Freud. Therefore, he was perhaps less inclined than others to remain in the role of disciple and less needy of mentorship. However, his quarrel with Freud had to do with very fundamental matters of basic principle. As Freud expanded on the role of the unconscious in explaining behavior and on the causal role of sexual impulses in early childhood, Adler felt out of place. Adler was more attuned to the interpersonal origins of psychopathology, proposing that neuroses (relatively mild forms of psychopathology not involving extensive loss of contact with reality) could be caused by individuals feeling that they are inferior to others. Foreshadowing the social-cognitive approaches that were to become popular a half-century later, Adler also believed that people's self-concepts and basic beliefs about other people could lead to neurosis. Freud and the Freudians dismissed the interpersonal approach as superficial, as many psychoanalysts still do (Ansbacher and Huber, 2004; Bergmann, 2004; Runyon, 1984). Jacob Moreno (1839–1974), another contemporary of Freud, went much further in his thinking about the social origins of psychopathology. Moreno was never a disciple of Freud. Indeed, his flamboyant, theatrical style suggests that he was an unlikely candidate for the role of anyone's disciple. An immigrant from Romania to Austria, then to the United States in flight because of the Nazis' persecution of Jews, Moreno was very influenced by the tense political climate between the two World Wars. It is said that Moreno met Freud only once, when he asked Freud a question at a public lecture. Moreno's expansive theory was developed with the objective of repairing the relationships between groups and nations by repairing one by one the social relationships within them. To achieve this, he developed the technique of psychodrama, which can be considered in some ways almost the diametric opposite of psychoanalysis. In psychodrama, people express their conflicts with others, sometimes on a theater stage. In Vienna, this was done in a purpose-built theater open to the public, unthinkable in psychoanalytic circles. Other "actors" would portray the people involved in the disputes and help resolve them, often by helping understand how each person involved in a dispute might see the situation differently. "Auxiliary" actors helped bring in aspects of the conflicts that the "protagonist" was unaware of. Moreno is also the father of sociometry, a technique used to determine how an individual is perceived by the other members of his or her social groups (Marineau, 1989; Moreno, 1953). At first Moreno developed his "theater of spontaneity" with children he met on the streets of Vienna, attempting to learn how to get them to interact in new, creative ways to which they were unaccustomed. Only later did he apply psychodrama to his adult patients (Moreno, 1947; Nuffield, 1988). Nowadays, psychodrama is applied mostly to adults but sociometry has become a mainstay of research on the peer relations of children with various forms of psychopathology, as will be detailed in Chapter 7. However, some principles adopted from Moreno's psychodrama have survived in their influence on group therapy, which is conducted with children, and especially with adolescents (Hoag and Burlingame, 1997).

Perhaps no other movement objected to the emergence of medical models of mental illness as strongly as the interpersonalists led by the American psychiatrist Harry Stack Sullivan (1892–1949). Sullivan's illustrious career included positions as psychiatric consultant with the US military and appointments as chief psychiatrist at leading hospitals in Baltimore and New York. Much of Sullivan's thinking was undoubtedly shaped by his personal experiences of loneliness. He grew up in an isolated farm community, the son of Irish Catholic immigrants in an anti-Catholic town. He was also lonely as he could not publicly reveal his sexual attraction to other men because of the repressive climate of the times, even though he did eventually develop a long-term close relationship with a younger man who was known to the public as his adopted son (Evans, 1996; Perry, 1982; Wake, 2008).

According to Sullivan, most psychological disorders are caused by psychosocial factors, principally unfavorable social conditions and/or poor parenting. He also emphasized the consequences on an individual's adjustment of not having benefited from close friendship, especially during the early adolescent and adolescent years. He believed that mental disorders did not have sharp boundaries as proposed in the classification schemes that were becoming prevalent during the years of his practice. He maintained, for example, that, just as psychotic people are not psychotic much of the time, non-psychotic people may have some small psychotic episodes on occasion. Sullivan did not believe in the promise of objective definition of mental disorders, believing that the most important information was to understand the perceptions of each suffering individual. In his view, each individual's difficulties were unique and their causes somewhat idiosyncratic. Finally, years before such criticisms were first leveled at classification schemes such as the DSM (see Chapter 3), Sullivan observed that the diagnostic distinctions that preoccupied many of his colleagues did not provide information useful for therapeutic treatment (Evans, 1996).

Child "symptoms" seen as symptomatic of family psychopathology

The idea that child psychopathology might be caused by improper discipline or guidance by parents can be traced back to ancient times. By the 1950s, some radical practitioners altered this age-old perspective by considering the family itself, rather than the child or any other family member, as the "patient." In tracing the early history of systemic family therapy, Broderick and Shrader (1981) regard the emergence of this new modality as inevitable. By the beginning of the twentieth century, social workers and counselors visited US families in their homes to provide advice. They could not help but notice that, very often, the child who displayed atypical behavior was not the only family member to do so. At the suggestion of pioneer social worker Mary

Richmond (1868–1924), professional social workers began to take copious notes on the behavior of all members of the families they worked with. This was to become part of a process called *social diagnosis*, introduced by Richmond in a book with the same title (Richmond, 1917; Broderick and Shrader, 1981).

By the 1950s, a minority group of mental health professionals in the United States began to work with whole families together, focusing on family process rather than the psychopathology of any individual family member. A dynamic and daring, interdisciplinary group working in Palo Alto, California introduced revolutionary ideas based on communications theory. The Palo Alto group – Gregory Bateson (1904–80), Jay Haley (1932–2005), John Weakland (1919–95), Don Jackson (1920–68) and Virginia Satir (1916–88) – developed radical new ideas about the origins of psychopathology and dramatic techniques (that some might call histrionic) for its treatment. In its purest form, systems theory can be interpreted to reject the idea that psychopathology resides within the child or any other member of his or her family – it is the whole family system that is pathological. The most loyal practitioners of this approach use the term "identified patient" to refer to the child or the adult family member who has been referred for assessment or treatment (Beels, 2002; Broderick and Shrader, 1981).

The systems theorists observed that families operated in ways that maximized *homeostasis* or steady state. In doing so, they stubbornly repeat the same "games" that keep the family in a stable but unsatisfactory state. Any change in one part of the family system could threaten other parts as well as the stability of a system. For example, a family member's depression might serve some function within the system, perhaps maintaining the depressed person in a weak position that enables other members to dominate (Nichols and Schwartz, 1991). Strengthening the depressed person might affect the balance of the system, perhaps diminishing the power of another member or members. Systemic family therapists typically work with the entire family at one time, often using strong, almost

theatrical techniques to get the family to understand how it works and, hopefully, change. One of their best-known techniques is *paradoxical instruction* – telling the family to do the exact opposite of what they should. They developed these techniques based on knowledge of mechanisms of human influence, including hypnotism. Techniques known as *positive connotation*, introduced by the Milan school of family therapy (see below), consist of praising, paradoxically, elements of the family system that maintain homeostasis, even though the therapist's intention is to change these elements. For example, they might praise a sibling who sacrificed his or her own welfare to provide for a brother or sister who decided to leave home, rather than encouraging that sibling to make sure that his or her own needs are looked after as well (Palazzoli Selvini, et al., 1978).

The original work of the Palo Alto group focused on the family roots of schizophrenia. In one of the most daring theories about the workings of human systems, since discredited, Bateson and his colleagues introduced the concept of the *double bind*, in which a family unwittingly treats the "sick" "identified patient" as incompetent. They remind the family *scapegoat* that he or she is incompetent by sending mixed messages, for example messages indicating that the person is both loved and unloved, wanted and unwanted, needed and imposing an excessive burden on the family (Bateson et al., 1963). These mixed messages were linked to the onset of schizophrenia (Beels, 2002; Broderick and Schrader, 1981). The double-bind hypothesis has since been discredited; research has revealed quite clearly that communication of this type is not a cause of schizophrenia (Koopmans, 2001). It is worth noting that the history of thinking about psychopathology is marked by repeated dismissals of attempts to attribute schizophrenia to psychological causes. Adolf Meyer, whose work is discussed earlier in this chapter, maintained in the early 1900s that schizophrenia occurred in individuals who were subjected during their adolescent years to so much stress that their natural processes of resistance could not overcome it (DeVylder, 2013).

As time went on, the systemic mode of thinking and delivering therapy achieved some degree of acceptance. Many social workers, trained to attend to the social context of individual behavior, were amenable to seeing the family as "the case" (Beels, 2002; Haley, 1973). Originally dismissed as a highly intellectual therapy, it was adapted successfully to members of the lower socio-economic classes and to ethnic minorities by Minuchin (1974), who worked with families from the poorest neighborhoods of Philadelphia.

It is probably no coincidence that systemic thinking about families developed in parallel among professionals in Milan. The family has always been considered a major socializing agent and home base for Italians, and its importance remains fundamental in the psychological lives of Italians despite marked urbanization and modernization. Italy was undergoing considerable social change in the 1960s and 1970s, with frontal attacks by intellectuals on many social institutions they considered elitist. The psychoanalytic belief that pathology resided within the individual had become inconsistent with the personal philosophies and political principles of many Italians. By the 1970s, international communication had improved to the extent that professionals could collaborate actively across borders; the Milan Family Therapy group worked in close collaboration with systems theorists in the United States, some of whom were brought to Italy as consultants (Boscolo et al., 1987).

The behavioral revolution

Most of the therapies discussed until this point left an important step untaken: reconciling clinical diagnosis and therapy with the empirical roots of the profession of psychology. The therapeutic application of the scientific principles of learning theory constitutes a radical departure from the psychotherapeutic and diagnostic methods used before it. Laboratory research on human learning processes progressed simultaneously in the United States and the Soviet Union at the beginning of the twentieth century. In the United States, John B. Watson objected to the non-scientific basis of the main psychological theories of the time. He criticized most of all the methods used to develop and validate them, insisting that introspection was a respectable activity but one that should be relegated to philosophers, not psychologists. Watson and his successors in the behaviorist movement insisted that in order to discover the scientific rules of human behavior, psychologists should study that phenomenon by itself – behavior. They saw no basis for explaining behavior by invoking inner motives, unmet needs, drives, impulses or repressed memories. These internal processes were thought to reside in a "black box" because their existence and workings could never be proven scientifically, not that they saw any real reason to try. Watson initially saw little application for his theories in the assessment and treatment of child psychopathology. However, in 1920 he published a case study showing that fearful behavior could be induced in the laboratory; he trained Little Albert, a healthy 11-month-old infant, to become afraid of white rats and other furry animals. A few years later, a colleague published a case study showing that fears could be *un*trained in the laboratory: a little boy named Peter was "cured" of his fear of rabbits (Jones, 1924; Kazdin, 1984; O'Leary and O'Leary, 1972; Watson and Raynor, 1920). Ivan Pavlov's (1849–1936) parallel work in Russia was based on very similar principles, perhaps articulated less forcefully. Pavlov's research was highly regarded by the Soviet authorities in the first years after the Russian Revolution, to the point that they changed the name of a city in his honor. Pavlov offered some suggestions as to how his theories might be applied to promote better schools and institutions (Zagrina, 2009). For the most part, however, the applications of early behaviorism were confined to the laboratory and to writings on psychological theory. Nevertheless, these contributions can be seen as playing an important historical role by constituting a very cohesive opposition voice to the two mainstream movements of the time, which focused on the development of "disease" models of psychopathology and "romantic" Freudian psychoanalysis, respectively. In counterpoint, they gave rise to a distinct, independent psychological perspective, seen by some as releasing clinical psychology from the role Graziano (1975) called "peripheral psychiatry."

In the 1960s, behaviorism was called into service by clinical psychologists working on many types of child psychopathology. The philosophical groundwork for applied behavior analysis had been accomplished by the eminent psychologist B. F. Skinner (1904–90), who, in a novel entitled *Walden Two*, unveiled in 1948 his daring dream of a Utopian society that would operate totally on the basis of positive reinforcement (Skinner, 1948). In recalling the social climate of the 1970s, scholars have invoked the shock reaction in the United States to the achievements of the Soviets in science, culminating in their launch of the first satellite, Sputnik, into outer space in 1957. There was an unprecedented emphasis on science in the United States and lingering doubt about the efficacy of the educational system in producing great scientific minds. Behavioral methods have been seen as consistent with the social demands of this era – they provided treatment that was scientifically valid and easily shown to be effective (Graziano, 1975; Portes, 1971).

Between the 1950s and the 1970s, behaviorally oriented psychologists developed and evaluated techniques grounded in learning theory to help remediate various forms of children's atypical behavior. For the most part, these techniques involved parents and teachers, who were taught to change their typical patterns of reward and punishment into systematic patterns that would extinguish the problem behaviors and reinforce appropriate alternatives. Probably the most comprehensive and meticulous work in applying behavioral principles to improve atypical child behavior has been conducted by Gerald Patterson (1895–1967) and his colleagues at the Oregon Social Learning Center. In their longitudinal studies,

Patterson and his co-workers identified the ways in which adolescents "coerce" their parents into yielding de facto power, resulting in an escalating cycle of youth violence and family misery. They provided parents with the behavioral techniques needed to reverse this cycle (Patterson, 1982).

In some institutions, larger-scale "token economies" were put into place, with the institutional caregivers in charge. Children received tokens for positive behaviors; the tokens could later be redeemed for privileges or prizes. Thus, the behaviorists provided treatments that were effective without recourse to considerations of the psychic causes of the condition treated or its diagnostic status, which both psychoanalysts and proponents of disease models regard as anathema. Behavior therapy cannot proceed, however, without a careful *behavioral assessment* of the conditions in the child's environment that sustain the problem behavior (DiLorenzo, 1988; O'Leary and O'Leary, 1972).

By the end of the 1970s, enthusiasm for behavior modification waned. Some critics contended that token-economy environments stifled children's intrinsic interest in their tasks and activities. Others discovered that the results persisted in the controlled environment that provided the systematic reinforcement prescribed by the behavioral psychologists, but did not transfer or generalize to other settings in the children's concurrent or subsequent lives. In response, behaviorists countered that neither of these contentions are consistent with research. Those debates continue until the present day (Ogilvie and Prior, 1982; Wakefield, 2008). In any case, the behavioral revolution had lost much of its steam.

Behavioral techniques are still used widely in some situations. Faced with what appears to be a rapid and unexplainable increase in the prevalence of autism, many parents and professionals today ask of behaviorists what the American public asked of them in the 1960s – for techniques that are clearly effective and not clouded by "fuzzy" theories about the hidden causes of the problem. As in the 1960s, there are also many people who still insist on delving into what they believe to be the hidden causes.

Classical behaviorism overthrown by the cognitive revolution

As noted earlier, Alfred Adler introduced the idea that people's thinking about themselves and others could influence their feelings, behavior and adjustment. This idea was reinforced by subsequent research by the Soviet psychologists Alexander Luria (1902–77) and Lev Vygotsky, who showed how children use verbal instructions from others and their own internal dialogue to direct their behavior. One of the reasons why these ideas appealed to research-oriented child psychologists in the 1970s and afterwards may be their desire to offer some treatment directly to the child, building the child's repertoire of skills to cope with the environment (Philips, 1978). *Cognitive-behavioral* or *social-learning* methods satisfy this desire much better than classic behavior modification, in which the therapist works through mediators in the child's environment. As time went on, many practitioners found that adequate control over the environment can be difficult to achieve. Parents and teachers may also have come to expect some direct work with the child. This does not at all mean that the cognitive-behavioral therapists who practiced in the 1970s did not work, or did not want to work, with the environment. Indeed, they soon discovered that working only on thinking or language processes was often not sufficient to effect change. Cognitive methods had to be combined with behavioral methods, hence the term "cognitive-behavioral therapy."

Thus, many former behaviorists began to delve into the previously forbidden "black box" of inner thoughts that mediate the link between environmental stimuli and the child's learning. They came to believe that mediating cognitive processes could explain psychopathology better than considering only the contingencies of stimuli and responses, as in operant learning or behavioral theory. Cognitive social learning theories are based on the assumption that learning depends fundamentally on how the individual receives and cognitively processes stimulus and consequence information. They further assume that any therapeutic gain is caused by producing change in the cognitive events or processes that produce behavior (Foster, 1988). Many of these ideas derive from the theories of Albert Bandura (born 1925), who disputed the contention that behavior was shaped exclusively by the environment, although he very definitely did recognize the role of the environment in shaping both normal and abnormal behavior. Bandura posited a reciprocal process, in which environmental influence is complemented by information processing systems within the individual and by feedback processes linking these internal mechanisms with the outside world. His *social-learning theory* is thus based on *reciprocal determinism* (Bandura, 1969; Foster, 1988). As summarized concisely by Bandura (1969, p. 46): "persons, far from being ruled by an imposing environment, play an active role in constructing their own reinforcement contingencies through their characteristic modes of response." For example, a child who is disliked by his classmates comes to believe that no one wants to associate with him. Based on that belief, the child behaves in an unresponsive, cold manner, strengthening his belief that he or she is disliked, leading to further rejection by peers. As time goes on, the child may develop diagnosable social anxiety (Kendall, 1985). Thus, where a classic behaviorist would explain this behavior as a simple function of the punishing behavior of the peer group, which Bandura would not deny, Bandura would insist that considering the child's internal processing of the information received from peers – and its consequences – provides a more complete explanation (Foster, 1988; Kendall, 1985).

Social-learning theorists have also focused on a number of other cognitive mechanisms, all of which may operate simultaneously. Among these is the tendency to ignore or misinterpret important stimuli received from the environment. For example, a person might only classify people and their behaviors as entirely good or bad, remaining unable to process the various gradations in between that form the foundations of most interpersonal relationships. Both socially withdrawn and aggressive children and youth have been found to misinterpret vague information received from other people as indicating that the other people intend to harm them (Dodge, 1985; Foster, 1988).

Yet other cognitive-behaviorists base both their explanations of dysfunctional behavior and their methods of correcting it on the processes of *modeling* and *imitation*. This approach considers not only what is shown to the child but also how the child receives and processes the modeled behavior. Their therapies involve presenting the child with a model – live, videotaped or role-played – of appropriate behavior, often in combination with the opportunity for the child to practice imitating the model and to receive feedback on the practice. Derived more directly from the work of Luria and Vygotsky is *self-instruction training*, in which the therapist guides the child in using internal language to regulate his or her behavior, typically to remain calm rather than act aggressively out of anger (Foster, 1988; Kendall and Braswell, 1982).

Cognitive-behaviorists did not discard at all the emphasis on empirical research that is the foundation of classic behavioral approaches. The fact that their explanations and therapies are in widespread use today derives from the extent that social-learning approaches have been subjected to scrutiny in high-quality research, and deemed effective. (A more detailed description of social-learning theories of childhood depression and of how they are being tested by researchers appears in Chapter 11.) It is in the area of depression that cognitive-behavioral therapies and the theories on which they are based have been subjected to the most rigorous empirical scrutiny. However, cognitive-behavioral theories are also applied extensively to current work on social anxiety, aggression and other forms of child psychopathology.

Concluding remarks

The second half of the twentieth century brought not only the behavioral and cognitive revolutions but also, with and because of these new approaches, a substantial reconciliation between the practice of child-clinical psychology and the empirical roots of the discipline of psychology. Research in the field has expanded greatly in the past 30 years or so, with more articles published in a single month these days than in several years of the first half of the twentieth century. Despite the burgeoning interest in the field, many if not most of the questions first asked decades or centuries ago about the nature and origins of children's psychological problems have yet to be answered completely.

Another very substantial accomplishment of the years since World War II is the expansion of the scope of the child-clinical psychologist beyond the walls of hospitals and psychologists' offices. The child in distress is now much more likely to be understood and helped with due attention to the social context in which the child lives, including the family, school, community and culture.

Summary

- Prior to the nineteenth century, little attention was paid to child psychopathology.
- The writings of Hippocrates indicate that the Greeks traced mental disorders to four "humors" – blood, phlegm, yellow bile and black bile, imbalances of which affected mind and body. Mental disorders were classified as epilepsy, paranoia, mania and melancholia.

- The ancient Greeks are sometimes portrayed as cruel to children with unusual or disorganized thoughts or behavior.
- Parts of the Old Testament appear similarly unmerciful to children, including the stoning of unmanageable sons in Deuteronomy. However, in Genesis there is a reference to the importance of treating children well and in Psalms (127:3) they are called a "gift from God."

- Roman and Athenian fathers had the power to sell atypical or difficult children into slavery. Romans have also been criticized for overindulging children's desires for games and sports and not focusing on their moral education.
- In the Middle Ages, the Catholic Church believed in original sin and educated children to overcome their perceived inherent evil. A misbehaving child could be put in front of the Inquisition, possibly resulting in burning as a witch or a lifetime of servitude to the Church. Exorcism was also a possibility.
- In medieval times, monastic doctors were creative and benevolent in their care of children experiencing mental distress.
- Doubt has been cast on the cruelty of the Middle Ages toward the mentally ill, since most documents pertain to Church authorities or nobles. Local churches were kind to the mentally ill. Adults and children were both cared for by their families.
- There were two diagnoses: idiocy – now known as intellectual disability; and lunacy – psychosis or schizophrenia. Idiocy was deemed incurable and would result in property confiscation. Lunacy was seen as curable.
- Thomas Phaire included some aspects of child psychopathology in the first English textbook of pediatrics, considering children's diseases separate from adults'. He argued against overtreatment. Problems he referenced included nightmares and bedwetting.
- Jean-Marc Gaspard Itard wrote a famous case study on the benevolent taming of a "wild child" using therapies that showed that atypical children were not inherently evil.
- In colonial North America, atypical children and adolescents were sometimes suspected to be witches.
- Cruelty to children with psychological problems abated by the early nineteenth century. Isolation and exile became the norm, to asylums or workhouses, or out of their native countries. This was seen as benevolent behavior.
- The mid-nineteenth century saw rapid advance in scientific and social progress, and the French and American Revolutions brought increased interest in the welfare of the downtrodden. Novelists raised awareness of the plight of the less fortunate, including children. Child labor laws resulted, as well as compulsory education in many Western nations. By the beginning of the twentieth century, the child welfare movement began in the United States.
- Concern grew over the unsuitability of urban climates for raising children and the problem of massing "idle" youth. Juvenile courts were established, with the aim of limiting exposure of young offenders to vices such as smoking and alcohol in pubs. Most concern was over the socialization of boys – there were few young female offenders, though they seem to have been treated more harshly, as some say they still are.
- Compulsory, free education emerged sporadically from the 1600s, in places such as Scotland, Prussia and some colonies in North America. Over the nineteenth century, schooling became more uniform in the United States and UK. It was not until well into the twentieth century that these laws were extended to completely include children with many serious forms of psychopathology.
- Locke and Rousseau, whose theories were cornerstones of the French and American Revolutions, were influential to the emergence of childhood as a distinct stage of development. Locke argued against the idea that an individual's nature was innate, and Rousseau introduced a model explaining qualitative differences between a child's thinking at various stages of development. Rousseau believed children were inherently "noble savages."
- Many practitioners disagreed with Rousseau's emphasis on environmental factors, believing in genetic causation of psychopathology.

- In the nineteenth century, authors such as Dickens and Daudet began writing representative, benevolent depictions of children in their novels.
- Concern over the unsuitability of children to factory life was seen as the cause of child psychopathology. Socioeconomic class is still correlated with many forms of mental illness.
- Renewed scientific interest was applied to studying children in the late nineteenth and particularly the early twentieth century. Observations of children's behavior, such as Darwin's 5-year compilation on his son and other "baby biographies," emerged, as part of studies on evolutionary processes.
- Stanley Hall began the child study movement in the 1880s using questionnaires concerning child development. Hall reconciled biological and social influences on development and adjustment and promoted adolescence as a separate and important stage of development. He called adolescence a time of "storm and stress."
- In the early twentieth century the Child Study Movement and the Rockefeller Foundation established laboratory schools where children could be observed. The movement wanted to form and revise theories of development.
- Family life and work locations changed, increasing demands on parents to shape children's development and character.
- The eighteenth and nineteenth centuries and the 1950s to 1970s were characterized by the "intrusive," "socialization" and "helping" modes of parenting, respectively. Parents increasingly turned to guidance clinics, which some professionals say excessively blamed mothers.
- Increased incidence of working mothers, and school and state influence has further changed Western family life. The effects of these changes have been the subject of some studies.
- The 1930s Cambridge-Somerville study featured a control group and longitudinal follow-up. Boys of 5 to 11 years old were assigned counselors and offered medical care, recreation opportunities and summer camps. Thirty years of study revealed that the control group had fewer criminal convictions and lower rates of psychopathology, perhaps due to dependence on their counselors.
- After World War II, it was apparent that there were more children needing help with mental health than was available, attracting more adherents to mental health prevention.
- Binet introduced systematic assessment techniques. He is best known as the father of intelligence testing. Binet worked fervently to capture the diversity of children's development and adjustment, but his work is often misconceived as reducing "intelligence to a single number," which has resulted in a number of abuses.
- Binet was concerned with extending education to children with atypical behaviors, whom he believed required special techniques. He differed from contemporaries, such as Cesare Lombroso, who grouped low intelligence, criminality and psychopathy within the same condition. Binet tried to find treatments that would enable "abnormal children" to best use their capacities.
- Reverence for the natural process of development caused considerable resistance to the classification of children's psychological problems. Reconciling the advantages of classification with variations in development remains a challenge today.
- The decision that some disorders previously only thought to occur in adults could occur in children ultimately won the day for classification.
- In the 1930s, disease models were applied to children's mental health disorders, focusing on schizophrenia. Pediatricians began recognizing childhood psychopathology as a debilitating condition.
- By the early twentieth century, most psychiatrists preferred the medical model, believing a diseased brain was the primary cause of psychopathology. However, Janet emphasized sociogenesis, the social origin of higher psychological processes,

- believing they developed in interpersonal relationships prior to being internalized.
- Though no longer well known, it has been argued that Janet was more the father of psychoanalysis and psychotherapy than Freud. He inspired Soviet Vygotsky, who went further than Janet in explicating how learning acquired in interpersonal relations is internalized by a child. Contemporary educationalists find his work highly insightful.
- The biopsychosocial theory of Adolf Meyer postulated that psychopathology is the reaction of the entire organism to unfavorable environments and stressful experiences. Far-fetched theories appeared in the nineteenth century, including excessive masturbation leading to schizophrenia and immoderate use of intellectual faculties leading to neurosis, especially in girls and women.
- By the end of the nineteenth century, psychopathology was understood to be caused by brain dysfunction. Freud's emphasis on the causal role of developmental stages of childhood sexuality and experiences was revolutionary. His work bridged the divide between those with and without biological training.
- Despite the importance with which childhood experiences were viewed, the psychoanalytic field at the time was "child phobic". Freud himself only analyzed one 5-year-old, now called "Little Hans," to confirm his own theories, concluding he learned "nothing new."
- Associates of Freud were more interested in developing child psychoanalysis. His daughter was accused by Melanie Klein of diluting the experience of therapy for children by spending too much effort on building a rapport, failing to interpret negative aspects of the therapist's relationship with the child and dwelling too much on the child's relationships with his or her parents. Nevertheless, the tradition of child psychoanalysis was established.
- Children were seen as ill-suited to the same psychoanalytic techniques as adults, due to the difficulty of arranging frequent sessions of sufficient length and their changing and weak ego structures. Psychodynamic therapies for children focus on loosening fixations and increasing the child's capacity for reality testing. Play therapy tries to use play to help the child achieve self-acceptance. Developed by Axline, play therapy helps the child by providing positive regard and reflecting the child's feelings back to him/her.
- Following World War II the influence of psychoanalysis declined.
- John Bowlby noted that Freud neglected many possible parent-related factors in the Little Hans analysis.
- Bowlby believed that children build a basic understanding of close interpersonal relationships from interacting with their caregiver, then use this understanding to explore other relationships.
- Menninger created a diagnostic scheme in which some disorders were seen as environmentally caused and others caused by stressors. His work would be the foundation for the first Diagnostic and Statistical Manual.
- Freud and Adler, though both psychoanalysts, disagreed on basic principles: Freud believing in the unconscious origin of behavior, Adler focusing on interpersonal origins. Freud and many psychoanalysts to this day consider Adler's approach superficial.
- Jacob Moreno developed psychodrama, focusing on interpersonal relationships and socio-cultural influence. Members of the public served as actors, who portrayed the people involved in stressful incidents experienced by the individuals who came to the theater for help in resolving their conflicts with others.
- Interpersonalists, led by Harry Stack Sullivan, objected strongly to the emergence of purely medical models of mental illness.
- Sullivan emphasized psychosocial factors as causes of psychological disorders, principally especially difficulties in forming intimate

interpersonal relationships during early adolescence. He placed importance on close friendships in adolescence.

- By the 1950s, the entire family would sometimes be treated as the patient. The Palo Alto group pioneered in the application of systems theory. They rejected the idea that psychopathology resided in an individual, in favor of the view that it was within the whole family.

- Systems theorists note that families tend to stay in a static state. Aiding a distressed family member requires working with the entire family to adjust to the new dynamic.

- The Palo Alto group had a now-discredited double-bind hypothesis, in which mixed messages about whether family members loved, needed and felt burdened by an individual caused schizophrenia.

- The Milan school is noted for dramatic techniques in assessing and treating dysfunctional families, including paradoxical instruction.

- John B. Watson and his successors insisted a more scientific method must be used to develop psychological theories, by studying behavior directly and exclusively. Inner motives, unmet needs, drives, impulses and repressed memories were seen as inaccessible. Watson showed that fearful behavior could be induced in the laboratory and a colleague showed that fears could also be "untrained." Pavlov's work, perhaps less forceful, was based on similar techniques. B. F. Skinner provided the philosophical groundwork for behavioral analysis.

- Between the 1950s and 1970s, parents and teachers were taught by behaviorists to alter patterns of reward and punishment to extinguish problem behaviors. Gerald Patterson and his colleagues completed longitudinal studies on adolescents coercing their parents resulting in cycles of youth violence and misery, and they helped parents reverse these cycles.

- In "Token economics" children are rewarded for positive behaviors. Careful behavioral assessment of children's environments.

- By the end of the 1970s, behaviorism was less popular. Token economies were criticized as stifling children's interest in their tasks and activities. Results were said not to transfer outside of controlled environments. Debate over this persists.

- Behavioral techniques are still used, especially in treatment of autism (see Chapter 17). The inattention to hidden underlying causes that typifies the behavioral approach is valued by some but decried by others.

- Luria and Vygotsky showed that children use verbal instructions and internal dialogue to direct their behavior. Cognitive-behavioral or social-learning methods satisfy a desire to offer treatment directly to children, more so than behavior modification, which is based on re-engineering of the reinforcement patterns of human environments. Such control of human environments is often difficult to achieve.

- Albert Bandura posited that environmental influence is complemented by information processing systems and feedback processes linking them to the outside world. His social-learning theory is based on reciprocal determinism.

- Social-learning has focused on a number of simultaneously operating cognitive processes, among which is the tendency to ignore or misinterpret stimuli. Both socially withdrawn and aggressive children and youth misinterpret vague information as indicating another person is a threat.

- Modeling and imitation constitute a corrective process for dysfunctional behavior, in which children are presented with a model of appropriate behavior and allowed to practice it, with feedback. Self-instruction training involves guiding the child to use internal language to regulate behavior.

- Since World War II, child-clinical psychologists have moved beyond hospitals to family, school and community environments.

Study questions

1. How do philosophical and religious ideas about the fundamental nature of the child affect beliefs about psychopathology and its treatment?
2. For what important reason have many scholars who emphasize the distinct nature of development during childhood resisted the diagnosis of children's mental health problems using standard categories?
3. What is the fundamental difference between Axline's play therapy and child psychoanalysis?
4. What is the basic distinction between Harry Stack Sullivan's conception of abnormal behavior and Freud's?
5. State one important difference between applied behavior analysis and cognitive-behavior therapy and one important similarity between them.

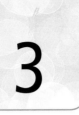

3

Classification of children's psychological problems
Pseudoscience or fundamental part of the helping process?

Classification, compassion and science: a historical perspective

Throughout most of history, psychological problems were not differentiated in any way. All individuals suffering from "idiocy" and "lunacy," as the combined condition was known in seventeenth-century Britain, were lumped together to be scorned and ridiculed. Some of the madhouses of the time had separate sections for the "mad" and the "foolish." Showing more insight and sympathy than most of their contemporaries, some writers from ancient Greeks through Shakespeare portrayed "fools" as displaying keen insight that was expressed in a confusing but highly perceptive manner (Andrews, 1998). Such undifferentiated concepts of mental illness did not die as recently as is sometimes thought: The US census of 1840, in one of the earliest attempts to determine the prevalence of mental illness, included only a single category "idiocy/insanity," which was only replaced 40 years later with seven types of mental disorder (Mash and Barkley, 2002).

Whatever the limitations of the *medical model* that is at the core of much contemporary practice in the mental health professions, this way of looking at psychological disorder, with the image of being sick that comes with it, is undoubtedly more benevolent than the previous image of being simultaneously deranged and dimwitted. The term "medical model" has surely been defined more frequently and probably more clearly by its critics than by its proponents. However, it is fair to say that its assumptions include, first of all, that mental disorders and distress function in much the same way as physical diseases. Hence, once the exact disease has been identified from among those that are known, the condition needs to be treated in a more

or less standard way that is prescribed by qualified professional experts (these features are delineated in somewhat disparaging language by McCready, 1986).

This chapter begins with consideration of the importance of classification to the sciences in general and to thinking and practice in medical science specifically. The core of the chapter is devoted to the organizational structures of the two most prevalent classification systems, the DSM and ICD, and to the advantages and disadvantages of these systems as they are used in contemporary mental health practices. The next section is devoted to the different ways in which classification systems of mental illness can be organized and structured: Is there a clear dividing line between normal and abnormal? The important distinctions in the way disorders can be classified are much more than semantic. They reflect very fundamentally the way disorder is understood. The section includes deliberation about the inherent differences between classifying the psychological distress of adults and children. The chapter continues with a description of the underlying principles of the new DSM-5 as applied to children and adolescents. The chapter concludes with some thoughts about the responsible, ethical use of diagnostic systems.

Classical beliefs about the structure of mental illness

Since ancient times, dividing mental illness into different subtypes has been a fundamental part of efforts to understand and treat psychological distress. It is possible to trace the need to generate subtypes back to the ancient Greeks, whose teachings included the observation that diseases consist of clusters of symptoms that typically occur together, constituting a *syndrome* (Pichot, 1994). The ancient Greeks, led by the physician Hippocrates, classified temperaments, or *humors*, into melancholic (sad, contemplative), sanguine (outgoing, friendly), phlegmatic (relaxed, content, shy) or choleric (hard-driven, ambitious; Pinault, 1992). An excess of any of these humors was thought to lead to mental distress. Interestingly, this notion – of mental illness occurring at the extreme of a behavioral dimension that need not be pathological – is still evident in current classification schemes, as will be discussed later in this chapter.

The prominent seventeenth-century English physician Thomas Sydenham, the grandfather of medical science in his country, is considered the first major advocate of classification of diseases as fundamental in modern medical practice. He and other pioneers of classification systems were inspired by the taxonomies that had emerged in the field of botany (Pichot, 1994). Sydenham maintained that nature works in virtually the same way in producing diseases in different people. Therefore, when the same disease occurs in different individuals, the symptoms and their progression are very similar (Payne, 1900; Pichot, 1994).

A century later, classification had become central in all the natural sciences, led by botany. Scientists argued with each other about the more general applicability of classification models developed to distinguish plants. An important transformation occurred in the eighteenth and nineteenth centuries, when scientists began to go beyond observable behaviors in constructing their taxonomies, focusing as well on internalized *essences*, which included the internal working mechanisms of the observable features (Pratt, 1977; Jensen, Hoagwood and Zitner, 2006). By the nineteenth century, psychiatrists in France, such as Philippe Pinel, Jean-Étienne Esquirol and Étienne-Jean Georget, began to work with children who suffered mental disorders. In doing so, they distinguished between several fundamental types of disorder, differentiating, for example, between disorders that they believed to be the result of brain lesions and those that they believed were not (Pichot, 1994).

The foundations of current classification systems were laid by Émil Kraepelin, an influential nineteenth-century German psychiatrist and author of seminal textbooks. A strong believer in the biological origins of mental disorders, he sought passionately to apply the basic methods of natural science to the diagnosis and treatment of mental disorders. Even though he refrained from proposing definitive lists of the symptoms that characterize each disorder, as in the current DSM schemes discussed later in this chapter, Kraepelin was criticized for imposing more order on his typology of mental disorders than actually occurs in real life (Jablensky, 1999). His colleagues also disputed the extent to which specific disorders can be traced to specific dysfunctions of different areas of the brain, a controversy that continues to this day. Summarizing the objections very philosophically, Jaspers (1963, cited by Jablensky, 1999) remarked that: "the idea of the disease entity is in truth an idea in Kant's sense . . . the concept of an objective which one cannot reach . . . but all the same it indicates the path for fruitful research and supplies a valid point of orientation for particular empirical investigations." Contextualizing Kraepelin's work within the philosophical debates of his time, Radden (1996), in a perceptive paper entitled "Lumps and Bumps," noted that Kraepelin was a "lumper" – a scholar who wanted to group symptoms together into syndromes – as opposed to a "splitter" – a scholar who wanted to expand the number of categories. Importantly, Kraepelin aspired to use empirical data to justify the categories he proposed (Jablensky, 1999). As will be discussed in detail later in this chapter, the premise that the categories can be justified scientifically is central to the diagnostic systems that prevail nowadays.

An important precept of the medical model and its most convincing justification is that the identification of the specific illness leads to specific and therefore optimally effective treatment. However, as recently as 50 years ago, the treatment provided for the mental health problems of children and adolescents tended to be very non-specific, vaguely psychoanalytic and plagued with the ritualistic blaming of parents, according to the observations of esteemed British child psychiatrist Michael Rutter. Probably for that reason, differential diagnosis (i.e., identification of the specific illness) was not a major concern of the mental health professionals of the time (Mayes and Horwitz, 2005; Rutter and Stevenson, 2010). Precision in diagnosis became more important as professionals struggled to adapt their practices to new advances in theory and research regarding the origins of several disorders. Rutter and Stevenson cite, among other landmark developments, Kanner's detailed description of autism in the 1940s. At the same time, longitudinal studies were beginning to demonstrate that several different but identifiable patterns could be observed in the emergence of psychopathological symptoms. Intuitively, understanding the pattern that corresponds to the specific symptoms and their future course seems valuable if not essential.

Causes of mental illness as elements of classification schemes

Even as recently as 50 years ago, classification of mental disorders involved not only the classification of symptoms but also the classification of their supposed causes. In practice, that classification of causes, especially as applied to child psychopathology, never progressed beyond the most general enumeration of a few possibilities, mostly environmental. In DSM-I, a classification scheme that appeared in 1952, the child and adolescent disorders were largely undifferentiated and were called "reactions." However, better scientific data were already appearing that led many to question such simplistic notions of causation. It became apparent that, as methodologists have long espoused, a simple correlation between a parenting practice and a child's problem does not constitute scientific proof that the parents caused the problem in question. The scientific community realized that the parent may also have been reacting to a problematic child or adolescent behavior that was already there. Most contemporary authorities do not attempt to decide which came first, the child's problem or the parenting practice associated with it, recognizing instead the *bidirectionality of*

influence (Bell and Harper, 1977; Rutter and Stevenson, 2010).

A related challenge to the then-common practice of attributing the cause of children's problems to some aspect of their environments came from the perceptive and highly influential observations of American psychologist Paul Meehl (1959; in Meehl, 1973, pp. 225–302, Chapter 13). He ridiculed what he saw as flimsy thinking in which it is believed that major, long-lasting mental health problems result from trivial events in a child's early life. Meehl lambasted clinicians who believed in what he dubbed the "spun-glass" theory of the child's mind. Fortunately, children's psyches are not as fragile as spun glass; they are equipped to resist long-term damage from the relatively trivial events that Meehl's colleagues discussed as causes of enduring psychological distress.

At the same time, longitudinal studies on the emergence of psychopathology began to encompass multiple factors, biological and social. It became apparent that there were not only a number of negative influences that might cause a disorder but also *protective factors*, positive processes and events that helped the individual become resilient to the negative influences. These protective factors include positive interpersonal relationships and the intellectual ability and flexibility needed to succeed in school and to solve problems (Kohlberg, LaCrosse and Ricks, 1972). The major theorists in the field came to realize that this multidimensional causal etiology is usually too complex to be tracked accurately in an individual case. Therefore, although there was greater awareness of the complexity of mental disorder, "big theories" of personality, which attempted to provide explanations of virtually all aspects of behavior in ways that are too complicated to ever be proven, were increasingly discarded (Rutter and Stevenson, 2010).

For all these reasons, causal inferences have been essentially eliminated from contemporary classification schemes, including the new DSM-5. This constituted a return to classification based entirely on observable phenomena, which has a long history in biology among other disciplines.

The elusive quest for objectivity

By the 1970s, the subjectivity of the diagnostic process was widely decried. What one professional called depression another called anxiety; yet another diagnosed it as masked aggression. Public awareness of this problem undermined confidence in the mental health professions. Mass media raised awareness of the imprecision in mental health diagnosis by publicizing the results of the famous and bold Rosenhan experiment. Rosenhan (1973) sent well-adjusted confederates, including several psychologists, a psychiatrist and a psychology student, to the emergency rooms of psychiatric hospitals. The students were told to respond honestly to the questions asked of them by the attending clinicians except for a few vague words about hearing voices and not having a clear sense of their places in life. All of the confederates were diagnosed as schizophrenic and admitted to hospital. Clearly, the stage was set for change. Change did come by the 1980s, as will be detailed shortly.

Basic functions of classification

The act of diagnosis itself is sometimes seen as therapeutic by some proponents of the medical model, who see the diagnosis as providing meaning and understanding of the patient's problem (Brody and Waters, 1980). Taylor and Rutter (2010) outline succinctly some of the basic functions of classification systems in the field of mental health. One of the most fundamental is to provide for clear communication among professionals, be they practitioners or researchers. If the scientific community is to digest and synthesize the results of a dozen studies on the family relations of children with depression, for example, it is important that the participants in each study be depressed according to the same criteria. Similarly, a professional contemplating a treatment program for a child with autism should choose from among treatments that have established effectiveness for that specific disorder. In gauging the effectiveness,

it is important to peruse the results of evaluations of the treatments contemplated. This task is nearly impossible if the evaluations are not conducted with similar populations. Such clarity is also imperative in communicating information about child psychopathology to non-professionals, especially parents, who can become valuable allies in the treatment process. Reliable diagnostic terminology enables epidemiological studies in which researchers establish how common a particular disorder is; this is important for public policy and for the allocation of professional resources. Very importantly, the use of standard terminology facilitates access by professionals to literature on a particular condition. This standard use of diagnostic terms is seen as enabling scientifically based predictions about the course of disorders. It should also facilitate the formulation of new theories regarding disorders (Blashfield, Keeley and Burgess, 2009).

Another important function of classification systems, as detailed by Taylor and Rutter (2010), is to facilitate the efficient delivery of assessment and treatment services to children and families. Professionals and institutions use diagnostic categories in their record-keeping. Depending on the organization of the health-service systems in their countries, states and provinces, many professionals use these categories when seeking payment from their government health systems or insurance companies. Of course, critics of contemporary service delivery do not regard this as an advantage.

Finally, accuracy in terminology is essential in order to establish how common a problematic condition is among the general population. Efforts to determine the extent of mental illness can be traced back to the London Bills of Mortality in seventeenth-century England (www.who.int/classifications/icd/en/HistoryOfICD.pdf, retrieved November 9, 2010) and to the US Census Bureau since the early nineteenth century. Epidemiologists nowadays cannot do their jobs effectively without confronting issues of terminology and consistency of usage. Thus, all of these advantages of classification are predicated on the scientific validity of the classification system, which, as will be discussed later, should not be taken for granted.

DSM overhauled: a victory for science?

At present, there are two major diagnostic systems for mental disorders in widespread use: the *Diagnostic and Statistical Manual*, in a fifth edition released in 2013 (American Psychiatric Association, 2013; the Arabic numeral is used starting with the fifth edition to accommodate future revision – DSM-5.1, etc.), and the mental health section of the International Classification of Diseases, tenth edition (World Health Organization, 1996). DSM-5 is used almost exclusively in North America. DSM-5 co-exists with ICD-10 in many other parts of the world. At this point, the conceptual bases of the two systems are very similar and emerge from a drastic revision to the DSM that began with the publication of DSM-III (American Psychiatric Association, 1980) in 1980. Although the two systems are now quite similar in structure and underlying philosophy, their delineation of the specific disorders and the criteria they use for diagnosing them are not identical. These differences may appear minor against the backdrop of the overall systems. However, what first appears to be a minor detail may result in consequential differences between the systems in both the nature and extent of the diagnosis of individual disorders. Therefore, many leaders in the field are calling for increased compatibility in the future (First, 2009; Taylor and Rutter, 2010), which is indeed likely to emerge.

The DSM-III was the result of a far more elaborate and reasoned examination of the ways in which mental disorder can be classified than was evident in predecessors such as DSM-I and DSM-II. Many of the world leaders in developmental psychopathology were involved in the process, which included working groups assigned to deliberate the specifics of the diagnosis of individual disorders. These working groups based their decisions to some extent on empirical field trials of the new diagnostic criteria. However, the consensus of experts' opinions was the basis of the interpretation of the data from these field trials and of many decisions that were not based on the field trial. Over time, such consensus decision-making came to be criticized for many reasons, not the least of which is the weight unwittingly assigned to the personal values and quirks of the experts chosen (e.g., Caplan, 1995). Nevertheless, the process for the development of the new DSM-5 was quite similar.

At the time of its release, DSM-III was hailed by many prominent psychiatrists in the United States (Mayes and Horwitz, 2005), who declared "victory for science" (Klerman et al., 1984, p. 539) and rejoiced in the "triumph for science over ideology" (Sabshin, 1990, p. 1,272). They considered their profession transformed, redeemed and rejuvenated by the new classification scheme even though the developers of DSM-III, most of whom were also psychiatrists, considered their product tentative and imperfect. As detailed later in this chapter, the victory call may have been somewhat premature. However, the DSM has become the standard tool of a discipline that has expanded rapidly since its creation, perhaps in part because of it.

The International Classification of Diseases shadows the DSM

The International Classification of Diseases – 10 (ICD-10) is a complete classification system for all diseases and causes of death, not just mental disorders. First introduced in 1900, it is the official system for the classification of diseases endorsed by the World Health Organization. Unlike DSM-5, the complete system is available for consultation online without cost at http://apps.who.int/classifications/apps/icd/icd10online/. Until its most recent editions, the ICD differed in many fundamental ways from the versions of the DSM available at the time of their appearance. More recently, however, an intentional rapprochement of the two systems has emerged, with each successive version of the ICD becoming more similar to the DSM (Pitzer and Schmidt, 2000). This is very evident in the most recent revision of the ICD, the tenth edition published in 2007 and will surely be even more evident in the new version slated for 2015.

The language of the ICD is somewhat less oriented toward empirical precision and more oriented toward professional judgment, in the tradition of European psychiatry. Some important conceptual differences do remain. For example, in the ICD-10 section on "disorders of psychological development," specific guidelines are included to prompt the diagnosis of the most frequent co-occurring (comorbid) disorders (Schulte-Markwort, Marutt and Riedesser, 2003).

Basic features of DSM-5 and ICD-10

DSM-5 and ICD-10 are, for the most part, categorical systems. This means that the particular condition, such as depression or anxiety, is either present or absent. The decision as to whether the particular condition is present or absent is based on diagnostic criteria, which consist of observable behaviors. In most cases, the observable behavior must be present for a specified period of time, often 3 or 6 months. Many of the conditions that occur frequently, such as enduring personality problems and social anxiety, are normally diagnosed only in individuals above a certain age. In most cases, several but not all of the observable behaviors in a list of diagnostic features must be present. Thus, few discrete behaviors are considered *pathognomonic*, that is, as automatic indicators of a particular condition whenever they occur. The diagnostic criteria for the specific disorders are presented in Chapters 12 through 24, which pertain to the major forms of child psychopathology.

Dissent and disillusionment about classification and classification systems

Despite the undisputed contributions of the DSM in terms of improved (if not perfect) reliability of diagnosis and the resulting enhancement of communication, there remains an overall "air of disquietude" (Jensen, Hoagwood and Zitner, 2006, p. 25) in the field about these systems. In attempting to identify the basis of this disquietude, Jensen, Hoagwood and Zitner (2006) describe a nagging feeling that the disorders described do not exactly fit most of the cases that are referred to mental health professionals. This disquietude may be growing among professionals who subscribe to the basic principles underlying DSM and ICD but who are disappointed with the systems, which have emerged as not delivering everything that they were supposed to. These disenchanted "fellow travelers" are joined by professionals with more fundamental objections to the basic foundation on which the DSM and ICD are constructed.

Conceptual and definitional problems

The complete title of DSM is Diagnostic and Statistical Manual of Mental Disorders (American Psychiatric Association, 2000). Controversy begins with the title itself, largely because of the term "mental disorders." Ironically, despite the invocation of the notion of disorder and its near-synonym "disease," the biological foundations of child psychopathology are negated to a considerable degree by the adjective "mental." As discussed in Chapter 1, many psychiatrists regret the choice of the adjective because it implies a mind–body dichotomy. They point out that no known disorder is entirely "mental," as will become apparent in the subsequent chapters on the physiological correlates of child psychology and on the disorders themselves (Frances, 1994; Jensen, Hoagwood and Zitner, 2006).

Diagnosis seen as excessive reductionism

Although most professionals probably appreciate the virtues of agreement among themselves in their use of terminology, not all agree with the steps that are likely necessary to achieve this goal. For example, Mirowsky and Ross (1989), in an essay entitled "Psychiatric Diagnosis as Reified Measurement," observe that using diagnostic systems like the DSM entails overlooking the fact that psychological problems are not discrete and do not fall into distinct categories. In order to achieve reliability of measurement, clinicians, first of all, have to give up the individuality in their diagnostic procedures and employ instead highly structured interview procedures. These structured procedures focus on a limited range of the important issues in clients' lives, namely the features that happen to be listed in the criteria for the diagnosis of certain disorders.

Similarly, there has been some condemnation of the abandonment of the rich if subjective language derived from theories that are not easily reduced to concrete behavioral descriptors. For example, psychoanalyst and social critic Philip Cushman, decrying what he calls "psychology's assault on personhood" remarked that the DSM:

is a kind of tinker-toy self, composed of concrete, singular behaviors that can be easily disconnected and reconnected to one another in order to form the larger – but momentary – self-configurations. There is little that is complex, indeterminate, and ambiguous, let alone anything that refers to deeper, darker, unseen forces that form a larger, entangled pattern or style of personality or type of character. [It] is a self of parts, not wholes; behaviors, not personalities; concrete observations, not artistic interpretations; conscious speech, not unconscious dreams; surfaces, not depths; incontrovertible data points, not ambiguous narrative; cleanliness, not messiness. (Cushman, 2002, p. 108)

Comorbidity: reflections on a reality

As winter approaches, magazines and websites provide information useful in helping individuals decide whether they or their children have a cold, the flu or an allergy. The distinction among these conditions affects treatment in the most fundamental ways, including in many cases the basic decision as to whether the individual should see his or her physician. In many other situations, however, two physical illnesses can co-exist. The medical term *comorbidity*, introduced by Feinstein (1970), refers to the co-existence of illnesses, be they physical, mental

or both. For example, a person might have both liver cancer and heart disease. Similarly, it is very common for physical disease, for example heart disease, to co-occur with a psychological disorder such as depression (e.g., Taylor, 2010). In many cases, the two conditions affect each other. Their simultaneous presence must be considered when contemplating treatment (Feinstein, 1970; Zachar, 2009). The term *comorbidity* is often used interchangeably with the terms "co-occurrence" and "covariation." The latter terms, however, do not imply a connection between the two conditions, unlike many uses of the term comorbidity (Baldwin and Dadds, 2008).

Since the appearance of DSM-III, the rates of comorbidity in diagnoses have increased drastically in the diagnosis of both adult and child mental disorders. In the cases of the most common children's psychological disorders, that is, disruptive behavior disorders, attention deficit disorders, anxiety and depression, there are, according to many reports, more children diagnosed as having two or more disorders than children diagnosed as having only one. This results in a confusing set of combinations. There could be and often are combinations of the ten most frequent symptom patterns (i.e., anxiety, inattention, obsessive-compulsive, depression, bipolar, attention deficit, conduct disorder, oppositional defiant disorder [ODD], tics, autism and substance abuse), resulting in a total of 10^2 or 1,024 patterns that a professional working in the field of child mental health would have to recognize and treat. For these and other reasons, it could be argued that knowledge and clinical practice are not really advanced by current diagnostic systems, which force users not to "look deeper" into children's psychological distress but to remain close "to the surface" (Jensen, Hoagwood and Zitner, 2006, p. 25).

It is often believed that individuals who suffer from comorbid disorders are more "ill" and more difficult to treat than their counterparts who are diagnosed as having only a single disorder. This has only sometimes emerged in the limited research on this issue. In a systematic review of the literature on the responsiveness to treatment by children diagnosed as having attention deficit/hyperactivity disorder, Ollendick and his colleagues (2008) discovered that, in most cases, comorbidity was unrelated to treatment outcome.

Some have seen this increasing pervasiveness of comorbid diagnoses as a "crisis of comorbidity" (Zachar, 2009, p. 14). There are several possible explanations for the exploding rates of comorbidity. A very common explanation, the *artifactual hypothesis*, is that the DSM and ICD systems are flawed, particularly because they have introduced too many categories that do not really represent distinct disease entities (Aragona, 2009). This, of course, constitutes an argument for fewer categories or perhaps subcategories grouped hierarchically into larger categories, as discussed later in this chapter. However, it has also been argued that comorbidity is part of the essential nature of mental health disorders. This might be, first of all, because many different mental disorders share similar or identical causes, be they genetic, physiological or environmental. It is also possible that certain disorders now considered separate are related temporally, that is, one disorder may be an early form of another (Caron and Rutter, 1991). More globally, according to the *vulnerable population hypothesis*, certain people may be particularly vulnerable to psychological problems, perhaps because of environmental and social conditions, perhaps because of personality or temperament problems, perhaps because of physiological factors, or perhaps because of any combination of these risk factors (Zachar, 2009). Thus, there may be no crisis of comorbidity at all and the burgeoning comorbidity rates may not necessarily invalidate the DSM or ICD systems. High comorbidity may reflect no more than an emerging generation of diagnosticians who are trained to recognize the multiple conditions affecting the psychological well-being of the people they treat. On the other hand, what some see as a crisis of comorbidity may be no more than increasing recognition that the conceptual basis of the diagnostic system is not built on a solid

foundation because, as some critics of the DSM have pointed out, "disorders might merge into one another with no natural boundary between them" (Kendall and Jablensky, 2003).

Scientific, philosophical and political assaults

Behavioral attack (or counter-attack)

As mentioned earlier, the major diagnostic systems in current use, the DSM and ICD, were refined substantially in the 1960s and 1970s, thus coinciding with the heyday of behaviorism in North American psychology and the emergence shortly thereafter of social-learning models. In many of the criticisms of the DSM offered by sociologists and others, the advent of DSM-III was seen as a rejection of psychoanalysis in favor of behaviorism. Ironically, behaviorists have expressed many reservations about the new diagnostic system as well. As summarized by Andersson and Ghaderi (2006) and Hickey (1998), behaviorists vary in their objections. True to the empirical roots of the behavioral movement, many object to the delineation of disorders on the basis of the consensus of expert opinions rather than on research supporting the clustering of symptoms and the differentiation of conditions. Although many of their non-behavioral colleagues think that the theory underlying the DSM is behaviorism, that is not the perception of most behaviorists. Despite the claim made by its developers that the DSM is atheoretical, many behaviorists see the underlying theory as the medical model.

Accordingly, many prominent behaviorists and social-learning theorists expressed a number of vociferous criticisms of the "disease" model of mental illness, especially as it is applied to children. Their objections were articulated very clearly by Bandura (1969), the renowned pioneer of social-learning approaches to psychopathology and psychotherapy (see Chapter 2). He observed that the labeling as diseases of behavioral patterns that differ from accepted social and ethical norms has resulted in the modification of social deviance being considered a medical specialty. As a result, he argued, there is an excessive reliance on chemical and physical remedies. An unintended consequence of disease models, he maintained, is that the people suffering from the "diseases" become reluctant to seek treatment because they fear they will be stigmatized as ill or crazy. This is especially problematic, he wrote, because it chases away people whose atypical behavior is not dysfunctional enough to necessitate intensive intervention while many of their more minor difficulties may be quite easy to treat. The adjectives "healthy" and "sick" have even come to be used in reference to societal processes and social phenomena in general, not just individuals who display atypical behavior. He remarked that the process of deciding what constitutes a symptom of a disease is arbitrary and subjective, despite efforts at standardizing the basis of such inferences. For example, some parents might encourage aggressiveness in their sons whereas school personnel might regard the same behaviors as symptomatic of a mental disorder. He further maintained that the degree to which a particular atypical behavior inconveniences others is much more likely to cause the behavior to be labeled "sick" than other atypical behaviors that are easier for others to tolerate. Finally, applying to the case of children's psychological difficulties a criticism leveled by behaviorists at personality theorists, Bandura invoked Mischel's (1968) work on the situational specificity of behavior. From that perspective, an important error in the medical model is the belief that an individual's behavior, in this case atypical problem behavior, is similar across various social contexts. Mischel's position is that much more behavior is specific to the situation in which it occurs than is commonly believed. The corollary is that there is less cross-situational consistency in behavior than would be needed to validate both "big" personality theories and medical models of mental illness, both of which are based on the assumption that individuals behave in similar ways in multiple contexts.

It might be expected that behaviorists, who are often known for their disavowals of unnecessary

theory and their focus on observable phenomena, would applaud the adaptation of an atheoretical stance that began with DSM-III. However, behaviorises objected to the lack of scientific precision as strongly as psychoanalysts deplored the loss of the psychoanalytic wisdom. Bandura (1969) suggested that scientific theories be allowed to compete with each other and that the theory or theories that emerge from research as most congruent with problem behavior be adopted as a reference for the diagnostic process. The claim that the DSM-IV is atheoretical has been widely questioned and not only by behaviorists and social-learning theorists. Many insist that no diagnostic system can be completely atheoretical (Sadler, Wiggins and Schwartz, 1994).

Classification schemes and the "turf battles" of mental health disciplines

Whether that is their fundamental purpose or not, classification systems delineate the boundaries of mental health disciplines. According to many observers, including a condition in the classification system used by a particular profession amounts to that profession staking claim to the "territory" of diagnosing and treating that disorder (Blashfield, Keeley and Burgess, 2009). There are many accusations insinuating that the profession of psychiatry uses its diagnostic system to expand its authority and, indeed, its revenue. For example, Houts (2002) attributes that motivation to the rapid expansion of the number of diagnostic categories that appear in successive editions of the DSM. Houts disagrees vehemently with what he sees as the common myth that the new categories have emerged from advances in scientific research. He maintains that scientific research would be more likely to result in the consolidation of categories, with categories that would each have enhanced empirical support, as has emerged in the classification of physical illnesses. Categories of physical illness have been reorganized on the basis of research but their number has remained stable for many decades.

A tool that increases stigma

Critics contend that the price of this expansion of the realm of mental illness is widespread stigmatization. The preamble to the DSM-IV (American Psychiatric Association, 2000, pp. xxii), the predecessor to the current DSM-5, indicated that the system is intended as a classification system for disorders, not for the people who may have them. It is difficult, however, to see how these categories could be used in practice without diagnosing people. Were the creators of the DSM unaware of this? Probably not: the preamble is included as a reminder that the distinguished professionals who constructed the system were aware of many of the scientific realities that could not be reflected in a system they considered workable. The Introduction to DSM-5 contains no such injunction, consistent with the candid recognition of the limits of the system that are recognized in the new version.

Feminist critique: diagnosis as blaming the victim

As aptly summarized by Eriksen and Kress (2005, p. 81), "the field of abnormal psychology has . . . had a troubled and troubling relationship with women." Although many of the feminist critiques of DSM pertain to adult disorders, there have been some vehement condemnations of the gender imbalances in the rates of diagnosis of children as having, especially, attention deficit/hyperactivity disorder and disruptive behavior disorders. As detailed in the chapters devoted to those disorders, boys constitute the overwhelming majority of children who receive these diagnoses. However, this depends on the age at which the children are diagnosed; the gender differences are unsubstantial before the beginning of elementary school. The sudden surfacing of gender differences has been interpreted, first of all, as indicating that diagnosis and ensuing treatment are used as control mechanisms by school systems to achieve compliance with their traditional organizational structures. It is also possible that adults become insensitive to girls' problems as they

dwell on the adjustment of boys (Caplan, 1992; Keenan and Shaw, 1997; McDermott, 1996).

Some feminists have objected intensely to the existence of diagnoses for the difficulties suffered by victims of physical, emotional or sexual abuse. According to these critics, the anger, depression or anxiety they experience should not be considered psychopathology because such reactions are perfectly normal in the context of such abuse.

Diagnosis seen as cultural imperialism

Many critics have seen the DSM/ICD models as reflecting the core cultural values of Western culture, especially the majority culture of the United States. In addition to these criticisms of cultural bias in the content of diagnostic systems, there are also criticisms about cultural bias in the ways they tend to be used. These issues are considered in Chapter 8.

Diagnosis seen as diminishing attention to other important aspects of treatment planning

Another problem with the way the DSM and ICD schemes are commonly used, if not with their basic structures, is that the diagnosis of disorder has moved to the forefront of contacts between members of the public and many mental health professionals. As noted earlier in this chapter, many of the leaders of the field describe the pre-DSM era in psychiatry as one in which diagnosis was unimportant and "loose." Some critics maintain that the field has now gone too far in the opposite direction (Wykes and Callard, 2010). Individuals' strengths are not highlighted as much as they could be in contacts with mental health professionals. This is unfortunate given the fact that longitudinal researchers have elucidated both risk factors for child psychopathology and potent protective factors that promote resistance to psychopathology among individuals who are otherwise vulnerable (e.g., Ingram and Price, 2010). The social context, with the resources it might provide to support the treatment of the individual, is not necessarily considered as part of the assessment of an individual's difficulties. These shortcomings are particularly salient in an era during which, in parallel to the burgeoning literature on psychopathology, seminal writings on positive psychology have received widespread attention (Seligman and Csikszentmihalyi, 2000).

Inconsistency in nomenclature and unreliability of diagnosis: shaking the foundation of the DSM

As detailed in the chapter to this point, the conceptual limitations of the DSM and many of the categories included in it have been widely lambasted. Nevertheless, the prevailing impression is that the system is beneficial primarily because it has brought uniformity in the use of terminology and consistency in diagnostic practice. A pillar of current classification systems is the agreement between one clinician and another about the correct identification of the disease or disorder that affects an individual (*inter-rater reliability*). The fact that diagnosis is not as reliable as it is supposed to be threatens the foundation of DSM and, in the minds of many, the very basis of its existence. As a very crude but visible yardstick for gauging how much progress has been made, it may be useful to reflect about what would happen if the confederates who participated in Rosenhan's pseudo-patient experiment, discussed earlier in this chapter, went to psychiatric hospitals today. Several similar experiments have been conducted more recently. For example, the British Broadcasting Corporation's *Horizon* science program conducted an experiment in 2008 in which ten volunteers were sent to mental health professionals (November 29, 2008, entitled "How Mad Are You?"; Hammond, 2009). Five of the volunteers had histories of chronic mental illness; five had no history of mental illness. Two of the ten were diagnosed correctly by the professionals they saw. This represents greater accuracy than in Rosenhan's time but by no means the precision anticipated when DSM-III and DSM-IV were released. Hopefully,

greater precision will be revealed once more research is conducted on the reliability and validity of DSM-5.

A succinct review of the evidence of DSM-IV's reliability in the diagnosis of child psychopathology was compiled by Kirk (2004). He begins by reviewing the statistical indices relevant to this issue. A perfect system would be one in which every instance of a particular disorder would be identified by different diagnosticians of the same case, with no cases of another child being identified as suffering from that disorder. Since it is not reasonable to expect perfect agreement, "errors" or disagreements are measured in terms of the number or percentage of *false positives* –individuals who are diagnosed with a particular disorder who do not really have it. If there are many false positives, the category or instrument is one that lacks *specificity*. There are also *false negatives* – cases that should have been diagnosed with the disorder but who are missed. If there are many of them, the diagnostic category is one that lacks *sensitivity*. Another important issue related to specificity is the rate of *comorbidity*: If, for example, 90 percent of cases diagnosed as having one disorder are also diagnosed as having another, the category is not only non-specific but probably not useful. Such almost unanimous agreement between raters would also be reflected in a ceiling-level *kappa statistic*. Cohen's kappa is based on the number of agreements between observers, considered as a proportion of the total decisions made (i.e., agreements + disagreements), corrected for the number of agreements between raters that might occur purely by chance. Of course, such perfection is never encountered. An agreement rate of about 80 percent, resulting in kappa of .70 or more (after correction for random agreement), is usually considered acceptable from a scientific viewpoint. A final consideration is the number of cases identified, which should match the known prevalence rate for the particular condition. If half the children in a population are diagnosed as having a specific form of mental illness, the category or the diagnostic procedure is not effective as an identifier of pathology because it is probably not useful to think of that many as being "sick." In order to avoid these errors, structured interviews for parents have been developed so as to standardize the diagnostic information sought by clinical interviewers and to make sure that they do not overlook information about some of the symptoms that might lead to accepting or rejecting a diagnosis. These interviews, of which the Diagnostic and Interview Schedule for Children-IV (NIHM DISC-IV) is the best known, typically last for several hours.

Pending new research on the reliability and validity of the DSM-5 categories, research on this issue has been conducted on the reliability and validity of the DSM-IV diagnostic categories. For example, DISC-IV interviews were used to validate clinician's diagnoses in the field trials that were used by the DSM-IV commission to validate the diagnostic categories for oppositional defiant disorder and conduct disorder (see Chapter 12). The kappas for inter-rater agreement never exceeded .59 and were sometimes as low as .20, which indicates little more than random agreement (Lahey et al., 1994). Using a different methodology, Kirk and Hsieh (2004) presented clinicians with written vignettes containing a case history that clearly corresponded to the DSM-IV criteria for the diagnosis of conduct disorder. Fewer than half of the clinicians who participated in that study made the diagnosis that was indicated.

A somewhat different picture, but unfortunately not one that suggests satisfactory validity, has emerged from research on the DSM-IV criteria for attention deficit/hyperactivity disorder (see Chapter 14). Kirk (2004) reanalyzed data from a study by Streiner (2003) to provide an estimate of the rate of false-positive and false-negative diagnoses. In a population of 1,000, about fifty children would be expected to have ADHD using the epidemiological information reported in the DSM-IV manual. The data indicate that most of these would in fact be correctly identified using the criteria, 45.5 of the 50, or 91 percent. The remainder, or 9 percent, would constitute a fully acceptable rate of false negatives. However the rate of false positives would be gargantuan: An estimated 370.5 of the

non-disordered children, over a third of the total population, would be diagnosed as having ADHD. This is not only an unacceptable rate of false positives but an unacceptable rate of diagnosis.

The symptoms of internalizing disorders, such as depression and anxiety, are not as apparent or intrusive as those of externalizing disorders such as aggression or attention problems. Therefore, it comes as no surprise that the validity and reliability of the DSM-IV categories for depression and anxiety among children and adolescents are no better than the corresponding statistics for aggression and ADHD, examples of which were provided in the previous paragraphs. Here again, specificity is a major concern.

There is so much overlap, for example, between anxiety and depression that some experts regard them as aspects of the same disorder or as subtypes of a larger overarching disorder (Goldberg et al., 2010). It has been established that better reliability and validity are more likely with a system that features fewer, larger categories, or, perhaps, larger categories that are divided into subtypes (Achenbach, 1966; Taylor and Rutter, 2010). This would make the classification system *hierarchical*, as advocated by Thomas Achenbach, developer of some of the most widely used rating scales for the diagnosis of many childhood disorders (Dumenci, Achenbach and Windle, 2011).

In contrast with the extensive literature on the reliability of DSM or the absence of it, relatively little attention has been devoted to many aspects of its validity. *Predictive validity* refers to the ability of an instrument to predict, for example, the future course of a condition, including its amenability to treatment. The lack of validity data is unfortunate, because, as noted by Berrios (1999), a useful system of classification of mental disorders must not only "pigeon-hole without error" (1999, p. 148); the system must also display predictive power. As discussed earlier, this requisite probably exceeds what can be expected of categorical systems with their arbitrary cut-off scores delineating what is diagnosable and what is not.

Moving beyond a categorical model to more complex ways of understanding disorder

A classification system can be much more than a list of disorders. As described in this section, there is a widespread feeling that a dimensional model will help resolve many of the concerns about current diagnostic systems. At the most general level, there are three types of models that can be used when classifying disorders of childhood: *categorical*, *dimensional* and mixed *categorical-dimensional*. Specific emphasis is placed on the implications of categorical and dimensional models to classify the disorders of children and adolescents. For example, instead of having to decide whether or not an individual suffers from major depression, the clinician might be asked to rate how depressed the individual is, perhaps, for example, on a scale of 1 to 10. These issues reappear at the end of the chapter because they are fundamental in the upcoming revisions of the DSM and ICD.

There are some important assumptions inherent in the decision to use *categorical*, *dimensional* or *mixed* models (Sonuga-Barke, 1998). A simple categorical model only allows the diagnostician to indicate the total absence or presence of a problem condition, not to indicate the degree to which an individual's problems correspond to the condition. This, obviously, is based on the postulate that disorders vary by type rather than degree, that disorders are at some level discrete entities and individuals with disorders differ from others qualitatively rather than quantitatively. Second, categorical models are predicated on the assumption that *impairment* of the individual's functioning, which may be listed as one of the symptoms leading to a diagnosis, invariably accompanies diagnosis. Third, they presume that disorders are *endogenous*, that is, that they are located within the individual. The assumptions of categorical models of classification are problematic when the model is used for classifying childhood psychopathology.

The first assumption states that individuals with mental illness differ from non-afflicted individuals qualitatively; they do not simply display too much or too little of a normative trait. Accordingly, the disorder itself takes on a status in reality as a discrete disease entity, like pneumonia or asthma. The introductory material indicates that the diagnostic entities in the DSM are not necessarily discrete and that the population of people with a specific diagnosis may be very heterogeneous. Unfortunately, this epigrammatic disclaimer at the front of the book is usually overlooked, largely because it does not correspond with the diagnostic system that follows or any real-life way of using it. The assumption of discrete disease entities is particularly problematic for childhood disorders because many of these disorders are non-normative representations of otherwise normative behavior (Drabick, 2009). Most young children have difficulty focusing their attention. It is only after a certain limit that it is considered a disorder. For example, uncontrolled urination is normative before age 5 but not after (APA, 2000) and is considered a disorder, termed enuresis, if it persists. In both these cases, the boundary lines between disorder and non-disorder are quite arbitrary. A convincing argument for a dimensional system, which would allow the clinician to indicate the degree to which the behavior constitutes a serious problem, could be made. Looking at the scientific basis of an all-or-none, have-it-or-not-have-it categorical model, it has been observed that the evidence supports such categorical distinctions only for some disorders, although the limited research to date is not entirely consistent as to which disorders those are. There may be strong support for the categories of autism and schizophrenia (Jensen, Hoagwood and Zitner, 2006). However, dimensional models seem to describe attention deficit disorder and post-traumatic stress disorder much better than categorical models (Coghill and Sonuga-Barke, 2012).

When applied to any disorder, a categorical model, by definition, includes a cut-off point between diagnosable and non-diagnosable. For example, the cut-off point may be 2 weeks of symptoms rather than three or four, and five out of eight of the symptoms listed for a disorder rather than four or six. In theory, any such cut-offs should have some basis (American Educational Research Association, American Psychological Association, National Council on Measurement in Education , 1999). A cut-off for a disorder, for example, six of the nine symptoms in a list, might be justifiable if it would be demonstrated clearly that children displaying six symptoms have a clear negative outcome, such as not being able to function in regular elementary-school classes, that is not common among children who display only five of the symptoms on the lists. Such empirical support for cut-off points is very rarely available for most of the disorders. However, it is important to remember that the current versions of DSM and ICD can be seen as having taken the first steps in moving beyond simple categorization with these very lists of symptoms. By their very nature, this feature implies recognition that all conditions that are subsumed under the same diagnostic category are not necessarily identical (Regier, 2008). DSM-5 does allow for differentiation of disorders, which can be achieved by adding *specifiers.* Specifiers are used to make internal distinctions within diagnostic classifications, such as the degree of severity, age of their appearance or overlap with some symptoms of other disorders.

The second assumption of categorical models of classification is that impairment of functioning is an integral feature of disorder. In the case of child psychopathology, however, both the disorder and the afflicted individual are in flux as the child grows and develops. Therefore, it is not surprising that the nature and degree of impairment experienced by an individual with mental illness vary by age (Pine et al., 2010). Moreover, changes in environments can moderate impairment in children quite significantly, much more than in adults, suggesting that impairment is not necessarily inherent in dysfunction in childhood at a specific point in time (Pine et al., 2010). Indeed, impairment in childhood may be context-specific, may not persist for a long enough time to be considered dysfunctional, or may be marked by discontinuity.

Developmental issues in applying categorical and dimensional models

From the perspective of developmental psychopathology, there are many problems in the application of categorical models to the psychological difficulties of children and adolescents. Some disorders of early childhood and adolescence are merely non-normative forms of behavior that are otherwise normative. The non-normative forms deviate from normal patterns of development in terms of either degree or timing. This reality is probably represented best in dimensional models. (Drabick, 2009; Maser et al., 2009; Pine et al., 2010).

Another problem in applying categorical models to child psychopathology pertains to the assumption that disorders are endogenous, that is, internal to the individual. As noted in Chapter 1, this notion is particularly challenging when applied to children because the problem behaviors of children may be far more intrinsically embedded in environments such as homes and schools than are the psychological difficulties of adults. For all these reasons, categorical models have serious disadvantages, some of which are more consequential in applications to children than to adults. Although it could be argued that the same diagnostic system cannot possibly work with children and adults equally well, there are few contemporary advocates of a separate diagnostic system for children and adolescents.

A categorical system for developmental psychopathology cannot accommodate the fact that the developing brain is subject to drastic changes in anatomy, physiology and function as it develops, resulting in a wide range of behavioral manifestations that cannot be represented well in a "one size fits all" system. Perhaps related to these neurobiological factors are the wide age and gender differences in the diagnosed mental disorders of children and adolescents; these gender differences are often much larger than gender differences in diagnosed adult disorders. A dimensional scale might allow for the representation of difficulties in one gender or in certain age groups that are now considered subclinical (just below the cut-off points for diagnosis) in the categorical DSM and ICD systems (Hudziak et al., 2008). According to Achenbach (2009), it is highly unlikely that the same symptom thresholds are valid across the lifespan to the degree that they are used in that way in the current DSM systems. For example, there is no basis for requiring that the same number of symptoms be present for the same period of time (i.e., 6 months) to diagnose attention deficit/hyperactivity disorder at all ages from preschool through adulthood. Therefore, it is necessary to rethink the concept of "threshold," or, at the very least, justify the thresholds presented at the various ages at which they are to be used. Achenbach also disputes the use of impairment criteria to make a diagnosis. Indeed, some disorders may exist before they cause significant impairment; it could be argued that it is these disorders that require much more of the attention of mental health professionals than they have received to date. Finally, in a plea for precision, Achenbach objects to the inclusion in diagnostic systems of criteria that require the diagnostician to decide whether symptoms caused impairment years before the diagnostician's current contact with the child (e.g., a diagnostic system in which symptoms must have been present before a specified age [Achenbach, 2009], such as 12 years, as is specified in some places in DSM-5).

Hudziak, Achenbach, Althoff and Pine argue that a dimensional approach to classification would enhance the agreement between teachers and parents who participate in ratings of children's typical and atypical behaviors (2007). In a completely categorical system, these two essential sources of information may be seen as disagreeing with each other with regard to a cut-off score for diagnosis when, in fact, one of them may indicate a score just below the cut-off, while the score for the other source is just above the cut-off. Summarizing the current unfortunate state of diagnostic instruments intended for different informants De los Reyes and Kazdin (2005) remind

us that, "despite many efforts to improve agreement, differences between informants' reports remain among 'the most robust findings in clinical child research'" (De Los Reyes and Kazdin, 2005, p. 483).

As limited as categorical models of classification may be for the diagnosis of the mental disorders of school-age children and adolescents, their incongruence with the developmental process is certainly more graphic when applied to preschool children. Consequently, mental health professionals working with preschool children have developed a number of alternative classification systems for psychopathology during the preschool childhood and adolescent years. Of course, these systems have not been validated as extensively as the DSM or ICD and are not used as frequently (e.g., Drotar, 1999; Postert et al., 2009). It should be noted that in DSM-5, there are separate criteria for diagnosing children and adults as having disorders with the same name, including social anxiety disorder and gender dysphoria. As with many other features of DSM-5, this indicates awareness of the problems inherent in minimizing developmental differences, even if the DSM-5 Commission was unable to resolve these problems in a fundamental structural manner.

Moving away from a completely categorical model: An unreachable dream?

Thus, replacing categorical models with dimensional models or partly dimensional models would probably allow the diagnostic process to better reflect the realities of child development and the environmental embeddedness of children's lives. In dimensional models, there is not a discrete boundary line between disorder and non-disorder. The problem behaviors are seen as a continuum, with the individual's behavior situated along the continuum ranging from mildly problematic to highly disordered.

Thus, adopting a dimensional model of classification for disorders of early childhood and adolescence would be quite tempting due to both the weaknesses of a categorical model and the strengths of dimensional models. In theory, a dimensional model of classification would improve both specificity and sensitivity of diagnosis (Carrey and Gregson, 2008). Psychiatrist Helen Chmura Kraemer (2008, p. 9) remarked:

When is a dimensional diagnosis unneeded or impossible? The brief answer: Virtually never. The only situation in which a dimensional adjunct would not add quality to the categorical diagnosis is when there is no meaningful clinical variation among those who are diagnosed positive on the categorical diagnosis and no meaningful clinical variation among those who are diagnosed negative on the categorical dimension.

Such situations are virtually non-existent. Kraemar acknowledges, however, that sometimes dimensional diagnosis would be ideal but may not be possible or practical.

Some authorities, however, do believe that dimensional models of classification have some significant disadvantages. One possible shortcoming of dimension systems is a corollary of their most significant advantage, namely that they do not delineate clearly the boundaries of discrete disorders. Because of this, many authorities believe they would significantly hinder communication (Carrey and Gregson, 2008; Sonuga-Barke, 1998; Helzer et al., 2008). Disorders of childhood can be difficult for laypersons to understand, making clear and efficient communication systems particularly essential. Furthermore, a dimensional model could lead to more individuals being seen as in need of professional mental health services whose problems now fall just below the cut-off point for diagnosis. Such services might be helpful but might also stigmatize them.

It has been argued that obscuring the demarcation between children who do and do not suffer from some form of psychopathology may unwittingly compromise the help they receive. Many of these disorders require schools and other institutions to allocate resources to help individuals suffering from psychopathology. For example, individuals diagnosed with learning disabilities may require additional help such as special tutoring or adaptation of the methods used by schools to evaluate learning. Categorical

models of special education have emerged in parallel to categorical models of psychopathology, evoking parallel controversy in the field of education (e.g., Kavale and Forness, 1999). In some jurisdictions, including many US states and Canadian provinces, a child with a learning problem has no legal right to special help unless he or she has been diagnosed. More generally, if a diagnosis cannot be clearly communicated to non-mental health professionals, the value of the diagnostic system as doorkeeper to helping resources may be seriously undermined.

Another possible limitation of dimensional models, again an artifact of their many advantages, is that they operate under the assumption that individuals differ from non-disordered individuals by degree rather than by type (Drabick, 2009). Implying that disorders are not discrete entities may make it difficult to explain why symptoms tend to co-occur with one another and why symptom clusters often exist in a non-linear relationship with other clinically meaningful information.

Responding to these skeptics are many authorities who insist that clinical practice would in fact be advanced by including dimensional features within a system that is basically categorical. For example, Hudziak et al. (2008) point out that many standardized rating scales of children's behavior problems, attention deficits, autism and social responsiveness feature continuous (dimensional) measurement within scales that correspond quite well to categorical DSM diagnoses. These scales have become mainstays of research and empirically oriented clinical care.

Combining categorical and dimensional approaches might result from allowing the data available about a given disorder to decide whether the disorder should be diagnosed using a categorical or dimensional model, as proposed by Meehl (1992, 1995). He suggested that if the statistical information about a disorder indicates that it is a discrete disorder that can be separated empirically from other disorders, a categorical system is appropriate. Conversely, if the data do not point to a discrete disorder, as is almost always the case in child psychopathology, a dimensional system is more appropriate. A corollary of Meehl's proposal is that it is more important for diagnostic systems to be useful in describing the true nature of a disorder (its *ontological status*) than to be user-friendly. It should be noted that this *bottom-up* procedure would be the opposite of that used in validating DSM-III, DSM-IV and now DSM-5, in which the categories are first sketched on in a *top-down* manner on the basis of experts' opinions, then validated in empirical field trials.

Of course, while this data-driven decision-making would deal with dimensionally based disorders ontologically, it does not address any practical limitations inherent in dimensional models of classification. To address the pragmatic issue of communication, psychological science would have to decide on a cut-off score even on dimensional scales; individuals with difficulties that meet or exceed the score would be deemed as requiring treatment and individuals falling below the score would not. Importantly, the cut-off score would have to be derived from relationships with other clinically meaningful information; otherwise it would be seen as arbitrary and culturally determined, as the DSM often is. Alternatively, one could use a cross-cutting dimensional-categorical approach in which disorders are organized categorically and specific features (such as suicidality) are measured dimensionally to increase the information in a clinical profile. In speculating on the optimal way of combining categorical models, Achenbach (2009) reminds his readers of a basic mathematical property: Dimensional data can be reduced to categorical data by establishing an appropriate cut-off point, whereas categorical data cannot also be used as dimensional data.

DSM-5: a downgrade from bible to dictionary?

DSM-5, released in May 2013, is closer to a periodic tune-up of the DSM than a total overhaul. The most important changes desired by mainstream mental health practitioners working with children and adolescents were articulated by Friedman, Sadhu and Jellinek (2012). Their wish list was not unsubstantial, even though it was recognized that it is difficult to "carve nature at its joints" (2012, p. 164). Reliability in diagnosis had to be improved. The diagnostic categories would have to be bolstered by improved validity. There would have to be lower rates of comorbidity because diagnostic categories would no longer be artificial constructs. Most importantly, they called for diagnostic categories that lead to interventions specific to them. They expressed the hope that the changes to the basic structure of the system would make it more sensitive to developmental issues. There were widespread calls for greater recognition of the continuous rather than categorical nature of mental disorder. In response to such demands, a developmental task force worked to find ways of improving the fit between the emerging diagnostic system and the psychological, social and biological processes that influence both typical and atypical behavior during childhood and adolescence. Other task forces worked on the delineation and diagnostic criteria of specific disorders. Extensive field trials were conducted to determine in a preliminary way the reliability of diagnosis and the clinical utility of the diagnostic criteria. In the end, DSM-5 turned out to be a revision, not a conceptual overhaul. Its brief Introduction is almost apologetic in tone. The limits of a categorical system are acknowledged. The extensive overlap among the different disorders is noted. The Commission members are clearly scientists at heart. The science for them to work with simply does not exist. There is some recognition of the enormous overlap of the disorders in the different "specifiers." In DSM-5 specifiers are features of a disorder that are not included in the main diagnostic criteria but that may apply to a common variant of the disorder. Although the distinction between a specifier and a subtype is quite subtle, the term "specifier" is less suggestive of a discrete disorder. For example, a clinician diagnosing bipolar disorder can specify if it is a bipolar diagnosis with anxious features or with psychotic features. There is also provision for the delineation of mild, moderate and severe forms of some disorders by the use of specifiers. The inclusion of the specifiers has done little to satisfy the many critics who were hoping for a truly dimensional system that is informed by developmental science.

Although many experts felt that the DSM-5 Commission did the best it could, there was considerable dissatisfaction particularly among many research-oriented experts who had been clamoring for a diagnostic system with a better research base. Little had changed since DSM-III. The categories listed in DSM-5, like those in its predecessors, are based as much on the consensus of the opinions of experts as on strong empirical data. Some critics began to express doubt that even that consensus has always been illusory. The most damning criticism came from Dr. Thomas Insel, Director of the important National Institute of Mental Health in the United States. In the Institute's blog dated April 29, 2013, Insel remarked that:

While DSM has been described as a "Bible" for the field, it is, at best, a dictionary, creating a set of labels and defining each. The strength of each of the editions of DSM has been "reliability" – each edition has ensured that clinicians use the same terms in the same ways. The weakness is its lack of validity . . . Patients with mental disorders deserve better. (www.nimh.nih.gov/about/director/2013/transforming-diagnosis.shtml, retrieved June 27, 2013)

The National Institute then abandoned its practice of organizing the research it funds around DSM categories.

Structural changes in DSM-5

DSM-5 did abolish two structural features of DSM-IV that turned out to be less useful than they were intended to be. First, the distinction between Axis I and Axis II disorders was eliminated. That distinction was introduced in DSM-IV in order to ensure that clinicians pay due attention to enduring conditions and disabilities that may underlie in a subtle way a problem presented by a client. This dichotomy has been criticized for arousing excessive pessimism about the Axis II disorders, which included intellectual disabilities as well as maladaptive adult personality styles.

There is no longer a separate section devoted to disorders usually first evident in childhood or adolescence. However, disorders that usually emerge early in life appear earlier in the volume than others without any formal delineation of a special section. The previous structural differentiation was not very useful because of the many disorders that are common to both children and adults. In many cases, there are provisions for some differentiation of the criteria depending on whether they are applied to children or adults. Experts versed in the field of child development would have preferred that disorders such as anxiety and depression be understood in more distinct ways when they occur in children. There is some substantial recognition of the developmental process in DSM-5. For example, there are some diagnoses that can only be used with adults. A new and very controversial category, mood dysregulation disorder, can only be applied to school-age children and adolescents. This disorder, discussed in Chapter 20, is characterized by recurrent fits of temper that are out of proportion to anything that might have provoked them.

The changes in the delineation of the disorders and in their criteria are summarized in this book in the chapters relevant to their disorders. However, relevant to the discussion here of the changes made in DSM-5 is the fact that in some disorders, such as attention deficit/hyperactivity disorder, the criteria for diagnosis have become less stringent. This incurs the accusation mentioned earlier in this chapter that psychiatrists do everything in their power to increase the number of people who can be considered psychiatric patients. This concern was expressed in no uncertain terms by the British Psychological Society: "A major concern raised in the letter is that the proposed revisions include lowering diagnostic thresholds across a range of disorders. It is feared that this could lead to medical explanations being applied to normal experiences, and also to the unnecessary use of potentially harmful interventions" (www.bps.org.uk/news/society-statement-dsm-5, retrieved June 17, 2013). There is no doubt that current scientific knowledge is insufficient to support a truly reliable, valid, comprehensive diagnostic system. Given that fact, is it too outrageous to speculate that it might have been better to create an authoritative, first-rate dictionary? A dictionary cannot do everything a good diagnostic system can do, of course. A good dictionary can, however, be very useful.

Responsible, ethical use of the DSM and ICD: an oxymoron?

It is important to make a distinction between the conceptual underpinnings of classifications of mental disorders and the ways in which these classification systems are used. Unfortunately, there has been relatively little research on how clinicians use classification systems (Hill and Ridley, 2001). Responsible, ethical use of diagnostic systems depends, first of all, on the users being aware of both the strengths and limits of the systems they are using. To start with, users, including, especially, professionals in training, should not ignore the preamble to the DSM, which states rather succinctly what the system purports and does not purport to be (Marecek, 1993). Indeed, the DSM-IV contained dimensions that could be used by clinicians to code the severity of the child's or adolescent's symptoms and the degree of life impairment they caused; clinicians generally ignored those dimensions (Friedman et al., 2012). Finally, users should remember that the system provides for situations in which the clinician is not certain of the diagnosis, although use of those provisions may be inconsistent with practice in jurisdictions where payment for psychological treatment is dependent on a diagnosis.

When classification systems emerged in the sciences during the eighteenth and nineteenth centuries, the ability to classify was seen as a God-given gift and talent (Berrios, 1999). Cambridge University psychiatrist German E. Berrios (1999) remarked that the fact that we have the ability to classify does not mean that we should use it. On the other hand, he also commented that the failure of mental health professionals to learn how to classify disorders well does not mean that we should stop classifying. Hopefully, as helping professionals continue to exercise that ability and test its limits, they will discover new ways to channel its application more exclusively to the purposes for which it was granted.

Summary

- Historically, little effort was made to classify psychological problems, and those suffering from them were generally viewed with derision. The modern "medical model" is undoubtedly more benevolent, regardless of its limitations.
- The ancient Greeks believed that psychological distress stemmed from an imbalance of four "humors" (black bile, yellow bile, phlegm and blood). A similar system could be found in ancient India. This persisted until the seventeenth century, when Thomas Sydenham and his contemporaries began modeling classifications of diseases after those used in botany.
- During the eighteenth and nineteenth centuries, classification became increasingly prevalent in the natural sciences, and eventually emerged in clinical psychology.
- The foundations of current classification systems were laid by Kraepelin, an influential German psychiatrist who worked at the end of the eighteenth century and beginning of the nineteenth. Though criticized by some

contemporaries, his categorization of mental disorders according to empirical evidence, is central to modern diagnostic systems.

- The medical model's most important goals are to predict, once a disorder is identified, the course of symptoms and ultimately provide the correct treatment.

- Into the mid-twentieth century, classification of disorders according to their supposed causation by environmental factors was a widespread practice. Disorders, called "reactions," were generally blamed on poor parenting. In contrast, most contemporary authorities emphasize multiple causation of disorders.

- Influential American psychologist Paul Meehl rejected the idea that minor events could lead to major psychological disorders, as studies revealed that psychopathology is the result of both social and biological factors that may be both negative and protective.

- Despite such rejection by the scientific community, it is still common for the lay community to make these sorts of causal inferences based on little evidence. This led to skepticism about the diagnostic process. The Rosenhan experiment highlighted immense problems with the diagnostic system, leading to changes in the 1980s.

- It is important to use consistent criteria in diagnosis. Among the reasons for this is the need to focus on similar populations in evaluating the effectiveness of treatment.

- Standard terminology helps to ensure consistent, clear communication between professionals and institutions and helps assess the prevalence of conditions.

- The two major diagnostic systems in use are the Diagnostic and Statistical Manual – fifth edition (DSM-5), and the mental health section of the International Classification of Diseases, tenth edition (ICD-10). Both emerged from the dramatic revision of the DSM that began with DSM-III; they now use similar structure and there is pressure to increase compatibility. A new version

of the ICD, the ICD-11, is expected in the next few years.

- DSM-III was released in 1980, the result of deliberations by leading researchers and practitioners collaborating and building consensus.

- ICD is the creation of the World Health Organization. It is often considered more oriented toward professional judgment than the DSM.

- Both DSM-5 and ICD-10 are used mainly to decide whether a condition is absent or present, based on criteria. Many critics would prefer a system in which a disorder would be diagnosed along a continuum of maladjustment.

- The full title of DSM (Diagnostic and Statistical Manual of Mental Disorders) is sometimes seen as problematic in that it suggests mental disorders do not have a physical component, with diagnosis seen as reductionist, sometimes forcing psychological problems into categories.

- Since the introduction of DSM-IV, comorbidity, the diagnosis of multiple conditions, has increased drastically. Children with common disorders are more likely to be diagnosed with more than one.

- Individuals with comorbidity are often seen as more "ill," though this is not always the case.

- It has been argued that DSM and ICD have too many categories, which leads to diagnosis of comorbid disorders, and that these should be consolidated.

- It has also been argued that comorbidity may simply be the nature of mental disorders, and diagnosticians are only now adept enough to properly evaluate it.

- The advent of the DSM has been criticized as the rejection of psychoanalysis in favor of behaviorism, though behaviorists have reservations as well.

- Behaviorists and social-learning theorists argue that the "disease" model of mental illness has led to excessive reliance on chemical and physical remedies. The stigmatization of individuals as "sick" is seen as problematic.

- Though DSM claims to be "atheoretical," this is widely questioned.
- The specification of classification schemes has been seen as the psychiatry profession staking claim to the diagnosis and treatment of disorders.
- Feminist critics have objected to the classification of anger, depression and anxiety resulting from abuse as psychopathology.
- The DSM/ICD models are criticized as being biased by Western culture.
- Despite its strengths, diagnosis has been criticized as diminishing other important aspects of treatment planning.
- Despite limitations, DSM is recognized for providing uniform terminology that should enhance communication among professionals.
- Reliability of diagnosis is the foundation of the DSM model. An experiment similar to Rosenhan's early research shows that professionals still disagree very frequently about the diagnosis of people's problems.
- Ideally, classification systems should lead to diagnostic practices with high specificity (diagnosing the exact disorder rather than similar disorders), sensitivity (not missing diagnoses of problems that really exist) and agreement among different diagnosticians about the diagnosis of the same individual.
- Under very specific conditions only, DSM-IV has shown high reliability and validity for use with children, but not more generally. New research using DSM-5 criteria has begun.
- Research has been done on the effectiveness of the DSM in facilitating the clinical care of children. The results have not been promising. Hopefully, data on the usefulness of DSM-5 will yield better results.
- The DSM is often seen as leading to the excessive diagnosis of many disorders, including attention deficit/hyperactivity (ADHD), depression and anxiety.
- Little work has been done to evaluate the ability of the DSM to predict the course of disorders.

- A problem with categorical systems is that they assume that disorders consist of unique traits and not simply the excesses or deficits of normative traits.
- Categorical systems indicate the presence or absence of a disorder based on the presence of a minimum number of specified features. This idea has little empirical support.
- The assumption of impairment is not as valid in child psychopathology as it is for adults, as child impairment is not as consistent due to development and changing situations.
- In child psychopathology, mental illness may represent failed maturation. Some forms of psychopathology are non-normative forms of otherwise normative behavior. This implies that disorders are probably dimensional in nature.
- The assumption that disorders are located within individuals is problematic since disorders in children are strongly embedded in their social environments.
- The developing nature of children's minds and wider gender and age differences make categorical systems less applicable. A dimensional scale would better represent groups with symptoms considered subclinical, and could be superior to the system of thresholds.
- A dimensional system might increase parent–teacher agreement in ratings of children's behavior.
- Categorical systems are often seen as even less applicable to preschool children than they might be for school-age children and adolescents.
- Although dimensional classification may represent reality very well, it is sometimes not possible to develop a practical dimensional categorical system.
- Dimensional models do not have clearly defined boundaries and could result in too many individuals being seen as needing professional help and/or being stigmatized.
- A blurring of the line between children with and without disorders, as might happen with a dimensional system, may compromise the ability to receive help.
- DSM-5 has eliminated some structural features of its predecessor, the DSM-IV. These include a

separate axis for disorders that are considered lifelong and inherent to the individual.

- In DSM-5, there is no longer a separate section for disorders usually first seen in childhood and adolescence. However, disorders that usually appear early in life are listed first, without being identified in a separate section.

- Initial reaction to DSM-5, which was released in May 2013, was more negative than expected. Many critics were anticipating a more fundamental overhaul of the system based on new research. The introductory material includes a statement that the research needed to do this simply does not exist.

Study questions

1. What is the difference between a "lumper" and a "splitter"?
2. What are the major functions of standard diagnostic systems that are intended by their developers?
3. In what important way or ways could diagnostic systems hinder the well-being of individuals in distress?
4. What is the major difference between early diagnostic systems, such as the DSM-I, and the more recent DSM-III, DSM-IV and DSM-5?
5. What are the major advantages and disadvantages of dimensional (as opposed to categorical) models of classification?

4 Genetics and psychopathology

There is a substantial genetic basis for most of the childhood mental disorders described in this book, even though many psychologists may prefer to ignore this reality. Before considering the implications of genetic causation, however, the manner in which genetic causation may occur will first be discussed. As detailed herein, knowledge in this area is increasing rapidly. Direct examination of genetic material is becoming increasingly feasible.

Emergence of genetics in the nineteenth century

Human behavioral genetics, the scientific study of heritability in individual differences in human behavior, is thought to have begun with Charles Darwin's cousin Sir Francis Galton (1822–1911) (Rushton, 1990), who provided the first evidence that individual differences in intelligence and behavior are heritable. Galton was also the first to promote the use of twins to disentangle the effects of genetic (or heritable) factors and environment on inter-individual differences in behavior.

The human body consists of approximately one trillion cells. Most human cells contain forty-six *chromosomes*. Each chromosome is a long, extremely thin *DNA* (deoxyribonucleic acid) molecule that consists of two parallel, intertwined chains of nucleotides in a double helix. One chain is inherited from each of the two biological parents. Four nucleotide varieties exist, differing in their nitrogenous base: adenine (A), guanine (G), thymine (T) and cytosine (C). Each chain is made up of hundreds of such nucleotides (i.e., gene sequences) and each gene has a designated place on every chromosome, called a *locus*. By way of various intermediate steps,

each gene communicates how to make a particular protein to the cell to carry out specific cellular functions. There are approximately 24,000 protein-encoding genes in humans. The complete set of DNA sequences in a human cell nucleus constitutes the *genotype*, which can only be measured using molecular analyses. In contrast, the *phenotype* is the outward manifestation of the genetic information contained in the cells and refers not only to the person's physical appearance, but may also refer to cognitive functioning and behavior. Notably, the DNA content of all the cells in the human body – that is, the *genetic code* or *genome* – is pretty much identical, regardless of whether they are skin cells, blood cells or brain cells. However, in each cell only a portion of the genes are "turned on" (i.e., activated or "expressed"). Some genes, called housekeeping genes, are activated in all cells because they influence general functions such as protein synthesis. Other genes are only activated in specific body tissues or during specific developmental periods, distinguishing them from other cell types. The same gene can therefore have multiple effects, depending on whether it is turned on or off and what other genes are activated at the same time. This is referred to as *pleiotropy*. The complete pattern or "blueprint" of tissue-specific gene-activation, which is determined during the development of the embryo, is called the *epigenetic code* or *epigenome*.

The 24,000 protein-encoding genes constitute only about 2 percent of DNA sequences in chromosomes. The remaining 98 percent of DNA sequences have sometimes been referred to as "junk DNA," but recent research has revealed that at least part of them play an important role in regulating how and when the genetic information is used – that is, whether a specific gene is "turned on" or "turned off" (Mattick, 2005). As will be discussed later, another source of influence on the selective activation of specific genes can come from the environment. Moreover, processes such as mutation or copy errors during reproduction can modify one or more nucleotides, leading to a slightly altered version of a gene that is then passed on to the next generation. Different variations of the same gene are called *alleles*. Many have no adverse effects on the individual and occur with fairly high frequency in the general population. Such gene variants are called *polymorphisms*. Although the occurrence of a different gene variant may either have no negative effect on cell functioning or possibly lead to an improvement, it can also cause problems. Most diseases, however – including psychopathological disorders – are likely the result of a complex array of allelic polymorphisms. To further complicate matters, genetic effects can also interact with each other. One type of gene–gene interaction is due to the fact that some alleles are dominant over other, recessive, alleles. For example, the allele for brown eye color is dominant over the recessive allele for blue eye color. If a person inherits a dominant allele from one parent and a recessive allele from the other parent, the dominant allele will be the one expressed. In addition to this *dominance* gene-interaction effect (involving the interaction between different alleles at the same gene locus), the effect of a gene on one locus can be modified by another gene on a different locus, called *epistasis*. For example, the gene causing albinism would hide the expression of the gene that controls the color of a person's hair.

In light of the complexity of genetic mechanisms, the effect of a single allele on a particular psychological disorder is not likely to be large. Hence, psychopathologies involving complex social behaviors (e.g., conduct disorder or anti-social personality disorder) are likely to be influenced by a multitude of different genes (Rutter, Moffitt and Caspi, 2006).

Overview of the quantitative genetic method

The vast majority of empirical evidence for genetic effects on mental disorders in humans originates from *quantitative genetic studies* (for an overview, see Jang, 2005). In contrast to *molecular genetic studies*, which attempt to identify specific genes related to a phenotype, quantitative genetic studies do not explicitly measure specific genes. In fact, many of them also do not include any specific measures of environmental influence. Instead, quantitative genetic studies statistically infer the relative strength of genetic and environmental effects by examining the phenotypic similarity of family members with varying degrees of genetic similarity. This can be accomplished using several different designs, most notably adoption designs and designs using twins reared together. Common to all quantitative genetic study designs is the assumption that inter-individual differences (or variability) in a measured behavior (i.e., a phenotype) are attributable to the sum of the genetic (G) and environmental (E) differences between people, in addition to differences caused by the interplay of genetic and environmental factors (GE), and measurement error (Falconer, 1960). The inter-individual variability due to genetic influences, G, is represented in quantitative genetic studies by the broad heritability coefficient, h^2_B, encompassing *additive* or *direct genetic* effects (h^2_a), interactive effects between alleles at the same gene locus, known as *genetic dominance* effects (h^2_d) and interactive effects between genes at different loci, called *genetic epistasis* effects (h^2_i). Environmental sources of variance, E, can be distinguished according to whether they are common (or shared) between members of a family or whether they are non-shared (i.e., *unique* to the individual). *Shared environment*, represented by the statistic c^2, refers to environmental factors – both inside and outside of the family – that make members of the same family unit living together similar to each other. Shared environment encompasses geographical or social neighborhood characteristics (e.g., crime level), family characteristics (e.g., socio-economic status, parental mental health), school-related characteristics (e.g., academic track) and other features of the physical and social environment that members of the family are jointly exposed to. In contrast to shared environment, *non-shared environment* factors (denoted as e^2) refer to experiences within the family or outside the family that make children of the same family grow apart. For example, although siblings may be raised together in the same family, parents may treat them differently (Dunn, Stocker and Plomin, 1990). Siblings' differential treatment by parents has been related to differences in siblings' behavior (e.g., Lam, Solmeyer and McHale, 2012). The most important non-shared environmental influences, however, are likely those experienced outside the family (Dunn and Plomin, 1990), especially experiences with peers, as many children do not affiliate with the same friends as their co-sibling (Pike and Atzaba-Poria, 2003; Rose, 2002; Thorpe and Gardner, 2006). Depending on the study design, different approaches are used to yield estimates of h^2_B, c^2 and e^2. The following sections describe the two most frequently used approaches in quantitative genetic research: the classical adoption design and the classical twins design (or, the twins-reared-together design).

The classical adoption design

In the classical adoption design, h^2_B is estimated by examining the degree of similarity (i.e., the phenotypic correlation) of children who were adopted at birth and raised by foster parents (with whom they are genetically unrelated) to their biological parents (with whom they share on average 50 percent of genes). If biological parents are not available, comparisons can be made between biological siblings, who also share approximately 50 percent of genes, and who have been placed in different adoptive homes. Any similarity between the adopted children and their biological parents or siblings can only be due to the genes they share, thus providing a direct estimate of h^2_B, with $h^2_B = r^2$. For example, if the phenotypic correlation between adopted children and their parents is $r = .70$, this would indicate that 49 percent of inter-individual variability is due to genetic influences. Environmental factors cannot explain the similarity between the adopted children and their biological relatives because the children were raised by members of an unrelated family.

Instead, environmental influences – more specifically those that are shared by family members growing up together (i.e., c^2) – are those that make adopted children similar to their foster parents or foster siblings. Because they have no genes in common, any similarity can only be due to the fact that they are exposed to similar environmental experiences. The value c^2 in adoption designs can be estimated simply via the phenotypic correlation between adoptees and their foster parents or siblings. The validity of the estimates for h^2_B and c^2 in this kind of adoption design rests on several assumptions, however, most notably that there is no genetic relatedness between adoptees and their foster parents, and that adoptees had no contact with their biological relatives, both difficult to ensure due to modern adoption laws.

The classical twin design

The twins-reared-together design is based on the comparison of identical or *monozygotic* (MZ) pairs and fraternal or *dizygotic* (DZ) *twin* pairs, where both members of a pair grow up in the same family. Monozygotic twinning occurs when one egg fertilized by one sperm then splits after conception into two genetically identical halves. These twins presumably share all of their genes and are the same sex. Dizygotic twinning occurs when two eggs are released and fertilized by two separate sperms. Like other biological siblings, dizygotic twins share on average half of their genes and can be the same sex or opposite sex. One advantage of the twin design over the classical adoption design is that twins have the same age, which eliminates age difference as a potential source of variability. Genetic and environmental sources of phenotypic variability can be estimated by comparing within-pair similarity of MZ twins and DZ twins (Falconer, 1960). Thus, genetic influences are indicated when the phenotypic similarity (i.e., correlation) of MZ twin pairs, who are assumed to be genetically identical, is greater than the phenotypic similarity of DZ twin pairs, who on average share only 50 percent of their genetic material. Genetic effects can be approximated with $h^2_B = 2(r_{MZ} - r_{DZ})$. For example, if the phenotypic correlation between MZ twins is r = .60 and the correlation between DZ twins is r = .40, then the genetic effect h^2_B on this particular phenotype is estimated as 2(.60 − .40) = .40. In other words, approximately 40 percent of the inter-individual differences in regard to the phenotype under study are due to genetic influences. Shared environmental influences, c^2, are indicated (a) when MZ pairs as well as DZ twin pairs are similar to each other *and* (b) when the degree of similarity among DZ twins is comparable to that of MZ twins. As such, the similarity between MZ twins would be attributable to the fact that both members of each pair share similar environmental experiences (as do DZ twins) rather than to the fact that they share 100 percent of their genes. Shared environment effects can be estimated by subtracting the MZ correlation from twice the DZ correlation, $c^2 = (2r_{DZ} − r_{MZ})$. Using the twin correlations from our previous example, the shared environment effect, c^2, would be estimated as [(2 × .40) − .60] = .20. In other words, approximately 20 percent of the inter-individual differences in regard to the phenotype under study are due to shared environmental influences. Finally, since MZ twins "share" the same home and 100 percent of their genes, any remaining within-pair differences among MZ twins can only be accounted for by non-shared environmental factors, e^2. An estimate of e^2 can be approximated by the extent to which the MZ correlation is less than 1, $e^2 = (1 − r_{MZ})$. Based on the twin correlations from our example, the non-shared environment effect e^2 would be estimated as (1 − .60) = .40. In other words, approximately 40 percent of the inter-individual differences in regard to the phenotype under study are due to non-shared environmental influences. However, in addition to reflecting non-shared environmental influences, estimates of e^2 also include measurement error that may have contributed to an artificially inflated difference between the two members of a twin pair. The twins-reared-apart design is based on the assumption that twins are representative of the general population (i.e., comparable to single-born children), that

MZ twins are genetically identical and that individuals do not systematically select a mate with similar genetic history (*assortative mating*). The *equal environment assumption* dictates that the environment in which MZ twins are raised must not be qualitatively different from the environment of DZ twins. This assumption is threatened if MZ twins are treated by their social environment (e.g., parents, peers, teachers) more similarly than are DZ twins. In this case, any greater similarity of MZ twins compared to DZ twins may be partially due to environmental, rather than genetic, influences.

Over the past decades, the rapid development of statistical software capabilities has allowed researchers to extend quantitative genetic analyses beyond the simple calculation of main effects. Thus, using structural equation modeling techniques, the original formulation of variance decomposition proposed by Falconer (1960) has been expanded to incorporate multivariate data (Neale, 2009; Neale and Cardon, 1992). This makes it possible, for example, to address questions concerning the underlying causes of comorbidity (i.e., whether or not the same genetic and environmental factors influence disorders that often occur together, such as anxiety and depression) or questions concerning developmental (i.e., age-related) changes in the relative influence of genetic and environmental factors on mental health. As discussed in more detail below, the inclusion of measured environmental variables is particularly useful for testing various theoretical models of gene–environment interplay in the etiology of psychopathological disorders.

Genetic effects on externalizing and internalizing psychopathology: findings from quantitative genetic studies

Findings from quantitative genetic studies almost unanimously suggest that all major psychopathological disorders occurring in childhood and adolescence (as well as in adulthood) have some genetic basis. For example, a meta-analysis of thirty-eight twin and adoption studies of children, adolescents and adults (Ferguson, 2010) revealed that individual differences in the broad category of "anti-social personality and behavior" (which includes aggression, delinquent and criminal behavior and conduct disorder) are explained by genetic effects (56%), shared environmental influences (11%) and non-shared environmental influences (31%). Although specific effect sizes vary across studies, twin and adoption studies largely produce similar results. Whereas the magnitude of both genetic and shared environmental effects on anti-social behavior seems to decrease with age, the magnitude of non-shared environmental influences increases. Nevertheless, genetic factors seem to be the main contributor to the stability or chronicity of anti-social behavior over the course of development. Consistent, strong genetic effects are also found for attention deficit/hyperactivity disorder and for oppositional defiant disorder. For ADHD, genetic factors account for 60 to 91 percent of the variance in the general population, and inattentive and hyperactive-impulsive subtypes seem to be largely influenced by the same genetic factors (for reviews, see Nikolas and Burt, 2010; Thapar, Langley, Owen and O'Donovan, 2007). Findings from longitudinal twin studies have also shown that it is mainly genetic influences that account for the stability of ADHD symptoms over time. Although studied less often than other externalizing disorders, moderate to strong genetic effects of around 20 to 60 percent have also been reported for ODD (Hudziak et al., 2005; Tuvblad et al., 2009). Finally, there is also evidence for a genetic basis of alcohol and illicit drug use and abuse (Korhonen et al., 2012).

The most consistent evidence for the heritability of depression and anxiety comes from twin studies. Heritability estimates for depressive symptomatology range from 30 to 50 percent, but some evidence suggests that genetic factors are less important in explaining depressive symptoms prior to puberty than later on in adolescence (Burt, 2009b; Rice, 2009). For both depression and anxiety, the variance in heritability seems to be explained more by non-shared than by shared environmental influences.

There is considerable comorbidity among the externalizing disorders, such as conduct disorder, attention deficit/hyperactivity disorder, oppositional defiant disorder and substance use in childhood and adolescence. Multivariate genetic research suggests that this comorbidity is primarily due to a common underlying genetic liability, even if there are also some genetic effects that are specific to each disorder (McAdams et al., 2012; Tuvblad et al., 2009). In contrast, environmental influences seem to show only little overlap among these different disorders. A review of twenty-three twin studies and twelve family studies reveals that a common genetic liability primarily accounts for the comorbidity of depression and anxiety and that much of this common genetic liability may be mediated via the personality trait of neuroticism (Middeldorp et al., 2005). Some scholars therefore suggest that etiological research should focus on a broad index of externalizing (or internalizing) psychopathology, instead of separately examining the different disorders that constitute the spectrum of externalizing (or internalizing) psychopathology (Krueger and Markon, 2006).

Overview of molecular genetic study designs

In contrast to quantitative genetic studies, which employ a top-down approach by using specific measured phenotypic differences between individuals to infer latent (i.e., unmeasured) genetic effects, the *molecular genetic approach* uses a bottom-up approach: Here, specific measured genes constitute the fundamental unit of analysis, and the goal is to link inter-individual variations on a specific gene to inter-individual differences in observed behaviors (see Table 4.1). Individual genetic information is usually obtained via blood or saliva samples, from which DNA is chemically extracted (Jones, 2009). Potential relations between the obtained molecular

Table 4.1 Main features of quantitative and molecular genetics research compared

	Quantitative genetic studies	Molecular genetic studies
Rationale	• Infers genetic effects *indirectly*, by examining the phenotypic similarity of family members with varying degrees of genetic relatedness • Genes do not have to be measured specifically	• *Directly* examines the effect of specific, measured genes
Methods	Twin design: • compares the degree of phenotypic similarity between members of *identical* twin pairs to the degree of phenotypic similarity between members of *non-identical* twin pairs Adoption design: • compares the degree of phenotypic similarity of *adopted children* with their adoptive siblings and their adoptive parents to the degree of phenotypic similarity of *biological siblings* with each other and with their biological parents	Linkage method: • uses locations of known genes as a marker to help identify *unknown* genes that may be related to a particular phenotype (e.g., a disorder) • examines whether certain, potentially disease-causing genes are more often present close to the marker gene in family members that are affected by the disorder than in non-affected family members Association method: • a priori selects a *candidate gene* that is likely related to a particular disorder. Candidate genes are selected from a pool of *known* genes, whose biological functions are known • examines whether the candidate gene is found more often in affected than in unaffected individuals (these need not be members of the same family)

genetic data and observed phenotypic data are then analyzed using one of two principal approaches: the *linkage* method or the *association* method (for a review, see Eley and Rijsdijk, 2005).

The linkage method

In the linkage method, the locations of known genes on a chromosome are used as a marker to help identify unknown genes that may be related to a particular disorder or disease. Specifically, if the unknown disease-causing gene is believed to be on a specific chromosome, the location of a known gene on that chromosome is selected as a marker. Notably, the marker does not have to be itself related to the disease. If the disease-causing gene is far apart from the marker gene, it is unlikely that the two would be transmitted together from parent to offspring. If, however, the disease-causing gene is in close proximity to the marker gene, they are likely to be transmitted together (in other words, they are *linked*). This method works best, of course, for genetic mapping of single-gene diseases. For more complex, multiple-gene disorders, evidence of linkage would be indicated if two family members that are both affected by the disorder show a larger number of similar alleles around a particular marker (marker-allele sharing) than two family members where one has the disorder and the other has not.

The association method

A better-suited method for identifying susceptibility genes that are implicated in complex disorders or behaviors but have smaller effect sizes is the association method. In contrast to the linkage method, the association method does not require data from affected as well as unaffected family members. Instead, the association method uses population-based data and simply examines whether the hypothesized susceptibility gene can be found more often in affected than in unaffected individuals. Also in contrast to the linkage method, the hypothesized susceptibility gene (called the *candidate gene*) is selected a priori in the association method, based on its functional relevance to the phenotype under study. An important advantage of the association method lies in the fact that the phenotype under study can be categorical (e.g., presence versus absence of a diagnosis of major depression) or continuous (e.g., higher versus lower values on a continuous measure of depressive feelings). Since continuous measures cover the whole range of phenotypic variation, the chances of finding associations with candidate genes are sometimes greater than when using categorical all-or-none traits (Eley and Rijsdijk, 2005). The gene loci that contribute to the variation of a continuous – or quantitative – trait are known as *quantitative trait loci* (QTL). The success of association studies depends on the selection of an appropriate candidate gene. However, a vast number of candidate genes may be functionally relevant for a given phenotype. An alternative method is therefore a *complete genome scan*. This approach consists of systematically scanning a fixed number of genes on each chromosome across the complete sets of DNA of many people to find genetic variations associated with a particular disorder. Because the whole genome is scanned, analyses are not limited to a pre-specified set of candidate genes, nor are they limited to

protein-coding genes only, which increases the chance of finding associations with a disorder.

Genetic effects on externalizing and internalizing psychopathology: findings from molecular genetic studies

Given consistent findings from quantitative studies that both externalizing and internalizing psychopathologies are at least partly heritable, researchers initially expected to identify a relatively limited number of abnormal mutant genes that caused mental health problems (Rutter et al., 2006). However, the hunt for single mutant genes linked to specific mental health problems has so far met with little success.

As mentioned, findings from quantitative genetics suggest that diverse forms of externalizing psychopathologies share a common underlying liability. Neurobiological research indicates that this common liability is expressed in part through brain mechanisms related to cognitive control, impulsivity and reward sensitivity, that is, the cholinergic, serotonergic and noradrenergic systems in the brain. The hunt for specific genes related to externalizing problems has thus focused on genes implicated in these systems. One of those genes is GABRA2, which codes for a receptor for the inhibitory neurotransmitter GABA in the mammalian brain. Several studies have found an association between GABRA2 and alcohol and illicit drug dependence as well as anti-social personality disorder in adults (Dick, 2007). Another gene that has been linked to generalized externalizing psychopathology in younger and older adults is the cholinergic muscarinic 2 receptor (CHRM2) gene (Dick et al., 2008). CHRM2 has been related to memory and cognition in some studies (Deary, Johnson and Houlihan, 2009) – functions that are impaired in many psychiatric disorders. Monoamine oxidase A (MAO-A) is another candidate gene frequently used in the study of psychopathological disorders and behaviors. The MAO-A gene encodes the MAO-A enzyme, which metabolizes neurotransmitters such as norepinephrine, serotonin and dopamine and plays an important role in regulating behavior following threatening stimuli (Shih, Chen and Ridd, 1999).

Neurophysiological data suggest that MAO-A deficiency may lead to aggression through a heightened sensitivity to negative socio-emotional experiences such as interpersonal rejection (Eisenberger et al., 2007).

The cholinergic, serotonergic and noradrenergic systems also play an important role in affect regulation. These systems are described in more detail in Chapter 5. Not surprisingly, the genes implicated in the functioning of these systems have not only been linked to externalizing but also to internalizing psychopathologies. Other genotypes that have been examined as candidates for a specific link with internalizing problems include polymorphisms in the serotonin transporter promoter region. The serotonin transporter promoter region is involved in the reuptake of serotonin at brain synapses and is the target of certain types of antidepressant medication (i.e., selective serotonin reuptake inhibitors). Among the polymorphisms in this region that have received particular attention is 5-HTTLPR. Several studies suggest significant yet small associations between the S-allele of 5-HTTLPR and bipolar disorder, suicidal behavior and anxiety- and depression-related personality traits such as neuroticism (Gonda et al., 2011). Another gene in the serotonin transporter promoter region that has been frequently examined for a possible association with internalizing problems is the brain-derived neurotrophic factor (BDNF), which codes for a protein that stimulates the growth of sympathetic and sensory nerve cells. Some genetic association studies have suggested a role of specific BDNF genetic variants in depression. For example, Hilt and colleagues (Hilt et al., 2007) found that young adolescent girls who carried two copies of the Val allele of BDNF (i.e., who had the Val/Val genotype) had more depressive symptoms and higher rumination scores than girls who carried

only one copy (i.e., who had the Val/Met genotype). Furthermore, rumination – repeating pondering something, turning it over and over in one's head (a frequent symptom of depression) – mediated the relationship between genotype and depressive symptoms. Overall, while there is seemingly some support for an association between specific gene variants and both externalizing and internalizing psychopathologies, findings are often inconsistent across studies. The observed associations between specific gene variants and psychopathologies are usually small, which is to be expected. On average, specific genes explain no more than 1 percent of the variance of quantitative traits and increase the odds of any given disorder by no more than 30 percent (Kendler, 2005).

Mechanisms of gene–environment interplay

While gene–environment interplay is a rather general term that covers different concepts (Rutter et al., 2006), three genetic-environmental mechanisms may be of specific relevance for the development of mental disorders. The first involves *gene–environment correlations*, where genes predispose to disease indirectly by leading to increased exposure to risk environments. The second concerns *gene–environment interactions*, where, for example, genes moderate individual sensitivity to risk environments. The third refers to environmentally triggered epigenetic mechanisms that alter gene expression.

Gene–environment correlation (rGE)

Several of the personal characteristics and behaviors that may shape environmental experiences (e.g., aggression) are partly heritable and the environment becomes as a result itself influenced by genetic factors. This phenomenon is called gene–environment correlation, or rGE. Gene–environment correlations may come about through either the parents' genes or the child's genes. With this distinction in mind three forms of rGE have been described that reflect different causal mechanisms underlying genetic influence on environment: "passive," "active" and "evocative" rGE (Plomin, DeFries, and Loehlin, 1977; Jaffe and Price, 2012). *Passive rGE* occurs when the environment parents provide for their children (e.g., parenting style, enrolment in after-school activities, etc.) is influenced by parents' personal characteristics (e.g., mental health problems, intellectual qualities), which are partly determined by genetic factors. This type of rGE is called passive because the child's environmental experiences are not elicited by the child's own behavior, but rather by parental behavior that is itself genetically influenced and heritable. For example, parents with a history of mental health problems such as anti-social personality disorder or major depression (both of which are moderately heritable) are more likely to show hostile or neglectful parenting behavior than healthy parents (Bifulco et al., 2002; Serbin and Karp, 2004). As a consequence, the child's genotype, which is inherited from the parents, becomes correlated with the environment he or she grows up in. In contrast to passive rGE, both evocative rGE and active rGE involve environmental features that are shaped by the child's own – not the parents' – characteristics. *Evocative (or reactive) rGE* arises when the child's genetically influenced characteristics provoke a specific reaction from the social environment. For example, depressed children's interactive behavior with others is often characterized by more conflict and less collaboration than the interactive behavior of non-depressed children. Finally, *selective (or active) rGE* occurs when individuals select or actively shape their own environments, based on their genetically influenced personal characteristics. An example for a selective rGE would be when anti-social children (whose behavior may in part be genetically influenced) actively seek out friends with similar behavioral characteristics. According to Scarr (Scarr and McCartney, 1983), the relative importance of the three types of rGE should change over the course of development. Specifically, whereas the influence of the passive kind should decline from infancy to adolescence, evocative and selective rGE should become increasingly important with age.

Empirical evidence for rGE from quantitative genetic studies

Existing empirical evidence for gene–environment correlations mostly comes from quantitative genetic studies by showing that many presumably "environmental" features that are associated with the development of externalizing and internalizing mental health problems are themselves partly influenced by genetic factors. The list of genetically influenced environmental experiences ranges from exposure to warm or hostile parenting, deviant peer affiliation, friendship quality and popularity among peers to behavior-dependent life circumstances and events such as high school graduation, romantic-relationship quality and duration, and social support in adolescence and adulthood (for reviews, see Brendgen, 2012; Brendgen and Boivin, 2008). Passive rGE can best be tested through a parent-based design where the parents vary in the degree of their genetic relatedness, such as MZ twins and DZ twins who are parents (Jaffe and Price, 2012). By applying the usual MZ–DZ comparison to the phenotype of the rearing environment provided by these twin parents (e.g., the degree of physical punishment or cognitive stimulation), it is possible to estimate to what extent the parents' genes influence how they parent their own children. Using this design, evidence for passive rGE has indeed been found in some studies. For example, Neiderhiser and colleagues (Neiderhiser al., 2004; Neiderhiser et al., 2007) found moderate to large genetic effects indicative of passive rGE on positive as well as negative self-reported parenting behaviors, such as positive affect, coercion and monitoring. A research design that is particularly conducive for testing evocative rGE is an adoption design that includes information about the children and their adoptive parents as well as their biological parents. Using this design, Riggins-Casper and colleagues (Riggins-Caspers et al., 2003) found that adolescents at genetic risk for opposition and conduct problems were significantly more likely to receive harsh discipline from their adoptive parents than adolescents not at genetic risk, indicating evocative rGE.

These findings provide some evidence for passive and evocative rGE as possible mechanisms that link maladaptive parenting and anti-social behavior in the child. However, valid information on evocative rGE pertaining to environmental experiences outside the family that may be related to psychopathology, such as popularity or rejection among peers, is scarce. Ideally, the reaction of the social environment would have to be measured directly in order to deduce evocative rGE. The few quantitative genetic studies that have made use of this approach show modest but significant rGE in regard to peer rejection and peer victimization in young children (Brendgen et al., 2009; Brendgen et al., 2011; Boivin et al., 2013). Finally, a systematic test of a potential developmental change from passive to evocative or selective rGE, as hypothesized by Scarr, is also still outstanding. Nevertheless, some indication for a developmental change from passive to evocative or selective rGE is provided by findings that a global measure of behavior-dependent negative life events (e.g., being dumped by a friend, failing an exam) seems to be more substantially influenced by genetic factors in adolescents than in children (Rice, Harold and Thapar, 2002).

Empirical evidence for rGE from molecular genetic studies

In contrast to the considerable, yet unspecific, evidence for rGE from quantitative genetic studies, matching evidence from molecular genetic studies is still scarce. Rutter and colleagues have suggested that part of the reason for this lack of evidence may be that genes exert their "influence" on environmental experiences only indirectly, via their effect on individuals' behavior. These authors even suggested that "to search for genes coding for specific environments would be a totally misguided enterprise" (Rutter et al., 2006, p. 242).

Nevertheless, recent findings indicate that specific genes may indeed be related to specific environmental experiences, and that this relation is mediated by individuals' behavior (for a review, see Jaffee and Price, 2007). For example, individuals with the high risk variant of the GABRA2 gene have been found to be less likely to marry and to be more likely to divorce, in part because they are at higher risk for anti-social personality disorder (Dick et al., 2006). The most convincing finding to date comes from a study of 19-year-old males, who were asked to rate how much they liked or disliked their previously unacquainted peers (Burt, 2009a, 2008b). Boys who carried one or two copies of the G-allele of the G1438A polymorphism of the serotonin transporter receptor 2A (5HT2A) gene were significantly more popular than those who carried two copies of the A-allele. Moreover, rule-breaking behavior partially mediated the genetic effect on popularity, indicating evocative rGE. Intriguingly, however, the popular G-allele carriers showed more – not less – rule-breaking behavior. Burt explains this result by the fact that rebellious, rule-breaking behavior is often admired by older adolescents, particularly among males. Together, these findings appear to lend preliminary support to the idea that specific genes can predispose individuals not only to specific behaviors but also to the social consequences of these behaviors.

Gene–environment interaction (G×E)

Broadly speaking, gene–environment interaction, or G×E, refers to any situation in which (a) the effect of genes on a given phenotype varies depending on environmental circumstances, or (b) the effect of the environment on a given phenotype varies depending on individuals' genetic disposition (Shanahan and Hofer, 2005). In accordance with the suggestion by Rutter and colleagues that the principle of natural selection underlies G×E, genes are involved in the adaptation of organisms to their environment (Rutter et al., 2006). A gene–environment interaction (G×E) with respect to psychopathological behavior may arise through different processes (Shanahan and Hofer, 2005). A diathesis-stress process occurs when an environmental stressor triggers or exacerbates genetic predisposition for a specific phenotype, or when an environmental stressor only leads to a specific phenotype in individuals with a genetic predisposition. A suppression process of G×E arises when the presence of specific environmental conditions reduces the influence of genetic factors. Such environmental conditions may be clearly negative, such as war or famine, which may trigger psychopathology in individuals regardless of their genetic disposition. However, a suppression process can also involve environmental conditions that prevent or reduce the expression of genetic vulnerability for a psychopathology. These latter forms of suppression G×E have also been referred to as a compensation process (if environments are positive) or a social control process (if environments are restrictive), depending on the specific nature of the environment.

Empirical evidence for G×E from quantitative genetic studies

As is the case for rGE, most empirical evidence for G×E in regard to the development of psychopathological problems comes from research using twin or adoption designs. Adoption studies usually compare adoptees with and without genetic risk for a disorder (based on the presence or absence of disorder in their biological families) and examine whether conditions in the adoptive home moderate the effect of genetic risk on the adoptees' likelihood of developing the disorder themselves. As such, adoption studies are well suited to examine G×E that involves environmental conditions related to the familial rearing environment (e.g., SES, parental divorce). In contrast, G×E examination in twin studies may involve environmental conditions inside or outside of the home and can refer to environmental experiences that are shared or not

shared by the two twins in a pair. In twin studies, an individual's genetic risk for a disorder can be estimated based on (a) the presence or absence of the disorder in the co-twin and (b) the degree of genetic relatedness (i.e., monozygotic versus dizygotic) of the two twins (Ottman, 1994).

Evidence for G×E from quantitative genetic studies: externalizing psychopathology

As is the case for studies of rGE, the vast majority of quantitative genetic studies of G×E in regard to externalizing problems in children and adolescents (but also in adults) have focused on anti-social behavior and substance use (for a review, see Thapar, Harold, et al., 2007). Consistent with a diathesis-stress process of G×E, many of these studies support the notion that (a) negative features of the social environment can act as stressors that trigger genetic liability to externalizing psychopathology, or that (b) environmental adversity increases externalizing problems only or mainly in those individuals with a high genetic risk. G×E may also involve extrafamilial experiences. For example, using a sample of 6-year-old twins, Brendgen and colleagues showed that a genetic liability for physically aggressive behavior is much more likely to be manifested in children who affiliate with highly aggressive friends than in children who do not (Brendgen et al., 2008). Other adverse environmental features that have been found to trigger or increase the manifestation of a genetic liability to anti-social behavior as well as substance use in youth include such diverse aspects as academic problems, parent-child relationship problems, parental marital problems and divorce, as well as financial, legal and mental health problems in the family (Hicks et al., 2009). Evidence also exists, however, that the environment can reduce the effect of genetic liability for externalizing problems. For example, Dick and colleagues found that genetic influences on smoking were lower in adolescents who experienced greater parental monitoring and spent more time with their parents (Dick, et al., 2007).

A similar reduction of genetic influence was observed in regard to alcohol use when youth were raised in rural versus urban areas (Legrand et al., 2008).

Evidence for G×E from quantitative genetic studies: internalizing psychopathology

Interactive effects between genetic and environmental factors also seem to play an important role in the development of internalizing problems. Not surprisingly, adverse life events are among those environmental experiences that are particularly likely to interact with genetic vulnerability to trigger or increase internalizing problems (for reviews, see Rice, 2009; Rutter and Silberg, 2002; Rutter et al., 2006). In a recent study, Gheyara and colleagues (Gheyara et al., 2011) focused specifically on "independent" life events, that is, those that are unlikely to be brought on by the individual's behavior (i.e., death of a close friend or family member). They found that such life events were related to depression only in those adolescents with a genetic risk for such problems. Similar findings were reported in regard to anxiety disorders in children and adolescents (Lau et al., 2007). Of course, not all adverse environmental conditions that foster internalizing problems in genetically vulnerable individuals are independent of the individuals' behavior. For example, Eaves and colleagues (Eaves, Silberg and Erkanli, 2003) found that preadolescent girls with a genetic liability to anxiety were more likely to experience depression-inducing adverse life events later in adolescence (rGE). By the same token, the effects of these adverse life events on later depression were also stronger in the girls with a pre-existing genetic vulnerability to anxiety (G×E). Some environmental stressors may foster internalizing problems regardless of individuals' genetic vulnerability, however. Thus, Brendgen and colleagues (Brendgen et al., 2009) found that genetic factors play an important role in explaining depressive behavior, but only in children who are relatively popular among peers. In contrast, peer rejection is related to increased depressive behavior independent of children's genetic disposition.

Evidence for G×E from molecular genetic studies: externalizing psychopathology

With very few exceptions, molecular genetic studies investigating G×E effects on externalizing (or internalizing) psychopathology have focused on the effects of a maladaptive family environment (e.g., Bakermans-Kranenburg and Van IJzendoorn, 2006). In line with results from quantitative genetic studies, many of the findings are indicative of a diathesis-stress process. For example, in their seminal study with a sample of male children followed from birth to adulthood, Caspi and colleagues examined a possible interaction between MAO-A and childhood maltreatment with respect to four indicators of anti-social behavior (conduct disorder, convictions for violent offenses, disposition toward violence and anti-social personality disorder symptoms) (Caspi et al., 2002). Maltreatment experiences were unrelated to genotype, suggesting an absence of rGE. However, significant G×E was observed, such that childhood maltreatment was much more likely to lead to later anti-social behavior in boys with a low MAO-A activity genotype than in boys with a high MAO-A activity genotype. Positive environmental conditions may offset the effect of specific genetic risks, however. Such a compensation process of G×E was shown in a study that examined a possible moderating effect of parental monitoring on the association between GABRA2 and aggressive-delinquent behavior from early adolescence through young adulthood (Dick et al., 2009). The effect of GABRA2 on adolescents' externalizing behavior was much more evident under conditions of low parental monitoring than under conditions of high parental monitoring.

Evidence for G×E from molecular genetic studies: internalizing psychopathology

Some molecular genetic studies have also examined G×E effects with respect to internalizing problems. The first published study in this context came from Caspi and colleagues (Caspi et al., 2003), who

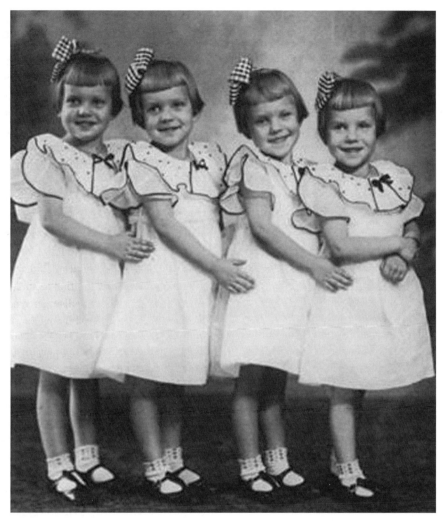

Figure 4.1 All four of the genetically identical Genain quadruplets developed schizophrenia, suggesting a genetic basis for the disorder.

focused on a potential G×E between life stress and the serotonin transporter gene polymorphism 5-HTTLPR. The findings showed significant main effects of both maltreatment in childhood and stressful life events in early adulthood on later depression, but no significant main effect for the serotonin transporter gene. However, in line with a diathesis-stress process of G×E, the effect of childhood maltreatment and of stressful life events in early adulthood on later depression was significantly stronger among individuals carrying at least one copy of the risk variant (i.e., the short allele) of 5-HTTLPR than among those who did not. The specificity of the genetic effect was tested by checking whether a similar G×E could be found with respect to the MAO-A gene, which was not the case. Although replications of G×E on internalizing psychopathology have not always been consistent, a recent large meta-analysis suggests that observed G×E of 5-HTTLPR and stressful life events are likely robust and do not reflect mere chance findings (Karg et al., 2011).

Epigenetic mechanisms

Since the DNA sequence is nearly identical in almost all the cells in the human body, the epigenetic code, that is, the pattern of activation of the different genes in the various body tissues, defines genome function and ultimately the phenotype. Notably, this selective activation of genes can be significantly altered by environmental influences through epigenetic mechanisms. In contrast to genetic mechanisms of change such as mutations, which alter the DNA sequence and hence the genes themselves, epigenetic mechanisms affect chemical processes that are implicated in the selective activation or deactivation of genes, and, thus, in gene expression (Berger et al., 2009). The two most frequently studied chemical processes underlying epigenetic changes so far are *DNA methylation* and *histone modifications* (Qiu, 2006). DNA methylation occurs when methyl molecules attach to certain DNA bases, which results in a suppression of gene activity. Histone modification occurs when a combination of different molecules attach to the "tails" of proteins called histones, around which the DNA strands are wrapped. These molecules play a role in determining whether genes are turned on or off (see Figure 4.2). Initially, scientists assumed that environmentally triggered epigenetic modifications of gene expression would be restricted to the prenatal period, because most of the epigenetic code is laid down during embryonic development (Razin and Riggs, 1980). However, the pioneering work of Fraga and colleagues (Fraga et al., 2005) has revealed that epigenetic patterns can also change later in life. Examining eighty identical (MZ) twins ranging from 3 to 74 years of age, these authors found that the two members of a twin pair were epigenetically indistinguishable from each other during the early years of life. In contrast, older MZ twins – especially those with different lifestyles – showed considerable differences in their patterns of DNA methylation and histone modification, both in specific body tissues and across the whole genome.

Epigenetically mediated environmental influences: evidence from animal studies

Over the past years, scientists have begun to identify specific environmental factors that lead to such epigenetic changes. Recent studies have shown that the social environment can influence epigenetic mechanisms and significantly alter the expression of genes relevant for social behavior and mental health (for a review, see Masterpasqua, 2009). The first evidence in this context came from a series of animal studies by Meaney and colleagues (Cameron et al., 2005; Champagne et al., 2004; Champagne et al., 2006; Weaver et al., 2004), who examined differences in the social behavior, neurophysiology and epigenetic patterns of adult rats that had received either high or low levels of licking and grooming (LG) from the mother during the first week after birth. Compared to rats who had received high maternal LG, rats who had received low maternal LG showed increases in hormonal stress reactivity of the hypothalamic-pituitary-adrenal (HPA) axis in adulthood. This increased HPA stress reactivity could be explained by decreases in the number and density of glucocorticoid receptors in the brain, which, in turn, could be explained by increased DNA methylation of the gene for glucocorticoid receptor expression.

Despite their potential heritability, epigenetic changes and their effects on gene expression are reversible. This was demonstrated in a study by Weaver and colleagues (Weaver et al., 2004), who injected a pharmacological substance known to reduce DNA methylation into the brains of adult rats who had received low maternal LG when they were pups. As a result of these injections, the DNA methylation levels of the low LG rats decreased significantly and became in fact indistinguishable from the methylation levels of rats who had received high maternal LG when they were pups.

Environmentally driven epigenetic changes seem to be reversible not only via pharmacological agents, however, but also via a modification of environmental conditions. Champagne and Meaney (2007) placed juvenile female rats who had received

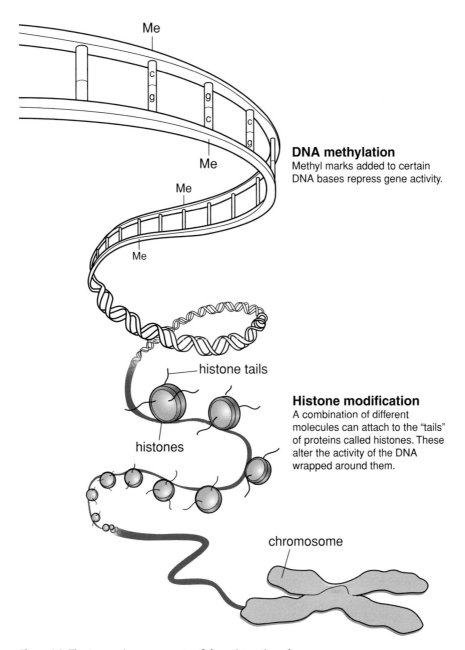

Figure 4.2 The two main components of the epigenetic code.
Source: Adapted by permission from Macmillan Publishers Ltd: NATURE, Qiu, Epigenetics: Unfinished symphony, copyright 2006.

either high or low maternal LG as pups into differing post-weaning environments: impoverished (i.e., housing in social isolation), standard (i.e., housing with a same-sex peer) or enriched (housing with multiple peers and toys). The authors found that the enriched post-weaning environment led to increased exploratory behavior and licking and grooming of their own pups in the offspring of low LG mothers.

In contrast, the impoverished post-weaning environment reduced the exploratory behavior and own licking and grooming behavior in the offspring of high-LG mothers. Remarkably, these effects were also transmitted to the next generation of offspring. This suggests that social environmental influences on phenotypic development are long-term and potentially heritable, yet also reversible by changing environmental conditions.

Epigenetically mediated environmental influences: evidence from studies with humans

Empirical evidence of social environmental influences on epigenetically mediated phenotypic changes in humans is still very rare and, due to obvious ethical restrictions, based on correlational rather than experimental research designs. Nevertheless, findings from a few recent studies indicate that epigenetic mechanisms may indeed play an important role in explaining how adverse environmental conditions may lead to psychopathology (for a review, see Champagne, 2012). First, compelling evidence in this context came from post-mortem studies comparing the brains of diseased persons who had suffered from mental disorders such as major depression, schizophrenia and bipolar disorder to the brains of unafflicted persons (Mill et al., 2008; Poulter et al., 2008). The results indicated that DNA hypermethylation in specific candidate genes may play an important role in the etiology of these disorders. Recent research even provides evidence for epigenetic mediation of specific environmental influences – notably maltreatment experiences during childhood – on mental disorder. For example, McGowan and colleagues compared the hippocampus brain areas of (a) suicide victims who had a history of child abuse, (b) suicide victims who did not have a history of child abuse and (c) control subjects who had died from causes other than suicide and who had no history of child abuse (McGowan et al., 2009). Increased levels of methylation in the gene for glucocorticoid receptor expression (which is implicated in the regulation of HPA reactivity) were found in abused suicide victims compared to non-abused suicide victims and controls, who did not differ from each other in this respect.

Because gene expression is tissue-specific, and because epigenetic changes of behavior-relevant gene expression are best observed in brain tissues, it is difficult to study epigenetic effects in humans while alive. It is also difficult in studies with humans to provide the experimental control necessary to separate prenatal, postnatal and genetic effects (Rutter et al., 2006). Nevertheless, a recent study offers important clues demonstrating how the prenatal environment may alter gene activity related to stress reactivity, which in turn may have important effects on the subsequent development of externalizing or internalizing mental health problems. Specifically, Oberlander and colleagues (Oberlander et al., 2008) examined DNA derived from the cord blood of newborns whose mothers were either (a) being treated with antidepressant medication during pregnancy, (b) not being treated for their depression or (c) not showing any depression symptoms. Controlling for mothers' prepartum use of antidepressants and their postpartum anxious-depressed mood, the authors found that mothers' depressed mood during pregnancy was related to greater HPA reactivity in the children, as assessed by salivary cortisol stress responses at 3 months of age. Moreover, this effect of prenatal exposure to mothers' depressed mood on stress reactivity seems to have been mediated by increased DNA methylation of the glucocorticoid receptor gene in the children. Findings from another recent study show that epigenetic changes in humans might also be triggered by the postnatal environment. Thus, Naumova and colleagues found increased methylation in the genes of children who were raised since birth in institutional care compared to children raised by their biological parents (Naumova et al., 2012). Most of these epigenetic differences were found in genes involved in the control of immune response, neural communication and brain development.

Although epigenetic research in general and with humans in particular is still in its infancy, the existing findings clearly suggest that adverse environments can lead to increased risk of physical and mental disorders by altering the epigenome. It is likely that epigenetic mechanisms of gene–environment interplay will prove to be important in a much wider range of environmental effects than those investigated so far. It is also probable that epigenetic mechanisms play a role in at least some of the different types of gene–environment interplay discussed previously, such as, for example, passive rGE and several forms of G×E (Rutter et al., 2006; Bagot and Meaney, 2010). In light of the rapid and potentially lasting epigenetic changes triggered by environmental influences, which often lead to an increased risk of disease, the question arises whether this adaptability of the organism can convey any evolutionary advantage. Several scholars indeed suggest that it can (Szyf, McGowan and Meaney, 2008). According to these authors, the epigenetic response to environmental adversity is not simply an accidental aberration leading to pathology but a biological mechanism designed to increase endocrine, cognitive and emotional responses to stress. Under conditions of environmental adversity, such increased preparedness of defensive systems may convey important advantages with respect to survival and reproduction – with the trade-off that it increases the risk of disease over the long term.

Future directions in genetics research

The past decade has witnessed an explosion of research in the genetic etiology of externalizing and internalizing problems. The findings show that genes play an important part in the development of mental disorder, even if they are unlikely to be sufficient or even necessary causes of psychopathology (Rutter et al., 2006). Genetic research has helped shift the blame for behavioral problems away from a sole focus on failures of the social environment. Still, much remains to be learned about the role of genes and their interplay with environmental influences in the development of psychopathology. One important issue concerns the fact that the genetic influences can change at different points during development as genes are turned on and off. Similarly, the same environmental conditions may have different influences on the course of psychopathology at different stages of development. Especially quantitative genetic studies have increasingly begun to use longitudinal data to assess genetic effects on behavior from a development perspective, although a similar approach is still largely lacking in molecular genetic studies. Longitudinal data are also crucial in order to disentangle the temporal relationships between exposure to environmental risk factors and onset of mental health problems. Moreover, longitudinal designs will be important in future research that examines environmental influences on epigenetically mediated changes in human behavior.

Going beyond the question of heritability and of identifying specific genes associated with mental disorders, an important challenge for future research will be to understand the actual pathways that link the genotype (and the epigenotype) to behavior. One step in this direction is the study of endophenotypes. Endophenotypes are intermediate phenotypes that are more proximal to the genes that influence a disorder than are the externally visible behavioral symptoms of the disorder (Gottesman and Gould, 2003). They include neurophysiological, biochemical, endocrinological, neuroanatomical, cognitive or neuropsychological functional processes. If endophenotypes are related to a disorder and both share the same genetic influences, this would provide evidence for a specific pathway from gene function to behavior. In recent years, an increasing number of studies have examined genetic associations of endophenotypes related to mental disorder, and functioning of the endocrine system may be a useful target for research on the mechanisms linking gene expression to internalizing disorders. Recently developed neuroimaging tools such as functional magnetic resonance imaging (fMRI) and positron emission tomography (PET) broaden the possibilities to study endophenotypes related to various aspects of brain functioning. Given their greater proximity to genes, studies of endophenotypes are also likely to produce greater gene effect sizes than studies that focus exclusively on behavioral phenotypes.

Clinical implications

One might believe that the only practical implication of genetic research is to identify susceptibility genes, which would make it possible to screen patients for genetic risk of psychiatric disorders and develop drug therapies to mitigate gene functioning. Genetic testing is already being used for patient screening with respect to a variety of heritable diseases, such as ovarian and breast cancer, and a similar approach could eventually be used for psychopathological disorders. However, despite the identification of candidate genes associated with specific psychopathologies, Rutter and Plomin (2009) cautioned that it still may take some time until molecular genetic findings translate into pharmaceutical treatment of such disorders.

Over the shorter term, the usefulness of genetic research on psychopathology is perhaps most evident for the development of psychosocial intervention programs. Although both internalizing and externalizing psychopathologies have a substantial genetic basis, findings consistently indicate that the environment also plays a crucial role. Heritability does not imply inevitability. Rather, genetic predispositions "establish a range of possible behavioral reactions to the range of possible experiences that environments can provide" (Weinberg, 1989, p. 101). At the individual level,

this means that genetic predispositions likely limit the extent to which a behavior change is possible. For example, a genetically vulnerable individual suffering from severe social phobia may be able to adequately function in most social interactions after treatment, but may never be comfortable giving a speech in front of a large group. An understanding of how genetic predispositions influence behavior under specific environmental conditions can thus help clinicians and their clients plan realistic treatment goals and develop effective strategies to reach them (Beevers and McGeary, 2012). However, as not every treatment plan is equally effective for every individual, and some recent studies show that genetic research can provide important clues about what type of treatment may be most beneficial for which client, depending on the individual's genetic propensity (Bakermans-Kranenburg et al., 2008; Eley et al., 2012). Eventually, this information can help tailor targeted intervention programs to individual needs, thus optimizing both efficacy and efficiency of treatments.

Perhaps a final question that needs to be addressed in this context concerns the ethical issues that are raised by finding genes associated with psychopathology. What about the danger of social stigma resulting from the identification of a genetic predisposition? This concern may be greatest for genetic risks related to psychiatric problems or undesirable behaviors, and may be especially pronounced in vulnerable populations such as children and adolescents (Burke and Diekema, 2006). As noted by Plomin and Davis (Plomin and Davis, 2009, p. 69), however, scientific knowledge alone does not account for societal and political decisions, but values are just as important in the decision-making process. As such, genetics could be used to argue for devoting more resources to help genetically at-risk individuals. While the societal implications and ethical issues of genetic research need to be carefully considered, there is also great potential for an invaluable contribution to the prevention and treatment of mental (and physical) health problems.

Summary

- Humans contain forty-six chromosomes in most of their cells, each of which consists of a double helix of complementary strands of DNA. The strands of DNA contain genetic material inherited equally from both mother and father.
- The same genes can have a range of effects depending on whether they are activated or deactivated. Two percent of DNA sequences are protein-encoding genes. At least part of the other 98 percent of DNA are involved in the process of turning genes on or off.
- Gene effects can depend on the effect of other genes. Such gene–gene interactions include dominance (where an allele, or DNA pair-member, of a gene is dominant over the other allele on the same gene locus) and epistasis (an allele on one gene locus affects the expression of a gene on a different gene locus).
- Complex psychopathologies such as conduct disorder, anxiety disorder or depression are likely to be influenced by a multitude of genes.
- Quantitative genetic studies do not directly measure genes but instead statistically infer the relative strength of genetic and environmental effects by examining the phenotypic (observable) similarity of family members who differ in their genetic relatedness with each other.
- The classical adoption design involves examining the phenotypic similarity of children raised in adoptive homes with their biological parents or biological siblings. Any observed similarity can only be attributed to genetic factors since their environments are different.
- The classical twin design involves twins reared together (often but not necessarily by their biological parents). Here, the degree of phenotypic similarity between monozygotic twins (MZ; sharing virtually all of their DNA) is compared with the degree of phenotypic similarity between dizygotic twins (DZ; sharing on average 50% of their DNA).
- Strong genetic influences can be inferred when the phenotypic similarity is higher in MZ twins than in DZ twins. Strong shared environmental influences can be inferred when the phenotypic similarity is high and very similar for both MZ and DZ twins.
- Quantitative genetic studies demonstrate that all major psychopathologies have some genetic basis. For instance, genetic factors account for 60 to 91 percent of the variance in attention deficit/hyperactivity disorder (ADHD), for 20 to 60 percent of the variance in oppositional defiant disorder (ODD) and for 30 to 50 percent of the variance in depression symptoms. The comorbidity (or co-occurrence) of different disorders such as ODD and ADHD is in large part due to an underlying genetic mechanism influencing both disorders.
- Molecular genetic studies attempt to relate specific measured genes to psychopathology.
- The linkage method of molecular genetics tests whether two family members that are affected by a disorder show a larger number of similar alleles around a particular marker gene than two family members where one has the disorder and the other has not.
- The association method of molecular genetics examines whether a priori selected susceptibility genes (candidate genes for the genetic influence on a specific psychopathology) can be found more often in affected than in unaffected individuals in a population.
- Substance dependence and anti-social personality disorder have been linked to the GABRA2 gene. The cholinergic

muscarinic 2 receptor (CHRM2) gene and the monoamine oxidase A (MAO-A) gene have also been implicated in general externalized psychopathology.

- Internalizing psychopathologies such as depression have been related to the CHRM2 gene. Depression as well as bipolar disorder, suicidal behaviors and neuroticism have also been linked to polymorphisms (specific variants) of the serotonin transporter and promoter genes, such as the S-allele of the 5-HTTLPR gene.

- Environmental experiences can be related to an individual's genetic susceptibility for psychopathology through a gene–environment correlation (rGE), whereby specific genotypes predispose an individual to experience certain environments.

- Passive rGE involves the influence of parents' traits (which are partially genetically determined) on a child's environment. Evocative (or reactive) rGE involves the influence of a child's genotype on the non-active evocation of certain reactions from their environment. Selective (or active) rGE involves a child's actively selecting, in accordance with his or her genotype, specific desired environments.

- Coming mostly from quantitative genetic studies, empirical evidence has been found for all three types of rGE. For instance, individuals at high genetic risk for externalizing or internalizing psychopathology are more likely to experience negative environments such as harsh parenting, rejection by peers, affiliation with anti-social peers and academic failure.

- Genes and the environment can work together to influence psychopathology through different forms of gene–environment interactions (G×E): a diathesis-stress process occurs when an environmental stressor triggers or exacerbates genetic predisposition for psychopathology; a suppression process occurs when environmental conditions reduce genetic influences. If these environments are positive, we also speak of a compensation process of G×E.

- Quantitative and molecular genetic studies have provided evidence for a diathesis-stress process whereby genetic predispositions for both externalizing and internalizing psychopathologies only become activated in certain aversive home and social environments. Research also shows that parental monitoring can suppress (reduce) the expression of a genetic susceptibility for externalizing psychopathologies such as substance use and delinquency.

- The development of psychopathological disorders may also be influenced by environmental effects on the epigenome (the overall pattern of gene-activation and deactivation in DNA). One epigenetic process is methylation, where methyl molecules attach to DNA bases to turn them off. Another epigenetic process, histone modification, occurs when molecules alter DNA histone protein tails, turning them on or off.

- Modifications of the epigenome through environmental influences can occur during embryonic development or later in life and can be reversed either through new environmental experiences or through pharmacological intervention.

- Evidence for epigenetic factors influencing psychopathology comes mainly from animal but also some human studies. For instance, children's exposure to adverse prenatal or postnatal environments has been linked to increased methylation in genes that are implicated in hormone regulation, immune response and brain development.

- One practical implication of genetic research is to identify susceptibility genes as well as the specific environments that moderate genetic risk. This could make it possible to screen individuals for genetic risk of psychiatric disorders and develop appropriate therapies that help mitigate the expression of a genetic disposition for psychopathology.

- Ethical considerations of genetic studies must be taken into account. Social stigma may result from knowing which children are genetically predisposed to certain psychopathologies. Policies need to be put in place to minimize such risk if genetic research is to optimally contribute to the prevention and treatment of psychopathological disorders.

Study questions

1. What is the essential difference between the methods used in quantitative genetic and molecular genetic studies?
2. What is the difference between gene–environment correlation and gene–environment interaction?
3. What is the difference between passive, active and evocative gene–environment correlations?
4. What is the essential difference between the linkage method and the association method in molecular genetics?
5. How accurate is it to say that psychological disorders of children and adolescents are primarily caused by genetic factors?

5 The physiological underpinnings of child psychopathology

As mentioned in Chapter 1, no "mental" health problem is exclusively mental. Every human action, thought and feeling is rooted in our physiology. This is not to suggest that the role of environmental influences in shaping children's behavior and development is minimal or can be ignored. The biological and environmental factors contributing to development are intricately intertwined and mutually influential. No biological event can lead to a behavior without the presence of an environmental context in which to enact that behavior, and no environmental event can elicit a behavioral response without also affecting biological functions. In this chapter, we review the neurophysiological, neuroendocrine and autonomic underpinnings of children's emotional and behavioral problems.

Some foundations

Currently observable patterns of feeling, thinking and acting can be attributed to the processes of natural selection that have shaped the evolutionary course of mammalian and human development. These processes have established interconnections between the limbic system, the prefrontal cortex and other neural areas (MacLean, 1990). Emotions and behaviors evolved and have been preserved because, throughout the evolutionary history of our species, they promoted adaptive responses to salient events (Johnson-Laird and Oatley, 1992; Lazarus, 1991). Many aspects of children's mental health problems stem from breakdowns in that normal, adaptive process (Frijda, 1994). The elicited emotion is not appropriate for the evoking stimulus, or it is felt too strongly or not strongly enough, or the bodily arousal it produces fails to

support the behaviors that would constitute an appropriate response.

Strongly tied into the perspectives of evolutionary theory and functional theory of emotion is the stress physiology of the *fight-or-flight response*. When a challenging or threatening event occurs, our bodies prepare to actively cope with the event by reallocating energy and arousal so that we are prepared to confront the event – *fight* (defend and overcome) – or escape from it – *flight* (withdraw and escape). Fight-or-flight responses were undoubtedly critical to the survival of our species in earlier evolutionary times, when predation and competition were regular life-threatening occurrences. The two key systems that control the stress physiology of the fight-or-flight response, and also stress-induced arousal in situations where fighting and fleeing would not be adaptive, are the hypothalamic-pituitary-adrenal axis system and the sympathetic-adrenomedullary system.

Two functionally related neural systems, though distinct from the fight-or-flight response, are important for guiding behavior according to the motivational theory proposed by American psychologist Jeremy Gray (Gray, 1982; Gray and McNaughton, 1996): the *behavioral activation system* (BAS) and the *behavioral inhibition system* (BIS). According to Gray, adaptive human functioning requires the appropriate balance of the motivations to defend and escape (fight-or-flight), to initiate active behavior (BAS) and to terminate ongoing behavior (BIS). The BAS motivates the drive to attain rewards, and thus is responsible for activating approach behavior in response to perceived desire. The BAS also activates avoidant behaviors when there are cues that punishment might occur but could be escaped. The BIS motivates the drive to avoid loss and harm, and thus is responsible for inhibiting ongoing behaviors in the presence of cues that suggest punishment is imminent, or that rewards are not available to be obtained. The BAS/BIS perspective has played an important role in research on behavior disorders, attention deficit and anxiety.

Our neurophysiology has evolved to support our advanced cognitive capabilities as well. The emerging discipline of *developmental cognitive neuroscience* emphasizes the *ontogenesis*, or progressive construction, of neural structures that support cognitive capacities (Johnson et al., 2005). The invention of such neuroimaging techniques as *positron emission tomography high-density event-related potentials* and *magnetic resonance imaging* has allowed researchers to examine the patterns of neural activity that accompany attention, memory, language and other abilities. Because these abilities and the neurobiology that supports them develop over a very protracted period in humans (infancy to early adulthood, and perhaps beyond), there are many opportunities for innate and external influences to affect their development. Paralleling this, there have been many research efforts to relate individual differences in neural activation patterns associated with cognitive abilities to children's normative versus problematic adjustment (Cicchetti and Posner, 2005). Knowing how processes typically function at varying ages can help to identify what has deviated in maladjusted children, but studying abnormal activity also can highlight previously overlooked aspects of the normal development of cognitive functioning.

The brain

With these theoretical foundations in place, let us now consider physiology more directly. First, we review basic neural anatomical structures, neural chemistry and some of the functions associated with input from specific brain regions. We then discuss a range of methods used to study the brain directly.

Basic neuroanatomy

The *central nervous system* (CNS), which includes both the brain and the spinal cord, provides humans with a complex communication system for processing various sources of information (e.g., sensory, motor, autonomic). To a large extent, the brain has a process-based role in this system by detecting, transferring, interpreting and integrating information. Three key functions needed in an optimal brain include speed, adaptability and the ability to respond to subtle environmental differences.

Two types of brain cells help facilitate these neural functions, *neurons* and *glial cells*. Neurons communicate within and between brain areas by using electrical impulses to receive and transmit information. There are approximately 100 billion neurons in the brain. A neuron contains three main parts that aid in its communication with other cells: a *cell body*, *dendrites* and an *axon* (Figure 5.1). Dendrites are the tree-like structure of a neuron that receives signals from other cells in the cell body; a given neuron can have many dendrites. The axon is a long and fibrous extension of the neuron that transmits electrical impulses away from the neuron and to another cell. A white, fatty substance called *myelin* wraps around the axon, both protecting and insulating the nerve fiber to ensure rapid transmission of nerve impulses. The other type of cell in the brain is the glial cell. There are approximately 1 trillion glial cells in the brain, roughly ten times more than neurons. Glial cells maintain homeostasis, form myelin and provide support and protection for the brain's neurons. White matter is mainly made up of myelinated nerve fibers. Gray matter encompasses the parts of the brain and spinal cord that are composed primarily of groups of neuron cell bodies. During the adolescent years, there is a decline in gray matter volume as unused neural pathways and connections are "pruned" away (Giedd and Rapoport, 2010).

The brain is parsed into three sections: the *hindbrain*, *midbrain* and *forebrain*. The hindbrain,

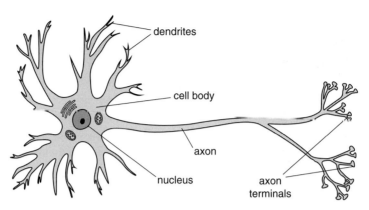

Figure 5.1 In a neuron, information travels from the dendrites to the cell body and along the axon, leaving through the axon terminals.

which includes the upper portion of the spinal cord, the brainstem and the cerebellum, controls vital functions of the body including heart beat and respiration. The cerebellum is located at the back of the brain between the cerebral cortex and the brainstem, and is responsible for motor control, coordination and balance. The cerebellum also supports the learning of rote movements, such as those involved in riding a bicycle. Below the cerebellum is the brainstem, a structure that allows the motor and sensory systems of the brain and cerebellum to communicate with the rest of the body. The brainstem is critical for modulating basic attention, arousal and consciousness, and acts as a conduit for all information going between the body and the brain. For example, the cranial nerves are in place to help deliver basic motor and sensory information from the brainstem to the brain. The brainstem also supports a concentration of monoamines (e.g., dopamine, norepinephrine and serotonin) to help modulate arousal. Further up the brainstem is the midbrain. The midbrain controls certain reflexes and plays a role in controlling eye movements as well as voluntary movements.

The forebrain (also called the cerebral cortex) is the largest, most developed part of the human brain and is the center of our most basic and most complex thoughts and emotions. The cerebral cortex and structures within it support a wide range of higher-order cognitive activities, such as storing memories, executing a goal or plan, paying attention to relevant information and generating imaginative thought. The cerebral cortex is divided into four lobes: frontal, temporal, parietal and occipital (Figure 5.2). These lobes are parsed into symmetric left and right hemispheres, which are separated by the corpus callosum. The corpus callosum is a mass of white matter that connects the left and right hemispheres to facilitate communication between them.

Located directly behind the forehead are the *frontal lobes*. The frontal lobes, also known as the frontal cortex, play a role in generating what are called *executive functions*. Executive functions include abilities such as making decisions and thinking abstractly as well as regulating and controlling one's behavioral and emotional responses. Abilities such as these allow humans to execute goal-directed behaviors and to adjust these behaviors to the situation at hand. The *prefrontal cortex* (PFC), which encompasses the largest part of the frontal lobe, is integrally involved in controlling executive functions such as planning, problem-solving, moral judgments, perspective-taking, controlling impulses and understanding consequences (Damasio et al., 2000; Goldman-Rakic, 1996). In addition, these higher-level cognitive functions play important roles in the conscious regulation of emotion as they are required for planning and executing complex

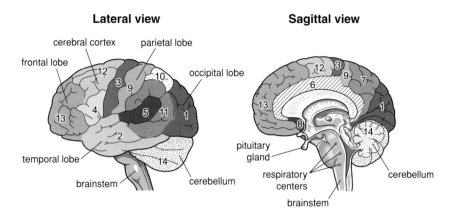

Lateral view

cerebral cortex   parietal lobe

frontal lobe

12

3 9   10

occipital lobe

13

4   5   11   1

2

temporal lobe

14

brainstem   cerebellum

Sagittal view

12 3 9 7

6

13   1

8   14

pituitary gland

respiratory centers

cerebellum

brainstem

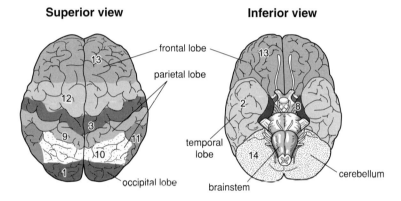

Superior view

13

frontal lobe

parietal lobe

12

3

9   11

10

1

occipital lobe

Inferior view

13

2   8

temporal lobe

14

brainstem   cerebellum

Functional Areas of the Cerebral Cortex

 Visual Area
Sight
Image recognition
Image perception

 Association Area
Short-term memory
Equilibrium
Emotion

 Motor Function Area
Initiation of voluntary muscles

4 Broca's Area
Muscles of speech

5 Auditory Area
Hearing

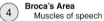 **Emotional Area**
Pain
Hunger
"Fight-or-flight" response

7 Sensory Association Area

8 Olfactory Area
Smelling

9 Sensory Area
Sensation from muscles and skin

10 Somatosensory Area
Evaluation of weight, texture, temperature, etc. for object recognition

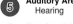 **Wernicke's Area**
Written and spoken language comprehension

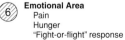 **Motor Function Area**
Eye movement and orientation

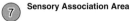 **Higher Mental Functions**
Concentration
Planning
Judgment
Emotional expression
Creativity
Inhibition

Functional Areas of the Cerebellum

 Motor Functions
Co-ordination of movement
Balance and equilibrium
Posture

Figure 5.2 Anatomy and functional areas of the brain.

behavioral sequences. The PFC also undergoes a prolonged period of maturation compared to other brain regions, reaching full functional status in late adolescence and early adulthood (Casey, Giedd and Thomas, 2000). Structural and functional maturational changes in the PFC are thought to underlie the dramatic developmental changes in emotional and behavioral responses that occur in adolescence (Casey et al., 2000; Nelson et al., 2005).

The PFC is further divided into three regions that serve different functions: the *dorsolateral PFC*, the *ventromedial PFC*, which is also known as the orbitofrontal cortex, and the *anterior cingulate cortex* (ACC). Researchers have found that input from the dorsolateral PFC is necessary for solving problems that involve manipulating information in one's mind "online" such that it is held in the working memory (Crone et al., 2006). The dorsolateral PFC is also recruited for retrieval of memories as well as verbal working memory (Owen, 2000). In contrast to the dorsolateral PFC, the orbitofrontal cortex is less involved in working memory aspects of reaching a goal or solving a problem but more involved in situations of social behavior (Blair and Cipolotti, 2000; Nelson and Guyer, 2011). A well-known case of orbitofrontal cortex damage involves a man named Phineas Gage (Damasio et al., 1994). After a railroad spike accidently shot up into his cheek and through his orbitofrontal cortex, the once-pleasant and responsible man underwent a drastic personality change into an impulsive and rude individual. Further research on the orbitofrontal cortex indicated that it indeed plays a major role in regulating social behavior, primarily through the ability to inhibit a response while considering potential options and choosing an alternative response that fits one's goals and plans. As discussed further below, the orbitofrontal cortex channels input to the *amygdala*, a region that facilitates immediate response to one's surroundings, in order to control emotional reactions, and thus is considered to play a pivotal role in emotion regulation.

Another area involved in emotion regulation and executive attention is the *cingulate gyrus*, which,

while not anatomically considered a part of the frontal lobe, is a section of the cortex that wraps around the corpus callosum. The frontal part of the cingulate gyrus includes the anterior cingulate cortex, which has been implicated in cognitive functions related to attention allocation, response selection, response conflict and error performance monitoring (Botvinick et al., 1999; Bush, Luu and Posner, 2000; Carter et al., 2000). The ACC, particularly in the rostral and ventral portions, has also been found to be engaged in a variety of emotional states and may play a role in various cognitive processes related to affective experience (Bush et al., 2000).

Several studies have indicated that the ACC plays an important role in emotion regulation (Etkin, Egner and Kalisch, 2011). Critchley et al. (2003) reported that activity within the ACC was related to transient task-related changes in activity controlled by the autonomic nervous system. These authors proposed that the ACC may serve as a regulator of autonomic functions such as heart and respiration rate. The ability to exert such top-down influence on lower-level neuronal subsystems is the kind of function that would be required of regions involved in emotion regulation. Indeed, the ACC has been linked to the ability to suppress and reappraise negative emotions (Ochsner et al., 2002) and studies indicate that individuals with mood and anxiety disorders show dysfunctions within the ACC (Phillips et al., 2003; Critchley et al., 2004).

The temporal lobe contains the *auditory cortex*, which is involved in auditory processing, the *hippocampus*, which is involved with long-term memory, and other areas that control visual and verbal memory as well as the discrimination of smells and sounds, hearing and speech. The temporal lobe also contains the *fusiform face area*, which is responsible for face recognition. The medial temporal lobe in particular supports the ability to recognize and learn the emotional meaning of stimuli. Within the medial temporal lobe, the hippocampus is critical in associating salient events with perceptual information about those events. That is, the hippocampus does not simply store memories in some type of memory bank. Rather, the hippocampus facilitates connections that are made among encoded pieces of information.

Also situated in the medial temporal lobe is an almond-shaped structure called the amygdala. The amygdala and associated projections function as a behavioral brake during the detection and evaluation of potentially threatening stimuli (Amaral, 2002; LeDoux, 2000). In the process of evaluating stimuli, activity in the amygdala determines the emotional response (conscious and preconscious) that the stimuli elicit. A great deal of neuroimaging work has focused on neural reaction to face stimuli displaying different emotions. For example, faces displaying fearful or threatening expressions have consistently activated the amygdala (Adolphs, 2010). Additional studies have shown reliable changes in amygdala activation when participants were asked to voluntarily enhance, suppress or maintain the emotion they were experiencing while viewing unpleasant and neutral pictures (Ochsner et al., 2002). As amygdalo-cortical fibers become denser during adolescence, better regulatory control with respect to harm-avoidant behaviors may be coming online (Cunningham, Bhattacharyya and Benes, 2002).

The *striatum* is a brain region that encompasses ventral and dorsal areas of the nucleus accumbens, caudate and putamen, with strong connections to frontal cortical regions, the hippocampus and the amygdala, and receives dopaminergic inputs from the ventral tegmental area of the midbrain (Schultz, 2006; Wise, 2004). The striatum is involved in associating emotionally salient environmental stimuli with anticipated outcomes to guide approach-or-avoidance behavioral responses (Berton et al., 2006; Schultz, 2006). As such, striatal circuitry has been highlighted in research on depression and substance abuse and addiction (Koob and Le Moal, 2001; Nestler and Carlezon, 2006). Striatal function also has been linked with responses to rewards and punishments (Breiter et al., 2001) and to the adjustment of behavioral responses based

on errant predictions of aversive and appetitive events (Seymour et al., 2004). In addition to non-social stimuli, a growing literature has focused on the role of striatal circuitry in relation to social cues and situations. In humans, neuroimaging studies have linked striatal regions to processes involved in attributing salience to social stimuli, such as human faces (Adolphs, 2003; Aharon et al., 2001), romantic attachment (Bartels and Zeki, 2000) and simulations of social cooperation (Rilling et al., 2002). Striatal response has also been documented when adolescents think about peers they would like to befriend (Guyer et al., 2009) and upon receipt of being accepted by peers (Guyer et al., 2012).

The parietal and occipital lobes provide critical input for cognitive functions but are less involved in emotion processing and regulation than the frontal lobe. In general, the parietal lobe supports integration of sensory information, such as movement, spatial orientation and navigation. It contains areas involved in speech, visual perception, recognition, perception of stimuli, and pain and touch sensation. The occipital lobe is the brain's visual processing center and contains the visual cortex which supports visual perception, visual-spatial processing, motion perception and color discrimination.

Neurobiological development from birth through adolescence is fundamental to the developing ability to regulate emotion. For example, excitatory systems (e.g., the sympathetic nervous system) are functional at birth whereas the development of inhibitory structures, such as the PFC, continues after birth (Thompson, 1994). During infancy and toddlerhood, myelination in limbic and cortical regions permits maturation of inhibitory cortical areas. Continued maturation of inhibitory cortical and parasympathetic structures balances the influence of subcortical and sympathetic structures on emotion regulation. In addition, the frontal lobes undergo increased maturation. During adolescence in particular, there is an increase in white matter, which consists mostly of myelinated axons, and a loss of gray matter density, which reflects increased synaptic pruning (Giedd and Rapoport, 2010;

Sowell, Peterson et al., 2003). These neurobiological changes contribute to greater inhibitory control and the ability to regulate emotional experiences. For example, negative emotional outbursts common at ages 2 and 3 (e.g., temper tantrums) tend to decrease as children are better able to regulate their emotions through inhibitory control.

Another way in which the brain plays a key role in how humans learn to regulate their own emotions stems from reading cues from those around them. From very early in life, the ability to detect and categorize faces is fairly mature and undergoes fairly limited changes in adolescence (Adolphs, 2001). For example, studies in infants have shown that face stimuli elicit specific patterns of electrical activity at the surface of the brain (Halit, De Haam and Johnson, 2003) as well as neural activation within the fusiform face area (Tzourio-Mazoyer et al., 2002). Thus, the early ability to respond to and categorize faces allows infants to initially rely on their caregivers to learn ways of modulating and regulating their emotions (Cole, Michel and Teti, 1994). In turn, by reading a child's cues, caregivers determine whether the child is in need of soothing or distraction from distress. Over time, these strategies assist children in developing ways to regulate their own emotions through processes such as self-soothing or gaze aversion (Buss and Goldsmith, 1998; Cole, Martin and Dennis, 2004).

Methods used to study the brain

One of the earliest ways in which scientists began to learn about the various functions of the brain was through the study of changes in behavior that accompany brain lesions. Brain lesions are considered a quasi-experimental method in which a given area of the brain is damaged or removed, with the concordant loss of a given function associated with that area. Lesions can occur in various ways such as through tumors, strokes, surgery and injury. A classic example of a lesion study comes from the case of H. M., who had both of his hippocampi removed as a way to stop epileptic seizures stemming from his medial temporal lobes. Following surgery, H. M.'s seizures ceased;

however, his ability to access or create new long-term memories was also lost. If H. M. learned a new person's name or read the morning newspaper, he was unable to remember these pieces of information minutes after learning them. Scientists studying H. M. were able to conclude that the hippocampus played a pivotal role in converting short-term memories into long-term memories.

X-radiation, or x-ray, is a form of electromagnetic radiation that was first used to create images of the brain before being replaced by more recent methods involving neuroimaging. Because x-rays are less effective at representing soft tissue than they are at taking pictures of bone, they do not generate very clear images of the brain. Additionally, x-ray is not safe for children as it relies on radiation emissions to take pictures of the brain and the iatrogenic effects of radiation on children are unknown. *Computerized tomography*, also called CT scan, is a series of x-rays taken from many angles that produce cross-sectional images of the body. These images can be used to create three-dimensional renderings of the brain or other body structures. The CT scan is a good method of studying the structure of the brain; however, it cannot determine the function of those structures and is not a viable method for studying brain activity.

Recent methodological advances have provided the tools necessary to more precisely study both the structure and the function of the brain's regions. The development of technologies such as *electroencephalograms*, positron emission tomography, *single photon emission computerized tomography*, magnetic resonance imaging (MRI) and *magnetic resonance spectroscopy* (MRS) has advanced the measurement of psychological processes at the neurobiological level.

Electroencephalography is a non-invasive test used to record the electrical activity of the brain. Electrodes are placed on specific regions of the scalp to record and create a graphical representation of spontaneous electrical impulses produced by the firing of neurons in the brain. Electroencephalography can be a very effective means of studying brain function, particularly in

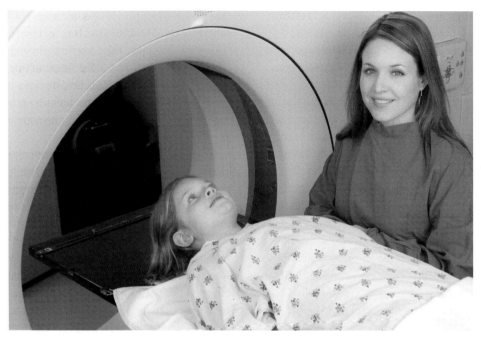

Figure 5.3 A magnetic resonance imaging scanner is used to create detailed pictures of the brain.

children. It is silent, has a high temporal resolution and is more mobile than other methods of studying brain function. Additionally, because the electrodes measure neuronal activity, research subjects do not have to create a motor response to stimuli in order to produce data. Electroencephalography does have some restrictions, however, such as its low spatial resolution and its need for simple study paradigms.

One type of brain response measured through electroencephalography is an *event-related potential* (ERP). An ERP is a brain response considered to be the result of higher cognitive processes, such as thoughts and perception. ERP indices can be useful when studying attention, memory, expectation and other advanced cognitive processes. As electroencephalography indiscriminately detects brain activity, it is impossible to determine an ERP from just one trial. Many trials need to be conducted to collect multiple responses that are then averaged, causing ERP brain activity to be noticeable against random brain activity. Because electroencephalography and ERPs capitalize on

electrical activity at the surface of the brain, the precision for identifying the involvement of exact brain regions is limited, particularly because large areas are usually mapped. In addition, electroencephalography does not allow for precise assessment of subcortical regions. Advances in electroencephalography technologies now make it possible to obtain high-density recordings using caps with a greater number of electrode contacts and to conduct more sophisticated data analyses of cortical activity than previously.

Positron emission tomography (PET) is a fairly invasive procedure that requires the injection of a marker substance, specifically radioactive glucose, to illuminate brain activation while a participant is engaged in a task; thus, PET scans can reveal functional processes. More active brain regions take up more of the marker substance; the concentration of glucose is then detected by the positrons emitted during radioactive decay. One of the strengths of a PET scan is that it can provide a lot of information about the localization of function. Drawbacks of using PET for the study of children and adolescents include its highly invasive procedures and the use of a radioactive substance. An extension of PET methodology is single photon emission computerized tomography, which integrates CT scans with a radioactive tracer, to show how blood moves through the brain and to assess brain metabolism regionally. In general, PET and single photon emission computerized tomography (SPECT) have not commonly been used to study developmental psychopathology in children because of their invasiveness.

Magnetic resonance imaging (MRI) is a non-invasive assessment of neural activity based on changes in blood oxygenation in the brain that can be used to produce images with great contrast between the different soft tissues in the brain. Higher measures of blood oxygenation indicate more blood in the measured region. An increase in blood to a specific region is an indication of more neural resources in that area, and thus enhanced activity in that area of the brain. MRI is a useful tool that has gained increasing popularity in neurological studies of children. There are many specialized types of MRI that are used in both clinical settings and research. *Structural MRI* (sMRI) measures and provides images of the size, volume and location of brain regions. *Functional MRI* (fMRI) provides measurements of the change in blood metabolism that is elicited when subjects perform some kind of a mental or motor task. Because fMRI does not provide an index of absolute activity, but rather a relative index of activity in one condition compared to another, fMRI analyses typically focus on comparing the neural response to an event of interest (e.g., reaction to a fearful face) to the neural response to a baseline condition (e.g., reaction to a neutral face).

Magnetic resonance spectroscopy is a neuroimaging technique that assesses electromagnetic properties of nuclei in the brain and the compounds to which they bind. This method provides a great deal of biochemical information about brain structure and composition of tissues; however, the sensitivity of magnetic resonance spectroscopy signals is limited to detecting large enough metabolic concentrations that are also

susceptible to the presence of the magnetic fields. Magnetic resonance spectroscopy has been more widely used to study child psychopathology such as depression, attention deficit/hyperactivity disorder (ADHD) and autism than to study typically developing children, but it is a promising tool for measuring neurochemical development in both healthy and ill children.

Another aspect of neurophysiology that scientists study is the brain's neurotransmitter system. The neurotransmitter system is one of the primary ways in which information travels through the brain. Chemical neurotransmitters are released by the axon of a neuron and sent across a synapse to receptors located on the dendrites of another neuron. Neurotransmitters are generally considered to be either excitatory or inhibitory in their influence on receptors, although some neurotransmitters have been found to serve both purposes. Assays taken of various neurotransmitters (often through cerebral spinal fluid) have provided a great deal of information about the different actions that neurotransmitters serve in relation to both healthy and pathological functioning. Key neurotransmitters include glutamate, gamma (γ)-aminobutric acid (GABA), acetylcholine, dopamine, serotonin and norepinephrine.

Glutamate is the main excitatory neurotransmitter in the brain and is synthesized from glucose (sugar). Glutamate travels along cells from the cortex to the brainstem for the purpose of triggering action potentials ("exciting") in motor neurons in order to produce muscle responses. In contrast, GABA, a product of glutamate, is the brain's primary inhibitory neurotransmitter and is used in almost every part of the brain. Many of the drugs that are used for sedating or tranquilizing work by strengthening the effects of GABA.

The neurotransmitter *acetylcholine* is used to stimulate muscles, and plays a role in autonomic nervous system functions such as heart rate, respiration and digestion. In the brain, acetylcholine is thought to support learning and alertness, which has been documented by observing deficits in thinking that result from drugs that block acetylcholine.

Dopamine is a neurotransmitter with several key functions in the brain's reward system for seeking out desirable stimuli. As such, the dopamine system has been a focus in research on mechanisms of drug abuse and addiction and has been considered important in the body's behavioral activation system (Gray, 1982; McNaughton and Corr, 2004). Not surprisingly, dysfunctional levels of dopamine are associated with depression given the symptoms of depression such as reduced desire for pleasurable stimuli and experiences. Disruptions to dopaminergic systems also have been implicated in ADHD.

The neurotransmitter *serotonin* plays a key role in regulating basic bodily functions such as sleep, appetite and temperature, as well as the cardiovascular and endocrine systems. Serotonin is further implicated in aspects of memory and learning and is considered to be part of the BIS that responds to feared or potentially harmful stimuli. Dysfunction in the serotonin system is associated with a range of disorders such as depression, anxiety, aggression and eating disorders.

Finally, *norepinephrine* is a neurotransmitter found in the CNS and the sympathetic branch of the ANS, which transmits impulse signals between neurons. Norepinephrine is released in times of extreme stress through the activation of a region in the brainstem called the locus coeruleus, which is a primary site from which many pathways stem and extend to locations in the cortex, limbic system and spinal cord. Norepinephrine influences the brain by influencing arousal, attention, focus and wakefulness. It also impacts the brain's "reward" circuitry. Because of these influences, many drugs that are used to treat ADHD and depression target levels of norepinephrine as well as dopamine.

Psychopathology and the brain

The effective regulation of emotion is crucial for maintaining a connection with ongoing perceptual and attentional processes, accessing a repertoire of adaptive and organized responses, and generating flexible and appropriate responses.

Regulatory processes can be voluntary or automatic, which underscores the difficulty in temporally distinguishing an emotion from the regulation of an emotion in the brain (Goldsmith and Davidson, 2004). Although some elements of emotion regulation require conscious effort (e.g., taking a deep breath and counting to ten to reduce anger), other aspects of emotion regulation are as automatic as the emotional reactions they regulate (e.g., experiencing a quickened heart beat in anticipation of a possible danger). Thus, both automatic and effortful processes typically operate in tandem in the regulation of even a single emotion, resulting in a continuous feedback loop.

The inability to regulate emotion can result in the misidentification of one's own emotions and the misdirection of one's emotional reactions, thereby hindering adaptive and appropriate functioning. Emotions such as fear, anxiety or sadness, for example, become dysfunctional or psychopathological when they bubble up in inappropriate contexts or when their valence or arousal is unpredictable or extreme and does not fit within the situational demands.

By using methods from neuroscience, we can gain a better understanding of the biological and physical manifestations of psychopathologies. Most psychiatric disorders involve disruptions in the ability to regulate emotion in appropriate ways and in appropriate contexts. The neurobiological characteristics of some of the more common types of childhood psychopathologies involving emotion regulation disruptions will be considered in the subsequent chapters devoted to disruptive behavior disorders, depression, ADHD and anxiety disorders (see Chapters 12 to 15).

Hormones

Endocrinologists study hormones, neuroendocrinologists study the interactions between hormones and the central nervous system, and *psychoneuroendocrinologists* study the roles played by hormones in

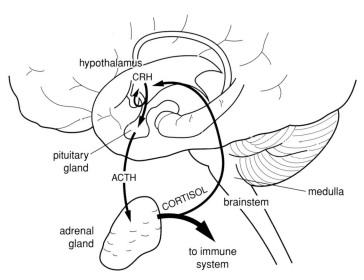

Figure 5.4 The hypothalamic–pituitary–adrenal (HPA) axis system is important for regulating response to stress.

the production and regulation of human behavior. Hormones are chemicals secreted by neurons in various brain structures, such as the hypothalamus, and other organs, such as the adrenal glands, that circulate through cerebral spinal fluid and serum (blood) in order to affect the activity of other cells and organs. These chemical messengers are often thought of as the "slow road" to regulation: Whereas the autonomic nervous system – the "fast road" – can directly stimulate target organs in a matter of milliseconds to seconds, hormones can take several seconds to several minutes to produce their effects. Much like the proverbial tortoise and hare, however, it would be a mistake to discount the contributions of the slower participant in the race to regulate bodily processes. Hormones are vitally important messengers and triggers for physiological and behavioral activity, affecting metabolism, growth, immune functions, arousal states, mood and other functions.

There are many hormones that affect human behavior and potentially are involved in emotional and behavioral problems. The neuroendocrine system that has garnered the most attention from researchers interested in developmental psychopathology is the *hypothalamic-pituitary-adrenal (HPA) axis*, which

is a major determinant of how humans respond to stress. Stressors include normal daily challenges like getting to school on time and arguing with a sibling, more threatening events like being victimized by a bully or growled at by a large, unleashed dog, and chronic stressors like living in poverty or having an abusive parent. Although experiencing some stress is a normal part of life, stress is also recognized as a powerful contributor to psychopathology in children and adults (Hankin and Abela, 2005). Understanding the physiology of stress, therefore, is essential for understanding the biological basis of children's emotional and behavioral maladjustment.

The hypothalamic-pituitary-adrenal (HPA) axis

The HPA axis system is considered to be one of the two principal stress response systems, along with the sympathetic-adrenomedullary system, which is discussed as part of autonomic physiology. The HPA axis functions through the coordinated activity of a series of organs within and outside the brain, which produce a cascade of hormones resulting in the release of *cortisol* from the adrenal glands (Figure 5.4) (Gunnar and Adam, 2012; Kaltas and

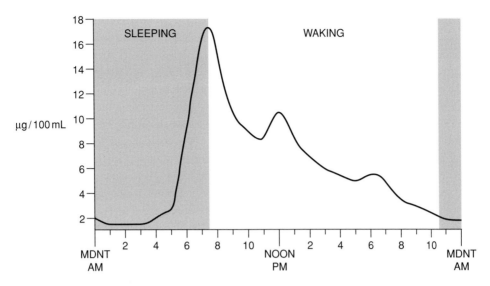

Figure 5.5 The diurnal cycle of HPA axis activity produces the most cortisol at waking and the least cortisol in the early hours of sleeping.

Chrousos, 2007). Activity of the HPA axis begins in the hypothalamus, as neurons in the paraventricular nuclei release corticotropin-releasing hormone and arginine vasopressin. These stimulate the corticotrophic cells in the anterior pituitary to secrete adrenocorticotropic hormone, which in turn crosses the blood–brain barrier, leaving the CNS and reaching the adrenal glands, which sit atop the kidneys. Adrenocorticotropic hormone triggers the adrenal cortex to release corticosteroids, including cortisol and dehydroepiandrosterone, into the serum of the circulatory system, where they are carried by the blood to targets throughout the body to produce a variety of effects.

It is important to know that the HPA axis is also a self-regulating system that decreases activity through a negative feedback loop. Cortisol can cross the blood–brain barrier to reach the CNS, and when it reaches a critical level, it signals the hypothalamus to reduce corticotropin-releasing hormone production in the paraventricular nuclei. As less corticotropin-releasing hormone is produced, the pituitary gland decreases its production of adrenocorticotropic hormone, such that the adrenal glands lose the signal to produce cortisol and dehydroepiandrosterone. This

self-regulation is a critically adaptive feature of the HPA axis, because too much cortisol can be harmful. Cortisol is a catabolic steroid, breaking down proteins to release energy. Although this is useful in the short term to support active coping with immediate challenges and threats, if elevated cortisol levels persist for extended periods of time – a condition called *hypercortisolism* – it can lead to a variety of harmful immunological, physical and psychological side effects. Cortisol is a prime example of how it is possible to have too much of a good thing.

The HPA axis is constantly active, to greater or lesser degrees. Over the circadian cycle of day and night, or waking and sleeping, normative cortisol production follows a predictable pattern (Figure 5.5) (Adam, 2012). Beginning a few months after birth (Gunnar and Quevedo, 2007), the normative pattern is for cortisol levels to be fairly high by the end of the sleeping period and to peak several minutes after awakening, which is called the cortisol awakening response (Chida and Steptoe, 2009). Circulating cortisol levels then drop rapidly over the morning, drop more slowly through the afternoon and are at their lowest in the evening, with temporary increases after eating meals (Gibson et al., 1999). Cortisol levels then increase again during sleep, until the waking level is reached in the morning hours. The waking (diurnal) rhythm constitutes "baseline" or "basal" HPA activity, representing the amount of cortisol that would be expected to be circulating through the blood at a given time of day, all other things being equal. Of course, all other things are rarely equal. First, there are large individual differences in cortisol production; whether due to genetics, temperament or early experience, some people produce more cortisol than others. Second, the diurnal rhythm itself can be weaker or stronger; some people have high peaks and low valleys (steeper slopes), whereas others have less extreme changes in their circulating cortisol levels over the course of the day (flatter slopes).

Third, healthy HPA functioning also supports appropriate responses to stress by changing its level of activity. Once the HPA axis begins ramping up its response to a stressful event, it typically takes about 20 minutes for the peak levels of circulating cortisol to be produced (Adam, 2012; Gunnar and Adam, 2012). Depending on the intensity and duration of the stressful event, it can take even longer for circulating cortisol to return to baseline levels, that is, the level that preceded the stressful event, or that would be expected in a calm child at that time in the diurnal rhythm. Curiously, early childhood might be a period of hyporesponsivity for the HPA axis (Gunnar and Quevedo, 2007). Compared to infants, older children, adolescents and adults, it can be challenging to elicit a large increase in circulating cortisol levels in young children (Gunnar, Talge and Herrera, 2009), although at this time it is not clear whether that is because young children are less responsive to stress or because researchers have not identified appropriate stressors to use in studies of young children. Either way, it is clear that basal cortisol levels rise over childhood, and as children begin to approach adolescence, their HPA axis responses to stressful events also strengthen.

Normal diurnal levels of cortisol are essential for healthy functioning. Temporary elevations in cortisol are generally seen as beneficial in the short term. However, cortisol elevations that are unusually prolonged can become harmful, as cortisol is catabolic, breaking down other tissues (Kaltas and Chrousos, 2007). An acute rise in circulating cortisol following a stressful event is associated with increased blood glucose levels and release of fatty acids (providing fuel for activity), increased respiration, heart rate and blood pressure (preparation for active coping), and heightened mental states, including attention, vigilance and anxiety (for monitoring salient cues in the environment that could signify danger). It also suppresses immune function. If elevated cortisol levels persist for hours, days or longer, however, the effects of hypercortisolism are neurotoxic: low energy, flattened emotions, proneness to infection, tissue damage and even neurostructural changes can occur. In fact, many of the short-term and long-term effects of cortisol have parallels in the symptoms of such mental health problems as depression and anxiety disorders.

It is worth noting how researchers study the activity of the HPA axis. Most cortisol that is produced by the adrenal cortex and secreted into serum gets bound to cortisol-binding protein and is rendered inactive. The remaining, unbound cortisol can have physiological effects on other organs and tissues. Unbound cortisol also gets secreted from serum through the salivary glands into saliva. The kidneys, which are responsible for cleaning the blood, break down cortisol and excrete it in urine. Thus, researchers can assess the activity of the HPA axis by measuring cortisol levels in blood, urine or saliva. Although there have been studies of all three of these bodily fluids, the majority of studies of children and youths have examined cortisol levels in saliva. Collecting saliva is practical (relatively easy and inexpensive) and ethical (non-invasive, not frightening and not embarrassing). The links between cortisol and children's psychopathology will be further considered in the subsequent chapters devoted to the specific disorders (see Chapters 12 to 15).

A brief note about other hormones

All of this attention to cortisol should not be taken to mean that it is the only hormone that matters for understanding developmental psychopathology. The other hormones produced by the HPA axis – dehydroepiandrosterone, corticotrophin-releasing hormone, and so on – also contribute to children's well-being. Moreover, although the HPA axis is a very important neuroendocrine system, it is not the only one. Perhaps most notably, during puberty the *hypothalamic-pituitary-gonadal (HPG) axis* is activated, which is responsible for the production of the sex steroids testosterone and estradiol, as well as other hormones. Given all of the physical, behavioral and emotional changes that occur over puberty, it is understandable that scientists also have been interested in examining the links between adolescents' psychological difficulties and their levels of androgens (e.g., testosterone) and estrogens (e.g., estradiol).

Autonomic nervous system (ANS)

Most studies on the connections between physiological activity and developmental psychopathology have involved measurement of peripheral systems, or autonomic and somatic activity. There are many reasons for this. The technologies to record heart rate, blood pressure, respiration, perspiration (sweating) and similar bodily processes are simpler and were developed earlier than effective and reliable techniques for hormonal assays or neuroimaging. Until very recently, measuring autonomic functions was also less intrusive than assessments of other physiological systems and therefore less frightening and potentially unethical for research with children. The preponderance of research on children's autonomic physiology has focused on one kind of developmental psychopathology: aggression and anti-social behavior.

The autonomic nervous system (ANS) is the information super-highway between the brain and the body. The central nervous system controls peripheral targets, like organs and muscles, by sending and receiving information through the ANS, the two main branches of which are the sympathetic (SNS) and parasympathetic nervous system (PNS). Most organs and peripheral systems are innervated (stimulated) by both the SNS and PNS branches of the ANS (Figure 5.6). The preganglionic neural synapses of both branches – that is, the communication links between the CNS and both the PNS and SNS neurons – primarily use the neurotransmitter acetylcholine. However, the SNS and PNS use different neurotransmitters for most of their postganglionic synapses – the communication links between the ANS branches and their targets. The SNS mostly uses the neurotransmitter norepinephrine (also known as noradrenaline) to trigger stimulation. (One notable deviation from this pattern, though, exists in the electrodermal system which controls perspiration, which we will review soon.) As norepinephrine is a relatively long-lasting agent, SNS activation can result in persisting autonomic arousal. The PNS exclusively uses the neurotransmitter acetylcholine as its communicative agent to trigger stimulation. Acetylcholine dissipates more quickly than norepinephrine, such that the autonomic effects of PNS stimulation are relatively quick.

SNS and PNS stimulation tend to have opposite effects on autonomic activity, with greater SNS activation accompanying increased autonomic arousal and greater PNS activation accompanying decreased autonomic arousal. Thus, the SNS and PNS are often portrayed as serving "on" and "off" functions, respectively. When an evocative, challenging or threatening event is perceived, the SNS stimulates greater autonomic arousal, and when the event is ended, the PNS stimulates subdued arousal. Thus, the SNS and PNS have often been seen as antagonistic, or as co-regulating each other through reciprocating dominance, reflecting the concept of homeostasis. As stimulation of one branch of the ANS moves the body into a state of greater (SNS) or lesser (PNS) arousal, the other branch of the ANS increases its activity in order to compensate and hasten the recovery of homeostasis.

This is too simplistic a portrayal of the dynamics of the ANS, however. Homeostasis is not the sole

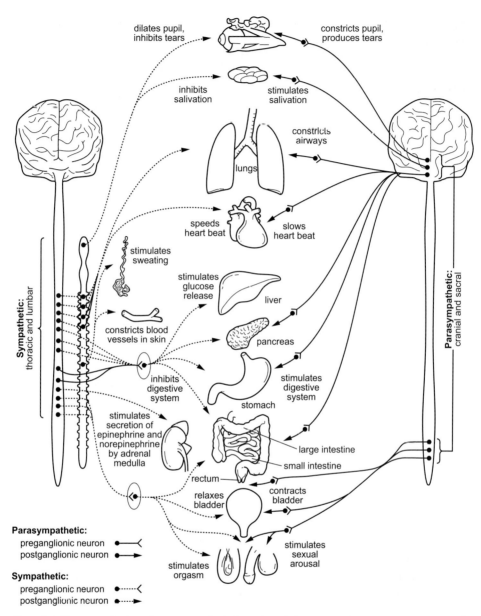

Figure 5.6 The sympathetic and parasympathetic branches of the autonomic nervous system control the activity of organs and systems throughout the body.

operating principle for autonomic control. The two branches of the ANS function reciprocally at times, but they can also be either independently active, or jointly co-active (see Table 5.1; Obradović and Boyce, 2012). Therefore, for example, the increases in heart

rate that accompany being exposed to something frightening might be the result of increased SNS activity, or the result of decreased PNS stimulation, or the result of simultaneous changes in the activity levels of both branches of the ANS. Intriguingly, the

Table 5.1 **The interactive effects of sympathetic and parasympathetic activation on states of autonomic arousal**

SYMPATHETIC RESPONSE	PARASYMPATHETIC RESPONSE		
	Increase	No Change	Decrease
Increase	Coactivation	Uncoupled Sympathetic Activation	Reciprocal Sympathetic Activation
No Change	Uncoupled Parasympathetic Activation	Baseline	Uncoupled Parasympathetic Withdrawal
Decrease	Reciprocal Parasympathetic Activation	Uncoupled Sympathetic Withdrawal	Coinhibition

Source: Berntson, G. G., Cacioppo, J. T. and Quigley, K. S. (1991). Autonomic determinism: The modes of autonomic control, the doctrine of autonomic space, and the laws of autonomic constraint, *Psychological Review*, *98*, 459–87.

interactive effects of SNS and PNS stimulation are *not* necessarily just additive. For example, there is evidence from animal research that increased SNS stimulation cannot markedly increase heart rate if PNS stimulation also increases, but PNS stimulation can produce greater decreases in heart rate when there is simultaneous SNS stimulation. Physiological researchers have coined the terms *autonomic space* and *allodynamic control* to characterize the simultaneous, interactive contributions of SNS and PNS stimulation to somatic activity. As constant as homeostasis is, it is not always efficient or effective. As we go about our daily activities, we are constantly being required to adjust our levels of arousal in order to respond to the changing demands of what we encounter. Constantly returning to a baseline state (homeostasis) would not be efficient or effective. Rather, adaptive functioning is maintained through continuing adjustments and fluctuations of physiological states (allostasis) (Berntson and Cacioppo, 2007; McEwen, 2012).

Because most organs are innervated by both branches of the ANS, it can be hard to determine the relative contributions of PNS and SNS activity.

Thus, knowing that children with disruptive behavior disorders, for example, tend to have slower heart rates than children without anti-social problems does not reveal whether anti-social children experience relatively weaker SNS stimulation, or relatively more PNS inhibition, of cardiac activity. (And of course, it is not as simple as one or the other . . .) Fortunately, some measures of autonomic activity have been identified that can be attributed specifically to one of the two branches of the ANS.

The PNS has long preganglionic neural fibers that extend from brainstem nuclei, such as the dorsal motor nucleus and nucleus ambiguus, to be in close proximity to the target tissue. Because of its long preganglionic and short postganglionic fibers, the PNS tends to have a shorter latency of action, or more rapid influence, than does the SNS. The tenth cranial nerve, or vagus nerve, exerts control over the heart, chiefly regulating the rate at which the heart beats (called chronotropic control), over which it has a more dynamic range of influence than does the SNS. One's heart does not beat at a constant rate; the fact that your heart rate is, say, sixty beats per minute does not mean that there is exactly 1 second between each consecutive beat – that's just the *average* of the sixty inter-beat intervals that occurred in that minute. *Heart rate variability* (HRV) is influenced by many factors, but one specific component of heart rate variability called *respiratory sinus arrhythmia*, or *cardiac vagal tone*, is under the specific control of the PNS via the vagus nerve. Respiratory sinus arrhythmia is a quantification of the changes in heart rate variability that occur at the frequency of the respiratory cycle. By measuring heart rate variability and isolating the frequency component unique to respiratory sinus arrhythmia, researchers can obtain a measure of the degree to which the PNS is exerting its influence over cardiac arousal.

Researchers in developmental psychopathology have found respiratory sinus arrhythmia to be a useful and non-invasive index because it appears to be a marker of children's ability to regulate their arousal levels. Stephen Porges (2011) developed the influential *polyvagal theory*, linking PNS control over cardiac activity to emotion expression and regulation. According to Porges, when children have higher baseline respiratory sinus arrhythmia, they seem to have greater capacity to regulate their emotional states and cope with challenges effectively. When situations are safe and comfortable, higher respiratory sinus arrhythmia helps children to calmly engage in positive social interactions. When a potentially important event occurs, a modest withdrawal of PNS influence, indexed by decreasing respiratory sinus arrhythmia, appears to be an effective regulatory response for increasing orientation and attention toward the event. A strong withdrawal of PNS influence, however, suggests that a child has responded to an event as a potential threat or challenge to which a large increase in heart rate would be needed, such as the fight-or-flight response. There has been quite a bit of research examining the relations between children's emotional and behavioral problems and their respiratory sinus arrhythmia at baseline and in response to various stimuli and challenges.

The sympathetic nervous system (SNS) and cardiovascular and electrodermal activity

Compared to the PNS, the SNS has shorter preganglionic fibers and longer postganglionic fibers. SNS fibers tend to branch toward multiple targets, producing more widespread effects, although both the PNS and SNS can activate differentially across organs (Vallbo, Hagbarth and Wallin, 2004). The SNS is part of the second major component of the body's stress response system, the sympathetic adrenomedullary system, after the HPA axis system. The SNS stimulates the adrenal medulla to release norepinephrine and epinephrine, which drive the fight-or-flight responses of many tissues, including release of glucose for energy, increased heart rate and blood pressure, blood flow being directed away from the skin and toward the brain and large muscle groups, pupil dilation and other effects. Although we saw previously that the PNS has relatively greater control over heart rate, the SNS has relatively greater control over cardiac flow (how much blood is pushed out with each beat) and blood pressure.

The influence of the SNS over cardiac flow has allowed researchers to develop another non-invasive measure that is appropriate for use with children. *Pre-ejection period* is a specific index of SNS influence over cardiac activity. A technique called *impedance cardiography* is used to assess changes in blood flow through the chambers of the heart during a heart beat. Pre-ejection period represents the number of milliseconds from the electromechanical signal that the left ventricle of the heart is about to begin contraction until the aortic valve opens (allowing the blood to be pumped out of the ventricle). Variability in that brief period of time is controlled by the SNS fibers that enervate the heart, with shorter pre-ejection period reflecting greater SNS influence over cardiac activity.

As a major driver of the fight-or-flight response, the SNS is closely linked to both anger and fear. Many childhood difficulties, particularly anti-social behavior and anxiety problems, are characterized by inappropriate anger and fear. SNS activity has also been related to both the activation and inhibition aspects of Gray's BAS/BIS theory (Fowles, 1988), although the research on this is not entirely consistent.

There are two other non-invasive ways to measure the activity of the SNS that are appropriate for developmental research. The first is by measuring *electrodermal activity*, or skin conductance. The SNS controls the eccrine sweat glands. Unlike almost all other SNS postganglionic connections, the SNS fibers that control eccrine gland activity principally use the neurotransmitter acetylcholine. SNS stimulation increases eccrine secretion, and the more people perspire, the more electrical current can flow across the surface of their skin. Psychophysiological researchers usually measure electrodermal activity by placing two electrodes on the palm of one hand and measuring the current flowing between them, due to the fact that eccrine glands on the palms are more responsive to psychological stimuli than to thermal changes.

The measurement of skin conductance can yield two pieces of information: the overall amount or level of current flow (sometimes called *tonic*), and changes in current flow (sometimes called *phasic*). Researchers alternatively refer to tonic current flow as electrodermal activity, or as skin conductance levels. Similarly, a phasic response reflecting an acute elevation in flow is referred to as electrodermal response, skin conductance response or galvanic skin response. Because electrodermal activity is easily measured and electrodermal responses are easily identified, skin conductance is a commonly used index of SNS activity. Electrodermal responses are relatively slow, typically occurring one to three seconds after an evocative stimulus occurs. Electrodermal responses can also occur spontaneously, and are called *non-specific electrodermal responses* because they do not seem to be produced in response to an identifiable stimulus. There is good evidence that electrodermal activity specifically reflects how SNS contributes to the inhibitory (BIS) side of Gray's motivational model

(Fowles, 1988), and thus, electrodermal activity and electrodermal responses are thought to reflect SNS contributions to threat avoidance and arousal due to punishment.

Another method for assessing SNS activity is by measuring the levels of salivary alpha-amylase, an enzyme that is produced in the mucosa tissue of the mouth whose principal function is to start the breakdown of starches. Although both the SNS and the PNS innervate the salivary glands, there is some evidence that increased secretion of alpha-amylase under stressful or challenging conditions is controlled by the SNS (Nater et al., 2005; Rohleder et al., 2006). The peak of salivary alpha-amylase production occurs several minutes after a stressful event is experienced, but the ease of its measurement is making salivary alpha-amylase an increasingly popular tool in developmental research. The links between ANS activity and developmental psychopathology will be further considered in the subsequent chapters devoted to the specific disorders (see Chapters 12 to 15).

Putting the pieces together

The following paragraphs summarize the ways in which multiple biological markers together constitute physiological bases for several of the most common forms of child psychopathology; detail will be provided in the subsequent chapters on the specific disorders.

Anxiety

The physiological basis of children's anxiety problems forms a clear pattern that is rooted in exaggerated and inappropriate fear responses. In response to stressful challenges, or even normal, minimally stressful daily events, anxious children react in ways that are consistent with the "flight" side of the fight-or-flight response, and suggest the inhibitory motivation of the BAS/BIS model is dominant over the activation motivation. This profile is manifested neurophysiologically as increased activation of the amygdala in response to emotionally salient stimuli, such as fearful faces or the delivery of peer evaluation, as well as patterns of greater asymmetry in psychophysiologic activity in the right frontal lobe, motivating greater avoidance or withdrawal behaviors. The HPA axis produces an acute stress response, producing more cortisol to prepare for flight. Heightened SNS stimulation produces bodily signs of distress, and the weakened regulatory influence of the PNS leaves anxious children unprepared to cope with their emotional arousal.

Depression

Depressed children and youths can be sad and disconsolate, lethargic, irritable and withdrawn from life's pleasures. It might be the case that when children experience depression there is a weakening of BAS, the motivation to actively engage and seek rewards. With respect to brain activity, depressed children and adolescents show decreased neural activity in the striatum and medial prefrontal cortex and decreased left frontal activity, possibly contributing to their low approach motivation. The HPA axis is chronically overactive, resulting in elevated circulating cortisol levels over the circadian cycle. This hypercortisolism likely depletes the resources of depressed children, yet they respond to stresses and challenges by producing even more cortisol. The influence of the PNS branch of their ANS is diminished, robbing them of another physiological resource to regulate their negative emotions.

Disruptive behavior disorders

In many ways, the physiological underpinning of children's disruptive behavior disorders looks like the antithesis of the biology of anxiety problems. The BIS is greatly weakened, with the BAS dominant, and they are poised for confrontation. The neurophysiology of anti-social children reveals an overall pattern of reduced activation in regions that guide emotion regulation and cognitive control. Emotion regulation deficits clearly appear to be reflected in their atypical respiratory sinus arrhythmia, indicating that PNS is not functioning normally. Activity of both the neuroendocrinological and the autonomic systems that drive stress physiology are attenuated in aggressive and anti-social children, so much so that they don't get those important somatic cues to alter their course of action in risky situations. When they get into a situation where a fight could ensue, or they could be arrested for their behavior, or they could provoke an adult caregiver's wrath, their low cortisol reaction and weak SNS activity fail to evoke that small fear response that would otherwise make them pause and reconsider. It may also be difficult for children and youths with disruptive behaviors to learn to change their anti-social ways, because any consequence, punishment or hurt they might experience also would be unlikely to provoke a stress response.

This interpretation of the affective, cognitive and behavioral consequences of reduced physiological reactivity is concordant with the fearlessness hypothesis of disruptive behavior disorders (see Chapter 12). An equally viable explanation for the association between physiology and anti-social behavior is the sensation-seeking hypothesis. Children and youths with low baseline or tonic physiology and reduced reactivity to the normative stresses of life might go through their days feeling relatively understimulated. Whereas dangerous or risky activities might elicit an uncomfortably high level of reactivity in most people, these understimulated youths might seek out such situations in order to experience some degree of physiological arousal.

Attention deficit/hyperactivity disorder

There is some support for the suggestion that children with ADHD have underactive BIS motivations (Quay, 1997), such that they are less able to inhibit their impulsive and inappropriate behaviors, but the research is far from consistent on this hypothesis. It is clear that they have poor self-control, and this is

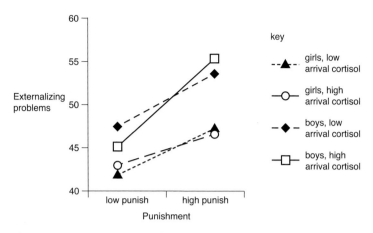

Figure 5.7 Young boys' levels of cortisol reactivity affect how strongly punishment by mothers predicts boys' externalizing behavior problems.

seen neurophysiologically in their under-recruitment of frontal-striatal input, which may be due to developmental changes such as cortical thinning. Their overall levels of brain activity seem to be lower or less mature. While they might not differ in HPA activity from children without ADHD, children with ADHD might experience diminished autonomic reactivity to stress and challenge. At present, it seems that this would have more to do with decreased SNS influence than with disruptions to PNS activity, but more research is needed to provide a more thorough understanding of the pathophysiology of ADHD.

Putting physiology into context

We began this chapter by stating that the focus on biological features of developmental psychopathology should not in any way suggest that children's life experiences are less important. Children's parents, families and home life, their friends and peers, the neighborhoods and communities they live in, and their broader cultural milieus are all important determinants of children's adaptive or maladaptive behavior, as biology and environment function together to shape children's development. Several researchers have found

that aspects of autonomic physiology were only associated with children's problems when children were living in particular family contexts. Indeed, children's adverse experiences might even be the causes of some of the disrupted physiological activity that accompanies their emotional and behavioral problems (Cicchetti and Rogosch, 2012; Strang, Hanson and Pollack, 2012).

Developmental scientists are becoming increasingly interested in examining and understanding the ways in which environment and biology are intertwined in the co-determination of children's paths toward healthy or unhealthy functioning (Hastings, Buss and Dennis, 2012). A growing number of *biopsychosocial* models have been proposed (Ellis et al., 2011; Rutter, Moffitt and Caspi, 2006; Sameroff, 2010), which seek to chart a more integrated and holistic perspective on developmental psychopathology. For example, Hastings and colleagues (Hastings et al., 2011) recently showed that the robust association between maternal punishment and young children's externalizing problems was particularly strong for boys who had stronger HPA reactivity to meeting strangers (Figure 5.7). This suggests that the neurobiological characteristics of children can moderate, or alter, the ways in which their social experiences shape their development. The information in this chapter is intended to stimulate thinking about the many roles that biological processes might play in children's development of mental health problems. Neurophysiology, neuroendocrinology and autonomic physiology are critical pieces of the puzzle and important to understand, but they are only some of the pieces.

How can an understanding of physiology be applied to working with children with problems?

Learning about the roles that physiology plays in the etiology and development of children's emotional, cognitive and behavioral problems is not solely an academic pursuit. There are a number of important implications of this research for clinicians. An integrative perspective that understands how deviations from normative and adaptive neurobiological regulation are associated with problems will be critical to ongoing efforts to enhance current diagnostic procedures, prevention programs and intervention techniques (Beauchaine, Hong and Marsh, 2008; Cicchetti and Gunnar, 2008; Greenberg, Riggs and Blair, 2007). For example,

distinct physiological correlates might be used to help determine which of two phenotypically similar disorders a child is manifesting. Examinations of multiple biomarkers, or *endophenotypes*, might also help to identify children and youths who are at greatest risk for the maintenance or exacerbation of problems over development, and therefore which youths are in greatest need of treatment. In accord with the principle of *multifinality*, it is widely accepted that superficially similar problems might have many diverse underlying causes, and it is likely that children with different sources for their problems would benefit from different, individually tailored treatments. Assessing the biological functioning of a child could help to identify the kinds of treatment procedures, both behavioral and pharmacological, to which she or he would be most responsive. As well, recognizing that neurobiological regulation is itself sensitive to and shaped by environmental influences (Cicchetti and Rogosch, 2012; Maheu et al., 2010; Strang et al., 2012), interventions might be aimed at the level of family, peer, school or neighborhood in order to alleviate the social pressures that could be disrupting children's adaptive physiology. As social experiences improve, effective physiological regulation might be re-established, contributing to the alleviation of children's psychological problems.

Summary

- According to both evolutionary theory and functional theory of emotion, certain emotions and behaviors develop and are preserved because they have at one point promoted positive adaptation for the human species.
- The neural representation of these learned behaviors and emotions relate to different brain systems responsible for automatic and stereotypic changes in arousal. In children with psychopathology, this process is disrupted and the response is not appropriate for the stimulus evoked.

- One such learned emotion/behavior is the fight (defend and overcome) or flight (withdraw and escape) response. The two key systems that control this response are the hypothalamic-pituitary-adrenal (HPA) axis system and the sympathetic-adrenomedullary system.
- Two additional neural systems, according to motivational theory, are the behavioral activation system (BAS) and the behavioral inhibition system (BIS). The former initiates active behavior (e.g., reward-seeking, punishment-avoiding), the latter inhibits ongoing behavior (e.g., avoiding

loss and harm, terminating reward-seeking when not obtainable). These have an important role in developmental psychopathology, especially behavior disorders, ADHD and anxiety.

- The discipline of developmental cognitive neuroscience focuses on the ontogenesis (i.e., progressive construction) of neural structures for cognitive abilities. Various neuroimaging techniques are used to study the associated patterns of behavioral and emotional processes, often with a focus on examining the cognitive differences between children with adjustment problems and those without.

- The central nervous system (CNS) includes both the brain and the spinal cord, and is the complex communication system for processing various sources of information.

- The approximately 100 billion neurons (brain cells) communicate within and between brain areas using electric impulses to receive and transmit information. A neuron is composed of a cell body, dendrites and an axon. Groups of neuron cell bodies constitute gray matter, which has been found to decrease in quantity in adolescence as unused connections are removed.

- The other type of brain cell is the glial cell. The approximately 1 trillion glial cells maintain homeostasis and provide support and protection for the neurons.

- The brain has three different sections: the hindbrain (which includes the spinal cord, the brainstem and the cerebellum) is responsible for the body's vital functions; the midbrain controls certain voluntary and involuntary movements, and the forebrain (also called the cerebral cortex) houses our most basic and most complex thoughts and emotions.

- The cerebral cortex is divided into four lobes (i.e. frontal, temporal, parietal and occipital) that are symmetrically parsed into two hemispheres, separated by the corpus callosum, a mass of white matter (nerve fibers) that connects these hemispheres to allow communication between them.

- The frontal lobe, of which the prefrontal cortex (PFC) is the largest portion, controls the higher-order executive functions in the brain. The maturation of the PFC, which takes longer than other parts of the brain, underlies the dramatic developmental changes in emotional and behavioral responses in adolescents. The PFC is composed of the dorsolateral PFC (responsible for working memory), the ventromedial PFC (also known as the orbitofrontal cortex; responsible for social behavior), and the anterior cingulate cortex (ACC; a portion of the cingulate gyrus responsible for attention allocation, response selection and monitoring of error performance). The ACC has been shown to also be involved with emotional regulation, particularly linked to mood and anxiety disorders.

- The temporal lobe contains the auditory cortex (involved in auditory processing), the hippocampus (involved in long-term memory, emotional memory and discrimination of senses), the fusiform face area (responsible for face recognition) and the amygdala (involved with emotional responses; develops during adolescence to regulate control of harm-avoidant behaviors).

- The striatum, involved in associating stimuli with a motivated response and linked to substance abuse and addiction, contains the nucleus accumbens, caudate and putamen, and connects to various areas of the brain, including the frontal cortex, the hippocampus and amygdala. Striatal circuitry has also been found to be involved with salience of human faces, romantic attachment, social cooperation and even situations of befriending in adolescence.

- The parietal lobe is responsible for processing and integrating sensory information received from the different areas of the brain, such as movement, orientation, speech, vision and tactile sensation.

- The occipital lobe, containing the visual cortex, deals with visual processing, including perception, visual-spatial processing, motion perception and color discrimination.

- Many neurobiological developments from birth to adolescence explain certain abilities for emotional regulation at different stages of life. This includes maturation of the PFC, myelination of inhibitory cortical areas and thus an increase in white matter, and a decrease of gray matter. Along the same lines, humans learn to regulate their emotions by reading cues from those around them.
- Brain lesions have been used as a preliminary method of studying brain functions. Through tumors, strokes, surgery or injury, when an area of the brain is damaged or removed, an associated function is often impaired or lost. H.M. is a well-known clinical example of this technique.
- X-radiation (i.e. using x-rays) and computerized tomography (CT scan) are early methods used to create images of the brain. The latter is a more comprehensive version of the former that is used to create three-dimensional renderings of the brain. These two methods cannot be used to determine brain function or activity, nor can they be used in research with children.
- More recent tools have been able to bring together both structure and function, leading to a more advanced understanding of the brain and more research on neurobiological foundations of emotion and cognition.
- One example of these tools, electroencephalography, maps the firing of neurons in the brain and can be used on children. Event-related potentials are a type of brain response that is considered to be the result of higher brain function, such as cognition or perception. Multiple trials are needed to distinguish these responses from random brain activity.
- Positron emission tomography is an invasive procedure using injected radioactive glucose to track brain function while performing a certain task. For these reasons, it is not often used in research with children and adolescents.
- Magnetic resonance imaging (MRI) is a non-invasive tool that relies on changes in blood oxygenation in the brain. Two types are used frequently in clinical settings: structural MRI (sMRI) and functional MRI (fMRI), which maps the structure and determines the function, respectively.
- Magnetic resonance spectroscopy is another neuroimaging technique that measures the electromagnetic properties of nuclei in the brain and the compounds to which they bind. It has been used to study child psychopathology such as depressions, ADHD and autism.
- Some additional tools have relied on diffusion of water in tissues to create images of white matter networks, while others have relied on changes in hemoglobin concentrations in the cortex associated with neural activity.
- Information travels through the brain by way of neurotransmitters, excitatory or inhibitory chemicals emitted by the axon that influence receptors located on the dendrites of an adjacent neuron. Important neurotransmitters include glutamate, gamma (γ)-aminobutyric acid (GABA), acetylcholine, dopamine, serotonin and norepinephrine.
- Glutamate is the main excitatory neurotransmitter; GABA is the main inhibitory neurotransmitter; acetylcholine stimulates muscles and is thought to support learning and alertness in the brain; dopamine is involved with the brain's reward system and is associated with depression at low levels as well as ADHD; serotonin regulates bodily functions such as sleep, appetite and temperature, is involved with memory and learning and is associated with depression, anxiety, aggression and eating disorders at atypical levels; and norepinephrine is found in the CNS, transmits impulse signals between neurons (such as arousal, attention, focus, wakefulness and the impacts of rewards) and is associated with ADHD and depression like dopamine.

- Emotional regulation can be both voluntary and involuntary, which is why it is sometimes difficult to distinguish an emotion from the regulation of that emotion, or exactly when the process of regulation begins. The voluntary and involuntary processes work together to regulate even a single emotion. An inability of the brain to manage the two may lead to misidentification of one's own emotion and misdirection of one's emotional reactions, resulting in emotions like fear, anxiety or sadness occurring in inappropriate contexts. This is the crux of many childhood psychopathologies.

- Hormones are chemicals secreted by neurons in various brain structures, such as the hypothalamus, and other organs, such as the adrenal glands, to act on other cells and organs via the cerebral spinal fluid tract or serum (blood) stream. With relation to the very quick autonomic nervous system, hormones take seconds to minutes to act.

- The HPA (hypothalamic-pituitary-adrenal) axis starts within the brain (hypothalamus) and ends in the adrenal glands releasing cortisol and dehydroepiandrosterone into the serum to act on the organs needed. A negative feedback loop exists so that when the cortisol reaches a critical level, it signals the hypothalamus to reduce production of the hormone cascade. Cortisol is a catabolic steroid, able to release energy in the short term to support fight-or-flight responses.

- Cortisol levels commence at their peak in the morning with the cortisol awakening response, then slowly drop over the course of the day and increase again while sleeping. Cortisol levels vary from person to person for a number of reasons: genetics, temperament and early experience are a few reasons. In addition, it has been shown that young children show less HPA reactivity than any other age group (sometimes called hyporesponsivity of the HPA axis).

- Too much cortisol in the body can lead to hypercortisolism, the effects of which are neurotoxic and parallel the symptoms of depression and anxiety.

- Researchers can measure cortisol levels in blood, urine and saliva, with saliva being the most practical and ethical of the three.

- The hypothalamic-pituitary-gonadal (HPG) axis is another important hormone cascade in adolescence leading to the production of the sex steroids testosterone and estradiol, among others. The link between this axis and psychopathology is another topic that has interested researchers for years.

- The autonomic nervous system (ANS), the channel through which the CNS controls peripheral organs and muscles, is comprised of the sympathetic nervous system (SNS) and the parasympathetic nervous system (PNS).

- Activation of the SNS leads to increased autonomic arousal, and activation of the PNS leads to decreased autonomic arousal. The former is activated when presented with a challenging or threatening event. The latter, when the event has ended. Thus, they work in tandem to maintain the body's homeostasis.

- In general, norepinephrine is a longer-lasting agent than acetylcholine, thus the SNS's postganglionic synapses, unlike its preganglionic synapses, use epinephrine resulting in a potentially persisting autonomic arousal. Both the PNS's preganglionic and postganglionic synapses use acetylcholine, thus its effects are relatively quick.

- Autonomic space and allodynamic control describe the fact that both the SNS and the PNS may be active simultaneously. Allostasis refers to the fact that the body may not return to a baseline physiological state, but it may fluctuate continuously throughout the day.

- The PNS has a more rapid influence than the SNS, due its longer preganglionic fibers and shorter postganglionic fibers. Researchers can use heart rate (and more specifically, the respiratory sinus arrhythmia) to determine the degree to which the PNS is influencing cardiac arousal.

- When children have a higher baseline respiratory sinus arrhythmia, they seem to have a greater capacity to regulate their emotional states and cope with challenges effectively.
- As part of the sympathetic adrenomedullary (SAM) system, the SNS stimulates the adrenal medulla to release norepinephrine and epinephrine, which drive the fight-or-flight responses in many tissues, releasing glucose for energy and increasing the heart rate and blood pressure. Compared to the PNS, the SNS has a greater control over cardiac flow and blood pressure.
- Appropriate for use in children, impedance cardiography is used to measure changes in blood flow through the chambers of the heart during a heart beat. It uses the pre-ejection period as a specific index of SNS influence over cardiac activity. The shorter the pre-ejection period, the greater the SNS influence. Behavior and anxiety problems in childhood are both characterized by inappropriate anger and fear, which is closely linked to the SNS.
- Electrodermal activity, also known as skin conductance or tonic current flow, is a non-invasive approach to measuring the activity of the SNS. Along with electrodermal responses (phasic responses), both are used to assess the SNS's contribution to threat avoidance and arousal due to punishment.
- A second method for assessing SNS activity is to measure the levels of alpha-amylase in saliva. The peak of the production of this enzyme occurs several minutes after a stressful event is experienced, and is relatively easy to collect.
- Anxiety in children is rooted in exaggerated and inappropriate fear responses. A weakened regulatory influence of the PNS and a heightened SNS stimulation leave children unprepared to cope with their emotional arousal.
- Depression in children is sometimes linked to a weakening of BAS, the motivation to actively

engage and seek rewards. Coupled with high cortisol levels and a decreased PNS, depressed children are sad, lethargic and withdrawn from life's pleasures.

- Disruptive behavior disorders (DBD) in children can be a result of a weakened BIS and heightened BAS (thus ready for confrontation), emotional regulation deficits, atypical respiratory sinus arrhythmia (decreased PNS), low cortisol levels and weak SNS. In a confrontation, these children do not consider the alternatives, and the consequences for their actions do not cause any increase in stress levels. This is consistent with the fearlessness hypothesis of DBD. A compatible hypothesis, the sensation-seeking hypothesis of DBD, can be explained physiologically by the fact that these children with low levels of cortisol may need to seek out risky situations to experience some degree of arousal.
- Research findings on the psychological underpinnings of ADHD are of not entirely consistent. While most agree that these children have poor self-control and perhaps lower and less mature levels of brain activity, some researchers have found a decreased SNS influence, whereas others have shown disruptions to the PNS activity.
- With respect to the integration of biological features and environmental influences to explain developmental psychopathology, scholars have found that deficits in autonomic physiology are only associated with child psychopathology when the children live in particular family contexts. With this, it is important to remember that a biopsychosocial approach will capture these issues the best.
- However, knowledge of the neurobiological and physiological foundations of developmental psychopathology is important for enhancing current diagnostic procedures, prevention programs and intervention techniques (both behavioral and pharmacological).

Study questions

1. What two key physiological systems control the fight-or-flight response in humans?
2. What are executive functions and what parts of the brain play fundamental roles in generating them?
3. What part of the brain is most closely associated with emotional responses to threatening stimuli?
4. What are the major functions of serotonin?
5. How do scientists study cortisol?

6

Family influences, family consequences and family interventions

When a child displays an atypical, maladaptive behavior, it is almost a reflex to ask what the parents did to cause it. The belief that parental upbringing is at the root of all positive and negative child outcomes is as old as history and deeply ingrained in religion, literature and people's belief systems. As mentioned in Chapter 2, this unrestrained attribution of child psychopathology to faulty parenting went unchecked in much of the scientific literature until the 1960s and 1970s. From that time on, however, understanding of the substantial heritability of most psychological disorders increased, which is not to say that genetic factors were not emphasized in earlier eras or that some degree of environmental causation has been excluded (see Chapters 2 and 4). Although the scientific community now recognizes the complex multiple etiology of children's mental disorders, it maintains its profound interest in parenting. Parents are responsible in all societies for the socialization of their children for successful functioning in society, guiding them from the totally dependent state in which they were born into an adult who can interact effectively with others and achieve prosocial goals (Baumrind, Larzelere and Owens, 2010). As such, they are the most appropriate sources of help and support for their children who experience problems in functioning successfully in society.

In this book, information about the family correlates of the various forms of child psychopathology appears in the chapters devoted to each specific disorder. The major purpose of this brief chapter is to sensitize the reader to the myriad ways in which families may influence and be influenced by child psychopathology, and how such knowledge can be used in treatment. This overview is also appropriate given the fact that many of the same aspects of family life have been found

to affect a variety of negative child outcomes. The chapter continues with a consideration, inspired by contemporary research and theory, of the different ways in which the family might influence child psychopathology, alone or in combination with causal agents outside the family. In this chapter, three different modalities of family influence are emphasized, together with the family interventions they have inspired. The first modality focuses on what parents *do* in their daily child-rearing practice. Many of the theorists and practitioners interested in child-rearing or *parenting style* bring with them background and interest in behavioral approaches. A very different vantage point is that of *attachment* theorists, who focus on the closeness and security of the relationships between children and their caregivers. Finally, *systemic* approaches to the family are considered. This intriguing way of looking at family life is inspired by systemic thinking in biology and cybernetics. Some consideration is also given to other modalities of family influence, such as the social support processes within and around the family, the implications of the family's economic resources and, subsequently, to the horrible sequelae of child abuse within the family. The final section consists of brief remarks about research methods used to study family influences.

Family factors in interaction with each other and with other possible causes of pathology

Different facets of family life that may trigger child psychopathology are considered in separate sections of this chapter. However, in real life, these aspects of family functioning are linked to each other.

Marital conflict can lead to depression in either or both parents. Conversely, depression can lead to unresponsiveness and thence to marital conflict. Financial stress can aggravate matters as, of course, can the challenges of dealing with a child of difficult temperament. In many cases, factors inherent to the child may interact with parental influences. For example, a child's *temperament* – best defined as "a distinctive profile of feelings and behaviors that originate in the child's biology and appear early in development" (Kagan, 2005) or "the behavioral response style of a person" (Chess and Thomas, 1996) may influence the parenting a child receives. It should be noted that while temperament is thought to be genetically determined, this is difficult to establish, especially in individual cases. Hence, in tracing the possible causes of children's mental health disorders, current scientific knowledge weighs in heavily on the side of studying simultaneously genetic and environmental factors and, especially, the interactions of the two.

Research methodologies for studying the multifaceted influence of the family have become increasingly sophisticated, making the parenting studies of 50 years ago, seminal as they have been, seem primitive. Before considering the different modalities of family life, this chapter begins with a brief summary of the major methodological considerations that differentiate more valuable research from well-intentioned but simplistic studies that may not present an accurate picture of the processes the researchers purport to be investigating. Optimal methods should ideally be mobilized in studying the interpersonal influences and correlates of psychological disorder during childhood. As with most treatises on research methodology, the prescriptions enumerated herein are not likely to correspond with the research methods used in any extant study. Therefore, they are presented for the reader's use in evaluating the research and for determining the level of confidence that is appropriate to bestow on any particular study.

Bronfenbrenner's (1986) ecological theory has been the most influential attempt at integrating and conceptualizing the multiple simultaneous influences of families on children and of the surrounding community and society on families. That theory has helped researchers move beyond the mother–child paradigm that dominated research until its emergence while at the same time incorporating the mother–child paradigm and placing it in context. As depicted in Figure 6.1, Bronfenbrenner's model starts with *microsystems* that represent environmental forces with which the child is in direct contact, including not only the child's relationships with his or her parents but also relationships with peers and teachers. Surrounding and influencing such direct contact are *mesosystems*, which represent such interactions as those between mothers and fathers or between parents and teachers. It is important to remember that Bronfenbrenner considered the interactions within mesosystems to be bidirectional, with children affecting parents as well as parents affecting children. The circle widens to include *macrosystems*, which represent the influence of the surrounding culture. *Exosystems* represent the effects of events occurring in a social setting just outside the settings in which the individual has direct contact. For example, parents' squabbles with their neighbors might indirectly affect the well-being of an infant. Not to be ignored are *chronosystems*, which represent changes over time in the systems already mentioned. Elements of this chapter that were inspired by ecological theory are the sections on social support and family poverty.

Child-rearing and child psychopathology

Deliberation about whether parents should be strict or lenient has preoccupied parents, philosophers and religious authorities since ancient times, based on the assumption that the outcome will determine how well adjusted the child will be. This debate continues in political circles in Western countries, where conservative politicians and their supporters abhor what they see as the devastating consequences of excessive permissiveness in child-rearing (Baumrind

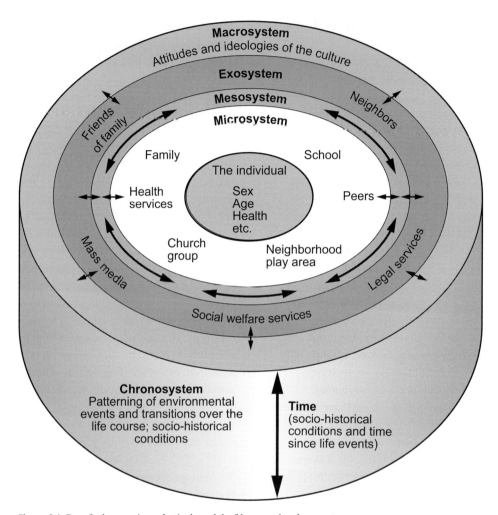

Figure 6.1 Bronfenbrenner's ecological model of human development.

et al., 2010). It is only recently, and largely as a product of the heightened interest in the outcomes of different modalities of parenting in the 1960s and 1970s, that empirical data can inform the discussion about how best to rear children.

Research designed to provide optimal answers to this question indicates that several dimensions of child-rearing must be considered simultaneously. Baumrind (1971, 1991, Baumrind et al., 2010), Maccoby and Martin (1983) have identified four major parent patterns that have been studied very extensively. These patterns are depicted in Table 6.1.

These patterns are based on two parenting dimensions, *responsiveness* and *demandingness*. *Authoritarian* parents are highly demanding but not responsive to their children. *Authoritative* parents are demanding of their children but also very responsive to them. *Permissive* parents are not very demanding but responsive, whereas *unengaged* or *rejecting-neglecting* parents, are not very involved with their children, and are neither demanding nor responsive.

The typology developed by Baumrind, Maccoby and Martin is not exhaustive. As research findings accumulate, it has become apparent that other important dimensions of parenting may be related to

Table 6.1 **Dimensions of parenting in Maccoby and Martin's model**

		Demandingness	
		High	Low
Responsiveness	High	Authoritative	Permissive
	Low	Authoritarian	Unengaged

Source: *Handbook of Child Psychology* (Vol. IV, p. 39), by E. M. Hetherington (Ed.), 1983, New York: Wiley. Adapted with permission.

children's mental health. For example, the methods that parents use to back up their demandingness may be very consequential. These methods can be classified, first of all, along the dimension of *power assertion*. Power can be asserted in an *unqualified* manner or it can be accompanied by reasoned explanations (Hoffman, 1988). *Confrontive* discipline, which involves reasoning with the child, can be implemented with different degrees of directness and firmness. In contrast, *gentle discipline* refers to discipline in which the lowest possible level of power is asserted. Asserting greater power, parents may use *coercive discipline*, in which they take advantage of their strength and positions of authority. Coercive discipline can also be implemented in several ways that may have very different implications for children's mental health. *Rational power assertion* (Hoffman, 1983) provides a predictable environment for the child, with clear information given about the parents' expectations and age-appropriate consequences for misbehavior. *Arbitrary discipline* is *not* predictable *or* appropriate to the child's age or personality, and may be inconsistent (Hoffman, 1983). Some parents implement coercive discipline by physical methods, others by forceful verbal interactions or that may induce shame or guilt. Baumrind and her colleagues now believe that, in exploring the outcomes associated with corporal punishment, it is important to discriminate between the spanking or smacking that unfortunately goes on in most homes and the severe physical punishment that causes injury and is considered a form of child abuse. They also insist on the important distinction between reprimands that do not assault the child's

self-image and hostile verbal criticism with demeaning "wounding words" (Baumrind, Larzelere and Owens, 2010).

The outcomes of different parenting styles have been studied extensively, with research ranging from many correlational studies to an influential multimethod longitudinal study in which the participants were tracked from preschool through adolescence (Baumrind, Larzelere and Owens, 2010). In general, the data indicate the superiority of an authoritative parenting style enforced in a firm, confrontive but supportive way. Specific research findings with regard to the parenting practices that have been linked with specific disorders are discussed in the chapters devoted to those disorders. Although the details contained in those chapters will not be repeated here, it is important at this stage to invoke the possibility that some parenting styles and their component elements may be differentially linked to different forms of child psychopathology. It should be noted that the studies on this issue are heavily weighted toward externalizing outcomes, that is, such problems as conduct disorder and attention deficit, together with associated school failure, school dropout and criminality. Many of the same dimensions of parenting are relevant to such internalizing disorders as anxiety and depression, as discussed in Chapters 15 and 13, although evidence of the parenting correlates of these problems is still quite limited. As detailed in those chapters, relevant aspects of parenting in the emergence of those disorders include parental warmth, restriction of the child's autonomy and encouragement of emotional expression by the child.

The cross-cultural applicability of the parenting models seen as optimal by US leaders such as Hoffman and Baumrind has been questioned. Several studies indicate that authoritarian parenting may cause no harm, and may actually facilitate child adjustment in traditional, family-oriented cultures, such as those of China and of the Arab population of Israel (Chao, 1994; Dwairy, 2008; Leung, Lau and Lam, 1998). In those cultures, it is parental inconsistency that may lead to the greatest child maladjustment (Dwairy, 2008). The dimension of parental autonomy-granting may be an important determinant of child outcome in cultures where some parents restrict their children in a various ways, such as the Hispanic and French cultures (Allès-Jardel et al., 2002; Domenech Rodriguez, Donovick and Crowley, 2009). In France, excessive restriction of children's freedom to explore their social environments has been found to be linked with less rewarding friendships (Allès-Jardel et al., 2002). However, as will be discussed shortly, excessive granting of autonomy, without monitoring the child's whereabouts in the community, can lead to juvenile delinquency. Recent research has explored cultural differences in parents' emotional expression. Studying the recollections of Americans of majority White, African and Asian heritage, Morelen et al. (2013) found that Asian-Americans recalled less positive emotional expression in their families than did the other participants. This perceived lack of emotional expression in early family life was not, however, correlated with subsequent psychopathology among Asian-Americans, as it was with the majority culture and Afro-American participants. Perhaps the expression of positive emotional expression is not normative among Asian-American families. If psychopathology emerges from parenting that is culturally non-normative, this absence of implications for mental health seems logical.

Interventions designed to assist parents in achieving optimal child-rearing have by far the greatest empirical support of any family intervention aimed at reducing child psychopathology (Eyberg, Nelson and Boggs, 2008; McMahon and Kotler, 2008), remembering, however, that, as mentioned earlier, most of the studies pertain to children with externalizing difficulties. Several of the better-established programs, such as the Triple P program developed in Australia (see meta-analysis by De Graaf et al., 2008) and the Incredible Years program developed in the United States (Webster-Stratton and Reid, 2011) have proven effective in a number of controlled studies using rigorous methodologies, including replication by researchers not affiliated with the laboratories where the programs were originally developed. Studies documenting their effectiveness have been conducted in cultures very different from those in which the interventions were first developed and tried, including, for example, a recent implementation of a parenting program based on cognitive-behavioral principles in rural areas of Lebanon (Fayyad et al., 2010) and a trial of the Incredible Years program in Jamaica (Baker-Henningham, et al., 2009). Standard, structured intervention to enhance child-rearing has proven superior to other forms of family intervention, including interventions aimed at reducing marital distress, in rigorous studies in which the two treatments were compared systematically with random assignment of participants to treatments (e.g., Bodenmann et al., 2008). Despite this success, it has been found that parenting interventions in developing countries vary widely in effectiveness, which is only rarely measured in this context with sound methodology (Mejia, Calam and Sanders, 2012). Thus, it is imperative to consider the cultural context whenever any attempt is made to "transplant" an intervention that has been successful in the First World to developing cultures that may be very different.

Parent training for improved child-rearing can be implemented in groups or with individual families. Some of the better-established programs offer a "menu" of interventions of varying intensity depending on the severity of the child's problem (e.g., Webster-Stratton and Reid, 2011). In an effort to deliver this form of intervention in an optimal but efficient way to families that need it, Dishion and Stormshak (2007) developed an effective technique known as the family check-up, in which the intervention starts with as little as three meetings with caregivers; a "menu" of follow-up interventions is available for those families who need and want more intensive work. In an even greater effort to reach parents who find it difficult to attend parent-group sessions, counseling by telephone and by electronic communication have been used successfully (Lingely-Pottie and McGrath, 2006).

Common elements in interventions aimed at optimal parenting include helping the parents set reasonable limits, communicate their rules clearly and enforce them consistently. The rules of the home are enforced by positive methods as far as possible. Practitioners in this field traditionally advocate a ratio of at least four positive interventions to one negative intervention (e.g., Power, Karustis and Habboushe, 2001). In these programs, negative interventions normally consist of sending the child for a few minutes to a time-out corner, where there is little in the way of enjoyable activity and where the child is not likely to receive attention. Some very recent behavioral work is aimed at achieving the same effect using positive methods only. Joseph Ducharme of the University of Toronto has reported considerable success with using positive behavioral interventions only, even for youngsters displaying very severe behavior problems. The term *errorless* refers to the use of structured behavioral methods using the very structure of the intervention, analysis of the setting in which the behavior occurs and positive reinforcement exclusively (Ducharme, 2008). Thus, the punitive methods that are used in some aspects of the classic behavioral tradition as a last resort when positive interventions failed may not be as necessary as was once thought.

Some of the parenting programs, such as Triple P, involve intervention conducted with parents only. An advantage of the Triple P program is that it contains graduated levels of intervention that can be matched to different levels of problem severity and parental needs for support. The intensities begin with Level 1, a universal program providing parenting information, often using printed information and videotapes. Level 2 is a very brief orientation to age-appropriate behavioral expectations, typically delivered in one or two sessions. In-depth parent training starts with Level 3, a four-session intervention, with a more intensive intervention for more severe difficulties at Level 4, which covers eight to ten sessions. Level 5, an extended, enhanced intervention, is provided to the families of children whose behavioral problems are chronic or who are facing both the challenges of a disruptive child and family distress from other sources. Telephone support is used to complement in-vivo care sessions in the standard program. In fact, there has been some success delivering the program by telephone only (Morawska et al., 2005). Several meta-analytic reviews have documented the effectiveness of the standard program Levels 4 and 5 (e.g., De Graaf et al., 2008). The effectiveness of the four-session Level 3 intervention was documented in a recent US study (Boyle et al., 2010).

Other programs, such as the Incredible Years, allow for the parent training to be complemented with interventions aimed at children directly and/or with teachers. Working with parents alone is quite effective according to the evaluative research, as mentioned earlier. The Incredible Years program, developed by Webster-Stratton and her colleagues (Webster-Stratton and Reid, 2003), combines parent training with simultaneous interventions for teachers and direct work with the child. Systematic research has demonstrated not only the effectiveness of the Incredible Years program but also the cost-effectiveness of adding the additional components (e.g., Foster, Olchowski and Webster-Stratton, 2007). The program addresses developmental issues by offering five different treatment packages for children of different ages, ranging from 1 month through 12 years old. There are two different parent training programs developed to address different obstacles to effective parenting and different levels of problem severity. The BASIC program focuses on basic child-management skills and understanding the expectations that are appropriate for children of different ages. BASIC is based in large part on social-learning theory and the findings of the Oregon Social Learning Center, discussed in Chapter 2. There is also the ADVANCE program, directed more at personal issues of the parents that affect their child-rearing, including depression, anger and inadequate interpersonal and problem-solving skills. Webster-Stratton and her colleagues have invested considerably in determining how best to deliver their intervention. Typically, parent groups meet weekly for about 2 hours each session. In addition to didactic presentation by the leaders, there is considerable group discussion. Participating parents are paired for mutual support. The group leaders complement the group sessions with weekly telephone support for each parent (www.incredibleyears.com).

The parent training component of the Incredible Years program is complemented by a classroom-based teacher-training program (Reid, Webster-Stratton and Hammond, 2003) devoted to the appropriate management of classroom behavior, forming harmonious interpersonal relationships with pupils and parents, and working as a "coach" to facilitate effective emotion regulation by pupils. The program developers report impressive evidence for the effectiveness of the teacher-training component. In randomized trials, the program has been found not only to be associated with reductions in pupil aggression but also with increases in pupil engagement with school activities, positive pupil interactions between pupils and more cooperative behaviors. Participating teachers were found to use more praise, less criticism and less punishment after the program.

The child-intervention component of the Incredible Years is the Dina Dinosaur series. There are two versions: one for universal classroom-wide delivery as primary prevention, the other for dedicated therapy groups. These contain a selection of the components of the best-known social skills, problem-solving and anger-management programs, which will be discussed shortly. The Dina

Dinosaur series has been found effective in reducing parent-reported behavior problems, whether implemented on their own or, as recommended, in combination with parent training (Webster-Stratton and Reid, 2003).

Research on less comprehensive clinic-based interventions also indicates that when a parenting intervention is used to complement a child-based intervention, the combination is more effective than either of the components alone (Kazdin, Siegel and Bass, 1992; Lochman and Wells, 2004; Spoth, Redmond and Shin, 1998). For that reason, Stormshak and Dishion (2009) admonish schools, which are normally most comfortable with interventions aimed only at pupils, not to shy away from outreach to parents in their efforts to help pupils at risk for mental health problems.

Child–parent attachment

Attachment theory offers a fascinating perspective on family life that is very different from the models of parenting proposed by socialization researchers such as Hoffman and Baumrind. Attachment-inspired interventions focus far more extensively on relationship bonds than behavioral interventions do. John Bowlby and Mary Ainsworth developed their theory around the premise that a close, intimate and trusting bond with caregiver(s) early in life results in the child developing a "working model" or mental image of close relationships as secure and trustworthy. The trusting, secure bond formed with the attachment figure serves as a *secure base* from which the child explores the surrounding world, and especially other people with whom close, trusting relationships might eventually be formed.

The best-known measure of attachment is the Strange Situation procedure, summarized in Box 6.1. Some degree of distress often occurs when the child is separated even temporarily from the attachment figure. If the distress is relatively mild and quickly resolved when the child and caregiver are reunited,

Box 6.1 | Ainsworth's Strange Situation procedure

The *Strange Situation* procedure was developed by pioneer attachment theorist Mary Ainsworth. It remains the best-known and most respected measure of child–parent attachment. First the mother and the child enter a playroom with a large variety of toys. This is followed by two brief separation sessions – when the mother leaves the playroom – and two brief reunions. Securely attached children welcome the mother warmly on her return. After they have settled again, they resume their exploration of the toys. In contrast, children who display avoidant attachment avoid contact with their mothers after her return, whereas resistant children display anger at those times (Ainsworth et al., 1978; Behrens, Parker and Haltigan, 2011). A fourth category, disorganized attachment, was added later to the system to represent children whose reactions to the separations and reunions do not follow a consistent pattern (Main and Solomon, 1990).

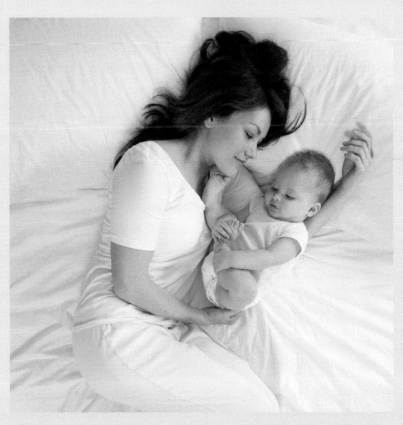

Box Figure 6.1 Secure attachment predicts the quality of close relationships later in life.

their relationship is considered one of *secure attachment*. However, if the child is very distressed when separated even briefly from the attachment figure, with the distress persisting even after the caregiver returns, and generally wary of strangers, his/her relationship is considered *insecure* and *ambivalent*. Another form of insecure attachment, *avoidant attachment*, occurs when an intimate bond between child and caregiver fails to emerge in the first place. Finally, *disorganized attachment* occurs when a child displays an inconsistent pattern of behavior when separated from the parent, wavering between ambivalent and avoidant styles. Further information about the categories of child–parent attachment appears in Table 6.2. Most writings on attachment theory focus on the bonds between the infant and mother. However, some attention has also been paid to attachment in relationships with fathers, foster parents, caregivers in crèches and daycare centers and schoolteachers. *Broad-band attachment* theory is based on the assumption that early attachment predicts a wide range of cognitive, affective and behavioral processes whereas *narrow-band attachment* theory focuses more specifically on the links between attachment and interpersonal relationships across the lifespan (Schneider et al. , 2001; Thompson, 2006).

A literal interpretation of attachment theory might suggest that insecure early attachment is likely to result in lifelong impairment, especially in the ability to form intimate relationships. However, other interpretations of the theory do not go that far, emphasizing that changes in attachment relationships do occur in many cases and that positive life experiences in general can affect the attachment style an individual is likely to follow (Schneider, 2006). In any case, correlations between ambivalent or avoidant attachment and subsequent psychopathology have emerged in some but not all relevant studies (for reviews see Greenberg, 1999). Many studies on the implications of insecure early attachment have not included disorganized attachment, either because this form of relating applied to very few study participants or because

the measures did not include this attachment style. This is being remedied in recent research. There are some indications that disorganized attachment in particular predicts various forms of psychopathology, including depression, inattention and anxiety (Borelli, David, Crowley and Mayes, 2010; Lyons-Ruth, 1996). Importantly, insecure early attachment does predict later difficulties in forming intimate bonds with friends. Friends provide social support; social support, in turn, builds resistance to psychopathology among children and adolescents at risk (Schneider et al., 2001).

Sensitivity to the child's needs is considered a major behavioral manifestation by many attachment theorists and researchers (Atkinson, Niccols, et al., 2000). Most interventions inspired by attachment theory aim to promote such sensitivity. Depressed mothers, many (but not all) of whom display some degree of insensitivity to their children's moods and feelings (Campbell, Shaw and Gilliom, 2000), have been targeted in many attachment-inspired interventions (Cicchetti, Toth and Rogosch, 2008).

On the surface, the roles of attachment figure and authority figure appear somewhat incompatible (see discussion by Bretherton, Goldby and Cho, 1997). Probably for that reason, it is rare but not unknown for both child–parent attachment and disciplinary practices to be included in the same study. Despite the difference in focus between the two schools of thought, there have been some preliminary efforts at combining techniques inspired by attachment theory with a focus on child discipline in preventive interventions (Dadds and Hawes, 2006; Mesmen et al., 2008).

Attachment during adolescence

Attachment is a lifelong process, with different manifestations of the attachment bond at different developmental stages. Adolescents are less explicit than younger children in their immediate reliance on their parents, for example, by seeking physical contact with them. Adolescents' attachment needs

Table 6.2 **The categories of child–parent attachment**

Ainsworth's classification of attachment

Classification	Behavior
Secure	Uses caregiver as a secure base for exploration
	Actively seeks contact or interaction at reunion
	Shows little or no resistance to contact or interaction
	If distressed, seeks and maintains contact and is soothed by caregiver's conduct
Anxious-resistant	Appears ambivalent about the caregiver
	Seeks proximity or contact, or resists release
	Shows open resistance to contact or interaction
	Tends to be very distressed during separations
	Shows little or no avoidance
	Shows generally maladaptive behavior
Anxious-avoidant	Shows little or no active resistance to interaction
	Often shows little or no distress during separations
	Often is affiliative toward strangers
	Displays little or no proximity-seeking to caregiver
	Displays little affective-sharing with caregiver
	Does not use caregiver as a secure base for exploration
Disorganized-disoriented	Displays disordered sequences of behavior (e.g., approach, then dazed avoidance)
	Displays simultaneous contradictory behaviors (e.g., marked gaze aversion during approach or contact)
	Displays inappropriate, stereotypical, repetitive gestures or motions
	Displays freezing or stilling behaviors
	Shows open fear of the caregiver (usually very brief)
	Directs attachment behavior toward the stranger when the caregiver returns
	Displays high avoidance and high resistance in the same episode
	Is depressed, dazed or disoriented or shows affectless facial expressions

Source: From Owens, *Child and Adolescent Development: An Integrated Approach w/InfoTrac*, 1E. © 2002 Wadsworth, a part of Cengage Learning, Inc. Reproduced by permission. www.cengage.com/permissions.

can be described as emotional rather than physical, but are no less crucial than the young child's need for immediate proximity to his or her trusted caregivers (Arbona and Power, 2003; Bowlby, 1977; Williams and Kelly, 2005). Although research methods for studying attachment during the adolescent years have been developed and refined, relatively little attention has been paid to the evaluation of attachment-inspired interventions for adolescents and their families.

Attachment bonds with fathers

As with most research on the family correlates of child psychopathology, many if not most of the studies on child–parent attachment have been conducted with mothers only. This is not surprising or totally inappropriate, given the fact that children in most societies spend much more time with mothers than with fathers. The quality of the time spent together by children and their fathers is known to vary enormously (e.g., Williams and Kelly, 2005). Many scholars bemoan the frequent absence of fathers not only from this area of research but also from the daily lives of their children. Many feel that fathering has very different implications for child outcome from those of mothering, but implications that are no less important. The different roles of mother and father attachment have been summarized by Richard Bowlby, son of John Bowlby, the pioneer "father" of attachment theory, and reported in an article by Newland and Coyl (2010). One attachment role, typically filled more by fathers than by mothers, is the provision of love and security. Another attachment role, frequently overlooked, is encouraging the exploration of the outside world and providing exciting and challenging experiences, which, Richard Bowlby maintains, is often the father's job. Thus, the typical father's role is much more than that of "secondary attachment figure" (p. 26). In helping their children prepare for interactions with the outside world, fathers may play a vital role in teaching the skills that are involved in adapting to new environments and in coping with adverse events (Williams and Kelly, 2005). Fathers encourage the exploration of the outside world by getting involved with their young children in physical activity and social play. In doing so, they assist their children in learning to take judicious risks. They continue this role with older children by bonding with them during leisure-time activities (Bretherton, Lambert and Golby, 2005; Paquette and Bigras, 2010). Related to the possibility that the father's role is less

anchored in reassurance and comforting than that of the mother, it has been found that fathers who occasionally engage in frightening play with their children may not damage attachment bonds with their children if they are generally sensitive in their interactions with their sons and daughters. This did not apply to mothers, whose frightening behavior has been linked with disorganized attachment bonds with children (Hazen et al., 2010).

For these reasons, it is commonly believed that father involvement is associated with positive outcomes for children and that father absence has devastating consequences. Although those contentions are supported by many relevant data the evidence remains very inconsistent. In an interesting study by Marcus and Betzer (1996), it was demonstrated that, in general, adolescents who enjoy positive attachment bonds with their fathers are less likely than adolescents whose relationships with their fathers are strained to exhibit anti-social behavior. That applied to attachment bonds with mothers and peers as well, although the influence of fathers was statistically stronger. However, this did not apply in one particular situation, in cases where the fathers were anti-social themselves. In that specific instance, sons and daughters are actually better off if their fathers are not involved with them. It is not surprising that these fathers with anti-social tendencies are more likely to transmit their anti-social inclinations to their children if they are extensively involved in their upbringing (Marcus and Betzer, 1996). In light of these and similar findings, Pleck (2007) argues that time spent with fathers is not by itself an appropriate variable that merits the attention of researchers. Researchers must go on to consider what the father brings to the relationship and how the time is spent. Summarizing the relatively few studies that have been conducted on the topic so far, Lucassen and her colleagues (2011) conclude that sensitivity to the child is not nearly as strong a correlate of attachment to fathers as it is of maternal attachment. However, fathers' sensitivity to the child might still be a useful basis for interventions because, according to some preliminary data, fathers are often more responsive to this kind of intervention than are mothers. In general, there has been very little systematic research on how the influences of mothers and fathers combine or interact in predicting child outcome. In a very preliminary study of general parenting style, Meunier, Bisceglia and Jenkins (2012) found some evidence that mothers' positivity may combine with fathers' positivity in a simple additive way but that the negative influences of mothers and fathers tend to compound in a multiplicative fashion. As well, the interactive effects of parenting by mothers and fathers in two-parent families differed somewhat according to the age of the child and the nature of the child outcome being predicted.

Needless to say, the literature comparing mothers' and fathers' roles is based on the typical if not stereotypical roles in Western society. It has been noted that in anywhere from 5 to 20 percent of cases studies, the father emerges as the child's preferred attachment figure even in the traditional sense of providing love and security (e.g., Freeman and Brown, 2001; Freeman, Newland and Coyl, 2010). Some authors recognize that there are now many blended families and single families as well as same-sex marriages and unions. They argue for focusing on the paternal figure or figures rather than the biological "father" (e.g., Coley, 2001). Going further, some of the sweeping changes in family constellation have prompted influential theorists to discard the "essential father theory," which pervaded scientific writings from the 1930s to the 1970s. That theory specifies that the father has a unique role in promoting appropriate gender identity in the developing child. Extensive, careful research on the children of two-parent lesbian families has shown conclusively that these families are no more likely than two-parent heterosexual families to have children with any known form of gender identity problem, maladjustment or psychopathology (Patterson and Chan, 1999; Pleck, 2007; Wainright, Russell and Patterson, 2004).

Attachment-inspired interventions

There have been some attempts at putting attachment theory to work in helping children and caregivers involved in insecure attachment relationships. Wisely, these interventions have targeted children in populations that can be identified by risk for subsequent psychopathology. Videotaped feedback for mothers is a prominent feature of many interventions inspired by attachment theory (e.g., Juffer, Bakermans-Kranenburg and Van IJzendoorn, 2008). This intervention is typically delivered during visits to the homes of mothers whose attachment bonds with their children are insecure. Thus, the intervention is targeted at mother–child dyads who are at risk for maladjustment but who have not been diagnosed with a mental health disorder. The core of the intervention consists of feedback from the therapists about the sensitivity and insensitivity of the interactions between the child and mother, brief segments of which are videotaped at the beginning of each visit. Post-treatment data indicate that the intervention tends to promote the mothers' sensitivity to their children. There is also some improvement in attachment security (Juffer et al., 2008).

A more elaborate attachment-based preventive intervention was developed by attachment researchers (Hoffman, Marvin, Cooper and Powell, 2006), illustrated in Figure 6.2. In contrast with the intervention developed by Van IJzendoorn and his colleagues, mentioned in the last paragraph, Circle of Security is delivered in small groups. The groups meet for twenty weekly sessions. Each group consists of six mothers or fathers of toddlers or preschoolers. Each parent reviews videotapes of his/her own interactions with his/her son or

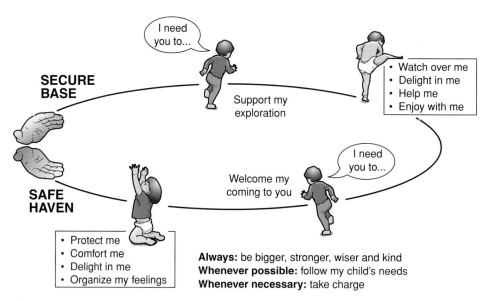

Figure 6.2 Circle of Security model.

daughter. However, the intervention protocol also emphasizes relationship education. In language accessible to them, the parents learn the basics of attachment theory using Ainsworth's concepts of Secure Base and Haven of Safety (Ainsworth et al., 1978). These are prominent features of the protocol. Participating parents learn the slogan: "Always be bigger, stronger, wiser and kind . . . Whenever possible, follow my child's need . . . Whenever necessary, take charge" (Marvin et al., 2002, p. 109). The parents discover internal needs that may lead to a *miscue*, or failure to recognize the child's emotional needs. For example, consider the situation of a mother and child whose interaction pattern is avoidant/dismissive. The child may learn that sending Mom a signal that he/she needs emotional support makes Mom uncomfortable and unresponsive. In response, the child learns to send an overt message that he/she wants to play, but without excitement or emotion, avoiding the mother's gaze. This miscue is seen as a result of the mother's avoidance of intimacy. The mother and child stay connected enough to meet the child's daily survival needs without being close enough for the child to feel

nurtured and loved. Without the secure base of nurture and love, the child develops a hesitation to explore relationships with other people and new experiences.

The intervention, prescribed in the procedures manual to ensure accurate implementation, is matched to the attachment profile of each dyad. As applied to the avoidant/dismissive type, for example, the specified goals are: (1) for mothers to gain an appreciation of how much their children need them; (2) for them to learn to recognize their children's subtle distress signals; and (3) to have the mothers use what they have learned to reduce miscuing at times when their children are in distress (Marvin et al., 2002, p. 115). The major learning tools are the videotaped vignettes. From the videotaped interchanges, the following sequences are selected: (1) the child is distressed and wants the parent, who does not respond; (2) the parent reacts competently and appropriately; (3) the parent seems to be struggling to respond properly; and (4) a happy, loving moment in the mother–child relationship (Marvin et al., 2002, p. 115). After viewing the videotapes together, all group members are invited to comment on what they have seen.

CASE STUDY: Paula, a toddler and her mother in an attachment-inspired intervention

Case example: Paula (Marvin et al., 2002). Paula is a 2-year-old who participated in the Circle of Security program together with her mother, Candy. During the initial session, Paula came with her mother, but, as soon as her mother put her down, she ran to the box of toys in the playroom, which became the almost exclusive focus of her attention. A few minutes later, she asked her mother if she wanted to see the toy rabbit. Mom replied yes but in a very timid voice. Paula kept playing with the toys, interacting very little with her mother. As part of the assessment procedure, the well-known Strange Situation procedure (see Box 6.1, above), Paula's Mom left the playroom briefly. Paula remained indifferent and kept interacting with the toys. Candy returned 18 minutes later but Paula kept playing with the toys. Mom asked Paula to put the toys away but Paula did not comply, defiantly picking up a new toy, a red plastic telephone. In the expanded attachment classification scheme developed by Marvin and his colleagues, these interactions were classified as not only disordered but also as controlling by the child and abdicating/role-reversed for the mother. The intervention team noticed that Paula's Mom was much more effective and enthusiastic when attempting to manage Paula's behavior than when Paula was enjoying herself on her own, although Paula and her Mom did enjoy reading together. Candy's depressive affect set the stage for Paula to assume control.

The intervention team set the goal of helping Paula's mother overcome her tendency to sit back and let Paula dominate the scene. They wanted to help Candy to assert authority but also to understand that her expressionless interactions with Paula deprived her daughter of the opportunity to learn how her mother was feeling. This is one of the things a child needs to learn in order to prepare for intimate relationships in later life. Having gathered extensive information from Mom about her own upbringing, the intervention team noticed parallels between the current child–mother interaction and Mom's recollections of her relationship with her own mother.

Candy and Paula participated in the Circle of Security program in a group of five mother–child dyads. At first, Candy was nervous about seeing her interactions with Paula on videotape. The group leader started by pointing out a videotaped segment in which Paula was enjoying playing with some "princess slippers." While playing, Paula glanced back at her mother and Candy responded with a smile. The leader asked the other parents in the group to help locate Paula's needs at that moment within the Circle of Security. Paula's needs were in the top half, exploration, "enjoy me" and "comfort me." Candy recognized this by responding with a smile, albeit a nervous smile. After showing Candy another clip, in which Paula was clearly taking charge of the situation, the group leader, sensing Candy's increasing discomfort, asked Candy what she thought was happening. Candy responded by expressing her accurate observation that Paula was dominating the interaction. As the weeks went on, Candy came to realize that her interactions with Paula were more like those of a sister rather than those of a mother.

At the end of the 20-week intervention, the Strange Situation assessment was repeated to evaluate the progress made. When Candy returns to the playroom after the brief separation that is a core feature of the assessment, she is able to interact warmly with Paula but nevertheless instruct her to pick up the toys. After the toys are picked up, she is able to deliver a warm congratulatory message: "Good job!" In the formal post-intervention classification of security types, the child was classified as secure with only some continuing disordered elements. The mother had progressed to the classification of ordered but borderline autonomous dismissing. Paula and Candy's results are not atypical for the Circle of Security intervention, which has been found to increase both parental sensitivity and child–parent attachment in a significant number of cases (Hoffman, Marvin, Cooper and Powell, 2006).

Social support within the family

Another important aspect of family relationships that affects adjustment and maladjustment is the social support provided by family members. *Social support* can be defined as giving and receiving communication that results in the individual belief that one is cared for and loved, esteemed and valued, and belongs to a network of communication and mutual obligations (Cobb, 1976). Social support is most consequential at moments of stress that could trigger or worsen psychological distress. Implicit in Cobb's definition are two distinct aspects of social support, the first being the objective existence of a network of supportive individuals who are in contact with an individual, especially at times of stress. This may be represented quantitatively by such indices as the number of individuals in a person's social support network and the frequency of his or her contacts with them. Equally important is the way in which the individual appraises the support he or she receives. There is not a one-to-one correspondence between quantitative indices of social support and individual satisfaction with the social support received. Social support can be provided by parents, siblings, friends, schoolteachers and religious leaders. Some authorities believe that it is an individual's personality, not only the actual support received by the person, that determines whether or not an individual feels supported (e.g., Pierce et al., 1997). Members of a person's social support network assist in many different ways, from providing emotional support to actual, concrete daily assistance with the tasks inherent in caring for and supervising children (*instrumental support*). Supportive communication can also consist of *appraisal support*, the provision of information, often of an evaluative nature, that helps the receiver maintain his or her self-concept (Brock and Lawrence, 2009).

Patterns of social support are determined somewhat by culture. In very family-oriented cultures, people assume that their relatives will provide support for them without the need to ask. In many traditional cultures, grandparents play a very important role in supporting children and grandchildren in many different ways. On the other hand, in Asian cultures where self-reliance is highly valued, people may be reluctant to seek social support even though it may well be available (Taylor et al., 2004). Although there are surely advantages in having a social support network that is readily available, there may be some advantage in having to seek support rather than receive it automatically from family members because one may then seek support of the type that is the most likely to lead to satisfaction with the advice and support received.

Children and adolescents in all societies rely on their parents as sources of social support, even though support may be expressed in different ways in different cultures (McNeely and Barber, 2010; Vitoroulis et al., 2012). Children and adolescents may derive different types of support from people of different ages and roles but, in general, different supportive individuals tend to act in concert to buffer resistance at moments of stress (Laursen, Furman and Mooney, 2006). Although the support of classmates and friends may be welcome, several studies indicate that support from age-mates cannot usually compensate for a lack of support from parents (e.g., Buchanan and Bowen, 2008; Schneider et al., 2008).

The family's financial status

Although money cannot of course buy mental health, financial hardship is clearly linked to the likelihood of children developing a psychological disorder. A glance at the subsequent chapters devoted to the specific disorders will indicate that low socio-economic status emerges frequently as a risk factor. The link between poverty and child psychopathology is also clearly demonstrated by a few more comprehensive studies that have considered multiple disorders as their dependent variable. In those studies, low socio-economic status emerges as a consistent and potent predictor of a wide range of disorders (e.g. Copeland et al., 2009; Morgan, Farkas and Wu, 2009).

There has also been some study of the reasons why poverty constitutes such a salient risk factor. There has also been some study of the reasons why poverty constitutes such a salient risk factor. One possibility is that financial stress interferes with the provision of consistent, authoritative child-rearing. In many families, financial stress and the parenting provided by families experiencing financial stress interact with biological risk factors such as difficult temperament (Flouri, 2008). Financial stress may also be reflected in inadequate nutrition, which probably has a long-term effect on children's well-being (Slopen et al., 2010).

The economic resources of the family also determine to a considerable extent the neighborhood in which the family lives. The concept of *social integration* can be seen as a community-level analogy to the concept of the social support network, which applies to individuals and groups (Berkman and Glass, 2000). If a family lives in a well-integrated neighborhood, its members will feel accepted and included. On the other hand, a neighborhood can also be not only poorly integrated, providing little social support for its residents, but also high in delinquency. Exposure to violence among children living in dangerous neighborhoods is a very strong predictor of externalizing disorders (Foster, Brooks-Gunn, Martin and Flannery, 2007). Thus, in many different ways that perhaps work together at the same time, the neighborhood in which the family lives may affect both risk and protective factors associated with child psychopathology.

Marital satisfaction and conflict

It is no coincidence that many of the squabbles between husbands and wives have to do with how to deal with their children. Although almost all couples experience immense joy when they first become parents, their marital relationship often deteriorates as they face the daily tasks of caring for an infant as well as massive changes in their own daily routines (Belksy and Kelly, 1994; El-Sheikh and Elmore-Staton, 2004). If conflict between parents remains high, the chances of a child displaying some form of maladjustment or psychopathology increase dramatically (e.g., Harold et al., 2004). Considerable research has been devoted to determining how children are affected. First of all, children and adolescents exposed to conflict between their mothers and fathers are likely to experience highly inconsistent and ineffective parenting (Benson, Buehler and Gerard, 2008). Parents unable to communicate well with each other and work well together are unlikely to offer their children warm, supportive child–parent relations combined with reasonable and consistent limit-setting, which together will best meet the needs of their new children (Dishion and Patterson, 2006; Shaw et al., 2004). Unfortunately, some children tend to blame themselves for the conflict (DeBoard-Lucas et al., 2010). Exposed to repeated negative displays of emotion, children may not learn appropriate ways of regulating their own emotions (Cummings, Papp and Kourous 2009).

Marital conflict is likely to increase when the parents must face the challenge of dealing with a child who is by temperament either withdrawn and unresponsive or difficult and agonistic (e.g., Pauli-Pott and Beckmann, 2007). This is unfortunate because children born with temperament-based risk factors are in particular need of the optimal parenting that might lead to social adjustment despite whatever limitations might be imposed by their genetic endowment.

Violence in the home

Family discord reaches the stage of physical violence in too many cases. In the United States, it is estimated that at least one child in twenty is a victim of severe physical assault and that physical assault has occurred within at least one in six couples (Straus et al., 1996). It is estimated that 28 percent of British women have experienced physical assault from male partners at some point in their lives (Walker et al., 2009). In addition, a very substantial number of men, constituting up to 40 percent of domestic violence cases in the UK, experience assault by their female wives or partners (www.guardian.co.uk/society/2010/sep/05/men-victims-domestic-violence, retrieved January 14, 2012). It is believed that the rates of domestic violence are higher than this in many countries of Africa and Latin America, where there are few social or legal sanctions related to it (Sokoloff and Pratt, 2005). All statistics on the frequency of domestic violence are suspect because many cases go unreported. In addition, many children in all countries are victims of emotional abuse, which is rarely reported. A sizeable number of children are both witnesses of domestic violence and victims of it; the rate of co-occurrence is estimated at 40 percent in cases brought to the attention of mental health workers because of either of these family problems (Appel and Holden, 1998). These children are known to be particularly vulnerable to various forms of psychopathology (Wolfe et al., 2003). Not surprisingly, domestic violence is related to many other problems in families. Abuse is linked to authoritarian, punitive child-rearing and to the lack of positive, affectionate child–parent interactions (Maikovich et al., 2008; Shaw et al., 2004). Domestic abuse occurs more frequently in homes where there is a depressed parent and in families living in poverty (Hay and Jones, 1994).

Domestic violence is associated with many negative outcomes for children. The harm to children may come about in several ways. Children who have witnessed or experienced physical violence often learn that violence is an acceptable form of human interaction (Black and Newman, 1996). They live with a persistent sense that danger is imminent. This has been likened to living in a war zone, where violence sometimes can be predicted but sometimes cannot (Margolin and Vickerman, 2007; Rossman and Ho, 2000).

The abuse, whether witnessed, received or both, is linked with profound effects on children's thinking about other people. They may overattend to cues that elicit anger and the belief that other people intend to harm them (Shackman, Shackman and Pollack, 2007). Exposure to abuse is thought to provoke physiological reactions as well. These and other implications of child psychopathology are discussed later in the chapters on mood disorders (Chapter 13) and post-traumatic stress disorder (Chapter 23).

The effects of parenting seen as non-linear

The growing literature on the effects of physical abuse has affected thinking about the effects of parenting in a more general way. Some authorities comment that the effects of different styles of parenting are not very strong in most cases as long as the parenting received by a child is "good enough." The effects begin at the extreme, once the parenting style crosses a threshold into abusive and harsh. This has important implications for research design and data analysis. First of all, sampling must allow for a wide range of parenting, including extreme styles. Secondly, the statistical analysis must be designed to accommodate effects that do not occur in a linear fashion, as in a product–moment correlation (Deater-Deckard and Dodge, 1997).

The family as a complex working system

Systems theorists conceive of the family as a complex system that consists of a number of mutually interrelated components that interact with each other. Complex systems are made up of multiple parts that have the capacity to communicate with each other, to assimilate and process information, which is used to modify their workings (e.g., Banathy, 1996). This understanding of family life is a specific application of systems theory or cybernetics, which has also enriched the fields of computer science, business administration, biology and sociology. Proponents of *family systems theory* would regard everything said so far in this chapter about family life as simplistic and "linear" because none of the approaches mentioned goes beyond a paradigm involving essentially only two members (e.g., mother and child) of a larger network of systems elements that affect the way in which these two members interact (Belsky and Fearon, 2004; Minuchin, 1985). Early systemic family therapists, who crafted this way of thinking in the 1960s and 1970s, believed that the system's dysfunction was the cause of the problems of one or more family members. More contemporary theorists, who embrace family systems theory as developmental psychopathologists (see Chapter 1) are more likely to think of the family process as moderating the course of psychopathology but not necessarily as its cause (e.g., Miklowitz, 2004).

Systemically oriented *family therapists* actively fight against the designation of the family member who is referred for psychological care as an *identified patient*. They believe that pathology lies in the family system, in which the identified patient may be a *scapegoat*. Scapegoating the identified patient serves some misguided purpose for the other members of the system. Each family system is characterized by a set of internal boundaries or unwritten rules that determine how power, social support and resources are distributed. In *cohesive families*, relationships are warm and supportive; there are clear but flexible boundaries that permit access to resources and support by children. In contrast, *disengaged families* are characterized by rigid boundaries and cold, unsupportive relationships among family members. Communication within the family is limited and ineffective. The family members may form *coalitions* in which some members habitually help each other and side with each other, often in opposition to other family members. A family therapist may try to *restructure* the family by loosening coalitions that are unhelpful. For example, Rivett and Street (2009) present the example of a mother who always answers questions for her adolescent daughter. The therapist asks the mother to use the therapy sessions to practice letting the daughter speak for herself. Finally, in *enmeshed* families, relationships between some of the members become entangled and stifling. Children may receive some affection and support, but in order to do so, they have to give up much of their autonomy and ally themselves with one subsystem in its hostility to another subsystem (Minuchin, 1974). This distinction among cohesive, disengaged and enmeshed families has proven useful in the prediction of children's maladjustment. For example, Sturge-Apple, Davies and Cummings (2010), in a 3-year multimethod longitudinal study conducted with children at the start of primary school, found that children from disengaged or enmeshed families had higher rates than children

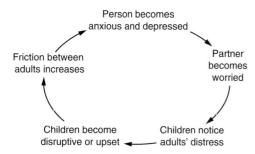

Figure 6.3 Individual symptoms seen in the context of the family system.

from cohesive families of several forms of maladjustment according to teacher reports. The difficulties experienced by pupils from disengaged and enmeshed families increased over the 3-year duration of the study.

Common to all forms of family therapy – and to many if not most other forms of therapy of any modality (Flaskas, 1992) – is the concept of *reframing*. Reframing can be defined as changing "the conceptual and/or emotional setting or viewpoint in relation to which a situation is experienced and to place it in another frame which fits the 'facts' of the same concrete situation equally well or even better, and thereby changes its entire meaning"

(Watzlawick, Weakland and Fisch, 1974, p. 94). This can be achieved without excessive risk by challenging the family's prevailing interpretation of a common theme, changing it from negative to positive. For example, in a situation where parents excessively restrict the community activities of an adolescent son or daughter, the therapist might propose an alteration of the prevailing interpretation of this behavior as a manifestation of the mother's neurotic need for control, suggesting that the restrictive parenting and detective-like questioning of the adolescent might be a manifestation of parental love. More dramatic and more controversial are reframing techniques that involve *paradoxical instructions*, instructions by the therapist for an "identified patient" to exhibit the symptoms that precipitated the referral for help. For example, a depressed adolescent might be told to look and feel as sad as possible and express as much negative emotion as possible; this is exactly the opposite of what the therapist really wants to see. The parents might be instructed to ask whether their son or daughter is really depressed. The success of such paradoxical commands varies widely (Shoham-Solomon and Rosenthal, 1987). Therefore, therapists are cautioned against using them excessively.

CASE STUDY: a Finnish 10-year-old boy and his family in systemic family therapy

Laitila et al. (1996) present an interesting case example of the use of systemic family therapy techniques with an enmeshed family. The six-session family intervention was conducted to help a 10-year-old boy who was referred to an out-patient psychiatric clinic in Finland because he was beginning to experience psychotic symptoms such as hallucinations. The therapists employed, first of all, a *reflecting-team* approach (see Anderson and Gehart, 2007). In that approach, the professionals of the team discuss what is going on in the therapy room among themselves, either in the presence of the family or by using a "bug in the ear" to communicate with the main therapist during the therapy sessions from behind a one-way mirror. The team discussed how the son might be using his symptoms to become excessively close to his mother, who clung to him during the initial sessions. In subsequent sessions, the therapist also used the technique of *family sculpture* (Duhl, Kantor and Duhl, 1973) to gain and deliver insight about the structure of relationships within the family system. Each family member was asked to create a "sculpture" of what the family might look like by directing the family members to position themselves in the ways that represent their roles in the family and to assume expressions that express their feelings about these roles. As the family learned more about itself from the reflecting team and family sculptures, they began to reconsider their boundaries and coalitions. Nearness replaced enmeshment and the "identified patient" became more independent and better adjusted.

In this case, the parents and the son attended the first session but the older sister attended subsequent sessions. The father contacted the team between sessions, which can be seen as undermining the open communication throughout the system that is the goal of family therapy. Family therapists typically work with the entire family together, making exhaustive efforts to *convert* a referral of an individual to a mandate to "cure" the family. Their dynamic, somewhat theatrical therapeutic techniques have captured the interest of child-clinical psychologists around the world. Devotion to systemic methods may be waning somewhat in recent years because, in spite of some empirical evidence for the effectiveness of systemic family therapy (e.g., Carr, 1991; Chamberlain and Rosicky, 1995; Cottrell and Boston, 2002), the empirical support for these techniques is not as extensive as for interventions focusing on child-rearing. Perhaps it is the "linear" nature of interventions aimed at improving child-rearing that makes them highly amenable to evaluative research. Rather than resisting this reality, some contemporary family therapists are suggesting at least a partial retreat from the ideological "purity" in adherence to systems theory, integration of systemic approaches with other modalities of intervention and heightened attention to empirical evaluative research (Rivett, 2008).

Methodological issues in linking family life to child outcome

As understanding has increased of the complex origins of child psychopathology, the methodological standards for inclusion of pertinent data into scientific knowledge have become more stringent than in the days when the literature consisted largely of simplistic correlational studies. The following checklist, which is not exhaustive, is offered as a guide in evaluating the evidence provided by research in this area.

1. Multiple sources of information should be used. The same informant (e.g., the mother) should not be the sole source of information about both the family variable and its hypothesized child outcome. When possible and appropriate for the variables being studied, self-reports should be complemented by observational data and/or ratings by other suitable informants.

2. Family interaction should be represented as close to "real time" as possible. Retrospective recollections of family life are subject to errors of memory and the intruding influences of

intervening events. This occurs to some degree when participants are asked to report on events occurring within the past month or year. More serious errors are inherent when, for example, university students are asked to report about the parenting they received as schoolchildren.

3. Multiple aspects of family life and parenting should be included as independent variables wherever logical and possible. This will help elucidate the unique predictive power of the aspect of family life in which the researcher is most interested.

4. Multiple outcomes should be considered whenever possible. Given the high rates of comorbidity among the different forms of child psychopathology, this will help avoid underestimating the influence of the aspect of family life being studied.

5. If clinicians' impressions are used, reliable scales for measuring them should be used or developed. If a standard diagnosis is the outcome variable, the reliability of the diagnosis should be established, usually by co-ratings of another trained clinician.

6. Longitudinal follow-up should be featured wherever possible. This will illustrate the long-term impact of the aspect of family life being studied. Statistical analysis using such techniques as structural equations modeling can be used with longitudinal data to make cautious inferences about the probable direction(s) of causality among the variables being studied.

7. Sampling should be consistent with the population to which the results are to be generalized. For example, conclusions based on data obtained from participants referred for professional care may not generalize to the population at large, and vice versa.

8. Interpretations of correlational data should include all possible causal directions. In many if not most cases, there are reasons to believe that child and parent behaviors influence each other in a *bidirectional manner*.

Conclusion: family interventions for prevention and treatment

Although blaming parents for their children's problems has hopefully fallen from favor, at least in professional circles, involving parents in preventive and therapeutic interventions certainly has not. The success of those interventions illustrates the value in working with parents or with whole families to prevent or ameliorate psychological distress during childhood, regardless of the cause or causes of the distress. It is likely that as awareness of the potential impact of working on parents' child-rearing increases, this preventive and therapeutic modality will not only expand but also be used in conjunction with other modalities, such as work with children either individually or in groups.

However, the data base that bolsters intervention work with parents, solid as it is, remains very uneven, with the most impressive empirical support for direct interventions inspired to a considerable extent by behavioral thinking that focuses on child-rearing. As well, the most substantial research conducted from that standpoint has been devoted to externalizing problems, especially disruptive behavior disorders. Indeed, when it comes to internalizing problems such as depression and anxiety, interventions conducted with parents are still in their infancy, with much greater empirical support for some forms of therapy that are delivered directly to children and adolescents.

More empirically oriented psychologists wishing to use the most effective interventions known can still profit from the wisdom of the more psychodynamic and systemic approaches. For example, even if a practitioner does not wish to implement any of the techniques that have been developed by systemic family therapists, the quality of the practitioner's care may nevertheless improve if he or she is aware of the family processes at work within the family that has come seeking help.

Summary

- Parents are the most important source of help and support for children who present difficulties functioning successfully in society.
- Both families and peers can act in numerous ways to influence child psychopathology, and can in turn be influenced by children displaying maladaptive behavior.
- Genetics play a large role in the etiology of child psychopathology, yet environmental factors (such as parental influences), and the interaction between the two, greatly affect the development of mental disorders as well.
- Different modalities of family influence include: parenting style, which focuses on parental behavior; attachment which focuses on intimacy and security between children and their caregivers; and systemic processes, with a cybernetic focus on communication and the roles played by family members. Many scholars advocate for more integration of these three distinct modalities in future research.
- Bronfenbrenner's ecological theory incorporates familial, communal and societal influences, beyond the standard mother–child relationship paradigm. At the center, the child's microsystems include the direct contact received from parents, peers and teachers. Mesosystems represent the interactions between these direct influences, such as parent–parent or parent–teacher relationships. Macrosystems refer to the influences of culture, and chronosystems refer to changes over time in any of these systems.
- Ecological theory emphasizes the roles of social support and family poverty.
- In studying family life and family interventions, researchers should: use multiple sources of information; ensure that recent family interactions are drawn on as often as possible; use multiple independent variables representing aspects of family life and parenting; consider multiple outcomes; establish reliable scales for corroborating clinician diagnoses; include longitudinal follow-up as often as possible, employ a representative sample of the population in question; and consider all possible causal directions for correlational data.
- The question of strictness or leniency in child-rearing has been an important issue that is based on the assumption that the child's adjustment is founded on the parenting style.
- Research identifies four major parent patterns based on two parenting dimensions: responsiveness and demandingness.
- Authoritarian parents are highly demanding but not responsive; authoritative parents are both demanding and responsive; permissive parents are responsive but not demanding; and unengaged/rejecting-neglecting parents are neither.
- An additional dimension of power assertion is often considered in recent studies. Power can be asserted in an unqualified manner or can involve reasoning with the child. Confrontive discipline involves such reasoning and can assume different degrees of directness and firmness, whereas gentle discipline refers to the lowest possible level of power assertion. Unqualified discipline includes coercive discipline, where parents use their strength and authority to their advantage. Coercive discipline can be split into rational power assertion, where the consequences are consistent and age-appropriate, and arbitrary discipline, where the consequences are not consistent or age-appropriate.
- Some scholars in this area encourage a distinction between severe, abusive, physical abuse and subabusive mild spanking, as well as the distinction between hostile, demeaning verbal criticism and reprimands that do not harm a child's self-image.

- Current research indicates the advantage of an authoritative parenting style enforced in a firm and confrontive, yet supportive, way.
- Parenting styles and their component elements may be related to different forms of psychopathology. Most studies focus on externalizing outcomes (e.g., conduct disorder and attention deficit, and their link to school failure, school dropout and criminality). Less research exists regarding the association of parenting style to internalizing disorders, such as anxiety and depression.
- Cross-cultural applications of parenting styles must be taken into consideration. Authoritarian parenting with consistency may not be harmful in some traditional cultures. In some cultures, parents' restriction of a child's autonomy may be a more serious problem than an authoritarian approach.
- Research on interventions aimed at assisting parents to optimize their child-rearing skills often provides considerable empirical support for this form of intervention. These interventions have often been shown to be superior to other forms of family intervention (e.g., reducing marital distress).
- The skills taught include helping the parents to set limits, communicate rules clearly, and enforce them consistently. Success has been achieved in behavioral work by using more positive than negative interventions. The errorless method involves complete elimination of punishment. Behavior analysis includes the structured measurement of reinforcing events.
- Interventions using both a parent-based component and a child-based component are often more effective than either used in isolation. For this reason, some scholars encourage schools to reach out to parents of children with mental health problems.
- Attachment theory is another important perspective with which to view issues within the family. According to attachment theory, close, secure and trustworthy relationship with caregivers aids the child in establishing a base upon which they can form their own relationships with others.
- The Strange Situation procedure categorizes the types of relationship a child may have with his/her attachment figure. A secure attachment is one where distress is mild upon separation; an insecure and ambivalent attachment is one where distress persists until even after reuniting with the attachment figure; an insecure and avoidant attachment occurs when the intimate bond between the child and the attachment figure never forms; and a disorganized attachment is one where the child displays an inconsistent pattern when separated from the attachment figure, often switching between ambivalent and avoidant styles. The attachment figure does not necessarily need to be the mother. Often, the father, foster parents or other caregivers are important attachment figures.
- Broad-band attachment theory refers to the idea that an early attachment predicts a wide range of cognitive, affective and behavioral processes. Narrow-band attachment theory refers solely to the links between attachment and intimate interpersonal relationships across the lifespan.
- Despite some interpretations of attachment theory, attachment style is not static and may change/modify based on positive life experiences.
- Correlations exist between ambivalent or avoidant attachment and psychopathology. An ambivalently attached child may have difficulty forming friendships, leading to poor social support. Disorganized attachment has predicted various forms of psychopathology, including depression, inattention and anxiety.
- Preliminary efforts to combine techniques of attachment theory with work on parents' disciplinary practices have emerged, but most studies have only focused on one or the other.

- Attachment is an important process that continues throughout an individual's life. Although attachment during adolescence is more emotional than physical, adolescents' needs are just as vital in development as those of younger children.
- Attachment theory as it relates to fathers is understudied. Fathers usually fill different roles than mothers for a child, encouraging exploration and adaptation and teaching coping strategies.
- Adolescents who enjoy positive attachment bonds with their fathers are less likely to exhibit anti-social behavior than adolescents whose relationships with their fathers are strained, unless the father is anti-social himself. Fathers are seen as having distinct roles in socialization connecting the growing child with the world outside the family.
- Many fathers are very responsive to attachment-inspired interventions.
- Research on the children of lesbian couples shows that a lack of father figure does not necessarily lead to any form of gender identity problem, maladjustment or psychopathology.
- In attachment theory-inspired interventions, efforts are made to target children with insecure attachment that are at risk for psychopathology. This includes videotaped feedback for mothers, increasing their sensitivity to their children.
- In some group interventions, such as the Circle of Security program, parents learn of their child's internal needs and when they are prone to a miscue, or a failure to recognize these emotional needs.
- Case studies show the success of interventions for children whose bonds within their attachment figures are insecure.
- Social support, another important aspect of family relationships that affects adjustment and maladjustment, refers to communication, both transmitted and received, that results in the belief that one is cared for and loved, esteemed and valued, and belongs to a network of communication and mutual obligations. Support is often most important at stressful moments when psychological distress can be triggered or worsen.
- Social support includes both the objective existence of support by parents, sibling and friends as well as the satisfaction of the individual receiving the support.
- Instrumental support consists of providing actual support (i.e. daily assistance with tasks inherent in caring for and supervising children), whereas appraisal support consists of providing information (usually evaluative) that maintains the individual's self-concept.
- In family-oriented cultures, social support from family members can be quickly called upon (e.g., grandparents); however, seeking support from people of one's own choosing often leads to higher satisfaction with the advice and support received.
- Parental support works in tandem with other support circles available to the individual, such as friends, although the latter cannot usually compensate for a lack of the former.
- Financial hardship is a risk factor for the development of psychological disorders in children. Reasons for this include: financial stress interfering with consistent, authoritative parenting; inadequate nutrition; and living in a poorly integrated and violent neighborhood.
- Marital conflict may affect maladjustment or psychopathology in children, for example, when parenting becomes inconsistent and ineffective. Additionally, when parents repeatedly display negative emotion, children do not learn appropriate methods of regulating their emotions.
- Violence in the home is an unfortunate factor that exists all around the world, ultimately leading to an increased risk for children to develop psychopathology. Children exposed to family violence may pay excessive attention to cues that elicit anger. They may believe that other people intend to harm them.

- Systems theorists conceive of the family as a complex system with a number of interrelated components that interact and communicate with one another. This perspective on family life is one of many applications of this theory, which is also used in biology, sociology and business administration. Family system theorists regard other family life theories as simplistic and "linear," as they often include, at most, two members (e.g., mother and child). Modern theorists in this domain would contend that psychopathologies are caused by multiple factors within and outside the family.
- Systemically oriented family therapists remove the label of identified patient from the family member who is sent for psychological care, and place the pathology in the family, referring to the patient as a scapegoat. Cohesive families comprise relationships that are warm and supportive and have clear boundaries for accessing support. Disengaged families comprise cold and unsupportive relationships among family members, where coalitions may be formed against one another. In enmeshed families, relationships between some of the members are stifling; children must choose sides and give up much of their autonomy.
- Reframing occurs when a concept or viewpoint is experienced in another frame of reference to fit the facts of the situation more positively. Paradoxical instructions are those that instruct the child or adolescent to exhibit the symptoms of their mental illness (e.g., an individual with depression acting depressed) or other instructions in which the therapist instructs the family to do things that are opposite to what the therapist really desires.

Study questions

1. How does intervening with families to prevent or treat child or adolescent psychopathology make sense in light of the fact that a very large part of such problems are attributable to genetic factors?
2. What is the essential difference between "errorless" interventions and other applications of behavior therapy to improve child-rearing?
3. In what ways are the implications of child–mother attachment for the psychological adjustment of children and adolescents different from the implications of child–father attachment?
4. Compare the objectives and basic format of behaviorally oriented, attachment-oriented and systems-oriented interventions with families.
5. In what important ways has contemporary knowledge about research methodology improved the quality of research on the family causes and correlates of child and adolescent psychopathology?

7

The helpful and harmful influences of peers, friends and siblings

A substantial portion of the professional and popular literature on the psychological problems of children and adolescents is devoted to family influences and to ways in which families can help their sons and daughters in distress. The famous nature-versus-nurture debate usually entails pitting family causation against genetics. However, "nurture" is not provided exclusively by parents. This chapter begins with a discussion of the relatively small professional literature in which family and peer influences are compared. The subsequent section is devoted to the basic characteristics and inherent features of relationships with peers and peer influence. A section on the distinction between close friendships and less intimate relationships with peer-group members follows. The dynamics of peer influence, an often-maligned phenomenon, are discussed next: Are peer-relations problems just a sign of general malfunctioning, a cause (or the cause) of the problem, or a mechanism through which problems can improve or worsen? Interventions designed to improve the peer relations of children and adolescents at risk for psychopathology are considered next. The chapter continues with a section on the much understudied role of the peers who typically live at home: one's siblings. A brief plea that interpersonal relationships be given greater weight in the basic understanding of psychopathology than in most contemporary thinking appears at the end of the chapter.

Peer and family influences – separately and in combination

The idea of an anti-social peer group negating the benefits of a warm, supportive family upbringing is undoubtedly the most familiar connotation of the concept of peer influence. However, as noted in the previous chapter, it is probably much more common for the families and peers of an individual to match each other in terms of supportiveness, warmth and enjoyable interaction. Peers are also more likely to affirm the authority of parents than to undermine it (Clasen and Brown, 1985). Satisfying bonds with parents are likely to co-occur with satisfying relationships with friends and peers. One obvious reason for this is that attachment theory, also discussed in the previous chapter, is in fact reflected in research results: Children and adolescents who experienced warm, trusting and secure bonds with their caregivers tend to end up with the ability to relate intimately to peers, especially close friends (Schneider et al., 2001). As well, the interests, characteristics and social skills that emerge from effective, authoritative parenting may be applied by children to their own interchanges with peers (Brown and Mounts, 2007).

Atypical as they may be, situations in which a child or adolescent is surrounded by a supportive prosocial family but an anti-social peer group, or the converse – a dysfunctional family and a supportive peer group – may have particular implications for the emergence of psychopathology and resistance to it. Interpersonal relationships sometimes provide a degree of protection from maladjustment for children and adolescents from troubled family backgrounds. However, no responsible theorist or researcher claims that a warm, supportive peer group can substitute for a warm, supportive family.

Given the frequent juxtaposition of parent and peer influences in both the professional literature and the thinking of many parents, comparisons of parent and peer influences are featured in many studies. The researchers' hypothesis is sometimes that peer

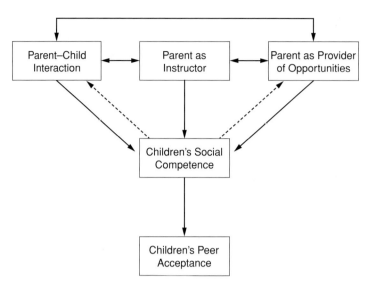

Figure 7.1 Parents may indirectly affect their children's peer relations in several ways.

influence explains at least part of the outcome (be it adjustment or maladjustment) over and above the influence of parents. In other cases, the researchers expect that parents and peers influence different types of negative outcome, often in different ways.

There is one notable exception to the prevalent attempts at delineating the different ways in which family and peer influence work together rather than pitting one against the other. American psychologist Judith Rich Harris (1995, 1998) debunks research on socialization by parents as methodologically and conceptually flawed. She argues that genetic factors and socialization by childhood and adolescent peers account primarily for how children turn out to be. Harris maintains that the role of peers in socialization is inherent in the human species, which is programmed to seek companionship. Hence, in their socializing role, peers are in essence acting in the service of genetics. Parenting, if not totally irrelevant, has surely been over-rated. Thought-provoking as Harris' observations may be, they have failed to spark substantial debate.

A developmental perspective is indispensable in understanding and comparing the influences of parents and peers. Parents influence their children at all ages, as do peers; toddlers form close relationships

with other toddlers as early as age 2 (Howes, 1983). However, the relative importance of the social support and socialization processes involving parents and peers varies by age, as described in Parke's tripartite model (McDowell and Parke, 2009). That model, illustrated in Figure 7.1, is very useful in explaining how three major forms of parenting differentially affect the interpersonal relations of children at different developmental stages.

During early childhood, parents' nurturance and warmth are paralleled in positive interactions between the young child and his or her peers. This has been demonstrated very well in observations of child–mother and child–peer interaction in several rigorous studies (Isley, O'Neil and Parke, 1996; Pettit and Harrist, 1993). At this stage, most parents have virtually total control over when and where their children will be in contact with peers and over the choice of peers with whom their children associate. However, the purpose of the natural process of development is to promote autonomy and the capacity to relate to others in an intimate way. As development proceeds through middle childhood and into adolescence, direct parental influence wanes as peer influence becomes stronger. Nevertheless, parents still affect their children's relations with others by virtue of their roles as instructors and as providers of opportunities (Gonzales and Dodge, 2009; McDowell and Parke, 2009). Even so, it is not clear that parents' advice to older children necessarily leads to better peer relations. In fact, parents have been found to give more advice to children who do not do well in relating to others. This may occur because the parents want to remediate social skill problems that they see in their children. Of course, these findings may also mean that the advice given is misguided or not received in the ways intended by the parents (McDowell and Parke, 2009).

By early adolescence, the peer group emerges as a major object of attention and source of influence. This brings a heightened need to conform to the attitudes and behaviors of whatever peer group or "crowd" the adolescent joins. This is thought to occur because of the value assigned by adolescents to their peers and not because they are unable to resist pressures coming from them to conform (Brown et al., 2008). Of course, the group norms to which the adolescent strives to conform may be prosocial or anti-social, conventional or simply faddish. Many scholars working with adolescents believe, in fact, that adolescent peer influence is usually positive. Peer influence provides and clarifies norms for behavior. The peer group is the "staging ground" in which adolescents practice social behaviors, learn about different social roles and consolidate their identities (Brown et al., 2008; Eder, 1995; Gonzales and Dodge, 2009).

Before adolescence, it is very unlikely that peer pressure will lead to anti-social attitudes, beliefs or behaviors. Such negative influence can and does happen from early adolescence onward (Cillessen and Mayeux, 2004), depending not only on the nature of the group but also on some factors that make a particular individual susceptible to negative influence. For example, adolescents who are vulnerable because of some form of maladjustment, such as anxiety, are known to be influenced by peers with a wide range of characteristics and popularity levels. In contrast, adolescents who are not anxious seem to be influenced more exclusively by peers

who are popular (Cohen and Prinstein, 2006). Some adolescents, especially adolescent males, develop a preference for risky behaviors of different kinds. This preference for risk is thought to relate to changing brain structure and function, with rewards bringing greater excitement while judgment is still immature (Gonzales and Dodge, 2009; Steinberg et al., 2009). Parents are unlikely to share or support embarkation in activities of ever-increasing risk but high risk-takers may find a common niche as a clique or crowd.

At whatever stage of child or adolescent development, family and peer influences are by no means totally separate, as explained by Brown and Mounts (2007). First of all, parents may (and, to the extent appropriate, should) regulate the contacts children and adolescents have with their peers. Hopefully, they do so without placing excessive restrictions on the child's exploration of the peer world or without monitoring the child's social activities enough to prevent contacts with young people involved in delinquency or substance abuse. Parents may also offer advice to their children about how to relate with peers. Parents may in fact "orchestrate" activities in which their children meet other children, for example by inviting other parents with children the same age to their homes. This has been shown to facilitate the social development of preschoolers (Ladd and Hart, 1992), but might not be appropriate for adolescents. Friends often get to know each other's families very well, sometimes to the extent of almost becoming members of each other's families. This occurs more often in some cultures than in others; it is common among African-Americans (Chatters, Taylor and Jayakody, 1994). In some cultures, friends may be formally inducted into the family as honorary cousins (Brown and Mounts, 2007).

Dodge and his colleagues propose a *dynamic cascade model* (Dodge et al., 2009; Gonzales and Dodge, 2009) to describe how parenting and peer relations affect each other reciprocally over time. While their children are very young, some parents may be harsh in their discipline and relate to their children without emotional warmth. For that reason, the children fail to develop the social and cognitive skills needed to relate to others. Seeing that their children lack social skills and get into conflicts with peers, the parents find it even more difficult to engage in warm, supportive parenting. The distance between child and parents increases over time. By early adolescence, the child can only find friends among groups who engage in anti-social behavior or substance abuse. This is abetted by the parents' failure to supervise the children's peer associations in the community at the very developmental stage when children need appropriate monitoring, supervision and guidance the most.

In some instances, which have clear implications for emerging psychopathology, the peer group can assume the role of the family or vice versa. In some urban areas of the United States, gangs assume many of the roles of families, with older members of the gang taking on some of the activities of parents. Conversely, some parents abdicate their parental roles and relate to their children as friends (Brown and Mounts, 2007). On the other hand, it has been shown that supportive parenting can help mitigate the negative effects of victimization by peers in the emergence of depression in school-aged children. Excellent evidence for this effect emerged from a longitudinal study using multiple sources of information by Bilsky and her colleagues (2013).

The interplay of family and peer influence is known to vary somewhat by culture although the developmental transition from total reliance on parents to increased investment in peer relations occurs everywhere. It has sometimes been found that relations with peers and friends are less intimate in cultures characterized by close relationships with members of one's extended family than elsewhere. An example is French's comparison of children's relationships in the United States and Indonesia (French, Pidada and Victor, 2005). However, in other cultures, the peer world has been found to provide young people with a valued respite from the intensity of collective life and a space to cultivate individual identities (see Schneider, Lee and Alvarez-Valdivia's [2012] exploration of friendships in Japan and Cuba).

Some inherent features of peer influence

Because much less has been written about peer influence than about family influence, many misconceptions abound about the ways in which peer influence operates. The most important inherent feature of peer contacts, as opposed to family relations, is that children and adolescents in most places, especially large schools and communities, are active in selecting the group, clique or "crowd" they wish to join. Therefore, adolescents prone to deviant behavior may seek out the company of other adolescents prone to deviant behavior. This *self-selection* means that the deviant behavior is not necessarily the result of influence by the peers who are involved in it. They may well have been interested in deviant behavior before they met and it may have been the pre-existing deviant behavior that brought them together (Gonzales and Dodge, 2009; Lazarsfeld and Merton, 1954). This self-selection factor must be considered in the design of any research on peer influence. The effects of peer influence and self-selection are best untangled with longitudinal data to which sophisticated statistical techniques, such as structural equations modeling, are applied. As time passes, though, even if the anti-social peers were originally brought together by common interests, the anti-social group or clique reinforces the propensity for anti-social behavior by talking about it, rewarding it and sharing thoughts about it (e.g., Dishion, Piehler and Myers, 2008).

Bakken and Brown (2009) enumerate a number of other interesting and important features of peer influence. Peer influence is often intentional: According to the very limited data available, adolescents appear to have the clear intention of influencing the behavior of their peers. Their reasons for being so intentional may be to enforce the prevailing group norms or rules. They may also actively attempt to influence peers in order to enhance the social reputations of themselves or, in a helpful way, the social reputations of the peers they are trying to influence. Peer influence can take many forms.

Peers can shape the behavior of a non-conforming peer by ridiculing him or her or by excluding him or her from group activities. Tactics ranging from friendly teasing to nasty verbal or physical aggression are within the repertoires of groups of children and adolescents. However, peer influence can also be very subtle. *Modeling* occurs when a person imitates the behavior he or she sees. Many children and adolescents copy the behavior, dress style or language of peers without the "model" doing anything other than appearing. As well, influence can only occur if the receiver is open to influence. This is a personality trait (Bratus and Davis, 1990). Certain individuals are more susceptible to influence than others. People in subordinate positions, which surely includes many children suffering from mental distress, are more likely to be influenced than others (Adler and Adler, 1998; Bakken and Brown, 2009). Perhaps people are most susceptible to influence at difficult moments in their lives, of which adolescence brings many. Finally, Bakken and Brown (2009) point out that multiple peer inferences operate simultaneously in many situations. Children and adolescents are often faced with the complex task of deciding whether to follow the advice or model of a friend who is involved in anti-social behavior or to listen to another friend who advises against participating in a collective anti-social act.

Thus, for the reasons outlined above, both peer rejection and peer acceptance can lead to psychopathology. As explained in the next section, peer rejection – being actively disliked by one's peer group – is associated with many indicators of maladjustment. However, because of the negative peer influence discussed above, being accepted by a peer group with deviant values is not necessarily more desirable. Whether it is better for a child or adolescent to have no friends or to have only friends who are negative role models is not known. However, in most cases, this is probably not a real choice. The literature on the emergence of juvenile delinquency, for example, indicates that most delinquents do have friends, often friends who are like themselves involved in delinquency. However, the friendships tend not to be of the type that provides the support,

security and trust that constitute the psychological benefits of the friendship bond, as discussed in the next section. To the limited extent permitted by extant research, it appears more likely that the negative influences of anti-social friends are stronger predictors of delinquency and other forms of maladjustment than any measure of friendship quality or than the fact of having, or not having, any friends (Brendgen, Vitaro and Bukowski, 2000; Knecht et al., 2010; Poulin, Dishion and Haas, 1999; Scholte, Van Lieshout and Van Aken, 2001).

Reputation in large groups vs. intimate friendship bonds

Peer influences occur simultaneously at different levels. Classroom groups are the least voluntary of the peer groups in which children interact. Children typically have somewhat greater choice of the peer groups they encounter during leisure-time activities such as sports, music and arts. It is in the choice of their closest friends that most children have the greatest freedom to select their associates. Rewarding relations with peers at each of these levels have implications for psychological adjustment, but in very different ways.

Classroom and school groups

At the large-group level, peer rejection – being actively disliked by one's daily associates in school, for example – has been studied very widely and is known to have devastating consequences. Children are known to reject their peers in many different ways, which have been grouped by Asher, Rose and Gabriel (2001) into six different categories: (1) exclusion of a child from social interaction; (2) preventing a child from having access to a friend; (3) using aggression of various types, be it physical, verbal or relational; (4) controlling and dominating; (5) expressing disapproval of the rejected child or his/her behavior; and (6) communicating rejection though a third party, e.g., saying negative things about the rejected child to another classmate while the rejected child is within earshot. Rejected status, unfortunately, is quite stable over time and has long-lasting consequences. Making matters worse, the exclusion experienced by rejected children limits their opportunities for developing and practicing the social skills they need for positive social action in the future (Rubin, Bukowski and Parker, 2006). Rejection and exclusion are known to affect emotion regulation (Baumeister et al., 2005), classroom participation (Buhs and Ladd, 2001) and academic achievement (Greenman, Schneider and Tomada, 2009). Thus, peer rejection may impair the academic success that can lead to satisfaction and well-being in many cases. The many longitudinal studies documenting the long-term implications of peer rejection in childhood for subsequent psychopathology are discussed later in this chapter. Importantly, however, not all children and adolescents are equally affected by peer rejection: Some children are more sensitive than others to being scorned by their schoolmates and it is those sensitive children who are the most affected psychologically and behaviorally (Downey et al., 1998).

After-school activities

Extracurricular activities are another arena in which children and adolescents encounter their peers. In many cases, involvement in sports or cultural activities is voluntary on the part of children and their parents. These activities probably provide invaluable opportunities for the development of social skills as well as skill at the activity itself. The activity, in turn, may open doors to new social contacts. The social interactions during extracurricular activities have not been studied extensively. It has been shown a number of times that children and adolescents who participate in them are less likely than others to develop some form of psychopathology. It is also known that children and adolescents with some form of psychopathology are less likely than others to participate in an extracurricular activity. However, research findings in this area are not entirely consistent, with some studies failing to show a clear

link between activity participation and adjustment (e.g. Urban, Lewin-Bizan and Lerner, 2009). Probably the most authoritative data on the implications of extracurricular activities for psychopathology are from a longitudinal study conducted by Bohnert and Garber (2007). Their longitudinal design, with measurement of psychopathology before entry to high school, provides a much clearer picture of the causal processes involved than correlational designs. Their results confirm that, after taking into account psychopathology before entering high school, participants who participated in extracurricular activities were less likely than others to develop an externalizing disorder. Similarly, a correlational study by Mason and colleagues (2009) indicated that adolescents involved in extracurricular activities display lower levels of depression than other adolescents. Focusing on preschool children, a recent Canadian study indicated that youngsters involved in sports are less likely than non-participants to experience early signs of anxiety (Findlay and Coplan, 2008). There has been some cross-cultural replication of research documenting the benefits of extracurricular activities in Spain (Molinuevo et al., 2010) and among African-Americans (Fredricks and Eccles, 2008). However, some studies indicate that sports participation increases children's aggression, even if the sport is not of a particularly combative nature such as handball, as demonstrated in a study of French male adolescents (Rascle, Coulomb-Cabagno and Delsarte, 2005). One recent study suggests that the benefits of extracurricular activities may depend on the characteristics of the friends who participate: The benefits of leisure-time activities will accrue if the fellow participants are supportive and prosocial (Simpkins, Eccles and Becnel, 2008).

Small groups and cliques

From middle childhood onwards, children feel the need to modify the relatively monolithic nature of interactions in large groups to allow for increasing individual differences in interests and identities. They begin to form well-defined *cliques*, which typically consist of three to nine children. Clique members are often each other's close friends. From the time at which the cliques emerge, they account for a very large proportion of the social interactions of their members. Clique activities are exclusive; non-members rarely participate in their activities or share in their communication. Cliques are formed on the basis of a shared characteristic. This may be an activity at which the clique members excel, such as academics or athletics. Cliques may also be defined according to their common position in the larger group, for example, isolates or popular children. They may also be identified on the basis of typical social behavior such as aggression or shyness/social withdrawal. Very often, the defining characteristic is known to both the members and their schoolmates, who may assign a nickname to the clique that reflects its defining feature (Cairns, Xie and Leung, 1998; Crockett, Losoff and Petersen, 1984; Kindermann, 1998).

Although most children are members of cliques, little is known at present about the ramifications of clique membership or non-membership for adjustment and psychopathology. In an interesting study conducted with almost 500 primary-school children in the United States, Kwon and Lease (2007) identified cliques who were formed on the basis of the typical social behaviors of their members and the activities at which they excelled. There was a clique of academically advanced pupils, and another of athletes. There were cliques of children known for their enjoyment of social activities. Interestingly, there were several different kinds of aggressive cliques. One clique was tough but effective and socially competent. There was also a clique of bullies. There was also an "incompetent" aggressive clique that was disliked by non-members. Finally, there was a clique of children who were socially withdrawn and shy. Members of both the socially withdrawn clique and the incompetent aggressive clique rated themselves as lonelier than others and higher in anxiety and depression.

Close friendship

In counterpoint with their peer relations in larger groups, children also form close friendships.

According to many philosophical writings as well as the findings of studies on what children expect of their friends, intimacy is the feature that distinguishes a close friendship from relationships with other peers. Children and adolescents also expect their friends to keep secrets, to provide social support at times of difficulty, to take their side against third parties and to resolve disagreements equitably and with minimal conflict. Children typically become friends with children they encounter at school, in their neighborhoods or in leisure activities, in other words, children who are available to enjoy common pastimes. However, according to the principle of *homophily*, it is often a shared characteristic that cements the friendship. This may be a physical characteristic, particular talent or strength, or a psychological or behavioral characteristic such as aggression or shyness. Psychologists once believed that children were incapable of close friendship until their cognitive development reached a stage at which they could understand how other children's thinking about a situation was different from their own. However, careful observational studies have revealed that children as young as 2 or 3 years form emotional attachments with friends long before they can verbalize any description of their friendships. At all ages, girls and women are more oriented to relating in intimate ways to close friends than are boys and men. However, boys and men also enter into close friendships that are important to them (Benenson, Apostoleris and Parnass, 1997; Berndt, 2004; Bukowski, Newcomb and Hartup, 1996; Schneider, 2000). Before deciding conclusively that intimacy is more of a girls' pursuit, it may be worthwhile to consider the possibility that boys express their needs for intimacy in subtle ways that differ from female expressions of closeness (Way, 2004).

The American psychiatrist Harry Stack Sullivan (1953) reconceptualized psychopathology in terms of interpersonal relationships. He emphasized the role of *chumship*, a close relationship with a friend during the early adolescent years, as preparation for satisfying intimate romantic relationships later on.

He also emphasized the role of peers as evaluators of young people's capacities and talents, enabling them to become less reliant than in previous years on the evaluations of their parents.

In theory, close friendship should provide support and companionship to many children with different forms of psychopathology who cannot achieve acceptance in larger peer groups. Unfortunately, this often does not happen because, as will be detailed in subsequent chapters, children in psychological distress very often fail to bring to their friendships the intimacy and mutual understanding needed to form close relationships with socially competent peers. They may, however, be able to relate to other children experiencing many of the same difficulties, as would be expected according to the principle of homophily. As detailed earlier in this chapter, children in psychological distress may be vulnerable to the influence of "bad" friends who will only aggravate their problems. Nevertheless, helping children with adjustment problems achieve rewarding close friendship may be a more viable objective for interventions than attempting to reverse their negative reputations in large groups.

In a very convincing illustration of the protective power of friendship, Bukowski, Laursen and Hoza (2010) followed 431 children each year during the first 3 years of primary school. They focused specifically on the participants who were found to avoid contact with peers and who were also excluded by their peers from group activities at the start of the study. In general, depressed affect increased dramatically over the 3 years of the study for members of the high-exclusion, high-avoidance group. Importantly, however, this effect was moderated by friendship: There was much less evidence of an increase in depressed affect among children of the high-exclusion, high-avoidance group who had friends. This study is particularly interesting because it demonstrates how one form of peer interaction, namely having a close friend, can protect from deficits in another aspect of peer interaction, that is, participation in the larger peer group and acceptance by its members.

Mapping the role of peers in the emergence of psychopathology

Peer rejection as marker of maladjustment

Providing a useful conceptual framework for research on the implications of peer relations for psychopathology, Bukowski and Adams (2005) group the studies into five categories (see Box 7.1). The first category consists of studies in which peer relations are conceptualized as *markers* of maladjustment, that is, as a sign, often an early sign, of broader dysfunction. This approach has a relatively long history, rooted in longitudinal studies started as early as the 1920s and, in many cases, spanning the life cycle from birth through adulthood.

Parker and Asher (1987) reviewed the results of the many longitudinal studies showing that peer-relations difficulties predict later psychopathology. Early problems in peer relations are clear and consistent markers of such difficulties during adulthood as schizophrenia, criminal behavior and alcoholism. The authors concluded that peer rejection – being actively disliked – is a far stronger predictor of lifelong maladjustment than is peer neglect – being neither disliked nor very liked, or being usually ignored. They also found that aggressive behavior during childhood is a more robust predictor of later maladjustment than is shy, socially withdrawn behavior. However, reflecting the increased interest in internalizing disorders in recent years, it has now been established that social withdrawal and shyness are linked to such forms of psychopathology as anxiety and depression (Deater-Deckard, 2005; Rubin and Burgess, 2001).

Parker and Asher conceptualize two different models that might explain the reasons behind the findings linking peer relations to psychopathology in many longitudinal studies conducted in many different countries. The two competing models are depicted in Figure 7.2. According to the *causal model*, it is the peer-relations deficits themselves that are at the root of subsequent processes that terminate in a diagnosable mental health problem. In contrast, the *incidental model* depicts peer relations as simply

Box 7.1 | How peer relationships may be linked to psychopathology

- *Marker* – Peer relations are a sign of a larger problem but not the cause or result of the problem.
- *Moderator* – Peer relationships increase or decrease the effects of another cause or other causes of the problem, such as improper parenting or genetic risk.
- *Mediator* – Peer relationships are a step in a complicated causal path. For example, overprotective parenting may lead to lack of experience with peers, which may lead to a lack of friends, which may lead to loneliness and depression.
- *Mechanism* – Some aspect of peer relationships may be a cause or the cause of the pathology. For example, pre-delinquent youth and their friends talk about aggressive behavior, making it sound legitimate. This may lead to conduct disorder.
- *Meaning* – The way a person interprets aspects of his or her peer relationships is linked to the problem. For example, believing that one loses friends because of one's own shortcomings may lead to avoiding people and becoming lonely and depressed.

Source: Based on Bukowski, W. M. and Adams, R. (2005), Peer relations and psychopathology: Markers, mechanisms, mediators, moderators, and meanings. *Journal of Clinical Child and Adolescent Psychology*, *34*, 3–10.

(a) Causal Model

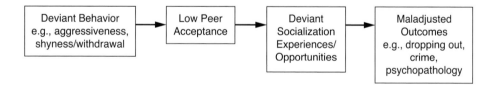

(b) Incidental Model

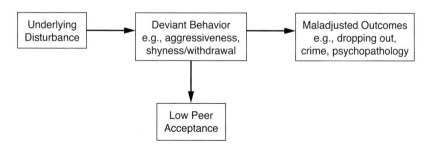

Figure 7.2 Causal and incidental models explaining how peer relations are linked to psychopathology.

one of many consequences of psychopathology that was already present. The peer group is, in essence, imposing the consequences that emerge from not meeting society's expectations about how people should relate to others (Masten, 2005).

Although far more limited than the studies of the long-term consequences of peer rejection, there has also been some longitudinal research on friendship. Longitudinal research on friendship is needed to provide empirical corroboration of Sullivan's theory on the developmental significance of friendship, discussed above. In a study that is ground-breaking despite its small sample size, Bagwell, Newcomb and Bukowski (1998) followed thirty participants from preadolescence into young adulthood. They found that being "chumless" in middle adolescence was associated with several aspects of psychopathology in adulthood. However, in some other studies, when peer rejection and friendship variables are studied together, friendship does not seem to predict the emergence of psychopathology beyond its correlation with peer rejection. This emerged, for example, in a Dutch study on the emergence of externalizing and internalizing symptoms 4 years after the initial data collection among children who had displayed peer-relations problems such as victimization by peers in the kindergarten year (van Lier and Koot, 2010). Clearly, more longitudinal research is needed, including research on the long-term implications of friendships of good and bad quality with friends who are models either of adjustment or maladjustment.

Moderating effects: peers as providing protection against mental distress

The second approach described by Bukowski and Adams is research designed to test models in which peer relations are seen as either strengthening or weakening the impact of another causal variable on a pathological outcome. As already mentioned, befriending anti-social peers could indeed amplify the effect of other risk factors, be they genetic or familial. However, in most studies, peer acceptance and friendship are seen as moderators that help

protect the child against pre-existing risk factors, especially dysfunctional parenting. The roles of peer relations in the etiologies of specific disorders are included in the subsequent chapters devoted to the disorders; only a few examples are included here to illustrate the concept of moderation.

Supportive friendship in wartime

Intriguing research has confirmed that friendship is a protective factor against post-traumatic stress disorder (PTSD; see Chapter 23) among children who have been exposed to war-related traumatic events. This was originally observed by Anna Freud in her work with English children who had been evacuated from bomb-ravaged London during World War II (Freud and Burlingame, 1943). This protective effect was studied in work with children who experienced the recent hostilities in the Gaza Strip, on both sides of the border. On the Gaza side, Peltonen and colleagues (2010) conducted a study with 227 Palestinian boys and girls aged 10–14 years. They found that war-related stress led to deterioration of relationships with both peers and siblings. The participants who managed to maintain high-quality relationships with their siblings were less prone to PTSD. Inconsistent with Anna Freud's finding, however, friendship did not serve as a protector for the participants. At the same time, data about the protective effects of social support were being gathered in Sderot, Israel, which was also bombarded during the same hostilities. Henrich and Shahar (2008) were able to collect data on the depressive affect of the early adolescent participants because a study was already underway when the bombardment began. Participants who reported that they were exposed to rocket attacks were less likely to display increased depressive symptomatology after the hostilities if they reported satisfactory social support prior to the exposure. Unfortunately, the small sample size precluded Henrich and Shahar from differentiating between social support from friends and from family members. In a later study in the same community it was determined that parent support was a protective factor whereas support from friends was actually associated with an increase in violent reactions (Brookmeyer et al., 2011). However, in another study after a suicide bombing in Dimona, Israel, support from friends was found to buffer negative reactions (Shahar et al., 2009). Given the inconsistent findings from both sides of the Israel–Gaza border, more research is needed to confirm Anna Freud's observations about the value of supportive friends for children who have experienced the stresses of war.

Protection against victimization by bullies

Bullying in schools is a relational problem that is linked with psychological maladjustment on the part of both the bullies and victims (see, e.g., review by Hawker and Boulton, 2000). Research on bullying in schools has repeatedly revealed that bullying is not only a phenomenon that involves the bully and the victim but also that bullying is influenced very strongly by other pupils who are present at the time. Those present may do nothing, intervene to support the victim, encourage the bully or report the incident to adults (e.g., Salmivalli et al., 1996).

There has been considerable research on the moderating effects of friendship for children who are vulnerable to victimization by school bullies. In a landmark study, Hodges and colleagues (1999) followed 393 children for a period of 1 year whose ages averaged 10 years. They found that both bullying and victimization were very stable. However, participants who appeared to be at risk for becoming victims at the start of the study were less likely to actually be victimized if they had reciprocal best friends (i.e., friends who also considered them as friends) in comparison to at-risk, friendless participants. Schwartz et al. (2000) confirmed the protective properties of friendship in a study conducted with a younger sample who began participating in the research as they began schooling. Once they had started school, children who had been exposed to harsh, punitive and hostile parenting tended to become victimized by bullies. This was less likely to happen, however, to participants at risk who managed to develop good friendships, perhaps

because they learned the skills involved in competent regulation of their emotions while interacting with friends. The findings about the protective properties of friendship in reducing the likelihood of being victimized by bullies have been replicated in many countries, including China and South Korea (Abou-ezzeddine et al., 2007), Japan, Portugal, Italy, Spain and England (Eslea et al., 2004). The early adolescent participants in an interview study conducted in Australia by Burns, Cross and Maycock (2010) reported that they would stop bullying if they knew that their friends opposed this kind of behavior. Some said that they would change their circle of friends if necessary to find a peer group that did not encourage bullying.

Impaired peer relations as mediating the emergence of psychopathology

Peer-relations problems have also been shown to mediate the links between poor parenting (in this case, lack of supervision and inconsistent discipline) and subsequent drug use in a study by Kung and Farrell (2000). A *mediating variable* is one that explains a correlation between two other variables. In this case, for example, lack of parental supervision leads to gravitation to an anti-social peer group, which in turn leads to drug abuse. Working with 443 American early adolescents from low-income homes, these researchers found that ineffective parenting was related to negative peer pressure, which, in turn, was related to drug use. Dill et al. (2004) provide yet another example of a mediational model in a study conducted with 296 elementary-school pupils finding that early shyness led to victimization by school bullies, which in turn led to feelings of depression.

Although there is no doubt that peers influence children and adolescents very strongly, not very much is known about exactly how this influence occurs. According to *deviance regulation theory*, two basic mechanisms are involved in the tendency to be influenced by peers. The first is the dynamic tension between individual needs to fit in and to stand out from the crowd and affirm one's uniqueness.

Individuals vary along a continuum ranging from total suppression of their individuality in the interest of conformity, to the healthy compromise, finally, to those who will fight steadfastly to be different from others. Secondly, there is an aspect of the normal socialization processes that results in most people being at least somewhat concerned about what others think of them (Blanton and Burkley, 2008).

Three hypotheses about the dynamics of peer influence have been proposed by Dishion, Piehler and Myers (2008). According to the *social argumentation hypothesis*, gravitation to an anti-social peer group may become inevitable once a child has been marginalized from the mainstream peer group, perhaps because of aggressive behavior. The marginalized child simply has no other potential friends. The *arrested socialization hypothesis* involves the assumption that gravitation to anti-social peers occurs because the child has grown up with a deficiency in some important aspect of cognitive and/or social development, such as the ability to appropriately regulate his or her emotions. Finally, the *intrasubjectivity hypothesis* focuses on the emergence of a shared understanding between friends of the social world and about how they should act on it. As their friendship continues, friends who are already prone to anti-social behavior collectively cultivate the beliefs that justify delinquency.

Brown et al. (2008) review the research strategies that have been employed to learn about exactly how peers influence each other. Classic laboratory studies (e.g., Asch, 1951) on conformity remain perhaps the best-known source of information. In those studies, children and adolescents are brought to the laboratory to participate in a task invented by the experimenters, such as estimating the exact length of a line. The participants were given such information as the estimates provided by friends or other children their age. Conformity to the responses of friends or age-mates was highest from early to middle adolescence, compared to younger children and older adolescents (e.g., Costanzo and Shaw, 1966) and in situations where other participants were going to

know the response given (e.g., Deutsch and Gerard, 1955). Importantly, participants who displayed some form of personal vulnerability, such as negative self-concepts, were more likely to conform than were others (Costanzo, 1970).

Over time, the scientific community became skeptical of experiments involving deception. The participants may not have been fooled. In later studies, for example, participants were presented with a vignette describing parents and/or peers attempting to exert influence and then asked how they would respond to the given situation. The results disappointed the researchers, who assumed in almost every study that parents and peers would provide opposite opinions; as noted earlier, this does not happen as often as many people assume. The identification of individuals who are particularly susceptible to peer influence has been a more fruitful outcome of research in which participants are asked how they would respond in a situation described. Children who are not supervised appropriately by their parents are among the most susceptible (Steinberg and Silverberg, 1986).

In recent years, there have been a few attempts at studying the processes of peer influence in conjunction with the emergence of psychopathology. These include studies by Allen, Porter and McFarland (2006), who observed how frequently participants yielded to their friends' position in a joint decision-making task. In longitudinal analyses, susceptibility to friends' influence was found to correlate with substance abuse and with increases in depressive affect. Researchers at the Oregon Social Learning Center (see Chapter 2) recorded conversations between boys displaying early signs of problematic aggression and their friends. They discovered that the friends "talked themselves" into delinquency, for example by responding positively to each other's remarks about the possibilities of engaging in delinquent acts (Granic and Dishion, 2003). There has also been some research on the cognitive aspects of susceptibility to peer influence, especially in the area of substance abuse and early involvement in risky sexual behaviors. Children and adolescents who tend to compare themselves, perhaps excessively, with peers, appear to be more likely than others to be influenced by peers into such forms of maladjustment (Gibbons, Pomery and Gerrard, 2008).

A final approach to research on the role of peer relations involves the way children understand their peer relations. It is often their misunderstanding of their peer relations that is considered a component of their psychopathology, whether the understanding of their own peer relations or of the feelings of their peers correspond to reality or not. Faulty attributions of hostile intent will be considered in the subsequent chapters on several major child mental health disorders. As will be detailed in those chapters, children with disorders as diverse as major depression, social anxiety and conduct disorder are known to believe that their peers do not want to associate with them and/or wish to harm them.

Interventions to enhance peer relations

Social skills training

Social skills training involves direct instruction in some of the skills involved in effective relating with others. These skills may be cognitive, such as appreciating the alternative available while solving a problem in a relationship with a friend or peer. Skills can also be overt and behavioral, such as knowing how to greet another child and ask in an appropriate way to join him/her in a game. Social skills can be taught in a variety of ways, to individuals known to lack them, to groups consisting of such individuals or to entire school populations. Cognitive skills tend to be taught by guided exercises in which, for example, children are taught: to (1) recognize when they are facing a problem; (2) think carefully about all possible solutions to the problem; (3) predict what would happen if they implemented each of the solutions; (4) decide which solution is best; (5) identify the steps involved in implementing that solution; and, finally, (6) evaluate how well they implemented the solution. This of course involves rational

thinking and forethought, which may tap the very cognitive skills in which children with many forms of psychopathology are deficient. Therefore, some social skills training programs focus on self-control. Children who are prone to immediate, impulsive responding are taught to use language to slow themselves down before reacting.

In contrast with cognitive approaches to social skills training, some interventions emphasize direct instruction in how to implement the socially competent behaviors that are typical of socially successful children. For example, the skill of disagreeing with a peer's opinion might be broken down into smaller steps, starting with the expression of one's esteem for the other child involved, then stating how one feels starting with the recognition that it is only an opinion. The trainer might model the skills step by step, ask the child trainees to imitate the model, and provide feedback and praise for accurate imitation. Arrangements are often made for an adult in the child's natural environment, such as a parent or teacher, to watch for situations in which the child might use newly learned skills, prompt them and reinforce successful use of them (Bienert and Schneider, 1995; Cartledge and Milburn, 1994; Dempsey and Matson, 2009; Schneider and Byrne, 1987).

Considerable enthusiasm greeted the advent of social skills training in the 1970s. At the time, children with various forms of psychological disorder were being integrated into regular school classes for the first time in many Western countries. The lack of social skills was seen as impeding their success. Considerable evaluative research has been conducted since then. Several meta-analyses have indicated some degree of success for many types of childhood disorder (Ang and Hughes, 2002; Losel and Beelmann, 2003; Schneider, 1992); therefore, this approach is certainly worth considering. However, social skills training has not fully lived up to the lofty expectations that surrounded its inception. All too often, the trainees master the skills during the training session but do not transfer them to their school and community environments for any extended period of time. Commenting on the applicability of social skills training for children with disruptive behavior disorders, Gresham and Elliott (1989) observed that in many cases, impulsive children do not really have any meaningful deficit in social skills. Their deficits are very often in *social performance*. In other words, children often fail to use the skills they already have because of some process at work in the immediate setting, be it impulsivity, anxiety or reinforcement for inappropriate behavior. Nevertheless, Gresham recognizes that social skills training does have a record of success and, therefore, he recommends its judicious use (Gresham et al., 2004). In recent years, social skills training has been applied extensively for disorders of which social skills deficits are a core feature, such as autism spectrum disorders.

Peers as intervention agents

Peer volunteers are increasingly involved in helping classmates with various psychological disorders. The peer volunteers range from preschool age through adolescence; they work on problems ranging from learning disability to conduct disorder to suicide prevention. A considerable literature has evolved regarding the selection and ongoing supervision of peer intervention agents as well as the ethical issues involved (see Rivera and Nangle, 2008 for a review). Although the main reasons for involving peers is certainly their availability and, in many cases, the responsiveness of one peer to another, a very substantial benefit is often improved peer relations. Not only may the peer helper bond with the child being helped, but the peer helper may also become a more helpful person and enhance the social reputation of the child being helped (Maher, 1984; Strain, 1985). Probably the most extensive involvement of peer helpers at this point is with children suffering from autism spectrum disorders; peer interventions for them are discussed in Chapter 17. A few other examples of the creative use of peer intervention agents follow.

Peer-led anti-bullying programs
Influenced by the extensive Finnish research on the vital role of "uninvolved bystanders" in

bully–victim encounters, Salmivalli and her colleagues (Karna et al., 2011; Salmivalli et al., 2011) trained early adolescents to function as peer counselors in implementing an anti-bullying program in Finnish schools. The peer counselors concentrated their efforts into an intensive 1-week campaign in the schools, during which they sensitized their fellow students to their own role in situations where they see other students being bullied. The program proved especially effective for girls, among whom it led to a clear reduction in bullying. Unfortunately, the effects were not as clear for boys (Salmivalli, 2001). Salmivalli and her Finnish colleagues are now working to combat school bullying in a more intensive program that still focuses on the "uninvolved bystander" but that is delivered by trained classroom teachers accompanied by information on bullying delivered by computer to primary-school pupils (the KiVa program, see Karna et al., 2011).

Working with peers on problems of playground aggression, Cunningham and his colleagues used a less didactic approach in their work in Canadian primary schools. Selected pupils were trained for 15 weeks to serve as conflict managers on the school playground. The conflict managers learned to intervene by using problem-solving skills to stop conflicts from escalating into serious fights. The program was highly successful. The conflict managers succeeded in resolving about 90 percent of the conflict. There was a significant drop in aggression, maintained at 1-year follow-up (Cunningham et al., 1998).

Sibling effects

According to a Vietnamese proverb, brothers and sisters are as close as hands and feet. The role of siblings in much of the literature in child psychopathology has been to help untangle the effects of genetics and of the environment, as discussed in Chapter 4. The many studies showing that siblings are likely to be similar to each other in problem behavior are generally difficult to interpret because the similarity may be due to shared genetic or shared environmental influences. Relatively little attention has been paid to how siblings affect each other's adjustment by means of their relationships. This gap in knowledge appears very gaping when one considers the extent to which siblings probably influence each other's development and adjustment. Ross and Howe (2009) emphasize the similarity between children's and adolescents' sibling relationships and their relationships with friends; sibling relations are much more like peer relations than are child–parent relations. Hence, children are likely to learn a great deal about how to manage friend relationships from their interactions with siblings. Furthermore, children are known to confide heavily in their siblings, constituting one of their earliest experiences of intimacy (Howe, Aquan-Assee and Bukowski, 1995). Siblings who share positive relationships are more likely than other siblings to spend time together and, therefore, to influence each other (Brody, 1998).

At the same time, sibling relationships are also characterized by considerable conflict. In middle childhood, this conflict often remains unresolved (Recchia and Howe, 2009). When siblings manage to learn to understand each other's perspectives on a social situation, they are likely to have fewer conflicts (Cutting and Dunn, 2006). Relatively little is known about how these aspects of sibling interaction are reflected in children's adjustment and psychopathology. However, the influence of siblings is probably quite strong.

Mature psychological separation from the family during adolescence includes some degree of separation from siblings as well as parents (Buhrmester and Furman, 1990). Nevertheless, siblings remain as very important sources of social support, often providing support in distinct ways that are not provided by either parents or friends (Lempers and Clark-Lempers, 1992; Seginer, 1992). Perhaps because siblings are relatively close in age, children are known to be particularly comfortable in seeking their support and advice (e.g., Moser and Jacob, 2002). It is not surprising, therefore, that some

research has elucidated parallels between the quality of sibling relations and psychopathology. Working with almost 300 Dutch two-child families, Branje et al. (2004) found that adolescents who were supported by their siblings were less likely than others to display externalizing symptoms. In contrast, adolescents who were in frequent conflict with their siblings were more likely than participants with less conflictual sibling relations to display internalizing symptoms such as depression or anxiety.

Interesting information also comes from a 7-year longitudinal study by Dunn and her colleagues (Dunn, Slomkowski and Beardsall, 1994), who followed a relatively small sample of thirty-nine sibling pairs for 7 years of their adolescent development. Siblings whose relationships were lacking in warmth, intimacy and friendliness were more likely than others to report high rates of both externalizing and internalizing problems. These findings suggest that sibling attachment may well merit much more attention than it has received. A model developed by Stewart, Beilfuss and Verbugge (1995) to describe adult sibling relationships may be a useful tool. These authors classify sibling relationships into the following categories: caregiver, buddy, critical, rival and casual. Just as different styles of parenting may have different effects on child adjustment, so may different ways of relating to siblings.

Going somewhat further, Yeh and Lempers (2004) conducted a 3-year longitudinal study with a larger sample (374 families) to learn more about some of the processes that may mediate the influences of siblings on adolescent adjustment. The analyses indicated support for the model: Adolescents who reported positive relationships with their siblings at the start of the study tended to report good friendship and high self-esteem the year after. In turn, friendship quality and self-esteem were negative predictors of loneliness and depression by the end of the study. Thus, the results suggest that the effects of the sibling bond on psychopathology may be mediated by the effects of siblings on adolescents' friendships and self-esteem. The interplay of sibling, parental and peer influences is depicted in Figure 7.3.

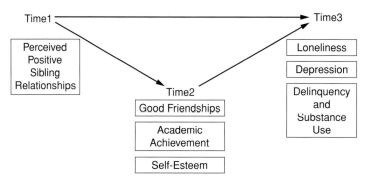

Figure 7.3 Siblings may indirectly influence adjustment outcomes in different ways.

Psychopathology redefined as a relationship construct

In contemporary scientific writings on child psychopathology, peers, friends and siblings have been being upgraded from the footnote status to which they were relegated in the early part of the twentieth century. As argued convincingly by Sroufe et al. (2000), relationships and problems in them can be: (1) features of disorders and criteria for their diagnosis; (2) risk factors for disorders; (3) protective factors in a resilience process that may prevent the onset of disorders; (4) moderators in the processes governing the appearance of disorders; (5) mediators in the processes governing the appearance of disorders; and (6) markers of subsequent disorder. Psychologists now recognize that much of what they call psychopathology is a process that occurs in relationships. Even psychoanalysts, who by definition are most interested in the goings-on within the individual psyche, are increasingly interested in the dynamics of interpersonal relationships, focusing on such issues as the use and abuse of power (Twemlow and Harvey, 2010). The challenge at this point is not only to refine the basic notion of psychopathology to reflect the extent that it is rooted in relationships but to apply that reality to assessment and diagnosis.

Summary

- Although the view that anti-social peer influences often negate the supportive influences of families is a common one, most often these two influences match with respect to their supportiveness, warmth and enjoyable interactions.
- Attachment theory can explain why children with secure bonds with their caregivers often end up with the ability to form intimate relationships with friends. Children can apply the social skills they have learned from their parents to these friendships.
- Peer relationships account for more of the adjustment or maladjustment of children than is often thought.
- The relative importance of parental and peer influences varies during childhood. In early childhood, parents are responsible for a large portion of their child's socialization, especially with regard to the companions with whom the children are allowed to associate.
- In middle childhood, peer influences become stronger as the child gains more autonomy. At

this stage, parents are still significant instructors and providers.

- In early adolescence, peer groups become the major influence for developmental learning, allowing youth the chance to practice social roles and behaviors and to shape their identities. It is during this stage that adolescents become particularly susceptible to peer pressure. In adolescent boys, changing brain structure and function can be related to risk-taking reward-seeking impulses grow while judgment is still immature. Peer groups are more likely to encourage risky behaviors than parents.

- Parents need to regulate their children's peer contact and find a healthy balance between excessive restriction and complete ignorance of their children's whereabouts.

- The dynamic cascade model describes the vicious circle child development undergoes when children are not provided with secure environments by the parents in early childhood. Ultimately, children do not learn the social and cognitive skills needed to relate to others, and parents find it more and more difficult to remedy the situation until adolescence when it is too late.

- Sometimes, the peer group can assume the role of the family, and vice versa. Very often, these are psychologically unhealthy situations.

- Several features of peer influence distinguish it from parental influence. Self-selection refers to the fact that children are responsible for choosing the peer group with which they will associate. A child may or may not display pre-existing deviant behavior before associating with a deviant peer group. Even if a child displays anti-social behavior before affiliating with an anti-social peer group, anti-social peer groups reinforce the propensity of anti-social behavior by talking about it and rewarding it.

- Peer influences are often intentional, in that children purposely modify their peers' behaviors for various reasons. Modeling occurs when a person imitates the behavior that he or she observes in another, such as a specific behavior,

dress or language. Certain individuals are more prone to peer influence than others due to their own personal problems.

- Thus, peer rejection and peer acceptance can both lead to psychopathology: Maladjustment is associated with being rejected by one's peer group, but peer acceptance into a socially deviant group also constitutes a risk factor.

- Cross-culturally, familial and peer influences can vary, although the switch from reliance on parents to investment in peer relations occurs everywhere. In collectivist, family-oriented societies, peer influences foster identity above and beyond the benefits of rich family life.

- Within classroom and school groups, peer rejection has long-lasting consequences, as rejected children have fewer opportunities to develop and practice positive social skills with their peers. Rejection also affects emotion regulation, classroom participation and academic achievement.

- Extracurricular activities play a large role in the socialization of children and adolescents, and can be a protective factor against the emergence of psychological distress, such as depression. However, some studies show an increase in aggression even among children who participate in non-combative sports. Others suggest that the benefits of these activities depend on the supportiveness of the other children involved.

- Cliques, small groups typically consisting of three to nine children often sharing a similar characteristic, have a very distinct role in the social development of the child. However, very little is known with regard to the consequences of cliques for child psychopathology.

- Close friendships differ from other peer relationships in terms of intimacy.

- Friends usually share some personal characteristics (principle of homophily).

- Intimacy is often incorrectly attributed solely to girls and women. However, boys and men may express their needs for intimacy in ways that differ from traditional female expressions of closeness.

- Chumship refers to a close relationship with a friend during early adolescence that serves as a preparation for the ability to form intimate romantic relationships later in life. Some theorists, especially Harry Stack Sullivan, believe that a lack of these relationships may lead to problems in close, intimate relationships later in life.

- Studies have shown that close friendship lessens the depressed affect seen in avoidant children that are excluded by their peers.

- Peer relations may serve as a marker (i.e., sign, see Box 7.1) of maladjustment and psychopathology. Early problems in peer relations are a clear and consistent marker of such difficulties during adulthood as schizophrenia, criminal behavior and alcoholism. In particular, peer rejection is a far stronger predictor of lifelong psychopathology than is peer neglect. Additionally, aggression is a stronger predictor of later maladjustment than shyness, although shyness has been linked to internalizing disorders such as anxiety and depression.

- The causal model refers to the idea that deficits in peer relations serve as precursors to psychopathology, whereas the incidental model depicts problems in peer relations as one of many consequences of a pre-existing psychopathology.

- Many but not all studies show that a lack of close friendships correlates with the emergence of psychopathology and other outcomes beyond the effects of general rejection by a larger peer group.

- Peer acceptance and friendship can help to a limited extent to protect the child against pre-existing risk factors, especially dysfunctional parenting.

- In some studies, friendship has been found to be a protective factor against post-traumatic stress disorder (PTSD) among children exposed to war-related traumatic events.

- Having a reciprocal best friend has been shown to be a protective factor for children at risk of becoming victims of bullies.

- Impaired peer relation can be considered a mediating variable (i.e., one that explains a correlation between two other variables). For example, lack of parental supervision can lead children to associate with anti-social peer groups, which, in turn, can lead to drug abuse.

- The deviance regulation theory describes two mechanisms that are involved in a youth's tendency to be influenced by peers: the dynamic tension between conformity and total expression of individuality and the normal socialization processes that result in youths being concerned about how their peers think of them.

- The social argumentation hypothesis is based on the idea that children, once rejected by the mainstream peer group, may associate with anti-social sub-groups or cliques.

- The arrested socialization hypothesis about the cause of deviant behavior centers around a developmental deficiency in cognitive or social processes which would normally allow the child to appropriately regulate his or her emotions, as being the main cause of deviant behavior.

- The intrasubjectivity hypothesis describes how children already prone to anti-social behavior collectively cultivate the beliefs that justify delinquency.

- In studies on conformity in childhood and adolescence, it has been found that participants with some form of personal vulnerability (e.g., negative self-image) are more likely to conform than were those without.

- Susceptibility to friends' influence may be correlated with increased substance abuse and depressive affect. Children and adolescents who excessively compare themselves to peers appear more likely than others to be influenced by peers into substance abuse and risky sexual behaviors.

- Another link between peer influence and psychopathology is found in the inaccurate perceptions that children may have about how their peers relate to them. Children and adolescents with major depression, social anxiety and conduct disorder are known to believe that their peers do not want to associate with them and/or wish to harm them.

- Interventions to enhance peer relations in children and adolescents with a psychological disorder may include social skills training (e.g., self-control, appropriate disagreement and interventions), using peers as intervention agents (e.g., peer-led anti-bullying programs).
- Many psychologists argue that psychopathology must be redefined with more emphasis being put on the interpersonal and relational aspects of the individual, with assessment and diagnosis to be changed accordingly.

Study questions

1. How typical is the situation often portrayed in literature and in the media in which positive family values are undermined by negative peer influences?
2. What age and cultural differences are thought to affect the extent to which the behavior of children and adolescents is influenced by their peers?
3. What is the self-selection factor in studies of peer influence and how does it affect the interpretation of the results?
4. What are the roles of peers in general and of "chums" specifically in the theory proposed by Harry Stack Sullivan?
5. Give at least one important reason why siblings may be more important sources of social support than parents in some circumstances.

8 Cultural dimensions of child psychopathology

Do as many children and adolescents of the Yoruba tribe in Nigeria get depressed as do children and adolescents in Norwegian fishing villages or members of street gangs in São Paulo, Brazil? If they do, are the features of their depressive episodes the same? Even if they are, can their depression be treated effectively by psychologists in essentially the same ways? Culture is so present in the thinking, feeling and behavior of individuals everywhere that its influence must be understood thoroughly when the causes, manifestations and treatment of psychopathology are contemplated (e.g., Hallowell, 1934).

In addition to the contact among cultures brought about by immigration, the influence of Western culture on non-Western parts of the world is also increasing because of the globalization of knowledge transmission in the sciences. Lambasting the ubiquitous Americanization of thinking about mental health around the world, Watters (2010) maintains that the wanton exportation of American thinking about mental disorder has resulted in the erosion of indigenous wisdom about psychological distress in other societies. Consequently, Western classification systems are applied to populations to which they may be inapplicable. Watters insists that non-Western people in some cases are actually beginning to suffer in ways that are being imported along with Western teachings about psychopathology.

This chapter begins with definitional and conceptual issues, starting with the definitions of culture itself. The chapter continues with a comparison of the universalist and relativist positions on the question of whether people in different cultures are similar enough to warrant ideas and categories of psychopathology that are applicable cross-culturally. Consideration is then given to the many mechanisms by which culture

may influence psychopathology, including shared values, religion, collective experiences of stress and beliefs about the determination of the fate of individuals. Subsequently, the vocabulary and tools of cross-cultural research are summarized, including the categories that researchers have developed for classifying cultures and the types of measures that are suitable for cross-cultural research. The growing place of culture in the DSM system is discussed next. The chapter ends with remarks about the need for cultural competence among child-clinical psychologists.

The concept of culture

Culture refers not only to the basic features of different societies but also to the values and beliefs of their members. Table 8.1 contains a selection of the definitions of culture that have been proposed by scholars of different disciplines. It should be noted that these definitions, heterogeneous as they are, have been criticized for placing culture within the individual, focusing on individual thinking and values. Lopez and Guarnaccia (2000) argue that culture is produced as much by action in the social and physical environment as by any process that occurs within the minds of individual people. Far from being something that individuals receive passively from their environments, culture is a dynamic, creative process that evolves from environmental features in interaction with individuals' responses to their social environments and their adaptation to changes in them. It is important to bear in mind that the definitions in Table 8.1 apply to the perceptions, thoughts, values and behaviors of groups of people at a given point in time. However, cultures change, sometimes radically.

Table 8.1 **Selected definitions of culture**

"Culture is defined as the shared patterns of behaviors and interactions, cognitive constructs, and affective understanding that are learned through a process of socialization. These shared patterns identify the members of a culture group while also distinguishing those of another group."

Center for Advanced Research in Language Association, University of Minnesota www.carla.umn.edu/culture/ definitions.html

"Most social scientists today view culture as consisting primarily of the symbolic, ideational, and intangible aspects of human societies. The essence of a culture is not its artifacts, tools, or other tangible cultural elements but how the members of the group interpret, use, and perceive them. It is the values, symbols, interpretations, and perspectives that distinguish one people from another in modernized societies; it is not material objects and other tangible aspects of human societies. People within a culture usually interpret the meaning of symbols, artifacts, and behaviors in the same or in similar ways."

Banks and McGee Banks, 1989, p. 367

"Culture: learned and shared human patterns or models for living; day-to-day living patterns; these patterns and models pervade all aspects of human social interaction. Culture is mankind's primary adaptive mechanism" (p. 367).

Damen, 1987, p. 51

"Culture is the collective programming of the mind which distinguishes the members of one category of people from another" (p. 51).

Hofstede, 1984, p. 51

"By culture we mean all those historically created designs for living, explicit and implicit, rational, irrational, and nonrational, which exist at any given time as potential guides for the behavior of men."

Kluckhohn and Kelly, 1945

"Culture consists of patterns, explicit and implicit, of and for behavior acquired and transmitted by symbols, constituting the distinctive achievements of human groups, including their embodiments in artifacts; the essential core of culture consists of traditional (i.e. historically derived and selected) ideas and especially their attached values; culture systems may, on the one hand, be considered as products of action, and, on the other, as conditioning elements of further action."

Kroeber and Kluckhohn,1952, p. 357

"Culture is the shared knowledge and schemes created by a set of people for perceiving, interpreting, expressing, and responding to the social realities around them" (p. 9).

Lederach,1995, p. 9

"A culture is a configuration of learned behaviors and results of behavior whose component elements are shared and transmitted by the members of a particular society" (p. 32).

Linton,1945, p. 32

"Culture ... consists in those patterns relative to behavior and the products of human action which may be inherited, that is, passed on from generation to generation independently of the biological genes" (p. 8).

Parson,1949, p. 8

"Culture has been defined in a number of ways, but most simply, as the learned and shared behavior of a community of interacting human beings" (p. 169).

Useem, Useem and Donoghue, 1963

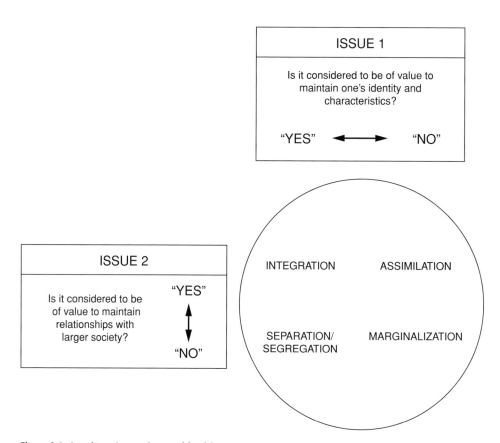

Figure 8.1 Acculturation and mental health.

Because of immigration, the media and education, contact between cultures in the contemporary world is very extensive. In general, this contact tends to make members of non-Western cultures increasingly familiar with Western culture and, in many ways, more similar to members of Western cultures.

Also worthy of attention is the fact that many large, industrial societies are complex and multifaceted. Within the same country, different ethnic groups may have their own cultures. At the same time, people of different socio-economic levels may have different values, priorities and norms, or, according to many of the definitions, their own cultures. Furthermore, members of immigrant groups may belong at the same time to both the culture of their countries of origin and the culture of the host country. Figure 8.1, based on the work of

Professor John Berry, depicts the different strategies immigrants may use as they contemplate their futures in their new countries. Immigrants from the same country to the same country may vary in terms of their *acculturation* – their voluntary or involuntary identification with the host culture. They may embrace their cultures of origin at times of stress or turn their backs on their cultures of origin to seek whatever relief they can obtain from Western science. Finally, because of intermarriage, many people have multiple cultural origins and belong simultaneously to different cultures. This unprecedented blending of the world's cultures is a source of richness and interest but can be, at the same time, a source of stress. Cross-cultural research in child psychopathology rarely if ever captures these complex realities.

Universalist and relativist positions on the cross-cultural similarity of children's mental disorders

As noted by Hooley, Maher and Maher (2013), what is considered normal in one culture may not be considered normal in another. For example, flagellating oneself with a whip may be considered a normal and laudable act of penitence in some religious groups but a pathological form of masochism by others. The globalization of concepts of child psychopathology can be considered at least partially legitimate if the basic structure of psychopathology, including the classification of the disorders, their definitions and core symptoms, their consequences for the people affected and the degree of overlap between different disorders are essentially the same for all members of the human species. Those are, in essence, the assumptions of the *universalist* position. The evidence supporting the universalist position and the basis of its opposite, the *relativist* position, is reviewed succinctly by Canino and Alegria (2008).

Perhaps the most useful clarification of the universalist position in Canino and Alegria's paper is their delineation of what the universalist position does *not* imply. They emphasize that even if the basic structure and definition of child mental disorders are universal, there may still be important cultural differences in the manifestations of the disorders. In other words, the ways in which a young person with conduct disorder displays the disorder may not be identical in every culture. His or her defiance may be more overt in one culture but might be displayed in a more passive way, but one that nonetheless involves defiance of authority, in another. The terms *ethnotypic consistency* and *heterotypic continuity* are used to describe the assumptions that what is referred to as the same disorder (e.g., depression or attention deficit) is actually very much the same in different cultures and/or at different stages of development, respectively (Weisz et al., 1997; Canino and Alegria, 2008). Canino and Alegria also explain that the universality of definitions of child normality and pathology are not negated by different *thresholds* in

different cultures for considering a child's behavior abnormal or problematic. Some cultures may be more tolerant than others of children's anxiety, social withdrawal or aggression.

There may also be differences among societies in the stresses of daily life that increase the risk for a particular disorder. These risk factors might include, for example, economic hardship or street violence. Conversely, daily life in some societies may result in more protective factors that reduce the risk of disorder, such as a supportive, effective educational system, good nutrition or opportunities for harmonious interpersonal relationships. Consequently, the rates of some disorders may be higher in some societies than in others. Nevertheless, differences between cultures in the incidence rates of specific disorders do not invalidate the universalist position because the basic definition and core symptom cluster overlap with other disorders, and outcome for persons affected with the disorders may remain invariant across cultures (Canino and Alegria, 2008).

In contrast with proponents of a universalist stance, many critics of current mental health practice insist that the influence of culture is so great that culture must be an integral part of the basic diagnostic process and of diagnostic systems. Accordingly, culture should determine in a fundamental way professionals' concepts of impairment and disorder, including the basic definitions of the disorders. Advocates of a relativist position disagree with the basic assumption in the DSM that disorder is largely located within the individual even though its outward manifestations may differ from person to person, place to place. The essence of the relativist position is that the basic understanding and definition of pathology must be conducted in reference to each culture and, hence, must be replicated in each culture. Therefore, neither current diagnostic systems such as the DSM and ICD nor any conceivable revisions can be considered applicable in all cultures, even if such systems allow minor modifications of the diagnostic process to accommodate cultural differences (e.g., Weisz, Jensen-Doss and Hawley, 2006).

The consensus of experts is that the debate between proponents of the universalist and relativist positions is to be resolved by more and better research (e.g., Nikapota and Rutter, 2010). Several scholars have specified exactly what would make the research better (Bird, 2002; Robins and Guze, 1970). First of all, helping professionals in different cultures should describe the disorder in essentially the same way (*face validity*). Secondly, the risk and protective factors that increase or decrease the manifestations of the disorder should be similar in different cultures. As well, the patterns of comorbidity between the disorder in question and other disorders should be similar across cultures. Furthermore, consequences for individuals affected by the disorder in terms of their physical and mental health should be similar. Finally, children in different cultures should respond in similar ways to standard treatments designed to alleviate the condition.

Complicating any effort at adjudicating between the universalist and relativist positions by empirical research is the fact that the instruments used for diagnosing disorder may not be equally valid in all cultures. Therefore, Canino and Alegria (2008) propose the additional criterion of cross-cultural validity of the measurement tools used in the diagnosis of the disorder in question. Indeed, there can be no meaningful implementation of the criteria proposed by Bird (2002) or by Robins and Guze (1970) in the absence of adequate instrumentation.

Using Bird's criteria, Canino and Alegria (2008) summarize the evidence available for evaluating the cross-cultural validity of standard diagnostic schemes for child psychopathology. They first address the issue of the face validity of the disorders in different cultures. The most extensive research on this issue conducted with children pertains to attention deficit/hyperactivity disorder (ADHD), and is reviewed by Bird (2002). The fact that there has been so much research on ADHD is certainly related to the accusation, discussed in detail in Chapter 14, that ADHD is a fabrication of North American society and its pharmaceutical companies. Despite these accusations, research conducted in such non-Western

countries as China, Japan, Brazil and South Africa reveals that parents and clinicians recognize the core DSM symptoms of ADHD as troublesome. The basic two-factor structure of the disorder (i.e., impulsivity and hyperactivity, see Chapter 14) also recurs in many heterogeneous cultures. Although the concept of ADHD does thus seem to be applicable to many cultures, its prevalence does vary from country to country (Polanczyk et al., 2007). This may occur because parents and teachers in some societies, such as those of East Asia, may be less tolerant of disruptive behaviors than are other parents (e.g., Ho et al., 1996).

However, recurrent symptom clusters not explained by the DSM or ICD have also been described in the research literature on children's difficulties in some non-Western cultures. Standard symptom checklists completed by Thai parents, for example, indicate that some groups of Thai children exhibit problematic patterns of behavioral immaturity, covert delinquency and preoccupation with sex that do not correspond with either patterns of parental responses in the United States or standard diagnostic classifications (Weisz et al., 1997). A common phenomenon in Latin America is *nerve attacks* (*ataques de nervios*), which is discussed in DSM-5 in the section on cultural issues to be considered in diagnosing anxiety disorders. It involves uncontrolled screaming, crying and trembling, sometimes accompanied by verbal and/ or physical aggression, fainting and seizure-like behavior. Canino et al. (2004) reported that 9 percent of the child population appears to experience *ataques de nervios* at some point. Another culturally related syndrome is *taijin kyofushu*, a form of anxiety that is very common in Japan and Korea that manifests itself as well among adolescents of East Asian background whose parents or grandparents have immigrated to Western countries. *Taijin kyofushu* involves an excessive fear of appearing offensive to others because of one's appearance, gaze or body odor (Kim, Rapee and Gaston, 2008).

Canino and Alegria (2008) remark that the current data base provides little reason to believe that there is substantial cross-cultural variation in the risk and protective factors that regulate the incidence of child mental health disorders in different cultures. In many cultures, boys are at greater risk than girls of the same ages for such externalizing conditions as conduct disorder and ADHD, whereas girls are somewhat more likely to be affected by depression and anxiety (Costello, Erkanli and Angold, 2006; Crijnen, Achenbach and Verhulst, 1997). A comprehensive meta-analysis of data from many countries indicates that adolescents in different cultures are much more likely than school-age children to suffer from depression (Costello et al., 2006). Harmonious family relations appear to function as protective factors that reduce the incidence of externalizing disorders among the US majority culture (Roberts and Roberts, 2007), in Puerto Rico (Bird et al., 2006) and in Cuba (Schneider, Lee and Alvarez-Valvidia, 2012). Thus, available data on the correlates of atypical child behavior and on the major disorders that affect children and adolescents, together with data on the workings of risk and protective factors, indicate little systematic cross-cultural variation.

Canino and Alegria conclude, similarly, that there is substantial consistency across cultures in the outcomes of the major mental disorders of childhood and adolescence and in the patterns of comorbidity among the disorders. For example, in most cultures, externalizing disorders such as conduct disorder and attention deficit are more likely than internalizing disorders to persist and lead to long-term maladjustment than are depression, social withdrawal or anxiety (Nottelmann and Jensen, 1995), which is not to say that these internalizing problems are not important and debilitating. The comorbidity rates for anxiety and depression are high in many cultures, and there is usually some co-occurrence of these internalizing problems and conduct disorder (Zoccolillo, 1992). Turning to the cross-cultural similarity in response to the standard treatment of the major children's mental health disorders, Canino and Alegria (2008) observe that the very few studies available have not detected any sizeable differences in response to treatment among different cultural groups in the United States or between the United

States and the other countries that have been studied, which include Australia, New Zealand, Norway, Spain and the UK. Obviously, this is a very limited sampling of the world's cultures. It is very possible that many treatments that work well in the United States may not be as successful in the Third World. For example, Schneider, Karcher and Schlapkohl (1999) argue that *cognitive-behavior therapy*, which features rational analysis of the social situations that the individuals in treatment find troublesome, is very heavily interwoven with the linear, rational mode of thinking that pervades Western philosophy and religion. Individuals who are influenced, for example, by the basic teaching of Hinduism or Buddhism may not find this form of analysis acceptable.

Other researchers place greater emphasis than do Canino and Alegria on the fact that some of the well-defined DSM "symptom" clusters may exist in some cultures but not cause marked impairment. One salient example is research published by Canadian researchers Vasey and Bartlett (2007), who gathered data in Samoa about *fa'afafine*, boys and men who displayed gender variance (see Chapter 24) but without the dysphoria needed to diagnose gender dysphoria in DSM-5. The male participants in their research dressed as girls, assumed girls' roles in pretend play and sometimes adopted a female identity during some of their formative years. Some of the participants did experience occasional dislike of their genitals and dislike of some of the roles expected for men in their society, such as physical labor. However, by and large, the *fa'afafine* did not report substantial distress because of their adoption of female roles and were in general tolerated quite well by the surrounding Samoan society. Only a minority of their parents made any sizeable efforts to discourage their feminine ways. Based on these observations, Vasey and Bartlett raise considerable objection to considering such gender-atypical self-presentations as forms of psychopathology. Their arguments may leave many skeptics unconvinced because acceptance of effeminate boys is so rare around the world that the Samoan example may be regarded as the proverbial exception that proves the rule. Another more global contribution of the Samoan research is to underscore the importance of understanding the cultural context of mental health and mental illness.

Far less dramatic but convincing in a very different way are other data showing that children and adolescents in some cultures are likely to exhibit many of the syndromes recognized in the DSM system at about the same rate as in the DSM field trials conducted in the United States. However, in many cases, the prevalence rates plummet when an *impairment criterion* is applied to filter out cases in which the symptoms are present but general life functioning is not markedly affected. This occurred, for example, in an epidemiological study conducted in Hong Kong by Leung and his colleagues (2008). The impairment criterion resulted in a dramatic reduction in the rates of diagnosable anxiety and substance abuse, with lesser reductions in depression and disruptive behavior disorders.

The bottom line offered by Canino and Alegria is that the evidence for the universalist and relativistic positions weighs in differently according to the specific disorder. Nevertheless, their review paper provides more evidence for the universalist position than is often recognized. It is important to remember that many relativists would dispute Canino and Alegria's contention that the different ways in which the disorders are manifest in different cultures and the differences in prevalence rates are but details that do not negate the basic similarity of the disorders across the human species. Cultural differences in the individual disorders are considered later in this book in the chapters devoted to them.

Mediating mechanisms: how culture shapes children's mental health and mental illness

Religion

Religion is a guiding force for many parents of non-Western cultural background. Their religious beliefs may or may not steer them away from seeking help for their children in distress from practitioners oriented toward the beliefs and practices of "First

World" psychology and psychiatry. As enumerated by Spika, Hood and Gorsuch (1985), religion may affect psychopathology in many different ways. In its most positive manifestation, religion can function as a form of therapy, curing the pathological condition. Religion may also lead the believer to suppress potentially deviant behavior that the religion would consider sinful. Religion may also function as a refuge in which an individual may conceal his or her psychopathology. It is also possible that the psychopathology may be expressed in some religious manner. Finally, in extreme cases, religion can be a cause of the pathology.

Many religions prescribe an ideal way of living, adherence to which may be seen as the path to recovery from mental illness. Conversely, failure to follow the prescribed way of managing one's life and/ or raising one's children may be seen as the cause of mental illness. This is evident in both Muslim and Jewish religious teachings. There is a biblical passage in Deuteronomy warning that those who turn away from the teachings of the Covenant "shall be mad for the sake of thine eyes which thou shalt see" (Deuteronomy 28:34). According to Buddhist teachings, mental suffering may emerge from the belief that the self is solid and unchanging. Distress may also be the product of unwholesome thoughts that are characterized by greed, hatred and delusion. The believer should not feel guilty about having those thoughts. However, dwelling on them, overidentifying with them and acting on them is seen as causing excessive rage, tension and anxiety. In order to avoid the resulting undesirable mental states, the individual should practice meditation in order to achieve the insight and mindfulness necessary for the elimination of maladaptive thoughts and their consequences. Understandably, an individual with such beliefs may be unenthusiastic about participating, for example, in a diagnostic interview with the purpose of determining where his or her distress lies within a diagnostic system like the DSM or ICD (Chawla and Marlatt, 2006). However, the observant client might be more responsive to a psychological intervention that included elements of spirituality. Religious beliefs may be inconsistent with the quest for objectivity that is the hallmark of diagnostic systems like DSM and ICD. For example, Hindu and Ayurvedic beliefs about the connection of the individual to the spiritual world have been seen as inspiring a greater emphasis on the subjectivity of human experience than is valued by practitioners who seek to reconcile their practices with scientific knowledge (Bhugra, 2007). Although the strict requirements of some traditional religions, in terms of both thoughts and practices, may cause stress for individuals who are not willing or able to comply, it is important to consider all aspects of the traditional religious doctrine and its application. For example, Rotenberg (2012), commenting on the education of young people in Orthodox Judaism, comments on the benefits of the intellectual exercise inherent in their study of the holy writings. In this context, different interpretations of the Bible are considered and debated. Such cognitive enrichment may in fact leave the young scholars cognitively flexible and, therefore, resilient to stress.

There have been many appeals to incorporate spirituality into the therapeutic process rather than having therapists compete with the religious beliefs of their non-Western clients. For example, mindfulness mediation has been employed, with some success, in the treatment of children's and adolescents' anxiety and behavior problems (e.g., Twohig et al., 2010). Rather than competing with practitioners of faith-based healing, it may be highly beneficial for clinical psychologists to encourage observant parents to complement the therapy delivered according to established mainstream procedures with the methods of healing prescribed by their religions.

Such understanding of the religious beliefs of individuals and families in distress need not, of course, be limited to persons of non-Western cultural background. According to a survey by Hathaway, Scott and Garver (2004), most practicing psychologists in the United States are somewhat aware of the role of religion in mental health but are not sure of how to apply these issues to their professional work. Miller and Kelley (2006) present an interesting argument for spiritually oriented psychotherapy with young people and their observant Protestant families in a chapter describing their experience with religiously observant adolescents of mainstream US culture. They insist that any inclusion of the spiritual dimension in the therapeutic context cannot and need not come at the expense of techniques or insights from the secular literature on psychopathology or psychotherapy. They also recognize that improvement obtained with conventional, mainstream methods can lead to spiritual growth as well as any technique rooted in spirituality or religion. Their own therapeutic work is based on a *client-centered framework* inspired by the psychology of Carl Rogers (Rogers, 1951). This therapeutic modality is based on heightened sensitivity to the client's feelings; it is devoid of the directive, instructional stance used by therapists practicing, for example, cognitive-behavioral therapy.

CASE STUDIES: Working with Sophie and Gillian to integrate religious beliefs with resolution of psychological problems

Miller and Kelley present two interesting case examples of their therapeutic work. The first case is that of Sophie, a 7-year-old with learning disabilities, especially in reading. Sophie was first taken to a conventional therapist who, after assessing Sophie, suggested a change of schools. In a more spiritually oriented client-centered intervention, Sophie's parents learned to reinterpret the nightly help with Sophie's schoolwork as an opportunity to connect with her rather than as a frustrating chore. The parents also learned to re-examine their values, rethinking what they came to see as their excessive emphasis on academic achievement at the expense of other important things in life.

The second case is that of Gillian, a 14-year-old having difficulty adjusting to the relatively impersonal environment of her secondary school after a transition from a primary school at which she was very comfortable and happy. She felt anxious and socially rejected in her new school. In spiritually oriented client-centered therapy it was discovered that Gillian engaged in moments of reflection and prayer in the morning that were very meaningful to her. In child-centered psychotherapy, Gillian learned to engage in a moment of spiritual reflection before entering school. When she found herself feeling alone and outside of the in-group, Gillian learned to remind herself that we are all children of God.

The refugee experience

Many children who have experienced the trials of war and of becoming refugees suffer severe psychological distress. Some of these children have immigrated to Western countries, where they face the dual challenge of adapting to very unfamiliar cultures and attempting to overcome the trauma of what they have lived through. Betancourt and colleagues (2009) interviewed children, adolescents and their adult caregivers in a camp for refugees in war-torn Northern Uganda. They discovered a wide range of psychological problems, only some of which could be explained by the diagnostic criteria for post-traumatic stress disorder in DSM-5 (see Chapter 23). Some of the children experienced a problem known locally as *two-tam*, having "a lot of thoughts," which involved poor self-esteem, feelings of hopelessness and poor concentration. Others suffered from a condition known as *kumu*, of which the central feature is persistent grief or sadness, often manifested by self-isolation, crying, loss of energy and many worries. In addition to these and several other local variants of mood and anxiety disorders, another group of refugee children displayed a form of oppositional defiant disorder or conduct disorder. Their symptoms ranged from rudeness, foul language and disobedience to deceitfulness and substance abuse.

When the traumata of the war and refugee experiences are compounded by the challenges of immigration, mental health problems abound. As detailed by Ellis and her colleagues (2010), who have worked with Somali refugee immigrants to the New England States of the United States, relatively few of the mental health problems of refugee immigrant children are ever brought to the attention of professionals. Many refugee immigrant children and their families receive help from religious leaders and from school personnel. However, and most unfortunately, most of the suffering is kept hidden. Among the reasons for this is the distrust by many refugee parents of authority figures, whom they associate even with helping professionals in their new host countries. As well, some parents may not wish to discuss – or have their children discuss – the terrifying experiences they have survived. It is encouraging that Ellis and her colleagues (2013) were able to implement a comprehensive prevention program with this population of Somali refugees. Through a combination of school-based group treatment and selective individual therapy, their mental health improved significantly, with these improvements maintained at 1-year follow-up.

Cultural beliefs about the causation of disorders

Culture often includes thinking about the origin of problems and about their resolution. Very often, these beliefs collide with the ways in which Western behavioral scientists understand the same phenomena. Many traditional Muslims, for example, believe that mental illness is linked with a failure to follow the healthy ways of living that are prescribed in the Quran (Ali, Milstein and Marzuk, 2005). At the same time, the family plays so fundamental a role in Arab culture that it is the family that is often charged with bringing about relief, with religious guidance (el-Islam, 2008). Parenting is considered so fundamental by many traditional cultures that children's psychological problems may almost invariably be attributed to faulty discipline or upbringing at home. However, some parents of Caribbean or Bangladeshi origin may believe that supernatural forces bring about mental illness (McCabe and Priebe, 2004). As a general rule, members of Western cultures with high levels of secular education are more likely than others to believe that mental health problems might be caused by biological factors. This is probably attributable in large part to the strong belief by members of non-Western cultures in other causal factors, including those mentioned earlier in this paragraph. However, there are important exceptions to the general belief among non-Western peoples in the environmental causation of psychopathology. In some cultures, having an environmentally caused psychological problem is a source of shame for individuals and their families. In those cultures, psychological difficulties may be presented to helping professionals in terms of their physiological manifestations. In fact, psychological stress may actually come to be expressed somatically to an astounding degree. It has been noted by professionals serving Chinese people, either in China or in Chinese communities overseas, that many individuals seeking help for somatic issues bring with them psychological problems that they have suppressed or do not want to recognize (e.g., Chun, Enomoto and Sue, 1996).

There are also many cultures in which mental illness is attributed to biological factors but where biology is understood in ways that differ from prevailing thinking in Western medicine. For example, in traditional Chinese medicine, the body and mind are treated together in a combined effort to achieve a balance of yin (negative) and yang (positive) energies (Hwang et al., 2008). Many Native Americans believe in the interconnectedness of humans, their fellows, the Creator and nature. Therefore, there can be no separation of healing

from spiritual belief or power. In many tribes, mental illness may be attributed to an imbalance among the spiritual, social, physical and mental interactions of an individual, his/her family or clan. Relief from mental illness is based on restoring the balance. Communities may play a primary role in bringing about the renewal of both body and spirit, often by participating in healing ceremonies for a community member in distress (Bennahum, 1998).

The skepticism of many non-Western persons about the biological origins of psychopathology is sometimes translated into low expectations for the success of treatment by medication. Expectation effects are very important determinants of the effectiveness of medication on psychological conditions, probably much more important than many practitioners who prescribe medication believe or want to believe. The general evidence for this is the very potent effect of *placebo* tablets, which look like actual medication but contain no active ingredients. Placebo effects, especially in the context of medication for child and adolescent psychological problems, are quite substantial in general (e.g., Cohen, D. et al., 2010). It has also been shown in some studies that placebo effects manifest themselves differentially in different cultures. There is even some suggestion in the literature that placebo pills of different colors evoke different expectations in different cultures (Buckalew and Coffield, 1982).

Culturally based doubts about the effectiveness of prescribed medication can lead not only to different placebo effects in different cultures but also to non-compliance with the prescription and to different side effects. Although the evidence is not entirely conclusive because of methodological problems in the research, it has been suggested that in very action-oriented populations, such as among English-speaking Canadians, agitation may be a more common side effect of sedative medications that are prescribed to bring relaxation and calm than in other groups such as French-speaking Canadians. Interestingly, the possibility that there is sometimes a genuine basis for culturally linked uncertainty about the effects of psychotropic medication cannot be totally ruled out. Because genetic endowment varies somewhat by country and community, genetic factors that may increase or decrease responsiveness to specific chemical compounds in different population groups are not totally inconceivable (Lin, Smith and Ortiz, 2001).

On the other hand, cultural factors may also clash head-on with Western scientific beliefs about the cognitive bases of psychopathology and treatments based on the modification of dysfunctional thinking processes. As mentioned earlier in this chapter, cognitive-behavioral therapy is firmly rooted in linear rational thinking. The individual is encouraged to keep things in perspective, consider a wide array of solutions to a problem and react in a controlled, systematic manner. This approach is antithetical to the concept of change in Eastern, particularly Buddhist, thinking, which, as mentioned earlier in this chapter, emphasizes awareness, spirituality and the cultivation of a pure, healthy lifestyle (Dwivedi, 2006; Schneider et al., 1999). Mental illness may be the result of lack of awareness of one's true place in the world and in the cosmos. Hence, "cure" may come about through experiences that heighten awareness, such as meditation, not from rational argumentation. Such spiritually oriented content is already being integrated with cognitive and relational approaches by therapists working with both Western and non-Western clients.

The self-system

Culture affects individuals' *self-construals* – the ways in which they interpret their own identities. These self-construals are thought to affect their understanding of the behaviors of people around them (Markus and Kitayama, 1991). Self-construals, according to influential theorists Markus and Kitayama (1991) may be either independent or interdependent. An independent self-construal emphasizes the autonomy of the individual whereas an interdependent self-construal emphasizes the individual's belonging to a larger social group. Unlike individuals with interdependent self-construals, people with independent self-construals may attribute

the behavior of another person or other persons to the individual's personality traits (Na and Kitayama, 2011). Interdependent self-construal may lead to excessive concern about violating perceived social norms, often resulting in anxiety (Essau et al., 2012).

Values and aspirations

Members of different cultures may regard certain child behaviors as normal or abnormal in light of their values in child-rearing and their aspirations for their children's futures. This may change in the same culture over time. Therefore, any given study of child psychopathology in a given culture is no more than a snapshot – a representation of things as they were when the study was conducted. A particularly interesting set of studies has been conducted in China concerning the social consequences of children's shyness and social anxiety. Early research by Chen revealed that, unlike schoolchildren in English Canada, primary-school children in China held shy children in very positive regard, reflecting the society's precept that modesty is a virtue, especially among children (Chen et al., 1998). However, more recent research conducted after the advent of a market economy and, surely, increased competition in schools, shows that, as in most other countries, shyness has become a reason for which children are rejected by their peers (Chen et al., 2005).

Recurring conceptual and methodological issues in cross-cultural research on child psychopathology

Culture as an independent variable

Whatever the objective of cross-cultural research in psychopathology, it is important for the researcher to measure directly the aspects of the cultures that are relevant to his or her hypotheses. For example, a researcher might hypothesize that learning disabilities constitute a greater impairment in China than in the United States because of Chinese parents' valuing of high educational achievement. In this situation, it is important for the researcher not only to collect data about the correlates of learning disabilities in China and the United States but also to collect data from the parents in each country about their values and their priorities for their children. Thus the data obtained from parents would serve, first of all, to confirm the researcher's assumptions about the two cultures. Furthermore, there will most likely be some variation in parents' emphasis on education within each country. With complete data, the researcher can confirm that differences *between* cultures are indeed bigger than differences *within* cultures.

Hypotheses about cultural dimensions of psychopathology often evolve from the rich vocabulary developed by cross-cultural psychologists to describe cultures. Many of the categories used in classifying cultures come from empirical research in which adults in different countries have described their values and priorities (Hofstede, 2003; Schwartz and Ros, 1995). The most important distinction emerging from this body of research is between individualism and collectivism. Members of *individualistic cultures* construct their self-identities as individual persons. They may value their autonomy to a great degree and believe that it is appropriate and important for people to be able to pursue their own goals. In contrast, members of collectivistic cultures derive much of their sense of identity from their belonging to larger groups such as their extended families, communities or nations. Although the distinction between individualistic and collectivistic cultures has been found in extensive research to explain many important features of societies and behaviors of individuals, some authorities believe that the value of this construct has been exaggerated at times (see meta-analysis and discussion of these issues by Oyserman and Lee, 2008).

As cultures evolve, some may retain their traditional collectivism in certain domains of life while becoming more individualistic in others. An important example of this is the contemporary culture of South Korea, where identification with the extended family group and society still prevails although it now co-exists with considerable individualism in the areas of education and work (Kim and Choi, 1994). In studying

the individualism or collectivism of other cultures, researchers from individualistic societies must discard some of their own values. It has indeed been found that the trait of individualism is not necessarily adaptive or healthy, even in societies that tend to be individualistic (Richardson, 1995)

The vocabulary for describing cultures includes other important elements in addition to individualism/collectivism that are overlooked all too frequently. *Power distance* refers to the degree to which persons of lower status in a culture accept and consider legitimate the authority of persons of higher status. The confusing term *masculinity/ femininity* includes the allowance for expressions of emotion and compassion in a culture. In cultures high in *uncertainty avoidance*, rules for behavior and expectations for compliance are very clear and strong.

These dimensions may predict how parents and teachers perceive the healthiness or pathology in children's behavior because parents tend to raise their children to function successfully in the cultures that await them as adults. Therefore, a parent living in a collectivistic culture with high power distance, masculinity and uncertainty avoidance, for example, may consider it normal and necessary for children to be polite, respectful and obedient. At the same time, a parent in an individualistic "feminine" culture low in power distance may consider it normal and desirable for his or her children to express their feelings and wishes and to learn to rely on themselves.

These and other dimensions of culture can inspire cross-cultural research in child psychopathology in several different ways. If a researcher wants to prove that the core features and correlates of a particular disorder are universal, as discussed later in this chapter, he or she might refer to these dimensions in selecting cultures that are as different as possible. If, however, the researcher wants to demonstrate that particular features of a culture are linked to patterns of child psychopathology in it (or their absence), he or she should sample as far as possible from societies that are known to vary in terms of the feature of interest.

Although descriptions of the core values of societies that may be found in literature or scientific writings are valuable, the usefulness of these descriptions by themselves as bolsters of the independent variable of culture in research design tends to be limited. Within a specific country or community, individuals are likely to vary in their core values, which may also change as societies change. Therefore, little may be achieved by describing the sample used by a researcher as individualistic or collectivistic, for example, on the basis of some reference to an outside source. It is far better to measure the core values of the participants directly, using instruments that are valid in the cultures being studied.

A study conducted in two different countries may not represent the true range of cultural differences between the countries. This desired comparison is only achieved if the samples of participants in the two countries are similar in education, income, age, family status and occupational prestige. Cultural minorities may not reflect the core values of multicultural societies. On the other hand, members of the traditional majority cultures of those societies may not represent the blend of cultures that now characterizes many large Western nations.

Dependent measures that may be associated with cultural variation

Like all other empirical research, cross-cultural research in child psychopathology can be no more useful than the soundness of the measures used in it. This means that the measurement tools must be reliable and valid in each culture being studied. This is a gargantuan challenge, made complex by the fact that most measures are developed in the Western countries where the profession of psychology is the best established. Not only are few measures developed or adapted in other places but the very fact of data being collected by an investigator about people's lives, problems and feelings may by itself lack ecological validity.

The cross-cultural literature contains extensive guidelines for the adaptation of questionnaires for cross-cultural research. Table 8.2 is a summary of the pertinent issues. The problems begin with the

translation of the items themselves. It is difficult to say enough about this issue. Pena (2007) outlines the criteria for the acceptable translation of research instruments. Some safeguards exist to ensure linguistic equivalence, such as having the translation checked by retranslating the translated items back to their original language and comparing the results with the original instrument. However, even if every word is translated accurately, the translated version may not sound the same as the original to native speakers of the two languages involved. The translated version, even if technically accurate, may evoke a stronger reaction than the original because of culturally laden associations that were not evoked in the original language. Furthermore, any psychological processes or psychological constructs, for example depression, must be equally familiar to readers in the different cultures being studied (Van de Vijver and Poortinga, 1997).

Psychometric equivalence

The translated items of a questionnaire are grouped together in ways that may function in similar fashion in different languages and cultures. The criteria for psychometric equivalence are described in a useful volume by Van de Vijver and Leung (1997). As detailed in that book, ideally, the statistical factor structure of the questionnaire should replicate in all the cultures studied. The items should be endorsed with the same relative frequency in each culture (in more technical terms, they should be of equal "difficulty"). They should also be equivalent in social desirability across cultures. In other words, the items should not evoke greater social stigma in one culture than in another. The response format (e.g., a seven-point scale) should be one that evokes similar response styles in different cultures, as opposed to a prevalence of extreme high or extreme low scores in one or more of the cultures involved. These standards are most often approximated in cross-cultural studies conducted with university students and/or business people, who, although more amenable to participating in research than many of their compatriots, may not represent their cultures very accurately.

Table 8.2 **Possible sources of bias in cross-cultural assessment**

Kind of bias	Source
Construct	– incomplete overlap of definitions of the construct across cultures
	– differential appropriateness of item content (e.g., skills do not belong to the repertoire of either cultural group)
	– poor sampling of all relevant behaviors (e.g., short instruments covering broad constructs)
	– incomplete coverage of the psychological construct
Method	– differential social desirability
	– differential response styles such as extremity scoring and acquiescence
	– differential stimulus familiarity
	– lack of comparability of samples (e.g., differences in educational background, age or gender composition)
	– differences in physical testing conditions
	– differential familiarity with response procedures
	– tester effects
	– communication problems between subject and tester in either cultural group
Item	– poor item translation
	– inadequate item formulation (e.g., complex wording)
	– one or a few items may invoke additional traits or abilities
	– incidental differences in appropriateness of the item content (e.g., topic of item of educational test not in curriculum in one cultural group)

Only a few researchers have managed to go beyond questionnaires in their cross-cultural explorations of child psychopathology, yielding very interesting results that would not have emerged had they not selected more intensive measurement strategies than are commonly used. In their comparisons of problematic child behavior in the United States, Thailand and Jamaica, Lambert, Weisz and colleagues have employed such techniques as vignettes containing descriptions of child behavior (Lambert et al., 1992) and logs of the problems that lead to the referral of children for professional help (Lambert, Weisz and Knight, 1989) as well as ratings by parents. In a particularly revealing study, noted both for its methodological implications and for its findings, Weisz et al. (1995) conducted direct observations of children at play in the United States and in Thailand. They discovered that there were many more instances of maladaptive behavior among the Thai children being observed. This is exactly the opposite of what they had found previously in a study based on parental reports. Their overall conclusion is that, although there may be more such behaviors as aggression or social withdrawal among Thai children, Thai parents have a higher threshold than that of US parents for considering such difficulties as serious and as warranting professional intervention.

Mixing qualitative and quantitative methods

It has been argued that researchers need to go beyond numerical representations of the world in order to meaningfully conduct research in cultures that differ from their own in fundamental ways that they may not understand completely. Yoshikawa and colleagues (2008) point out that the world can be understood not only by analyzing numbers but also by analyzing non-numerical ways of representing the world, such as words, texts, narratives and observations. They argue that judicious use of such *qualitative methods* will lead to more comprehensive understanding of complex causal mechanisms that underlie the phenomena being explored; these complex mechanisms may elude a purely quantitative approach. Despite their enthusiasm for mixing qualitative and quantitative methods, these authors disagree with the very informal sampling methods that are used in much qualitative research, arguing that systematic, purposive sampling of the population can and should be done in quantitative methods. Anthropologists have spearheaded comprehensive observational field work in cultures around the world for years. However, Yoshikawa et al. argue against the compartmentalization of researchers both by discipline and by methodological allegiance (2008). They call on psychologists to be more amenable than they have been traditionally to mixing qualitative and quantitative research strategies (i.e., to using *mixed models*) in order to better achieve their research objectives. Based on their opinion, the United States is in many ways an "outlier" compared to the cultures around the world to which US researchers hope to generalize their findings (p. 348). For that reason, they maintain that these mixed models are particularly applicable when researchers based in the United States conduct research in other cultures.

Researchers planning cross-cultural research and consumers who read and interpret the results must decide how much to heed the methodological caveats mentioned in this section, all of which are never overcome. Therefore, these methodological issues should be remembered when interpreting data, and not used to totally dismiss results that are based on methods that are less than perfect. Ultimately, in studying another culture, all researchers are biased by their own culturally based values to a lesser or greater extent, whatever quantitative or qualitative methods they apply.

Culture in the DSM and ICD systems

As introduced earlier, too much cultural variation can be seen as a fundamental threat to traditional classification schemes, which are based on the implicit assumptions that most disorders are universal and inherent to the human organism. Therefore, it is not surprising that recognition of cultural differences has been slow to emerge in the DSM and ICD. It was not until the development of DSM-IV in the 1990s that consideration was given to a serious role for cultural factors, as chronicled by Mezzich et al. (1999).

When DSM-IV appeared in 1994, it included the first explicit recognition of culture in a major classification scheme for mental disorders. Recommendations for the ways that culture should be considered in the DSM-IV were formulated by a Work Group on Culture and Diagnosis that cooperated and negotiated with the DSM-IV Commission as an independent entity. Only some of the recommendations of that work group were ever incorporated into the final product. The first important step was the reminder in the Introduction that the DSM is the work of professionals largely based in the United States, which undoubtedly reflects the cultural background of those who created it. In the Introduction, the clinician is reminded that culture must be considered when using DSM-IV in a multicultural society. These admonitions are brief and unelaborated but nevertheless notable because of their presence.

The DSM-IV and its successor DSM-5 also include some recognition of cultural considerations in the diagnostic process. It is recognized that culture may influence the prevalence of some disorders and it may also influence the symptoms of the same disorders that are manifested to different degrees by individuals in different cultures. Important as this initial recognition of culture has been, many experts on cultural factors in mental health have commented on their limitations. Nothing was included that might lead to a cultural challenge to the basic "architecture" of the system, perhaps implying that the structure of the system or its major diagnostic categories or its delineation of what constitutes a disorder might not be valid cross-culturally (Mezzich et al., 1999). Other critics have commented that the DSM, for the most part, considers culture as the range of cultural groups present in the United States, not around the world. Relegating culture-bound syndromes to the appendix has been seen as minimizing the more general role of culture and depicting it as "exotic" (Lopez and Guarnaccia, 2000).

Although general guidelines for clinical assessment were discussed in DSM-IV, the new DSM-5 also provides a very useful sixteen-point Cultural Formation Interview. The interview consists of questions about culture that can be interspersed into the normal diagnostic process. In administering the interview, clinicians formulate questions about, for example, the individual's cultural identity by asking directly about the individual's cultural background and the aspects of that cultural background that the person feels are most important. In another section, the interviewers ask about the causes that people who are close to the individual in distress believe to be at the root of the problem (American Psychiatric Association, 2013).

The section on cultural formation in DSM-5 concludes with a number of perceptive observations about culture. Clinicians are reminded, for example, that there is rarely a one-to-one match between cultural concepts of mental illness and DSM disorders. Furthermore, cultural concepts of mental distress may include worries that do not correspond to any diagnosable disorders. A cultural concept of a disorder, such as depression, may apply to more than one DSM-5 diagnosis; a person considered "depressed" in a cultural community may have disorders in addition to major depression (and may not have diagnosable major depression). The DSM-5 section contains a reminder that "like culture and DSM itself" (p. 758), cultural construal of mental illness may change over time (American Psychiatric Association, 2013). Unfortunately, these wise words appear in a section at the end of the DSM-5 manual that may not be part of the usual diagnostic process.

It should be noted that there are a few places in the world where the DSM and ICD are so alien to the ways in which mental health services are delivered that local mental health professionals have developed their own alternatives. These include the Latin American Guide for Psychiatric Diagnosis (Berganza, Mezzich and Jorge, 2002) and the Cuban Glossary of Psychiatry (Otero-Ojeda, 2002). Interestingly, these systems, which have had minimal impact outside their countries of origin, depart fundamentally from the basic assumptions of the ICD-10, on which they are based. The Cuban system, for example, has resuscitated the classic Freudian concept of neurosis. It describes the trajectories of many of the disorders so that their earlier forms, not yet warranting formal diagnosis, can be identified. Not surprisingly, given the prevailing ideology in the country, the Cuban system ascribes a major role to contextual factors in the etiology of the conditions it describes. Interestingly, these Latin American alternatives are built in large part from "the bottom up," that is, they start by classifying symptoms, then explaining what disorder might be behind them, rather than the "top-down" approach of classifying disorders and then specifying their symptoms. Unfortunately, no data are available to indicate whether these conceptual adaptations to the contemporary Cuban reality occur at the expense of objectivity and validity, which are the hallmarks of the latest revisions of the DSM and ICD.

Promoting the cultural competence of child-clinical psychologists

It is a sad reality that, despite the fact that members of minority cultural groups are subject to considerable stress, they often fail to seek help for their psychological problems or those of their children (Hwang et al., 2008). Recognizing this, the professional bodies that regulate the practice of psychology increasingly emphasize cultural sensitivity as an important and integral part of the training of psychologists (American Psychological Association, 2003; Australian Psychological Society,

2004; Fernando, 2005). Davidson (1999) described three fundamental aspects of cultural competence training for psychologists: knowledge, skills and awareness. One aspect of cultural competence training for psychologists involves knowing how culture affects the diagnostic and treatment process and learning in detail about the culture or cultures with which the future psychologists will work. In order to successfully take advantage of such knowledge, the psychologist must learn the skills needed to relate to clients of cultural backgrounds dissimilar to his/her own. This includes learning how to include assessment of the client's and/or the client's parents' cultural orientation into the helping process. Finally, the psychologist must learn to be aware of the ways his/her own culture affects all aspects of his/her diagnostic and therapeutic work. Considerable skill is required for a clinician to know when and how to apply these skills to an individual case, without either ignoring important culture issues that are relevant to clinical care or stereotyping the parents and children seeking help.

CASE STUDY: the *familismo* of Latin America and the depression and irritability of Jose, 8 years old

Zebracki and Stancin (2007) present an interesting case study that illustrates the way culture became an important part of the clinical care of Jose, who was an 8-year-old born in Puerto Rico but now living in the Midwest of the United States. Jose was referred by his family doctor because of depression and sleeplessness. Normally good-natured and well-behaved, Jose was beginning to become frustrated over many small things that happened in his daily life. He was also starting to argue with his mother and younger brother and disobey his parents.

It was obvious at the time of referral that Jose's behavior was related to his father's recent diagnosis of terminal brain cancer, even though the family had not told Jose the truth about what was behind the changes in family atmosphere that the child undoubtedly perceived. In seventeen sessions of psychotherapy, some with Jose, some with his mother, Jose was supported during the loss and bereavement process. A year later, all symptoms had abated despite the recurrence of occasional mild depressed feelings.

The first cultural issue discussed by Zebracki and Stancin is the timing of the referral and the fact that it took place. Although it had been suggested that Jose be seen for counseling at the time of his father's initial medical tests, Jose was not referred until a year after his father's diagnosis and only when his somatic problems brought him to the attention of his family doctor. Zebracki and Stancin speculate that parents of Latin American origin are reluctant to discuss personal problems with outsiders. Before any outside professional service is sought, members of this culture may wait until all family members are in agreement and until it is clear that the counsel of family members and clergy will be insufficient.

Culturally based fatalism, the belief that Dad's cancer was God's will, may have been a source of strength for the family, as was their belief that Dad would go to heaven. The authors believe that *marianismo* was a strong factor in Jose's mother's decision to conceal his father's diagnosis. Marianismo is an aspect of the female gender role in Hispanic society, where women are expected to be pure, passive but somewhat stoic, to care for others and to uphold high moral standards, perhaps higher than those of men (Stevens, 1973). Accordingly, Mom thought it best to bear the burden of knowing what would happen to Dad by herself and to continue looking after her children. In several sessions, the therapist encouraged her to be truthful with Jose. When she finally accepted this suggestion, Jose's problem behaviors diminished. However, after Dad's death, *Latin American machismo*, the cultural expectation that men be strong if not chauvinistic and hold their families together, probably emerged when the family started to expect Jose to help care for his younger brother and to provide emotional support for his grieving mother. The remaining challenge for the therapist was to reconcile Jose's new role as male head of his family with his need, as a child, to grieve.

Summary

- Culture, referring to both the basic features of different societies and the values and beliefs of their members, is an important influence on psychopathology.
- Many definitions of culture have been regarded as too focused on the individual and not enough on the dynamic aspects of social and physical environments, such as immigration, the media and inter-culture contact.
- Within the same society, different cultures may exist among socio-economic groups, ethnic groups and immigrant groups. Acculturation describes the voluntary or involuntary identification of immigrants from the same culture with the host culture to which they are immigrating.
- Due to intermarriage, many people have multiple cultural origins and belong to multiple cultures, a reality that has not been studied sufficiently in child psychopathology.
- Often, non-Western cultures are subject to the standards of psychopathology from the Western world, which may lead to the diagnosis of conditions that do not interfere with daily life.
- Cross-cultural studies in psychology have been motivated by attempts to specify the interactions

- of genetic and environmental forces in the nature–nurture debate.
- Cross-cultural research in the domain of developmental psychopathology is an ever-growing field. Scholars advocate precise methodological techniques to ensure that cultural differences are not overlooked.
- The universalist position refers to the idea that the fundamentals of psychopathology (classification, diagnosis, etc.), are the same for all members of the human species. There is a small section in DSM for disorders specific to certain culture.
- Proponents clarify the universalist position by emphasizing the fact that there may be different thresholds for diagnosis in different cultures, although ethnotypic consistency (i.e., similarity among cultures) and heterotypic continuity (i.e., stability across development) do exist regardless of these thresholds.
- Risk factors and protective factors may be quite different in different societies, which may lead to a higher or lower prevalence of diagnosable mental illness in some cultures.
- The relativist position contrasts with the universalist position by stating that the

assumption made in the DSM that disorders are located within the individual and not influenced by culture is incorrect. Thus, proponents of the relevant position maintain that no diagnosis can be applied universally in all cultures, even if cultural sensitivity is part of the diagnostic process.

- Cultural differences in maladjustment may vary depending on age group or historical era. More research is needed to understand both culture-specific and seemingly universal risk factors for children of different ages.

- Some major disorders that affect children and adolescents have been found to manifest themselves in similar ways across some cultures, such as the higher incidence of depression in adolescents than children and the finding that externalizing disorders are more likely than internalizing disorders to lead to long-term maladjustment in children and adolescents.

- An important issue to consider when conducting cross-cultural research is the impairment criterion, the requirement that the disorder must affect general life function regardless of the presence of symptoms. It has been shown that the same symptoms may lead to different consequences in different cultures.

- Religion can act as both a protective factor and a risk factor for psychopathology in a number of ways. It can act as a form of therapy, suppress potentially deviant behavior and act as a refuge from the pain that accompanies the disorder.

- Spirituality has been successfully incorporated into the therapeutic process, using, for example mindfulness mediation, in order to avoid competing with the religions of non-Western clients.

- However, some scholars insist that spiritual therapy must not reduce the techniques or insights from the secular literature on psychopathology or psychotherapy.

- A client-centered framework, where there is a heightened sensitivity to the client's feelings, has been adopted by some clinical psychologists working in cultures other than their own.

- Children who have suffered through war often develop various psychopathologies upon immigrating to Western countries and having to adapt to unfamiliar cultures and overcome their past trauma. Many of these problems remain undetected by professionals because they are kept private by families and communities.

- In general, members of Western cultures, which are more characterized by secular education than are other cultures, are more likely than members of non-Western cultures to believe that mental health problems are caused by biological factors.

- A problem with the use of medication in non-Western countries is skepticism about its effects. Placebo effects, for tablets that look like medication but have no active ingredients to alleviate mental illness, seem to vary across cultures.

- Some scholars have suggested that genetic factors that vary by country and community may actually account for increases or decreases in responsiveness to certain psychotropic medication.

- Cognitive-based treatments (e.g., cognitive-behavioral therapy), which often focus on linear rational thinking, may go against non-Western philosophies, in which awareness and spirituality dominate thinking.

- One important flaw in cross-cultural research may be resolved by directly measuring the features of the cultures that are thought to be relevant to the hypothesis.

- When comparing different cultures, participants must be similar in education, income, age, family status and occupational prestige.

- Linguistic equivalence (i.e., proper translations) and psychometric equivalence (i.e., equal difficulty and social desirability) must be verified to ensure valid measurement tools.

- Some researchers argue that there must be a proper mix of quantitative methods and qualitative methods (i.e., mixed models) to accurately describe the complex features and consequences of culture.

- The lack of cultural sensitivity in the DSM and ICD continues to be criticized widely.
- Cross-cultural researchers emphasize training for psychologists based on three fundamental aspects of cultural competency: knowledge, skills and awareness.

- The DSM-5 manual contains an interview for use by clinicians for learning about an individual's cultural identity and about the meaning of an individual's psychological problems in his or her culture. This interview appears toward the end of the manual as a supplement to normal diagnostic procedure.

Study questions

1. What is the most useful definition of culture for research in child psychopathology? Provide reasons for your choice.
2. What is the difference between individualistic and collectivistic cultures and what are the implications of this difference for psychopathology?
3. In what ways does culture affect the likelihood that a parent will seek psychological help for a child or adolescent?
4. Name some problems in using standard questionnaires developed in North America or Europe with Asian, African and/or Latin American populations?
5. In your opinion, is it reasonable to use the DSM or ICD in cultures around the world? Give the reasons for you answer.

9 Psychological assessment as part of the caring process

In the definition they propose of the psychological assessment of children, Ollendick and Hersen (1993) indicate what assessment should be and what it often but not always is: "an exploratory, hypothesis-testing process in which a range of developmentally sensitive and empirically validated procedures is used to understand a given child...and to formulate and evaluate specific intervention procedures" (p. 6). This image of assessment as the application of psychological science at the beginning of the helping process differs sharply from stereotypes and, to a considerable degree, from the routine testing that is a not uncommon vestige of earlier eras, as will be discussed later in this chapter. At its best, psychological assessment is the complete antithesis of the reading of tea leaves by fortune tellers. Children are not brought to psychologists to be "tested" like automobile batteries; they are brought so that the psychologist might engage with them and their parents in finding out what may explain the child's problems and how the problems might best be alleviated. Tests may be part of the process but tests constitute only some of the data that are used to confirm or disconfirm hypotheses that emerge mostly from an informed understanding of the problem that has brought the child and family to seek help.

Elaborating on the steps involved in conducting psychological assessment in such a therapeutic way, Finn (2007) enumerates several essential components of the process. First of all, clients (i.e., in the case of the assessment of children, parents, teachers and, to the extent their development permits, children) must be helped to formulate the questions they would like to see answered during the assessment process. The goals of the assessment are then specified collaboratively. Finally, the assessment results, including the information on which the psychologist's conclusions and recommendations are based, are discussed fully and empathically. Clients participate collaboratively in discussing what the results mean to them and in helping the psychologist make sense of them. Importantly, as noted by Johnston and Murray (2003), in hypothesis-based psychological assessment, the goal of the particular assessment should determine to a considerable degree the specific assessment measures that the psychologist uses.

An exhaustive list of tests, questionnaires and other assessment instruments is beyond the scope of this book. Excellent coverage of the various assessment instruments available to child psychologists is available in several recent texts devoted to psychological assessment, including the fifth edition of *Assessment of Children: Behavioral, Social and Clinical Foundations* by Sattler and Hoge (2006) and *Clinical Assessment of Child and Adolescent Personality and Behavior*, by Frick, Barry and Kamphaus (2010). An online database of psychological tests, PsycTESTS, was introduced recently by the American Psychological Association.

This chapter begins with a statement of the importance of using methodologically sound instruments in the assessment of children's psychological functioning. The next part of the chapter is devoted to a delineation of the different psychological processes that might be assessed by a child-clinical psychologist, such as intelligence, atypical behavior and personality. The methods used to understand these processes, such as standardized tests, interviews and direct observation, are compared. The chapter closes with some speculative remarks about the future of psychological assessment as part of the process of helping children and adolescents experiencing psychological distress.

Good measurement as part of good assessment

None of the previous discussion of collaborative, hypothesis-based assessment means that good measurement, including appropriate use of good tests, is no longer important. The proper place of measurement in psychological assessment is summarized by Cecil R. Reynolds, a prolific researcher on the assessment of children and editor of the very reputable journal *Psychological Assessment*:

If a thing exists, it can be measured – not always well, at least at first, but it can be measured. Measurement is a central component of assessment if we believe that fear, anxiety, intelligence, self-esteem, attention and similar latent variables are useful to us in developing an understanding of the human condition and leading us to ways to improve it. Clinical assessment…goes beyond measurement to deal with the development of a broader understanding of individuals and phenomena than measurement alone can provide. Yet without accurate, valid measurements, we are seriously handicapped in our clinical endeavors. (2010, p. 1)

Offering another very useful observation about the role of good measurement in good assessment, Reynolds (2010) remarked that a test by itself is not valid or invalid; it is the *use* of the test and the interpretations of the results that may be valid or invalid. This applies particularly to intelligence tests, which, as will be discussed later, are very valid for the purposes for which they were developed. However, some psychologists have reified these excellent instruments and used them for diagnosing virtually every form of psychopathology, often without satisfactory evidence of their validity.

A common pitfall occurs when the purported evidence for the discriminant validity of an instrument is that individuals who are known to suffer from the disorder typically perform differently from non-diagnosed individuals on the test in question. That happens very often: Clinical populations differ from non-clinical populations on many measures. It is necessary – and much more difficult – to prove that a measurement tool is valid in distinguishing different forms of psychopathology from one another (Reynolds, 2010). One way of reducing erroneous and excessive interpretation of assessment tools may be to focus more heavily on the theories that guide the development of these instruments. McFall (2005) remarks that a test or measure can be no better than its underlying theoretical and measurement models, just as water cannot travel higher than its source. He enjoins psychologists not to mimic the atheoretical approach taken, for example, by actuaries who determine the premiums applicable to insurance policies by calculating the statistical likelihood of an insured person encountering a particular calamity.

Beyond the issue of the validity of a specific test or tool for the purpose for which it is used is the question of how much a specific instrument may add to those already being used by an individual psychologist or clinic, its *incremental validity* (Johnston and Murray, 2003; Meehl, 1960). Incremental validity depends, of course, on the purpose of the assessment. A child's or adolescent's self-report of depressive feelings may be very sufficient for establishing a diagnosis of major depressive disorder. Ratings of the depression by teachers and/or parents may not add much useful information, which does not at all mean that those ratings are invalid by themselves. Self-reports by themselves are not as useful in diagnosing externalizing disorders such as disruptive behavior disorders or attention deficit. Incremental validity in these cases refers to the various tools available for obtaining information from adult informants and direct observation of the problem or problems.

A psychologist may be able to determine, for example, whether a child or adolescent has an attention problem from ratings completed by the child's teachers and/or parents. Observing the child in the classroom might be a valid way of assessing attention but it may not be worth the additional time and effort. However, if the goals of the assessment include finding out whether there is any way for the teacher to improve the child's attention, classroom observation may well pay off.

An assessment tool must be valid not only for the purpose for which it is being used but also for the population with which it is being used. The overwhelming majority of assessment instruments were developed originally in the majority cultures of Western countries. It is imperative that they then be validated in other cultures where they are to be used. Such cross-cultural validation has, fortunately, become standard practice among many of the major publishers of instruments for psychological assessment. It is important to safeguard as best as one can against language that might be interpreted as particularly stigmatizing in a specific culture and especially against examples of a disorder that are not applicable to the culture to which a measure is adapted. Considerable attention must be devoted to the thorny enterprise of translation. Words for describing emotions and states of mind are particularly difficult to translate. It has been noted that cross-cultural bias may be greater when symptoms are less severe than in cases where the pathology is so disabling that it is likely to be immediately evident in any cultural setting (e.g., Achenbach and Rescorla, 2007; Fields, 2010; Sabatier, 2003; see also Chapter 8).

Constructs that may be explored

Diagnostic status – structured diagnostic interviews

One common goal of psychological assessment is to determine the DSM or ICD diagnosis or diagnoses that correspond to the behaviors of the child being

assessed. Assessments focused on the construct of mental health diagnosis are most common in hospitals and psychiatric clinics. As detailed in Chapter 3, the most persuasive selling point of the most recent revisions of both the DSM and ICD systems is improved and more reliable diagnosis. Therefore, diagnostic interviews based largely on the symptoms specified for the disorders have been developed in conjunction with the diagnostic manuals. These interviews are usually highly structured: Typically, a standard series of questions is asked using the exact wording indicated in the protocol. "Probe" questions are added to obtain additional detail following certain pre-specified responses. Although structured diagnostic interviews for children exist, the parent is the interviewee in many if not most cases. The data from many of the structured interviews, which are usually tape-recorded, feed into statistical algorithms that indicate whether the disorder in question is applicable. These results indicate only that the data correspond to a diagnosis. As the results are not usually referenced to a normative population, one shortcoming of most structured interview methods is that no indication is provided as to how common or uncommon either a specific behavior or the complete diagnostic profile might be (Frick, Barry and Kamphaus, 2010).

The best-known example of a structured diagnostic interview for child psychopathology is the Diagnostic Interview Schedule for Children – IV (DISC-IV; Shaffer et al., 2000). A parallel instrument based on DSM-5 is being developed. The complete interview, which may take up to 2 hours, provides diagnostic data relevant to thirty-six mental health disorders; sample questions appear in Box 9.1. A self-administered version using automated voice prompts is in the final stages of development. Shorter interviews are available that focus on a narrower range of disorders. The time saving comes at a cost, however, given the known high rates of comorbidity among many of the disorders (Le Couteur and Gardner, 2010). Among of the best-known structured interviews that are designed for a relatively restricted

Box 9.1   **Example of stem/contingent question from DISC-IV
(Major Depression)**

I'm now going to ask you some questions about feeling sad and unhappy.

1. In the last year – that is, since you started seventh grade – was there a time when you often felt sad or depressed?

IF YES

A. Was there a time in the last year when you felt sad or depressed for a long time each day?

IF NOT, GO TO Q 2

B. Would you say that you felt that way for **most of the day?**
C. Was there a time when you felt sad or depressed **almost every day?**

IF NO, GO TO Q 2

D. In the last year, were there 2 weeks in a row when you felt sad or depressed almost every day?

IF NO, GO TO Q 2

E. When you were sad or depressed, did you feel better if something good happened or was about to happen to you?
F. Now, what about the **last 4 weeks?** Since the beginning of August, have you felt sad or depressed?

Source: Reprinted from *Journal of the American Academy of Child and Adolescent Psychiatry*, vol. 39, Shaffer, D., Fisher, P., Lucas, C. P., Dulcan, M. K., and Schwab-Stone, M. E., NIMH Diagnostic Interview Schedule for Children Version IV (NIMH DISC-IV): Description, Differences from Previous Versions, and Reliability of Some Common Diagnoses, pp. 28–38, Copyright 2000, with permission from Elsevier.

range of problems is the Kiddie-Schedule for Affective Disorders and Schizophrenia (K-SADS; Ambrosini, 2000), the Anxiety Disorders Interview Schedule – Child/Parent version (Silverman and Albano, 2004) and the Autism Diagnostic Interview – Revised (Rutter, Le Couteur and Lord, 2003).

Structured diagnostic interviews have generally been shown to achieve their stated purpose – reliability of diagnosis (Frick, Barry and Kamphaus,

2010; Le Couteur and Gardner, 2010). It should be noted that structured interviews do differ among themselves somewhat in terms of the degree of standardization in their intended use. The K-SADs protocol allows the clinician to select the questions to be asked; no such leeway is allowed in the DISC-IV (Le Couteur and Gardner, 2010). It is very possible that the degree of standardization involved in the DISC-IV is necessary to ensure that the questions needed to establish conclusive diagnoses are asked in a clear and understandable manner. Obviously, the rote administration of standard questions will differ from the personal conversational styles of most clinicians. There is a trade-off here: Asking questions in a standard way has been proven to be the best way of eliciting *facts*, whereas asking questions in an empathic personal style appears to be the best way of eliciting the expression of *emotion* (Cox, Rutter and Hollbrook, 1981; Le Couteur and Gardner, 2010). For that reason, structured diagnostic interviews are considered excellent for diagnostic purposes but certainly not a good way to develop rapport with clients or for establishing the working relationship needed for future collaboration in psychotherapy (Mash and Hunsley, 2005).

The amount of time taken to administer the entire sets of questions involved in structured diagnostic interviews has been questioned. Facilitative as they are of reliable diagnosis, there is some lingering doubt about their incremental validity (see above, this chapter). One criticism of the empirical status of structured interviews is that the interviews can be no better than the diagnostic categories to which they correspond (Frick, Barry and Kamphaus, 2010). As noted in Chapter 3, the internal consistency of some of the DSM diagnostic categories has been questioned. Hopefully, this issue will be less pertinent to DSM-5 and to the revision of the ICD that will appear in a few years.

One final criticism of structured diagnostic interviews is that the parent is very often the sole informant. This fits the hospital settings where many diagnostic interviews take place: Teachers rarely participate in diagnostic procedures there. However, information from teachers is invaluable in diagnosing and remediating the many maladaptive behaviors that are seen most often at school (Frick, Barry and Kamphaus, 2010).

Checklists and questionnaires

Paper-and-pencil checklists and questionnaires are used widely in psychological assessment, as will be discussed later in this chapter. Only occasionally, however, are they used to determine a DSM or ICD diagnosis. One important advantage of checklist/ questionnaire methods over structured interviews is economy. Portability is another advantage. A checklist can be completed while a family is in the waiting room of a clinic. A checklist can also be completed by people, such as teachers, who tend not to be physically present at the setting where the assessment is conducted, especially if it is a hospital, clinic or the office of a psychologist in private practice.

Unlike most structured interviews, the development of most checklists and questionnaires includes a standardization process that yields norms that permit comparison with other children and adolescents of the same age and sex. Other psychometric properties such as test–retest reliability are established. Individual items are scrutinized in a number of ways, to see how they relate to other items and scales and to the criterion, that is, diagnostic status. Responses to checklists and questionnaires can be examined for positive and negative *halo effects*, that is, indiscriminately describing the person being rated as either positive or negative in all respects. Other forms of *response bias*, such as avoiding the negative points 1 and 2 on a 1–5 scale, can be spotted, or avoiding the extreme points, 1 and 5. For example, the widely used Conners-3 scales, which are self-report, parent and teacher report scales for the assessment of attention deficit hyperactivity disorder (Conners, 2008) contain indices to indicate a tendency to project a general negative impression, positive impression, as well as general inconsistency in the responses.

Lost when a diagnostician opts for paper-and-pencil methods rather than interviews is the personal contact with the interviewer, which may yield invaluable diagnostic information that could temper the confidence placed in the actual data obtained. It can be argued that diagnostic interviews, especially when administered by computer, are more like questionnaires when the interviews are highly structured and standardized. Nevertheless, it is not considered responsible to base a diagnosis entirely on a paper-and-pencil instrument.

Although diagnostic status is sometimes inferred from questionnaires and checklists, these instruments rarely consist solely of items that correspond directly to the symptoms needed for DSM or ICD diagnoses. More often, the items represent a variety of descriptors of the disorder or disorders in question. Based on the data gathered during the development of the questionnaire or checklist, a cut-off point is often established, with scores above the cut-off point indicating the disorder. An example is the Social Phobia and Anxiety Inventory for Children (Beider, Turner and Fink, 1996). This scale consists of twenty-six items, each of which can be answered with scores ranging from 0 (never) to 2 (often). Thus, the maximum score possible is 52. Examination of the distributions of scores in several studies indicates that scores of 20 or higher are likely indicative of social anxicty (Inderbitzen-Nolan, Davies and McKeon, 2004; Morris and Masia, 1998). Of course, a cut-off score is only part of the information needed to make a conclusion about diagnostic status. It should be noted that among the prevailing ethical standards for the use of tests and other standardized instruments (American Educational Research Association, American Psychological Association, National Council on Measurement in Education, 1999) is the stipulation that when a cut-off score is used for decisions about individuals, the score must be justified by supporting data, as has been achieved for the Social Phobia and Anxiety Inventory for Children.

The best-developed and most comprehensive set of checklists for the assessment of child psychopathology is the Achenbach System of Empirically Based Assessment (ASEBA; Achenbach and Rescorla, 2000, 2001). This system includes separate rating scales for various age ranges starting with preschool. The parent and teacher rating scales are the most frequently used at all ages. In completing these scales, the parents and teachers indicate on a 0–2 scale how well the items describe the child. The items are descriptions of a large number (112 for the school-age versions) of problems such as "acts too young for his/her age" and "destroys his or her things." There is also a

youth self-report for adolescents. The scales yield scores for the broad dimensions of externalizing and internalizing as well as eight more specific scales: Anxious/Depressed, Withdrawn/Depressed, Somatic Complaints, Social Problem, Thought Problems, Attention Problems, Rule-Breaking Behavior and Aggressive Behavior. These are not exactly DSM categories but the scoring provides a way of using the items that are most similar to the symptoms specified in the DSM to achieve a DSM diagnosis. The ASEBA is one of the few instruments available with specific norms for multicultural groups, a guide for interpretation in several different cultures and translations into many languages (www.aseba.org, retrieved February 20, 2011).

Personality

The objective of psychological assessment may be to determine not the child's diagnostic status but to gather information about his or her personality or temperament. Frick, Barry and Kamphaus (2010) point out that assessing people's personality in an informal way is part of the daily modes of thinking and relating by most people. Parents – especially parents who have raised more than one child – often "assess" the temperaments of their children. The assessment of personality or temperament involves identifying *traits* that characterize the individual being assessed. Traits can be defined as "relatively stable dispositions to engage in particular acts ... or ways of thinking" (Frick, Barry and Kamphaus (2010, p. 4). For example, shyness, irascibility and outgoingness can be considered traits. The term *personality* is typically used in reference to the traits of adults; the term *temperament* is the parallel term used more often in reference to children. The pioneering research of Chess and Thomas has yielded a useful typology of children's temperaments (see Table 9.1), based on such dimensions as the child's activity level, the intensity of his/her reactions to stimuli, distractibility, reactions to approaches by other people, adaptability, mood and attention span. The temperament types

Table 9.1 Temperament types as delineated by Chess, Thomas and colleagues

TEMPERAMENTAL QUALITY	RATING	2 MONTHS	6 MONTHS	1 YEAR	2 YEARS	5 YEARS	10 YEARS
ACTIVITY LEVEL	HIGH	Moves often in sleep. Wriggles when diaper is changed.	Tries to stand in tub and splashes. Bounces in crib. Crawls after dog.	Drinks rapidly. Eats eagerly. Climbs into everything.	Climbs furniture. Explores. Gets in and out of bed while being put to sleep.	Leaves table often during meals. Always runs.	Plays ball and engages in other sports. Cannot sit still long enough to do homework.
	LOW	Does not move when being dressed or during sleep.	Passive in bath. Plays quietly in crib and falls asleep.	Drinks bottle slowly. Goes to sleep easily. Allows nail-cutting without fussing.	Enjoys quiet play with puzzles. Can listen to records for hours.	Takes a long time to dress. Sits quietly on long automobile rides.	Likes chess and reading. Eats very slowly.
RHYTHMICITY	REGULAR	Has been on 4-hour feeding schedule since born. Regular bowel movement.	Is asleep at 6:30 every night. Awakes 7:00 AM. Food intake is constant.	Sleeps after lunch each day. Always drinks bottle before bed.	Eats big lunch each day. Always has a snack before bedtime.	Falls asleep when put to bed. Bowel movement regular.	Eats only at mealtimes. Sleeps the same amount of time each night.
	IRREGULAR	Awakes at a different time each morning. Size of feeding varies.	Length of nap varies; so does food intake.	Will fall asleep for an hour or more. Moves bowels at a different time each day.	Nap time changes from day to day. Toilet training is difficult because bowel movement is unpredictable.	Food intake varies; so does time of bowel movement.	Food intake varies. Falls asleep at a different time each night.
DISTRACTIBILITY	DISTRACTIBLE	Will stop crying when diaper is changed. Stops fussing if given pacifier when diaper is being changed.	Stops crying when mother sings. Will remain still while clothing is changed or given a toy.	Cries when face is washed unless it is made into a game.	Will stop tantrum if another activity is suggested.	Can be coaxed out of forbidden activity by being led into something else.	Needs absolute silence for homework. Has hard time choosing a shirt in a store because they all appeal to him.

	1	2	3	4	5	6
NOT DISTRACTIBLE	Will not stop crying when diaper is changed. Fusses after eating, even if rocked.	Stops crying only after dressing is finished. Cries until given bottle.	Cries when toy is taken away and rejects substitute.	Screams if refused some desired object. Ignores mother's calling.	Seems not to hear if involved in favorite activity. Cries for a long time when hurt.	Can read a book while television set is at high volume. Does chores on schedule.
APPROVAL/ WITHDRAWAL — POSITIVE (APPROVAL)	Smiles and licks washcloth. Has always liked bottle.	Likes new food. Enjoys first bath in a large tub. Smiles and gurgles. Smiles and babbles at strangers. Plays with new toys immediately.	Approaches strangers readily. Sleeps well in new surroundings.	Slept well the first time he stayed overnight at grandparents' house.	Entered school building unhesitatingly. Tries new food.	Went to camp happily. Loved to ski the first time.
NEGATIVE WITHDRAWAL	Rejected cereal the first time. Cries when strangers appear.	?	Afraid when placed on sled. Will not sleep in strange beds.	Avoids strange children in the playground. Whimpers first time at beach. Will not go into water.	Hid behind mother when entering school.	Severely homesick at camp during first days. Does not like new activities.
ADAPTABILITY — ADAPTABLE	Was passive during the first bath; now enjoys bathing. Smiles at nurse.	Used to dislike new foods; now accepts them well.	Afraid of toy animals at first; now plays with them happily.	Obeys quickly. Stayed contentedly with grandparents for a week.	Hesitated to go to nursery school at first; now goes eagerly. Slept well on camping trip.	Likes camp, although homesick during first days. Learns enthusiastically.
NOT ADAPTABLE	Still startled by sudden, sharp noise. Resists diapering.	Does not cooperate with dressing. Fusses and cries when left with sitter.	Continues to reject new foods each time they are offered.	Cries and screams each time hair is cut. Disobeys persistently.	Has to be hand-led into classroom each day.	Does not adjust well to new school or new teacher; comes home late for dinner even when punished.

Table 9.1 (*cont.*)

TEMPERAMENTAL QUALITY	RATING	2 MONTHS	6 MONTHS	1 YEAR	2 YEARS	5 YEARS	10 YEARS
ATTENTION SPAN AND PERSISTENCE	LONG	If soiled, continues to cry until changes. Repeatedly rejects water if he wants milk.	Watches mobile over crib intensely. "Coos" frequently.	Plays by self in playpen for more than an hour. Listens to singing for long periods.	Works on a puzzle until it is completed. Watches when shown how to do something.	Practiced riding a two-wheeled bicycle for hours until mastered it. Spent over an hour reading a book.	Reads for two hours before sleeping. Does homework carefully.
	SHORT	Cries when awakened but stops almost immediately. Objects only mildly if cereal precedes bottle.	Sucks pacifier for only a few minutes and spits it out.	Loses interest in toy after a few minutes. Gives up easily if she falls while attempting to walk.	Gives up easily if a toy is hard to use. Asks for help immediately if undressing becomes difficult.	Still cannot tie his shoes because he gives up when he is not successful. Fidgets when parents read to him.	Gets up frequently from homework for a snack. Never finishes a book.
INTENSITY OF REACTION	INTENSE	Cries when diapers are wet. Rejects food vigorously when satisfied.	Cries loudly at the sound of thunder. Makes sucking movements when vitamins are administered.	Laughs hard when father plays roughly. Screams and kicks when temperature is taken.	Yells if he feels excitement or delight. Cries loudly if a toy is taken away.	Rushes to greet father. Gets hiccups from laughing hard.	Tears up an entire page of homework if one mistake is made. Slams door of room when teased by younger brother.
	MILD	Does not cry when diapers are wet. Whimpers instead of crying when hungry.	Does not kick often in tub. Does not smile. Screams and kicks when temperature is taken.	Do not fuss much when clothing is pulled over head.	When another child hit her, looked surprised, did not hit back.	Drops eyes and remains silent when given a firm parental "No." Does not laugh much.	When a mistake is made in a model airplane, corrects it quietly. Does not comment when reprimanded.

THRESHOLD OF RESPONSIVENESS	LOW	Stops sucking on bottle when approached.	Refuses fruit he likes when vitamins are added. Hides head from bright light.	Spits out food he does not like. Giggles when tickled.	Runs to door when father comes home. Must always be tucked tightly into bed.	Always notices when mother puts new dress on for first time. Refuses milk if it is not ice-cold.	Rejects fatty foods. Adjusts shower until water is exactly the right temperature.
	HIGH	Is not startled by loud noises. Takes bottle and breast equally well.	Eats everything. Does not object when diapers are wet or soiled.	Eats food he likes even if mixed with disliked food. Can be left easily with strangers.	Can be left with anyone. Falls to sleep easily on either back or stomach.	Does not hear loud, sudden noises when reading. Does not object to injections.	Never complains when sick. Eats all foods.
QUALITY OF MOOD	POSITIVE	Smacks lips when first tasting new food. Smiles at parents.	Plays with splashes in bath. Smiles at everyone.	Likes bottle; reaches for it and smiles. Laughs loudly when playing peekaboo.	Plays with sister; laughs and giggles. Smiles when she succeeds in putting shoes on.	Laughs loudly while watching television cartoons. Smiles at everyone.	Enjoys new accomplishments. Laughs when reading a funny passage aloud.
	NEGATIVE	Fusses after nursing. Cries when carriage is rocked.	Cries when given food she does not like.	Cries when given injections. Cries when left alone.	Cries and squirms when given haircut. Cries when mother leaves.	Objects to putting boots on. Cries when frustrated.	Cries when he cannot solve a homework problem. Very "weepy" if he does not get enough sleep.

Source: Thomas, A., Chess, S. and Birch, H. G. (1970). The origin of personality. *Scientific American, 111*, 102–9. With permission.

are: (1) *easy* – children who adjust well to new situations, adapt well to new routines and are cheerful and easy to calm; (2) *difficult* – slow to adapt to change, likely to react negatively and intensely; and (3) *slow to warm up* – difficult at first but adjust better with time (Thomas, Chess and Birch, 1970).

Learning about temperament can be helpful, for example, to a psychologist who is about to begin psychotherapy with a child or adolescent who is being assessed. This information may also be useful to a clinician who is providing advice to parents or teachers about their relationship with a particular child and management of his/her behavior. The concept of "goodness of fit" (Chess and Thomas, 1999; Coplan, Finlay and Schneider, 2010) refers to the matching of different temperament types to environments that maximize adjustment. For example, a difficult child may do best if enrolled in a daycare environment where routines are predictable, where the caregivers are stable and where the caregivers are readily available to the child, because of a favorable child–caregiver ratio or other reasons (e.g., De Schipper et al., 2004). Hence, one positive outcome of temperament or personality assessment could be recommendations pertinent to the choice of educational setting for a child in difficulty.

Personality has been measured with *projective techniques* throughout most of the history of psychology. These creative, intriguing tools provide ambiguous stimuli the responses to which are thought to reveal individual differences in personality and adjustment. The best-known projective technique is probably the Rorschach inkblots (Rorschach, 1927), which were originally made by folding paper in half after ink had been spilled, forming an image that can be identified in different ways. A standard series of ten printed "inkblots," with black and red "ink," is the basis of generations of theory and research. Inferences about personality can be made on the basis, for example, of what the person sees (e.g., a human being, a monster, a building), whether the respondent attends to minor detail or most of the blot, whether what the person sees is similar to what most other people see in the same blot or something very original, etc. Other projective techniques for children include the Children's Apperception Test (Bellak and Abrams, 1996), in which a drawing with animals is presented and the child is asked to make up a story about the people in the drawing. There is also a version for older children in which people, rather than animals, are depicted. Interpretation is based on the assumption of projection, that the main character in the story made up is the child being assessed. Sentence completion tasks (e.g. Rotter, Lah and Rafferty, 1992) involve children completing sentences like "The future seems . . . ." Drawings of the human figure and of the family can also be analyzed as projective techniques.

Although projective techniques have fascinated psychologists for decades, caution about the subjectivity in their use has increased in recent years. It is difficult for a psychologist to defend interpretations based on projective techniques, for example, in a juvenile justice situation or to a legal committee mandated to decide what educational or psychological services a child or adolescent should receive. Psychologists are encountering such situations with increasing frequency, together with greater demands for accountability. It has been argued that projective techniques remain a fertile source of new hypotheses and aspects of the child's thinking that are not evident in conversation or in more straightforward testing methods (Garb et al., 2002; McClure, Kubiszyn and Kaslow, 2002). However, critics argue that projective methods are likely to suggest much more pathology than really exists and that psychologists are no more immune than other people to seeing the sickness rather than the health (Hojnoski et al., 2006; Lee and Hunsley, 2003).

For these reasons, a contemporary assessment of child or adolescent personality or temperament is likely to be based on questionnaires and checklists. Complicating the assessment of children's personality is that the developers of instruments are not as certain as their counterparts working on adult personality as to what exactly they are seeking to measure. There is almost general consensus that a five-factor model (openness, conscientiousness, extraversion, agreeableness and neuroticism, remembered by the acronym OCEAN) can be used to describe the personalities of adults; no such consensus or prevailing model exists for child personality (Halverson et al., 2003). Interestingly, some recent initial research suggests that the parents' personalities should be assessed together with the child's because the effects of the child's personality seem to act interactively with those of his or her parents (Rettew et al., 2006).

Intellectual and cognitive development

Learning about a child's intellectual and cognitive development is a frequent objective of psychological assessment. It is important to remember that developmental disability and learning disabilities may co-occur with disruptive behavior disorders, substance abuse and other forms of psychopathology. Detecting the comorbidity (called *dual diagnosis*) has important implications for both understanding the individual and prescribing the optimal treatment. Dual diagnosis usually refers to some combination of learning and emotional/ behavioral disabilities. This concept has replaced the former trend of indicating what are supposed to be primary and secondary diagnoses, which all too often involved the implicit and unfounded assumption that the emotional or behavioral problem is merely a superficial manifestation of the learning or intellectual disability. Recognition of the very extensive co-occurrence of these disorders dictates increasing sophistication in both assessment and treatment procedures. Not only must the professional conducting the assessment be familiar with measures of both intellectual and behavioral functioning, but also be competent to assess emotional functioning with measures valid for populations of children and adolescents with intellectual and learning disabilities.

In the middle of the twentieth century, IQ testing was considered the hallmark and mainstay of the profession of psychology. No assessment would be conducted without it. Moreover, it is probably not much of an overstatement to assert that many assessments consisted of little more than IQ tests. Schools and institutions largely mimicked the US army's practice of classifying troops for types of service based substantially on IQ (see Gould, 1981 for a comprehensive and controversial chronicle of this practice). Many children from underprivileged homes in the United States, especially African-Americans, found themselves assigned to classes for the "educable mentally retarded" although in many cases there was no indication of intellectual disability other than IQ and poor academic progress. This history is important because it illustrates the extent to which IQ, which is thought to be based on inherent genetically determined ability, can be affected by inadequate educational experience. Such expeditious use of IQ scores was challenged successfully in the courts in California in the famous 1972 case of *Larry P. vs. Riles*. After 5 months of testimony and deliberation, the judge ruled that IQ tests could not be used as the basis of assigning a student of minority background to a special education program. As time passed, several legal challenges were launched. Assessment procedures were revised and improved, with IQ tests back in use as one of several sources of information. Despite these improvements, students of minority cultural origin are still represented disproportionately in special education classes in the United States (Hosp and Reshley, 2004). Contemporary assessment practice often includes IQ testing in a more reasoned and defensible manner than in the assessment procedures in which Larry P. participated. Greater attention is being paid in the norming process to the possibility of bias against minority groups. There is surely greater recognition of the need for the human examiner to consider much more than the raw

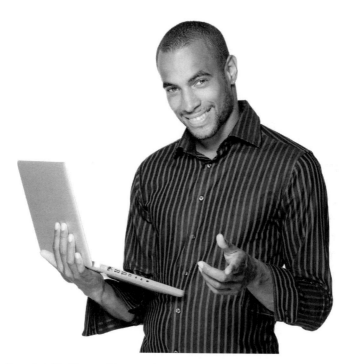

Figure 9.1 Vociferous objections have been raised about the misclassification of members of minority groups using IQ tests.

score of a specific test or of all tests in coming to a conclusion.

Reflected in the instruments used most widely in assessments nowadays is the discovery that intelligence is not a single entity but that there are multiple intelligences. One example of a multifactor conceptualization is Sternberg's *triarchical model*, in which intelligence is subdivided into: (1) *analytic intelligence*, the ability to process and analyze information and criticize; (2) *creative intelligence*, which applies to new material and unfamiliar tasks; and (3) *practical intelligence*, which represents learning the subtleties of the social world. Each of these three types is subdivided into subtypes (Sternberg, 1990). The most important difference between Sternberg's theory and many other multifactor models of intelligence is Sternberg's emphasis on the third factor, practical everyday knowledge of the workings of the social world.

The most widely used instrument for the assessment of the intellectual abilities of children

and adolescents is the Wechsler Intelligence Scale for Children – Fourth Edition (WISC-IV; Wechsler, 2003). It yields both a total IQ score and scores on each of ten core subtests and five supplementary subtests; see Box 9.2 for further information. The subtests are grouped into factors representing the component abilities of verbal comprehension, perceptual reasoning, processing speed and short-term working memory. The WISC-IV must be administered individually; group paper-and-pencil tests of intelligence are not useful in clinical assessment. The individual administration takes 1–1.5 hours. Contemporary intelligence tests like the WISC-IV are the results of a very thorough, sophisticated and painstaking process of development, including standardization with thousands of participants in several countries and very extensive validation.

Besides the information conveyed by the total IQ score, any discrepancies among the factors of verbal comprehension, perceptual reasoning, processing

Box 9.2 | The Weschler Intelligence Scale for Children

Introduced in 1949 and now approaching its fifth edition, this is the most widely used psychological test for children. It is designed to be administered on a one-to-one basis by a trained examiner. The development and standardization of this test represent years of work and methodological precision. The WISC-IV is designed for ages 7 through 16 years. Other versions of the Wechsler intelligence scales have been developed for children under 7 and for older adolescents and adults.

There are fifteen subtests in the WISC-IV, designed to assess different aspects of intelligence using different sensorimotor channels. A core of ten of the subtests is usually administered. The resulting subtest scores yield a number of composite scores, including the full-scale IQ, which is the best known.

The *Verbal Comprehension Index* consists of five subtests: Vocabulary (providing a definition for a word recited by the examiner); Similarities (saying how two words are alike); Comprehension (answering questions about social situations, rules and community institutions); Information (general factual knowledge); and Word Reasoning (identifying a concept based on a series of clues). Obviously, these abilities depend heavily on educational experiences.

The *Perceptual Reasoning Index* includes the Block Design subtest (arranging toy blocks to match a pattern shown by the examiner); Picture Concepts (matching pictures according to a linking concept); Matrix Reasoning (selecting a missing element that would logically complete a pattern); and Picture Completion (identifying the part that is missing in a figure drawing).

The *Processing Speed Index* consists of: Coding (a clerical task in which the child selects and writes the symbol associated with each number); Symbol Search (a picture matching game); and Cancellation (a timed hunt for all pictures of a given type among a larger array).

The *Working Memory Index* includes Digit Span (repeating series of numbers, in forward and backward order); Letter–Number sequencing (unscrambling a series of numbers and letters by repeating them in alphabetical and numerical order); and oral arithmetic.

Differences among the various scores that can be calculated are useful in understanding the intellectual functioning of individual children and, to some extent, designing educational programs for them. However, as noted in the text, these differences are sometimes interpreted clinically and educationally in ways that go beyond the supporting research.

speed and short-term working memory are certainly noteworthy in the clinician's understanding of the child or adolescent being assessed and in making recommendations to teachers. However, in order to make meaningful, informed recommendations, the clinician must supplement tools like the WISC-IV with other information, including assessment of achievement in academic subject areas. Given the amount of time psychologists have traditionally spent administering tests like the WISC-IV, it is not surprising that efforts have been made to use the resulting data more extensively in diagnosis than the supporting research permits. However, overinterpretation of the results of individual subtest scores has long been dubbed a prevalent "malpractice" (Hirshoren and Kavale, 1976).

In the hypothesis-based model of psychological assessment discussed at the beginning of this chapter, measurement of a child's intelligence may or may not be a worthwhile component of an assessment, depending on the purpose of the assessment. Accordingly, intelligence tests are one of the tools available for psychological assessment, to be used, like other tools, when they are useful. Perhaps contemporary clinical psychologists as a whole believe that IQ testing is still a good thing even if previous generations delivered too much of the good thing without enough other good things to go along with it.

Behavior

The purpose of an assessment may include the tracing of a picture of the child's typical behavior, of events that precipitate it and/or of the social environment in which it occurs. It is, unfortunately, rare for a clinical psychologist to have the time and mandate to observe child behavior directly in its natural setting. Le Couteur and Gardner (2010) enumerate some of the many advantages of direct observation when it is possible. First of all, direct observation can provide very useful detailed information about the behavior of children who cannot articulate their problems, such as young children and those with communicative disabilities. Observation may be the best way for a clinician to assess, for example, the stereotyped, repetitive movements and impaired social communication in autism spectrum disorder (e.g., Callahan et al., 2011; Perry et al., 2008). Direct observation can also provide information in which the clinician may have more confidence than in the results of rating scales in situations when paper-and-pencil instruments suggest some degree of bias or are inconsistent. However, despite the face validity of direct observations, it is important to remember that the presence of the observer does constitute a source of bias, one that cannot usually be avoided. Observation from a distance or from behind a one-way mirror is not always possible.

Perhaps the most important advantage of direct observation of behavior is that the observer derives information not only about the child being assessed but also about the social and physical environment in which problem behavior occurs. This contextual approach is particularly indicated when the purposes of the assessment include working, for example, with teachers, in improving problem behaviors that occur mainly in the classroom. Through observation, the clinician learns about the reinforcement patterns that may maintain the problem behavior in the classroom. An interesting case example is provided by Patterson (2009), who used the results of behavioral assessment to help a teacher reduce the problematic out-of-seat behavior. The intervention consisted of having the teacher greet the pupil upon arrival first thing in the morning with "small talk" – conversation about some daily event, for example – and deliver clear, consistent instructions about what the teacher expected to do that day. Patterson also used observational methods to confirm that the intervention procedure worked, which is standard in interventions emerging from the science of behavior analysis. As well as gaining useful insight about reinforcement processes that maintain problem behaviors and that may be manipulated to help eliminate them, the observer gains familiarity with the teacher's interaction style and the stressors he or she works under. This will hopefully make the clinician's recommendations more relevant and more effective. Observational methods can also be used to determine whether behavior has changed after an intervention. Whereas checklist and interview methods, for example, may not change because pre-treatment impressions of the child remain even after actual improvement, behavioral observations are known to be sensitive to treatment changes, especially if the observer is not informed about any intervention that has taken place (Dishion and Granic, 2004; Riley-Tillman, Methe and Weegar, 2009).

Direct observation in natural settings can usually be conducted only for a limited time. This can be unfortunate because many problem behaviors vary greatly from day to day and within school days (Briesch, Chafouleas and Riley-Tillman, 2010). A variety of well-developed coding schemes are available that provide detailed procedures regarding, for example, the definitions of the behaviors to be observed and coded systematically, the samples of time at which they should be observed and many other issues. One of the best-known coding schemes for the observation of parent–child interactions is the Dyadic Parent–Child Interaction Coding System by Eyberg and her colleagues (e.g., Callahan and Eyberg, 2010). Their coding system can be used in any setting where children and parents interact. It covers a variety of common positive and negative behaviors in parent–child interaction such as positive touch, compliance with the parents' instructions and yelling. In extensive research, the system has proven valid and reliable. The behavioral literature contains very extensive detail about the procedures for ensuring that observational methods are valid, including the important provisions for *inter-rater reliability*, confirming that separate observers witnessing the same event code it in the same way. Nock and Kurtz (2005) provide a very readable introduction to some of these requirements as they apply to observational assessments.

When time or access (e.g., to a home) preclude observations in a natural setting that provide adequate information about the problem being assessed, contrived or *closed-field* or *analogue* observation techniques can be used in an effort to optimize observation time. For example, the parents and child may be brought to a playroom in which toys are available. The parent may be observed while attempting to get the child to comply with an instruction or to clean up the playroom at the end of play. Families can also be observed while planning a family activity or solving a family problem. It is important for the task contrived to be representative of the child's or family's daily life, acceptable to them and likely to evoke the problem that has resulted in the referral for psychological assessment (Rhule, McMahon and Vando, 2009).

Of course, not all observational assessments conducted for the purpose of clinical assessment correspond to the rigorous traditions of the field of behavior analysis. More informal observations may indeed be more common and, when their results are interpreted in light of their nature, may be very useful. However, great caution must be exercised in interpreting observations conducted in unfamiliar settings. Perhaps the most overinterpreted behavioral observations in the psychological assessment of children are those conducted informally in the waiting rooms of the professionals conducting the assessments, an unfamiliar setting in which uncertainty about the upcoming procedures and the desire to convey a particular impression may unduly influence behavior.

Assessment of child psychopathology: current challenges and future directions

In reflecting on the current state of assessment in psychopathology, Kazdin (2005) offers several concise observations useful in achieving best practice in both research and clinical work. First of all, he notes that there is not really a "gold standard" against which measures can be validated. Because of the high rates of comorbidity among the disorders, the assessment process should include consideration of multiple disorders or symptoms.

Because informants (i.e., parents, teachers and youth) often disagree in describing a particular child, multiple informants should be used. The assessment should include information about the child's adaptive functioning at school, home and the community, not just information about dysfunction and disorder.

In contrast with the extensive research available on psychological tests and other assessment procedures, there has been very little research documenting the benefits of the entire process of psychological assessment (Hunsley, 2002). Research designed to make assessment more evidence-based lags well behind research pertinent to evidence-based intervention (Mash and Hunsley, 2005), which will be discussed in Chapter 11. Counseling psychologists Gelso and Fretz (2001) observed that "research in the coming decades will help decide whether psychological assessment is our dodo bird or a phoenix rising from the 'ashes' of the critiques of recent decades" (p. 400).

There are a number of encouraging trends indicating that many forward-thinking psychologists are advocating changes that will hopefully succeed not only in keeping psychological assessment alive but also in rejuvenating and revitalizing it. Some of these innovations do seem a bit contradictory but all represent contrasts to the mass routine testing that was both the mainstay of the psychology profession a generation or two ago and a blinder that prevented it from reaching its potential. One encouraging new approach, emphasized at the beginning of this chapter, is integrating assessment more fully into the helping process by making assessment more of a collaborative procedure taking into account the perspective and desires of clients. There appears to be no research documenting the feasibility and benefits of this approach in the psychological assessment of children and adolescents. However, a recent meta-analysis, based on seventeen published studies conducted with a total of 1,496 participants, confirms the benefits of working this way with adult clients (Poston and Hanson, 2010).

Other ways of renewing psychological assessment may involve squaring assessment practice with exciting recent findings in the field of neuropsychology and adapting to the increasingly technology-based character of contemporary life; these new modalities are discussed by Trull (2007). Benefits of two very distinct types can accrue from learning to apply up-to-the-minute technology. One area of benefit is making assessment more economical, efficient and authoritative without changing its essential nature. Computer-based interviewing (see above) and test administration bring gains in terms of clinical time. Hopefully, the clinician working with the child and family will complement computer-administered components with other assessment techniques that involve sensitive personal communication. However, in the case of assessment tools that relate to extensive research, computer scoring of the assessment protocol can connect the individual score profile to pertinent background research, assisting the clinician in the formulation of hypotheses.

The proliferation of handheld devices such as cell phones and smart phones can be an asset to the assessment process by enabling the inclusion of data on the experiences of the people being assessed in their own natural contexts and at various time points in their daily routines. *Experience-sampling techniques* (Hektner, Schmidt and Csikszentmihalyi, 2007), used up to now primarily as a research tool, involve individuals being contacted at different times to report on their feelings, moods and/or behaviors. Experience sampling involves daily diaries and logs of the occurrence of specific events or emotions; it is now carried out mainly by means of electronic communication including smartphones. These methods constitute a marked improvement over retrospective assessment (which involves, for example, asking a parent, teacher or child to recall how frequently a specific problem behavior or a troubling mood occurred during the week leading up to the moment at which a questionnaire is completed (Piasecki et al., 2007).

Revolutionary technological advances also permit increasing knowledge about the physiological processes that are known correlates of major forms of psychopathology, as discussed in Chapter 5. New methods permit increasingly direct access to biological processes as they occur. These methods include *ambulatory biosensors*, which are non-obtrusive devices that can measure cardiovascular, physical and/or chemical activity, carried by the people being assessed in their natural environments (Haynes and Yoshikowa, 2007). As already mentioned in several previous chapters, modern neuroimaging techniques permit direct observation of many of the workings of the brain that were previously the subject of guesswork, albeit educated guesswork. Despite the rapid improvement of imaging techniques, their application to the assessment of individuals remains unclear. Miller et al. (2007) caution against raising expectations that neuroimaging will reveal the hitherto unknown true cause of a psychopathology being assessed. They point out that the brain can be affected by a psychological state or the brain can be a cause of a psychological state. However, the main advantage they see in the judicious use of neuroimaging techniques in assessment is the possibility of discovering some process in action that was previously unknown to both the clinician and the person being assessed. If and when psychologists use neuroimaging technology in this way, they will be the first members of the profession who have achieved an ability often ascribed to them by uninformed persons: the ability to read other people's minds.

Summary

- Psychological assessment of children is an exploratory, hypothesis-testing process in which psychologists engage with children and their parents to attempt to explain a child's problems and alleviate them. It is not only a matter of "testing."
- Clients, teachers, parents and children being assessed should ideally formulate questions they would like to answer in assessment, and goals. Assessment results and their meaning for clients should be discussed empathetically. The measures used in assessment should be determined by the purpose of the assessment.
- Valid, reliable tests are essential to proper psychological assessment.
- Reynolds (2010) notes that tests are not invalid or valid; it is the ways in which they are used that are valid or invalid, particularly in the case of intelligence tests, which may sometimes be used for purposes other than measuring intelligence.
- Test results of clinical populations often vary from those of non-clinical ones in many ways. This is insufficient evidence of a test's discriminant validity for a specific form of psychopathology.
- McFall (2005) notes that a test is no better than its underlying models.
- The incremental validity is the added value of a given test over and above other measures already in common use.
- An assessment tool must be valid for its purpose and population. Cross-cultural validation is necessary when tests are used in cultures for which they were not developed.
- Structured diagnostic interviews are designed based on symptoms described in diagnostic manuals, such as the DSM or ICD to determine the diagnoses that correspond to a given child's behaviors. The Diagnostic Interview Schedule for Children is the best-known structured diagnostic interview for child psychopathology.

- Structured diagnostic interviews generally achieve reliable diagnosis. They vary, however, in their degree of standardization.
- There is some question about the incremental validity of structured diagnostic interviews.
- A criticism of structured diagnostic interviews is that parents are the sole informants. Teachers, who might provide valuable information, are excluded.
- Checklists and questionnaires are used widely in clinical assessment and research. Checklists are portable, economical and able to be completed by individuals who are not physically present for the assessment.
- Checklists provide results that can be compared to others for the same age group. Checklists can be examined for positive and negative halo effects and other forms of response bias.
- Paper-and-pencil methods cannot capture the information yielded by personal contact with the interviewer. When diagnostic interviews are highly structured and standardized, they might be considered more like questionnaires. It is considered irresponsible to base diagnosis solely on a paper-and-pencil instrument.
- Checklists rarely consist solely of items directly corresponding to symptoms needed for DSM or ICD diagnoses. Typically, they have a cut-off point, beyond which the results are considered indicative of a particular diagnosis. This cut-off point should be based on research, but often is not.
- The comprehensive, well-developed Achenbach System of Empirically Based Assessment has separate scales for various age ranges and for parents and teachers.
- Personality assessment does not determine diagnostic status. Personality (for adults) or temperament (for children) consist of traits characterizing the individual being assessed. Chess and Thomas (1999) developed a typology of children's temperament based on specific dimensions, which yields three types: easy, difficult and slow to warm up.
- "Goodness of fit" refers to the matching of temperament types to environments to maximize adjustment.
- Projective measures provide ambiguous stimuli, responses to which reveal differences in individuals' personality and adjustment. Methods include the well-known Rorschach inkblots, the Children's Apperception Test and Sentence Completion tasks.
- It can be difficult to defend interpretations based on projective techniques in a juvenile justice system or to a legal committee because of the subjectivity of the interpretations. Although projective tests are a fertile source of new hypotheses and aspects of children's thinking not otherwise evident, critics argue that projective methods suggest more pathology than actually exists.
- Assessment of a child or adolescent personality or temperament is likely to be based on questionnaires and checklists. These instruments are more objective than projective tests.
- Assessment often includes intellectual and cognitive ability, as well as the criteria for several DSM and ICD categories. Learning disabilities may co-occur with disruptive behavior disorders, substance abuse and other forms of psychopathology. Detecting comorbidity has become important because it may lead to more meaningful and effective treatment.
- In the mid-twentieth century, IQ testing was the mainstay of professional psychology, with some assessments consisting of little more than IQ tests. Many children of ethnic minorities were assigned to classes for the "educable mentally retarded," with no evidence except this IQ and poor academic progress. This practice was ultimately overturned in courts but, to this day, minorities are over-represented in special education classes.
- Contemporary measures of intelligence are based on a multifactor conceptualization,

such as Sternberg's triarchical model (1990), wherein intelligence is subdivided into analytic intelligence, creative intelligence and practical intelligence. Each type is further subdivided into subtypes. Sternberg's theory places more emphasis on the third factor, measuring practical everyday knowledge of social workings, than many other models.

- The *Wechsler Intelligence Scale for Children – Fourth Edition* is the most widely used. It yields a total IQ score and scores on ten subtests and five supplementary subtests. It is administered individually, taking 1–1.5 hours, and was developed in a thorough, painstaking process, with thousands of participants and very extensive validation.

- Discrepancies among factors of verbal comprehension, perceptual reasoning, processing speed and short-term working memory are useful in assessment and recommendations to teachers. However, tools like the WISC-IV must be supplemented. Overinterpretation of individual subtest scores has been dubbed "malpractice."

- Direct observation in a natural setting provides detailed information about children who cannot articulate their problems. Observation provides information in which the clinician may have more confidence, understanding of a teacher's interaction style and the stressors he or she works under, and information about the environment in which behavior occurs. Clinicians rarely have the time, however, for observational assessment.

- Time constraints on direct observation are unfortunate due to day-to-day variations in problem behaviors.

- Coding schemes, such as the well-known and methodologically sound Dyadic Parent–Child Interaction Coding System, provide rigorous procedures for recording behaviors.

- Closed-field or analogue techniques optimize observation time. They include observing a parent attempting to get a child to comply with instruction or a family planning an activity or solving a problem. The task must be representative of daily life, acceptable to those involved and must evoke the problem that resulted in referral for psychological assessment.

- Informal observations may be common and useful, but caution must be used in their interpretation. Perhaps most overinterpreted are observations of children in the waiting rooms of the professionals conducting assessments.

- Since comorbidity is common, the assessment process should include multiple disorders or symptoms. Informants often disagree in describing a child, so multiple informants should be used. Information about the child's adaptive functioning at school, home and in the community should be included.

- Little research has been done on the benefits of the entire process of assessment. Research to make assessment more evidence-based lags behind research on evidence-based intervention.

- Experience-sampling techniques have been expanded with the proliferation of cell phones. Individuals record their feelings, moods and behaviors at different times. This constitutes an improvement over retrospective assessment.

Study questions

1. What is incremental validity and why is it important when a child-clinical psychologist assesses the psychological functioning of a child or adolescent?
2. What are the advantages and disadvantages of standard diagnostic interviews?

3. In what ways can assessment of the temperament or personality of a child or adolescent be helpful in the treatment of psychological problems?
4. What is the current status of projective techniques in the psychological assessment of children and adolescents?
5. Is direct observation of behavior the best tool for the assessment of the psychological disorders of children and adolescents?

10 Prevention and mental health promotion

More mental illness than mental health professionals can manage

Compared to progress in the treatment of psychopathology that has already appeared, the psychology profession has lagged in developing effective prevention strategies. Serious consideration of prevention strategies in their own right did not begin until the 1960s, and this early attempt failed to make a considerable impact (Duncan, 1994; Hage and Romano, 2010). In the past half-century, however, prevention has begun to be taken seriously. The term *prevention science* has emerged to reflect an empirical perspective. In the area of child psychopathology, prevention initiatives are particularly important, first of all, because children who experience mental illness are more likely than others to experience mental illness in adulthood (Pine et al., 2010). Furthermore, many of the psychological resources that protect against mental illness are developed in childhood, making this period especially critical (Serna et al., 2003). Lastly, experiencing mental illness as a child costs the individual the enjoyment of his or her childhood. This alone is enough reason to consider prevention initiatives against childhood psychopathology.

This chapter begins with definitional issues, focusing on the thorny distinction between prevention and treatment. The important differences between universal prevention programs, that is, those addressed at entire populations or communities, and indicated programs, that is, programs intended for individuals who already show some signs of psychological distress, are considered next. The subsequent section is devoted to reasons for involving the community in the basic design of interventions, not just their delivery. A history of preventive mental health in North America and Europe appears next. The subsequent section is devoted to methodological issues in the evaluation of prevention programs. Guidelines for the successful implementation of prevention programs appear next, followed by several examples of successful prevention programs.

Defining prevention

Considerable energy has been invested in defining prevention and in delineating different levels of intervention that can be considered preventive. For a program to be considered preventive, it must: (1) be group-oriented; (2) be implemented before the targeted pathology becomes manifest; and (3) be intentional – that is, the purpose of the program must be explicitly prevention-oriented (APA Dictionary of Psychology, 2007; Cowen, 1996).

Although the difference between prevention and treatment may at first seem clear, at times it can be difficult to differentiate the two (O'Connell, Boat and Warner, 2009). This is largely due to the fact that experiencing a mental, behavioral or emotional disorder increases the risk of future dysfunction, and so from a developmental perspective, all treatment could be considered prevention because it prevents the individual's mental health from getting worse (O'Connell et al., 2009). In a report on mental health prevention in children and adolescents, O'Connell et al. (2009) discuss the differences between treatment and prevention. First, it is important to note that treatment and prevention are complementary and are both directed at reducing the long-term suffering caused by mental illness (O'Connell et al., 2009). Nonetheless, the two services are quite distinct: Treatment is directed at people already suffering from a disorder, with the intent of relieving, not preventing this disorder. It is most often directed at an individual, not a group.

Classifying prevention programs

The best-known taxonomy for classifying prevention as we understand it today was introduced in 1964 by Gerald Caplan, who proposed a three-tiered prevention model (Caplan, 1964). The first tier, *primary prevention*, involves an attempt to prevent occurrence of new pathology (i.e., reducing the incidence of a disorder in a population). The second tier, *secondary prevention*, focuses on early disease detection so that one can obstruct the development of the disease (i.e., reducing the prevalence of a disorder in a population). The last tier, *tertiary prevention*, consists of attempts to reduce the severity of impairment caused by a disorder that is already very evident, thereby preventing disability and incapacitation as far as possible. This model addresses preventive efforts at every stage of a disease: inception, development and lasting consequences. It also allows for prevention programs to begin even if sufficient understanding of the causes of different pathologies has not yet emerged. For instance, though the causes of autism spectrum disorder are not fully understood, Caplan's model allows for the conceptualization of programs that may prevent this disability and perhaps reduce the severity of symptoms. This model is also useful in cases where the causes of pathology are known but where no prevention initiative is feasible for it is too late to prevent the disorder; for example, tertiary prevention efforts can still be beneficial in cases of intellectual disability. Perhaps because of these strengths, Caplan's model has been widely embraced in both academia and clinical practice.

These tiers are the major elements of the standard nomenclature commonly used to describe levels of preventive programming. Despite its widespread use, critics have noted limitations with Caplan's model. Gordon (1983) argues that the model does not lend itself to preventing multidetermined disorders because it is difficult to decide when a multidetermined

disorder has begun, especially when its main causes are best measured dimensionally rather than categorically. In elucidating his argument, Gordon uses the example of prevention programs aimed at preventing myocardial infarction (heart attacks) by helping someone with high cholesterol. Gordon notes that Caplan's model cannot adequately classify this effort in any single tier. Although the person has not yet suffered a heart attack, one underlying element of the disease has already appeared, in this case, high cholesterol; accordingly one could classify the intervention as either *primary* or *secondary*.

Gordon and others have developed alternative frameworks for conceptualizing prevention strategies. Gordon's model (1983) considers three types of interventions based on the groups of people they address: *universal, selective* and *indicated. Universal* interventions are those that would benefit everybody. An example would be stimulating non-injurious exercise by healthy people. *Selective* interventions are those that would only benefit a subgroup of the population. For example, providing training to prevent the onset of post-traumatic stress disorder would only be beneficial for persons who have undergone a traumatic experience; it would not make sense to issue this training to everyone in the population. *Indicated* interventions target individuals who, upon examination, are found to manifest some trait that indicates sufficiently high risk to require the intervention. An example of this might be a program to help prevent heart attack in individuals with high cholesterol. According to Gordon, these initiatives are only preventive if they are applied to people who are not already demonstrating signs of illness or distress. Gordon's model provides well for the delineation of what can be considered prevention unfettered by the complicated issues of causality and pinpointing the onset of a disorder. Gordon's prevention model formed the basis for one of the largest conduct disorder prevention initiatives in North America: FAST Track (Conduct Problem's Prevention Research Group, 2011).

Mrazek and Haggerty's (1994) model has been embraced by both researchers and practitioners. The model is a reconceptualization of Gordon's

Table 10.1 **Models of prevention initiatives**

Caplan's Three-tiered Model	Primary	Prevents onset of disorder in *healthy* individuals
		Reduces the incidence of the disorder
	Secondary	Prevents the disease from becoming fully established by focusing on early disease detection and treatment
		Reduces the prevalence of the disorder
	Tertiary	Prevents disability and incapacitation
Gordon's Target-based Model	Universal	Targets and attempts to confer preventive resources on all persons in the population
	Selective	Targets individuals at elevated risk of developing the disorder
		Though theoretically anyone could benefit, its design is meant to address specific needs associated with the risk factors faced by the group to whom the intervention is targeted
	Indicated	Targets individuals belonging to a group who have some trait that indicates them to be at significant risk for developing the disorder
		The individuals are asymptomatic
Mrazek and Haggerty's Target-based Model	Universal	Targets and attempts to confer preventive resources on all persons in the population
	Selective	Targets individuals at elevated risk of developing the disorder
		Though the benefit could theoretically be for anyone, its design is meant to address specific needs associated with the risk factors faced by the group to whom the intervention is targeted
	Indicated	Targets individuals belonging to a group who have some trait that indicates them to be at significant risk for developing the disorder
		The individuals are either asymptomatic or *sub-threshold*

model (1983) and considers the same three levels of intervention. The key difference between the two models is that Gordon's model only applies to asymptomatic individuals, whereas Mrazek and Haggerty's *indicated* level is meant to apply to individuals already experiencing symptoms although they do not meet diagnostic criteria. Mrazek and Haggerty's model was created solely for classifying the prevention of mental disorders whereas Gordon's and Caplan's models were primarily designed to address physical disorders. For clarity, a summary of the different models is presented in Table 10.1.

The broader context of prevention: collaboration between professionals and the community

When attempting to understand prevention, it is not only important to consider *what* is being provided; it is also important to consider *where* and *how* it is being provided. For example, the intervention could be voluntary or involuntary; it could be implemented at schools, health centers, community centers or elsewhere; and the intervention could be provided by one agency or many.

Collaborating with the community is widely advocated as the optimal way of implementing a prevention program (Colby and Murrell, 1998; Griffin and Steen, 2010). When collaborating with community organizations and citizens, professionals and institutions must share their resources and decision-making authority. Thus, collaboration differs from more traditional approaches to mental health service delivery not only because it involves service taking place in the community but because the power, resources and authority are shared among all stakeholders. The stakeholders for mental health issues include a variety of people ranging from the person who is at risk to the major institutions within the community. Such partnerships have been successful in designing and implementing a wide range of prevention programs, from systematic efforts to enhance the social-emotional competence and health of young people (e.g., Weissberg, Kumpfer and Seligman, 2003) to teaching specific skills such as anger management, empathy and impulse control (e.g., Cooke et al., 2007).

History of mental health prevention

As with other ideas in the field of mental health, ideas about the prevention of mental illness necessarily occur in the context of the philosophies, beliefs and practices of the cultures in which they emerge. Because of the changing social and cultural contexts and the many changes in basic philosophy over

the course of this history, there have been many prevention movements that have failed to influence contemporary practice in meaningful ways. Although this section will focus on the history of prevention science as applied to disorders of childhood, important milestones in prevention science more generally are included because they inherently influence prevention in childhood disorders.

The origins of mental health prevention can be traced to ancient Greece. The ancient Greeks believed that a balanced lifestyle, participation in the community and refraining from consuming substances in excess would keep one's humors in balance (see Chapter 2) and would thus prevent mental health difficulties (Hage and Romano, 2010; Simon, 1992). Much like the history of psychopathology in general, the history of mental health prevention is fragmented and characterized by discontinuity; thus, the beliefs of the ancient Greeks were, by and large, lost to history. The story continues at the end of the Georgian era. During the 1830s, the Temperance Movement, which mounted an active campaign in all the major English-speaking countries against alcohol consumption, can be considered the first major modern attempt at preventing substance use disorder, which is now classified as a mental disorder (Blocker, 2006; Meyer and Quenzer, 2005). This idea re-emerged in the twentieth century.

As the nineteenth century progressed, superintendents of asylums were eager to see fewer young people ending up as miserable as their institutional charges. They began advocating for mental health prevention initiatives for at-risk groups, especially young children and children of parents with mental disorders. The enlightened attitude toward mental health problems that emerged in this era was discussed in Chapter 2.

Eugenics as attempted prevention

Looking back at the heyday of the *eugenics movement*, it is difficult to attribute anything other than sinister intent to its founders. However,

Main	0	1000	2000	
Ancient Greece				
• Hippocrates emphasizes benefits of healthy, balanced lifestyle				
• Plato emphasizes links between body and soul and proper care of both				
Enlightenment and Industrial Revolution			• Alcohol prohibition advocated by Temperance Movement in the UK	
			• Stanley Hall's child study movement provides practical tips to parents	
			• Parents' associations established in schools across the United States	
Progressive era			• Healy emphasizes social origins of juvenile delinquency and prevention	
			• Beers founds mental hygiene movement	
			• Eugenics Record Office established to prevent birth of children with disorders	
World Wars and inter-war years			• Mental hygiene movement expands to Europe, starting with Finland	
			• New York Hospital releases report emphasizing social origins of disorder	
			• Cambridge-Somerville study on preventing delinquency begins	
Cold War and space age			• Mental health needs of returning soldiers and their families inspire prevention	
			• Primary Mental Health Project started in Rochester, NY schools	
			• Enthusiasm wanes because of lack of evidence	
			• Head Start preschools established as part of Kennedy's War on Poverty	
Information age			• Start of FAST Track project, aimed at preventing problematic aggression	
			• Healthy Cities Project starts in Europe	

Figure 10.1 Major milestones leading to contemporary prevention.

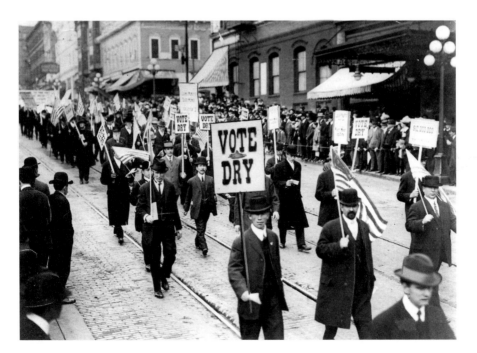

Figure 10.2 New York City policemen enforcing alcohol prohibition laws, which were enacted in part to prevent mental illness.

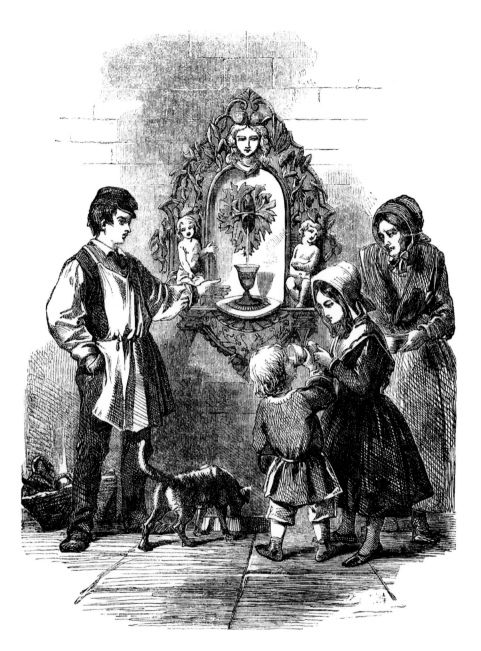

Figure 10.3 Victorian drinking fountain to encourage abstinence. Alcohol prohibition was intended as a primary prevention initiative.

the eugenics movement began in the nineteenth century as a sincere attempt at primary prevention (Simonsen, 2011; Spaulding and Balch, 1983; Trent, 2001). The rise of the eugenics movement at this particular moment in history can be seen as rooted somewhat in the accumulation of knowledge in the nineteenth century regarding the genetic basis of psychopathology, as detailed in Chapter 2. Eugenics was advocated by the fascist movement in Nazi Germany and is often linked, because of this association, with racism even though it does not necessarily have to apply to race (Dikotter,

1998; Simonsen, 2011; Trent, 2001). The eugenics movement primarily advocated *selective breeding* and forced immunizations as the most effective prevention strategies. This movement constituted a significant trend in mental health prevention from the 1860s through the 1950s. By 1935, twenty-seven US states had laws providing for forced sterilization; over 20,000 involuntary sterilizations occurred under these laws (Spaulding and Balch, 1983; Wehmeyer, 2003). In the 1950s, many scholars began to argue against eugenics because the cost–benefit ratio inherent in these practices seemed disproportionately harmful. The eugenics movement effectively came to an end. Nonetheless, practices that some believe to be reminiscent of forced sterilization are still used today to prevent recidivism in chronic sex offenders. An example is the use of antiandrogens to reduce sex drive (Polak and Nijman, 2005). Another possible perspective on this practice is that it prevents mental disorder in the potential victims of sexual violence. Additionally, advances in methods of detecting intellectual disability in the fetus have allowed families to decide to abort if intellectual disability seems likely (Alexander, 1998; Munroe, 2011). This practice differs from eugenics in two ways. First, the decision to terminate is not made by an institution, and second, the decision may be seen as directed at preventing a poor quality of life for the child rather than reducing harm to the gene pool of the society. Nonetheless, the influence of the eugenics movement is not totally absent from these practices. Although genetics still influences issues in mental health prevention today, the contemporary influences of the eugenics movement are minimal.

Community-based prevention of delinquency

Aside from eugenics, the first real prevention work began during the period of 1909 to 1917, when Dr. William Healy began studying the factors contributing to juvenile delinquency (Silk et al., 2000). He then developed a program to intervene early enough to hopefully prevent delinquent children becoming rooted in the criminal world. Originally these programs addressed children and youth who had already entered the criminal justice system in some way and, thus, were an early example of a *secondary-selective* prevention initiative. After working with and studying these children, Healy decided that there was not a single etiological pathway that could lead to a single prevention strategy, but, rather, a configuration of causative factors unique to each child (Silk et al., 2000).

Primary prevention became an important part of the discourse of the time. In keeping with the concern of the era regarding community health, the New York State Hospital recommended in 1918 as a means of preventing mental health difficulties that extreme poverty be eliminated (Spaulding and Balch, 1983; Stockdill, 2005). Indeed, poverty has been linked to many disorders of early childhood including oppositional defiance disorder and conduct disorder (Costello, Compton et al., 2003), as discussed elsewhere in this book. Nevertheless, the elimination of poverty is certainly too lofty an objective to be considered an element of the primary prevention agenda.

The National Congress of Mothers, founded in the 1890s, had 50,000 members by 1910; its name was changed to the current Parent–Teacher Association in the 1920s. Among the tenets of the movement was that childhood was to be valued for its own sake. The mothers' role was to enhance the potential that was inherently present in their children. According to Stanley Hall, a consultant and frequent speaker to the parent group, they should do this by being sensitive to their children's needs and following their parental intuitions. By Hall's time, most scientists and theologians concurred that the basic God-given nature of children is good, reversing the medieval belief discussed earlier. Hall's prescriptions were considered too permissive by most pediatricians at the time, leading to a resurgence of some degree of authoritarianism in the parenting of the 1920s (Brooks-Gunn and Johnson, 2006).

This was to be replaced down the road by the permissive "helping mode" of the 1950s through 1970s, in which parents are charged with raising their children in a way that will minimize their anxieties, satisfy their basic needs and maximize their potential. Books for parents provided advice on how children should be reared. Some how-to books appeared in the 1920s (e.g., Bruce, 1919, cited by Parry-Jones, 1989; Miller, 1923, cited by Parry-Jones, 1989). The most influential volume of its kind was Benjamin Spock's work, first published in 1946, originally entitled *The Common Sense Book of Baby and Child Care*; that tome is now in its eighth edition (Spock and Needlman, 2004). Parents increasingly sought advice from child guidance clinics about how to raise their children. Some of the clinical records from those clinics have survived since the 1930s. Looking at them now, some professionals consider the advice given as wholesale and gratuitous blaming of mothers for all their children's problems (Horn, 1989; Jones, 1999; Silk et al., 2000). Some feminist authors maintain that mental health professionals continue to blame mothers in this way (Caplan and Hall-McCorquodale, 1985; Faller, 2007).

Far from reserving the new science for people in therapy, mental health professionals began to transmit information about common psychological problems to parents and teachers. They shared some insights from psychoanalysis although the dynamics seem quite simplistic. An example is a volume entitled *Psychoanalysis in the Classroom* (1922), in which Green offered insight into the content of everyday children's daydreams. He insisted that all daydreams are egoistical, totally devoid of any moral purpose. Some involve a "fantasy of display" in which children perform wonderful feats that they could not achieve in real life. In some daydreams, children earn recognition for rescuing people in distress. In others, the dreamer occupies an exalted role, such as that of a deity or member of a royal family. In yet others, they earn the love of admired people by being of service to them. Thus, daydreams can reveal important information about the needs and desires of children. Green ventured that it was impossible to put an end to daydreaming in any way other than fulfilling the underlying needs expressed in the daydreams. Green (1947) went on to psychoanalyze the content of children's comic books,

warning of the grave harm that would befall children who read *Jungle Comics*.

Similarly, Harvey (1918) wrote about the phenomenon of children's imaginary playmates, which, he argued, relieved the loneliness of withdrawn children and children with no siblings. Robinson (1920) and Leonard (1920) offered explanations of children's telling of lies. Much of Robinson's insight is based on recollections of his own childhood, a method rarely used nowadays. In his fantasies, he displayed great skill at the game of baseball although he was not that good a player in real life. He himself stopped short of improving on his fantasy life by letting lies about false baseball prowess enter into his real-life conversation. However, he believes that many children improve on their fantasies in this way.

An "ounce of prevention" added to the field of childhood mental health

Taken together, the juvenile court movement and the parent–education movement constitute the most visible manifestations of yet another new line of thinking: that child psychopathology could be prevented. The founding hero of the early preventive mental health movement, then known as "mental hygiene," is Clifford Beers, a prolific, creative and troubled person. Beers was hospitalized in Pennsylvania for severe depression and paranoia in 1900, only 3 years after he graduated from university in science; all of his four siblings also suffered from mental illness. He was shocked at the mistreatment he witnessed in mental hospitals. He articulated his views on mental health in an autobiography entitled *A Mind that Found Itself* (Beers, 1981), a highly unusual step for an in-patient at the time. He also recounted his personal bouts with mental illness in his speeches and appeals for the funding of mental health research. In an additional effort to help prevent mental illness from reaching dimensions that entail hospitalization, he founded the first out-patient mental health clinic in 1913 and continued to direct it for over 20 years (Dain, 1980). Out-patient mental health clinics emerged as frontrunners in the prevention and early treatment of the mental disorders of both adults and children.

A pioneering large-scale prevention program designed to combat juvenile delinquency was introduced in the 1930s by psychologists working in the Boston area; it is known as the Cambridge-Somerville study, although the two communities that participated are not in fact Cambridge and Somerville. The Cambridge-Somerville study introduced important methodological interventions including a control group and longitudinal follow-up. Young boys, 5 through 11 years old, were assigned counselors with whom they developed special relationships. The counselors also arranged proper medical care, recreational opportunities and summer camps. The control group, matched for age and risk of delinquency, received no special treatment. The two groups were followed for 30 years by psychologist Joan McCord, who reported devastating results: Three decades later, the control group had fewer criminal convictions and lower rates of psychopathology (McCord, 1992)! These results, difficult to interpret, may have occurred because the boys had become dependent on their counselors but did not develop the life skills they would need to adjust to the challenges of life.

Needless to say, these results did little to inspire the psychologists of the time to devote their energies to prevention programs. After several more rounds of optimism and despair, the prevention of child psychopathology is now considered a very legitimate clinical and scientific activity, though its proponents maintain that it still struggles in the shadow of treatment facilities.

Based on the foundational work of William Healy, child guidance clinics emerged in many locations throughout the United States in an attempt to prevent juvenile delinquency (Silk et al., 2000; Spaulding and Balch, 1983). The child guidance movement was the first significant mental health prevention effort introduced by healthcare institutions and therefore constitutes a major milestone in the

history of prevention. Although these clinics were established to implement *primary* prevention (Lindt, 1950; Thomas and Penn, 2002; Spaulding and Balch, 1983), over time the goal of the centers became more modest, focusing on *secondary* and *tertiary* prevention (Lindt, 1950; Thomas and Penn, 2002). In 1923, Douglas Thom published a manual describing the methods of his "habit clinics," founded as alternatives to child guidance clinics. Habit clinics were founded to prevent maladaptive behaviors and cognitions from becoming engrained in the child's personality and, hence, from becoming cognitive causal factors in adult psychopathology (Jones, 2002; Spaulding and Balch, 1983).

By this point, concern over substance use disorders had persisted for almost 100 years. It is no surprise that they would be the next major mental health difficulty that would be targeted for preventive efforts. In the United States in 1920, the Eighteenth Amendment to the American Constitution was ratified, prohibiting the sale, manufacture, distribution, consumption and importation of alcohol (Meyer and Quenzer, 2005). Also in 1920, The Harrison Act (1914 [legislation requiring physicians to report their prescriptions of narcotics]) was reinterpreted by the Supreme Court to limit prescriptions to medical use, thereby making it illegal to consume opiates, cocaine and marijuana for recreation (Meyer and Quenzer, 2005). These laws were clear attempts to reduce abuse and dependence disorders. Although aimed at adults, they are relevant for children because these disorders have particularly high rates of transmission from parents to child, especially when reared in the same household (Merikangas, Dierker and Szatmari, 1998).

Prevention initiatives increase after World War II

Perhaps as a result of the Great Depression and World War II, there was no substantial work on preventing mental illness in childhood during the 1930s and early 1940s. However, in 1946, the US National Mental Health Act was enacted, encouraging the study and implementation of mental health prevention. This resulted in the establishment of the National Institute of Mental Health (Albee, 2005; Costello and Angold, 2000; Spaulding and Balch, 1983). Also in 1946, Thom undertook an organized effort to study the methods by which society in general, and the community in particular, could prevent mental health problems in the preschool child (Jones, 2002; Spaulding and Balch, 1983; for a more detailed history of mental health prevention in the United States from the end of World War II until the 1980s, please see Spaulding and Balch, 1983).

As detailed in Chapter 2, the 1950s can be characterized as a decade in which the environment was studied as a primary contributor to the pathogenesis of mental disturbance, stimulating major prevention initiatives. Accordingly, the *mental hygiene movement* prescribed a number of psychoeducation classes addressing sex education, human relationships, and pregnancy and mother education. The movement also advocated the establishment of nursery schools and marriage-counseling clinics (Jones, 2002; Thompson, 1950).

In 1957 the Primary Mental Health Project began as an attempt at early detection and prevention of school adjustment problems (Cowen, 1996; Cross and Wyman, 2006). Its emphasis on school programming to promote pupil adjustment, also targeting related areas such as academic achievement and behavioral adjustment, continues today, with large-scale programs and efforts such as the Head Start Program, a large initiative launched in the 1960s to enrich the early childhood education of poor children in the United States, and the Child Development Project, which will be discussed later in this chapter.

In counterpoint with this new energy and enthusiasm, the end of the 1950s saw increased criticism of prevention practices. In 1957, Gottlieb and Howell criticized the prevention movement of the time as lacking scientific validity. In another daring blow, they remarked that psychiatry, in all likelihood, lacked the knowledge to teach people how to raise children effectively – a major element of prevention programs of the time. They suggested that

instead of attempting to bring about broad-based environmental change, prevention efforts should be directed at specific proven factors in the etiologies of specific illnesses (Spaulding and Balch, 1983). In a similar vein, in 1961 the Joint Commission on Mental Illness and Health criticized the prevention movement as lacking sufficient empirical validation and as being too global and too optimistic. The Commission concluded that current efforts had failed to make any real change (Spaulding and Balch, 1983; Stockdill, 2005). Despite mounting criticism, the 1960s was a productive era for mental health prevention in terms of both policy and program implementation. In 1963, President Kennedy addressed the US Congress urging legislation that would promote the research and development of prevention programs (Cooper, 1990; Stockdill, 2005).

Unfortunately, the mounting interest of the 1950s and the fervent efforts of the 1960s did not result in mental health prevention programs consistent with the energy its enthusiastic proponents hoped to muster. Reflecting on the reasons for this, Duncan (1994) provides six explanations. First, prevention was never made a priority despite the fervent rhetoric. The law required that community mental health centers strive for five goals of which four were treatment-oriented, with only the fifth directed at prevention, though not explicitly. Given that the centers operated under constrained budgets, it was in their best interest to fund initiatives that would result in immediate concrete gains rather than investing in initiatives that might have some degree of general benefit in the future, especially when sufficient empirical evidence of the efficacy of preventive programming was lacking. Consequently, despite the best intentions, prevention research and programming only consumed 5 percent of the time of the national Community Mental Health Centers. Thus, the second reason why prevention failed to flourish in the 1960s is lack of funding.

The third reason is that these efforts, though intended as preventive, targeted individual behavior change. Emphasizing individual behavior change goes against a well-established public health maxim which states that the least effective strategies are those that rely on voluntary behavior change. Another reason why prevention failed to become commonplace is that the decision-makers were mostly mental health clinicians. Generally speaking, clinicians are interested in clinical methods and treatment, not social action and mass education. Furthermore, clinicians are chronically pressed for time. As well, prevention initiatives were probably expected to meet unreasonable goals. Lastly, the zeitgeist of the time presumed that psychopathology was a biological inevitability; environmental causation had fallen from favor. When psychopathology is understood solely through biological mechanisms, people begin to believe that mental illness is resistant to amelioration via psychosocial methods, especially those implemented at the community level.

Despite any waning enthusiasm in some circles within the medical community, the sustained interest in childhood as integral to successful prevention culminated in the Child Development Project in the 1970s. This project sought to improve school climate, thereby creating an environment that promotes psychological wellness (Cowen, 1996; Lewis, Watson and Schaps, 2003). It was based on *self-determination theory* (Deci and Ryan, 1985) and therefore sought to increase autonomy, belongingness and competence among the participating students. In this school-wide approach, children are given responsibility for following school rules. A cooperative learning program is utilized to minimize competition among students, including a peer-mentoring component. Outcomes from evaluations of this program suggest that program children became more cooperative, better able to defend their views regarding the handling of conflict, were more inclusive in their decision-making, had more friends and had greater self-esteem and empathy (Cowen, 1996; Lewis et al., 2003). School-based interventions of this nature, focusing simultaneously on academics, emotions and behavior, appear throughout the subsequent history of mental health prevention. In many instances, they combine a universal primary intervention aimed at

whole schools with a targeted, secondary prevention program for children already showing signs of maladjustment.

Aside from theoretical and methodological advances, the 1980s were characterized by increased research and by better dissemination of mental health prevention for women and minority groups. This mirrored greater sensitivity to the needs of these populations in society. As part of the same process, interest in social change re-emerged in thinking about ways to prevent mental health, emphasizing the role of schools, recalling the appeals made earlier in the century to eliminate poverty as a way of preventing mental illness. Albee (1998) noted that scientific discourse had switched from results-oriented discussions to discussions of the ethics, politics and ideology of prevention to which he contributed substantially (Iscoe, 2007; Trickett, 2007). Concerns about the influences of abuse, poverty and homelessness on mental illness became more vociferous. Some individuals argued for massive social reform to eliminate these stressors, whereas others insisted that increasing resilience in at-risk persons is a superior and certainly more feasible strategy (Albee, 1998; Iscoe, 2007; Trickett, 2007). The focus on resilience has remained strong to the present day. Calling for an end to the philosophical debate about what truly constitutes prevention, Cowen (1996) argued for a careful look at the few truly preventive programs that have worked, and building on them.

A brief European history

The history presented so far has been, primarily, an American history. However, mental health prevention has existed in other parts of the world since the turn of the nineteenth century. Indeed, the mental hygiene movement in Europe attended to preventive care as early as 1908 (Hosman, 1992). A more detailed history of mental health prevention in Europe is presented in a book entitled *Improving Children's Lives* (Albee, Bond and Monsey, 1992).

Although terminology differed from the prevalent vocabulary used in North America, ideas of primary, secondary and tertiary prevention, as well as mental health promotion, were featured in European textbooks on mental health as early as 1904 (Hosman, 1992). In 1917, Finland became the first European country to establish a mental hygiene association; which, like all European mental hygiene associations, placed an emphasis on prophylaxis rather than treatment. In the 1920s and 1930s, an international collaborative network of national mental hygiene associations was established and carried out regular meetings about prevention (Hosman, 1992). The prevention efforts of the time utilized a multidisciplinary and holistic approach reminiscent of contemporary practice (Hosman, 1992). Unfortunately, however, in the period from World War II until the 1980s, mental health prevention largely disappeared from the discourse of mental health workers in Europe (Hosman, 1992) at the same time as prevention achieved considerable prominence in the United States. Thankfully, the prevention movement in Europe was infused with new life in the 1980s, as more prevention programs began emerging in Great Britain, Norway, Germany, the Netherlands, the former Czechoslovakia, and Poland. Many of these preventive efforts were directed at children and adolescents (Hosman, 1992). Legislative changes facilitated the burgeoning child mental health prevention movement in Europe, with intra-European conferences being held on conventions for the Rights of the Child and the enactment of legislation enforcing these rights (Hosman, 1992).

The intellectual roots of contemporary mental health prevention in Europe go beyond what has been transplanted from the United States. One important approach to prevention in Europe was the *empowerment movement* of the 1980s and 1990s (Stark, 1992). This was a mental health promotion strategy that accepted, as a first principle, that individuals in society are able and responsible for taking control of their lives, which means taking control of their mental health (Stark, 1992). Although the empowerment process is complicated and difficult to achieve, the World

Health Organization's Healthy Cities Project facilitated a mental health promotion project based on empowerment in Munich. Entrenched in a model of community collaboration, citizens in Munich worked with administrative agencies to form a Self-Help Resources Center (Stark, 1992). Through this resources center, six task forces were created, each tackling a unique issue. These task forces sought to prevent mental illness by improving healthcare and nutrition, social environment and living conditions in the neighborhoods, environmental protection, schools, child advocacy and research (Stark, 1992). By empowering individuals to change their own environments and to take responsibility for their mental health and well-being, this project sought to promote mental health at an urban level.

Another important development in European mental health prevention emanates from the Netherlands, where mental health teams have been assigned to specific communities (Regional Institutes for Outpatient Mental Health Care). Each of these institutes includes, at minimum, one professional whose sole responsibility is prevention programming. The focus of that professional's activities is not standardized across the country, enabling, at least in theory, a match between prevention programming and the needs of the particular target community. The prevention programs tend to center around the following topics: parental education, the school system, sexual violence and incest, work and unemployment, divorce, ethnic groups, women, the elderly, suicide and social competence. The preventive functions of the healthcare institutes are required by law; this ensures that prevention will not be forgotten (Hutschemaekers, Tiemens and De Winter, 2007).

Recent methodological advances in prevention science

Arguably the most important development in the recent history of mental health prevention has been the emergence of research useful in rebutting the lingering contention that prevention simply does not work. This rigorous new research does not necessarily show that prevention efforts are always successful but that they sometimes are. The incipient rigorous methodology in studies on prevention has permitted the emergence of the term "prevention science," which reflects the empirical roots of many new prevention initiatives.

Some critics maintain that this rigor has come at too heavy a cost. Social critics with interest in prevention have not welcomed the advent of prevention science, which they see as ignoring broad social causes and focusing too heavily on individual diagnosable mental disorders (as opposed to distress in general), reduction of risk (rather than promotion of competence and resilience) and prioritizing random trials at any cost. In doing so, say the critics, prevention scientists are borrowing too heavily from the diagnostic categories developed by mainstream psychiatry in defining their target populations and objectives (Tebes, Kauffman and Connell, 2003).

In any case, rigorous empirical methods are available for studying the efficacy of prevention initiatives and for understanding why the programs achieve their levels of efficacy (e.g., Brown and Liao, 1999; Gross, Fogg and Conrad, 1993; Marchand et al., 2011). Population-based randomized prevention trials that span significant periods of time have become, in some circles at least, a gold standard (Brown and Liao, 1999; Marchand et al., 2011). Such trials might involve, for example, administering an intervention to different communities, selected at random, at different time points, enabling a comparison of the target community and the community that is placed on the "wait list." Figure 10.4 is a flowchart of the steps involved in a rigorous randomized clinical trial.

Another important advance has been a transition from atheoretical outcome-based approaches to theory-driven trials developed not only to investigate the efficacy of an intervention but to add at the same time to the body of knowledge about child development and the pathogenesis of mental disorder (Becker and Domitrovich, 2011; Koretz, 1991). The

developmental epidemiological framework (Brown and Liao, 1999) is based on three stages of systematic exploration. First, research is conducted to determine the levels of, and variations in, risk and protective factors for a given population before an intervention is implemented. Second, based on the developmental paths of the population, an intervention is created to target the risk and protective factors of the population in an effort to change the observed developmental trajectories. Third, the impact of intervention is evaluated based on the level of risk and protective factors faced by subgroups within the population, and this impact is considered both proximally and distally. This research method is best employed for universal programs or other programs whose outcome can be enumerated for all members in the population (e.g., rates of initial diagnosis of a disorder) (Brown and Liao, 1999; Marchand et al., 2011).

In a helpful review of evaluation methods for preventive interventions, Tebes et al. (2003) point out that the experimental approach to the evaluation of the primary approach provides only one of several possible methods, one that is derived heavily from logical empiricism. A "second generation" emerged in reaction to many perceived problems and limitations in applying such experimental paradigms. It had become apparent that many programs that had been verified in this traditional scientific way were for some reason never used. Increased focus was, therefore, placed on evaluation models, in which the way the program is used receives greater attention than what was done and what changes were produced. In many cases, the "second generation" methods were qualitative rather than quantitative, or some mixture of the two, unfettered by an overarching drive to achieve irrefutable scientific proof that the intervention works. In the current third generation, a more integrative model is based on developing the evaluative method in response to the purposes of the evaluation, which will vary from one situation to another. This entails a "menu" of different quantitative and qualitative methods that can be called upon as needed. In defining which of the multiple methods are selected, users

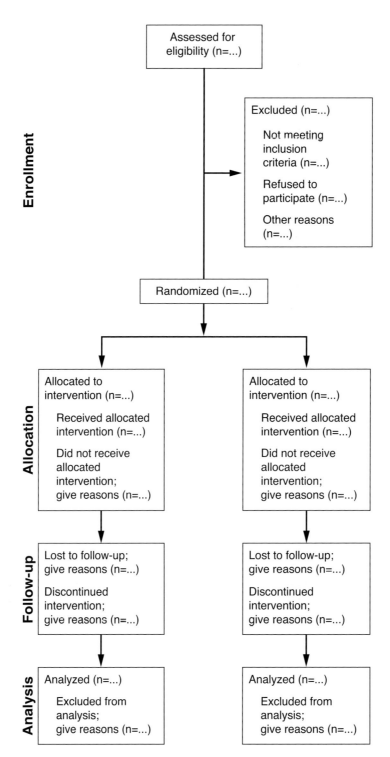

Figure. 10.4 The steps involved in conducting a randomized clinical trial.

of the program and interested stakeholders in the community should play an important role.

In outlining the stages of a comprehensive, meaningful evaluation, Tebes et al. (2003) emphasize "pre-design" considerations such as studying carefully the needs for a specific preventive intervention and the human and other resources that might be available for it. If necessary, the capacity in the community or organization to conduct a meaningful evaluation may have to be strengthened. It may be necessary to clarify the theory behind the model for all those concerned with it. This should be done collaboratively, in concert with defining clearly what the program is expected to achieve. *Formative evaluation* focuses on the process of implementing the program; formative evaluation may include data about the meaning of the program components for the people involved in it. It is complemented later on by *summative evaluation* or assessment of outcomes, as will be discussed shortly.

Once these preliminary steps have been followed, more formal data collection of various kinds may be implemented. Not yet considered is the impact of the program on the pathology it purports to reduce; at this stage, description is the main objective. The program may be described, for example, by means of case studies.

The next step is monitoring of the implementation of the preventive program. This step is essential so that whatever benefits emerge later on can be attributed to the intervention. Most prevention programs are implemented in the community by teachers, nurses and other community personnel, including volunteers. They may not always implement the program exactly as it was intended. Proper training and clear procedures manuals can facilitate *treatment integrity*. During an evaluation, integrity can be verified, for example, by videotaping the intervention sessions in progress and systematically checking that the prescribed procedures are present in the recordings. However, as with other applications of empirical methodology in prevention, some authorities in the field value individual and local adaptations of prescribed procedures more than others do (Dane and Schneider, 1998; Marchand et al., 2011).

Next, the outcome is monitored, attempting to demonstrate scientifically that the desired outcome can be attributed to the intervention. Random assignment is optimal in providing clear scientific evidence of success, but quasi-experimental design, in which groups are compared even though they were not formed by random assignment, may be appropriate and informative in situations where random assignment cannot be achieved. Time series designs can also provide very rigorous evaluation data. In essence, participants become their own controls; outcome is measured in terms of the difference between intervals of time during which the intervention was administered and other intervals during which no intervention took place. Sophisticated statistical techniques such as hierarchical linear modeling are useful in demonstrating the effects of an intervention over time when there have been a series of repeated measures (Tebes et al., 2003).

Goal attainment scaling provides an alternative to the traditional randomized clinical trial. This method is particularly applicable to prevention programs but is by no means limited to this area. *Goal attainment scaling* is a quantitative method for establishing that the goals of the intervention, which were established during the pre-design phase, have been achieved. Thus, an important part of the process is to assist the program developer or community agency in articulating clearly the goals for the program as a whole and for individual participants. Quantitative rating scales are used to assess how well these goals are achieved. Methodologists have developed sophisticated ways of analyzing the data obtained using these scales (Nuehring et al., 1983; Tennant, 2007).

Measurement of outcomes can be profitably combined with *cost–benefit analyses*. One of the major advantages of primary prevention, especially, is its low cost in comparison to the benefits it can potentially provide to at-risk individuals. Specification of the cost–benefit ratio can be invaluable in determining the cost of whatever positive outcomes emerge.

Finally, the evaluation of the intervention must be disseminated. There are indeed very reputable scientific journals devoted to prevention. However, consistent with the prevailing spirit in the prevention field, dissemination should ideally include community members and should be done in consultation with them (Tebes et al., 2003).

Successful prevention in contemporary practice

The growing data base on preventive mental health has converged to provide useful guidelines for exemplary practice. The characteristics of successful prevention initiatives have been identified in several review articles (e.g., Nation et al., 2003), and reviews of reviews (Bond and Carmola-Hauf, 2004, 2007; Hage et al., 2007). The features common to most successful prevention efforts include the following:

1. The initiative should be based on strong research and theory (Bond and Carmola-Hauf, 2004, 2007; Nation et al., 2003).
2. The program should focus on building strengths and protective factors as well as reducing risk factors (Bond and Carmola-Hauf, 2004, 2007; Hage et al., 2007).
3. The initiative should be sensitive to the context. This includes socio-political sensitivity, cultural sensitivity, sensitivity to the resources that might be available, sensitivity to the competencies (including developmental age) of active members and sensitivity to the abilities and needs of all stakeholders (Bond and Carmola-Hauf, 2004, 2007; Hage et al., 2007; Nation et al., 2003).
4. The initiative should function on many levels and in many systems; it should address both individual and systematic or contextual factors, and should address all mediators of the problem behavior (Bond and Carmola-Hauf, 2004, 2007; Hage et al., 2007; Nation et al., 2003).

5. The program should incorporate high-quality monitoring and evaluation in its structure and implementation (Bond and Carmola-Hauf, 2004, 2007; Nation et al., 2003).
6. The program should be addressed at problems that have been identified in research as predictable. In many cases, different problems are known to co-occur; the program should ideally target multiple, interrelated problems (Bloom and Gullotta, 2003).

The reviewers of the prevention literature also recommend ensuring that the purpose and goals are clearly defined (Bond and Carmola-Hauf, 2004) and that the program is sustainable, that is, likely to be continued in the community after the initial research on the program has been concluded (Bond and Carmola-Hauf, 2007). If skills are taught as part of the intervention, the reviewers recommend that a variety of teaching methods be employed (Nation et al., 2003).

The bottom line: does mental health prevention work?

Despite the tremendous methodological achievements of recent years, evaluation of prevention efforts remains difficult. One reason for this difficulty is the inability of the scientific method to demonstrate that something did *not* happen (Durlak and Wells, 1997). Accordingly, one requires a reliable and valid knowledge of the developmental psychopathological trajectory of the disorder under study to demonstrate the efficacy of a prevention program. Additionally, the heterogeneity among both the recipients and the different programs themselves makes it difficult to compare the efficacy of one program to another (Durlak and Wells, 1997). Nonetheless, in 1997, Durlak and Wells conducted an influential meta-analysis of 177 articles reporting on the efficacy of primary prevention programs. This meta-analysis remains the most comprehensive accounting of the effects of prevention programs on children's mental health (Kind, et al., 2010). The meta-analysts controlled for the limitations inherent in tallying the efficacy of prevention in a few ways. The first limitation, the inability to predict a lack of change, was overcome in two ways. First, they only used studies that included a control group of some kind. Second, rather than considering any specific disorder, which would require a sound knowledge of its etiology, the authors looked at all behavioral and emotional problem outcomes. To deal with the problem of heterogeneity in target groups in different studies, Durlak and Wells separated studies into *person-centered* (aimed directly at changing individuals) and *environment-centered* (aimed indirectly at changing individuals by changing the environments in which they live and work). The authors provide separate effectiveness statistics for transition programs (programs implemented during times of high stress, e.g., school transition), interpersonal problem-solving interventions and affective education (e.g., programs aimed at the appropriate expression of emotion). To further reduce the heterogeneity of the studies, they divided the programs by developmental level.

Among the results, they found that affective education programs were most effective for the youngest group, with diminishing returns for older child and adolescent populations. Interpersonal problem-solving programs were also more effective for young children than for older children. Nonetheless, older children (7–11) still benefited from these interventions. Impressive success rates were reported for behavioral person-centered interventions, school-based environment-centered interventions and transition programs.

On the whole, the programs had the dual benefit of reducing problems and increasing competencies. Thus, these meta-analytic data suggest that primary prevention programs are indeed effective. The authors recommend that future research investigate the specific attributes of effective programs. Although no similarly comprehensive meta-analysis of prevention programs has appeared since the Durlak and Wells report, there is no reason to think that the reported levels of effectiveness have not been at least maintained.

Selected examples of effective prevention programs

The following section provides examples of prevention practices that have proven efficacious. Examples of primary and secondary prevention programs will be provided, as well as for universal, selective and indicated programs within the primary level of prevention. Please note that the secondary level is included in the section on the FAST Track program, which includes both primary and secondary prevention components. Of course, these examples do not constitute a comprehensive representation of the many innovative programs that have been developed.

Primary universal prevention

As defined earlier in this chapter, *primary universal prevention* initiatives are provided to, and are planned to confer benefit on, all persons in the target population. The interventions are intended to target people before any symptoms become manifest. In one example from Norway, a group of researchers sought to reduce social anxiety by applying a *universal* prevention model (Aune and Stiles, 2009). The program was delivered over the course of 12 months; the first 4 months were used as a training phase and the last 8 months were a consolidation phase in which all participants were encouraged to practice the skills they learned. The intervention was instituted as follows. First, school and public health nurses participated in 1-day *psychoeducation* sessions to learn about anxiety, social anxiety and related phenomena. Second, a three-page overview of the information that would be given in the intervention appeared in local papers, which also included information about the study. Third, teachers and other school personnel participated in 90 minutes of psychoeducation at each school. Fourth, parents and guardians participated in 1 hour of psychoeducation at an evening meeting. Fifth, community health and welfare workers participated in 90 minutes of psychoeducation in a lecture format. Sixth, children participated in three consecutive

45-minute sessions of psychoeducation covering similar material. In addition, the program developers prepared a website and two booklets (one for students and one for parents) containing psychoeducational information that were created and distributed at the beginning of the program. The information focused on the principles of cognitive-behavioral treatment for anxiety disorders with an emphasis on social anxiety disorder. The booklets provided information on how thoughts and assumptions influence emotions and behavior. The content of all materials was tailored to the presumed needs of the audience. For example, nurses received more information on treatment whereas teachers received more information on classroom management.

In a randomized control trial of the intervention there were no differences between groups on level of anxiety before the intervention. However, at post-test the intervention group displayed significantly lower anxiety than the control group. Additionally, there was less anxiety after the intervention than before in the intervention group but there was no positive change for the control group. Within the intervention group, one less person had syndromal anxiety after the intervention as compared to before (thirty-eight individuals had syndromal anxiety before the intervention for the treatment group; after the intervention there were thirty-seven). In contrast, within the control group five individuals developed syndromal anxiety over the course of the wait period and no one improved (there were thirty-two people with syndromal anxiety before the intervention for the control group and thirty-seven after). This intervention was, therefore, demonstrated to be efficacious.

Other types of primary universal prevention programs include child abuse prevention programs and academic tutoring. Child abuse prevention can be considered a prevention initiative when it is intended to reduce psychopathology in the child; when its aims do not transcend simply preventing child abuse, however, it is not a prevention initiative in its proper sense (Compton, 2010; Cowen, 1996). Similarly, academic tutoring programs can be considered preventive when they are intended to prevent mental health difficulty but are not truly prevention programs when that is not their intent (Cowen, 1996). Of course, that does not mean that these interventions are not useful.

The FAST Track program in the United States is a primary universal prevention program complemented by secondary prevention initiatives with children at risk for disruptive behavior disorder. As part of the component PATHS (Promoting Alternative Thinking Strategies) curriculum, FAST Track seeks to increase self-control, emotional awareness and understanding, peer-related social skills, and social problem-solving (Conduct Problems Research Group, 2011). The curriculum is delivered by teachers in the classroom, who are encouraged to incorporate the content in their teaching throughout the day rather than relegating the intervention to an isolated block of time (Conduct Problems Research Group, 2011). In a longitudinal study of 2,937 children in the early elementary-school years, the FAST Track version of the PATHS curriculum was demonstrated to effectively reduce aggression, increase prosocial behavior and increase academic engagement over sustained periods of time (Conduct Problems Research Group, 2011). The FAST Track team has evaluated both the primary and secondary prevention components very thoroughly. The universal social-learning program consists of the PATHS curriculum plus consultation with teachers. The curriculum is delivered to the entire class by teachers who receive training and consultation from the FAST Track team. The lessons include such topics as self-control, awareness of emotion and appropriate ways of emotional expression, social skills in relating to peers, and social problem-solving (Kusche and Greenberg, 1995). Problem-solving training, discussed more fully later in this chapter, has been a mainstay of prevention programs for over 30 years. It typically consists of teaching children to recognize, first of all, when they are facing a problem. They then learn to generate multiple solutions to the problem and evaluate rationally the advantages and disadvantages of each. Subsequently, the children are guided through the systematic implementation of the solution they have selected. Finally, they learn to evaluate their own implementation of the solution without exaggerating their successes or failures.

After 3 years of implementation, there were some effects of the universal primary prevention program on several aspects of pupil adjustment according to the data for classes in the participating school. Most of the results, although not very large, reached levels of conventional statistical significance, averaging approximately 0.5 of a standard deviation. Importantly, both teacher and peer reports indicated some reduction in aggression and some increase in prosocial behavior. Teacher reports indicated greater academic engagement; peer reports mirrored this finding for boys only (Conduct Problems Research Group, 2011).

The secondary prevention components of FAST Track were delivered to children who were selected in their kindergartens at age 5 years on the basis of early signs of problematic aggression according to information obtained from both parents and teachers. Together with the adults who play important roles in their lives, they participated in a very intensive intervention, consisting of weekly sessions for parents focusing on child-rearing complemented by home visits by project workers, social skills training for the children and academic tutoring (Bierman, Greenberg and the Conduct Problems Prevention Research Group, 1996). The progress of the participating children has been tracked for a number of years, unlike most previous programs in which follow-up is reported for only one year or less following the program (Conduct Problems Research Group, 2011). There have been some significant improvements for the participants in the selective-intervention group, who were the 10 percent highest in aggression at the beginning of the study. Of that group, 37 percent showed no signs of problematic aggression after 3 years of participation in FAST Track, compared with 27 percent of the members of the control group, which received whatever services would have normally been provided by their schools and communities (Conduct Problems Prevention Research Group, 2002a, 2002b, 2002c).

In brief, the results of FAST Track, however sobering because it has not totally turned around these children's lives, should indicate to others contemplating new prevention programs that they may expect some return on their investment of effort but should not count on unconstrained success.

Like all other studies, the FAST Track research provides results that may be specific to the US context. There have been several successful attempts at adapting the program to other cultures. The Romanian government has financed a Romanian version, with outcome data reported by Stefan and Miclea (2013). The Romanians transformed all of the components of the FAST Track program, including the parent training and group social skills training, into a primary prevention package. Accordingly, the Romanian researchers opted not to provide separate group social skills training for at-risk children because their reading of the literature indicated that children showing early dysfunctional behavior do not benefit greatly from associating with each other. They learn more, the researchers maintained, from interacting with peers who are more competent socially. In Romania, the teacher-training component included not only classroom behavior management but also skills for the teachers to use in enhancing children's appropriate expression of emotion. In place of FAST Track's intensive parent training for the parents of children at risk, they opted for a shorter, four-session parent intervention that could be offered to parents of both high- and low-risk children. The intent of this change was to increase parent participation and reduce stigma. Compared to children in control-group classrooms, children participating in the prevention program improved in their emotional knowledge and problem-solving skills. The prevention-group participants also displayed fewer externalizing problems and fewer social-emotional problems than control-group participants according to most of the parent and teacher ratings. Only post-intervention results are reported in the article by Stefan and Miclea. Hopefully, follow-up data are forthcoming.

Primary-selective prevention

In Ontario, Canada, researchers sought to increase positive body image and appropriate eating behaviors in female athletes who are at especially high risk for developing eating disorders, in this case, female gymnasts (Buchholz et al., 2008). The program involved members of different professions (such as dieticians, body image experts, gymnastics coaches and others) in both the construction and dissemination of it. By involving individuals having different levels of contact with the targeted athletes in the creation and dissemination of the program, the intervention was thought to better address the needs and challenges of all stakeholders (Bond and Carmola-Hauf, 2007). The intervention itself consisted of psychoeducation pertaining to: eating attitudes, information about body health, individual differences in body size and shape, resisting pressures to diet, physical activity for enjoyment, self-esteem for female athletes, stress management and balance between sport and other activities (Buchholz et al., 2008). Because this program seeks to intervene in the key mediators of developing eating pathology, it can be considered a *primary-selective intervention.*

Peer mentoring and mediation programs can also be used for primary-selective prevention initiatives in light of the strong influence of peers, as discussed in Chapter 7 (Wright et al., 2007). One such program sought to prevent the development of anti-social behaviors in high-risk teenagers (Wright et al., 2007). The model included cooperative learning and classroom behavior management as well as peer tutoring, mentoring and mediation, thus targeting both the school climate and the individual (Wright et al., 2007).

Primary-indicated prevention

Primary-indicated prevention programs target individuals who show some symptoms of pathology but do not meet full diagnostic criteria for any pathology (Mrazek and Haggerty, 1994). A study conducted with Icelandic adolescents evaluated a prevention program for 171 14-year-old adolescents who either reported depressive symptoms or who displayed a negative attribution style (Arnarson and Craighead, 2009; see Chapter 13). The program consisted of fourteen sessions conducted during school designed to increase self-esteem. The intervention included an informative manual, homework assignments to challenge dysfunctional beliefs about oneself and other people, culturally relevant cartoons and videos, and relaxation exercises (Arnarson and Craighead, 2009). In a randomized control trial, this intervention was demonstrated to effectively prevent initial episodes of dysthymia and major depressive disorder in a significant number of participants.

Although this particular program was *indicated*, *universal* school-based prevention programs for major depression are common. A recent Canadian program in which prevention is approached from the perspective of mental health literacy is delivered both online and in a mental health magazine. Members are periodically encouraged to fill out surveys in which they track their positive and negative affect as well as risk behaviors. The at-risk youth are prompted to seek help and are provided with the information they need to do so (Santor and Bagnell, 2008).

The children of parents with mental illness are known to be particularly vulnerable. An example of a comprehensive and successful preventive intervention with that population is the Kanu program in Germany. This multimodal intervention includes: (1) help for the families in communication skills and facilitation of the children's understanding of their parents' problems; (2) matching the children with well-adjusted "godparents"; (3) parenting skills training; (4) group counseling for the children focusing on communication and social skills; and (5) training of the professionals who work with the family (Heitmann et al., 2012)

Conclusion: to what extent can mental illness be prevented in children and adolescents?

The aforementioned historic influences have brought preventive mental health into the new millennium as a more mature science, with many policy-makers and professionals recognizing its importance. Far more energy and far more resources are still needed for these ideas to be matched in practice. Ideally, successful primary prevention strategies will become the norm. Exclusive reliance on primary prevention, however, is likely to be insufficient. First of all, primary prevention requires a thorough understanding of the causes and trajectories of a given pathology to be fully effective; this level of knowledge has yet to be realized for most mental disorders. Furthermore, successful methods are only beginning to emerge

in preventing many of the causes of mental illness that have been identified. For the time being, then, it must be recognized that prevention science has not developed applied prevention programs effective in preventing all child psychology and is unlikely to do so in the future. Indeed, all child psychopathology is probably not preventable. Nevertheless, the enthusiastic contemporary advocates of prevention initiatives are likely to deliver a good return on the investment they seek in prevention, which at best is likely to constitute only a small fraction of the money and energy devoted to the treatment of full-blown child psychopathology. With increasing access to the internet, especially among young people, an effective and inexpensive modality for the delivery of some components of primary prevention programs has emerged over the past few years; its potential is just beginning to be tapped.

Summary

- Prevention strategies have lagged behind treatments for psychopathology. Serious consideration of prevention did not start until the latter half of the twentieth century.
- For a program to be considered preventive, it must: (1) be group oriented; (2) be implemented before the targeted pathology becomes manifest; and (3) be intentional.
- Treatment and prevention are considered complementary. In a way, all treatment is preventive, since it aims to prevent worsening of mental health. However, treatment is directed at people already suffering from a disorder.
- Gerald Caplan proposed a three-tiered prevention model, consisting of *primary prevention*, intended to prevent occurrence of a new pathology, *secondary prevention*, focusing on early disease detection and *tertiary prevention*, which attempts to reduce the severity of impairment caused by a disorder.

- Gordon's model consists of three types of interventions: *universal*, which would benefit everyone, *selective*, which only benefit a subgroup of the population and *indicated*, which target individuals manifesting a marker indicating high enough risk to require intervention. These measures are only preventive if they are applied to individuals not already demonstrating signs of illness or distress.
- Mrazek and Haggerty's model is a reconceptualization of Gordon's, in which the *indicated* level applies to individuals experiencing symptoms, but not meeting diagnostic criteria.
- The models represent an attempt to reduce the gray area between prevention and treatment when prevention programs target individuals.
- In understanding prevention, it is important to consider not just what is being provided,

but where and how. Collaborating with the community is widely advocated for the implementation of prevention programs. Power, resources and authority are shared throughout with stakeholders in the community, unlike traditional methods of delivering mental health services in most places.

- In ancient Greece, it was believed that a balanced lifestyle with community participation would ensure mental health. These beliefs were largely lost over time.
- Starting in the 1830s, the Temperance Movement, a campaign in all major English-speaking countries against alcohol consumption, can be considered the first major modern attempt at preventing substance use disorder.
- As the nineteenth century progressed, asylum superintendents advocated prevention initiatives for at-risk groups, particularly young children and children of parents with mental disorder.
- Eugenics was once promoted as mental health prevention. Eugenics has no role in modern mental health prevention.
- The first recognized prevention work began in 1909–1919 when Dr. William Healy began an early secondary-selective initiative designed to prevent repeat offending by children and youths.
- Substance abuse is a frequent target of prevention efforts. In 1920, the US ratified the Eighteenth Amendment, prohibiting the sale, manufacture, consumption and importation of alcohol, and the Harrison Act was reinterpreted to limit prescriptions to medical use.
- In 1946, the US National Mental Health Act was enacted, encouraging the study and implementation of mental health prevention, resulting in the establishment of the National Institute of Mental Health. Thom undertook a study of the methods by which society and community could prevent mental health problems.
- In the 1950s, the mental hygiene movement advocated psychoeducational classes addressing sex education, human relationships, pregnancy and mother education, as well as the establishment of nursery schools and marriage-counseling clinics.
- The Primary Mental Health Project began in 1957 to detect and prevent school adjustment problems, targeting academic achievement and behavioral adjustment.
- The end of the 1950s saw increased criticism of the prevention movement. Gottlieb and Howell said it lacked scientific validity and that psychiatry lacked the knowledge to teach people how to raise children effectively.
- Prevention went against a well-established public health maxim which states that the least effective strategies rely on voluntary change.
- In prevalent scientific thinking in the 1950s, psychopathology was seen as a biological inevitability.
- The Child Development Project, based on self-determination theory, was introduced in the 1970s. Using a school-wide approach, children were given responsibility for following school rules, and a cooperative learning program was introduced. Results show that children became more cooperative, better able to defend their views regarding the handling of conflict, more inclusive in decision-making, had more friends, greater self-esteem and greater empathy. Many similar programs subsequently appeared, usually combining a primary intervention for the whole school with secondary prevention for children showing signs of maladjustment.
- The 1980s saw increased research and better dissemination of mental health prevention for women and minority groups. Interest in social change re-emerged, emphasizing the role of schools, recalling earlier recommendations to eliminate poverty to prevent mental illness. Arguments were made for massive social reform to eliminate the influence of abuse, poverty and homelessness on mental health, but the focus has remained, to this day, on increasing resilience in at-risk persons.

- Critics have argued that prevention science focuses too heavily on individual disorders, reduction of risk and prioritization of random trials, while relying too heavily on diagnostic categories, as opposed to concern with broad social change, general mental distress and promotion of competence and resilience.
- Rigorous empirical methods, such as randomized prevention trials spanning significant periods of time, are used to study the efficacy of prevention programs and reasons why efficacy is achieved. These trials might involve comparing a community participating in an intervention with one that is not.
- The developmental epidemiological framework is based on three stages: determining levels of risk and protective factors, creating an intervention targeting those factors and evaluating impact. It is best used for universal programs, i.e. programs for all members of the population.
- A "second generation" of prevention programs has emerged, evaluating how the programs were used, rather than outcomes, often using qualitative or a mixture of qualitative and quantitative methods, with less focus on irrefutable scientific proof that the intervention works.
- Formative evaluation focuses on the process of implementing the program. Following this step, more formal data collection to assess the program may be implemented. The program may not be implemented exactly as intended. Treatment integrity can be facilitated with training using detailed manuals. Integrity can be verified during evaluation but some authorities value individual and local adaptations of procedures more than others.
- Time series designs can provide very rigorous evaluation data. Sophisticated techniques are used in demonstrating the effects of an intervention over time.
- Goal attainment scaling is a quantitative method for establishing that the goals of the intervention have been achieved. Quantitative rating scales describing how completely the goals are achieved are the main tools used in goal-attainment scaling. Methodologists have developed sophisticated ways of analyzing the data obtained with these scales.
- Cost–benefit analyses can be combined with measures of outcome. Prevention typically has low cost compared to its benefits.
- Dissemination results can be published in journals but results should also be disseminated to individuals in the participating community.
- Growing data on preventive mental health have revealed a number of features common to successful prevention efforts:
  - A strong base in research and theory.
  - Focus on building strengths and protective factors, as well as reducing risk factors.
  - Sensitivity to the context in which the initiative occurs.
  - Multilevel, multisystem functioning, addressing individual and systemic factors and all mediators of the problem behavior.
  - Incorporation of high-quality monitoring and evaluation.
  - Targeting of multiple interrelated problems.
- It is recommended that programs have clearly defined purposes and goals, be sustainable and, if skills are taught, use a variety of teaching methods.
- The US FAST Track program is aimed at children at risk for disruptive behavior disorder. It seeks to increase self-control, emotional awareness and understanding, peer-related social skills and social problem-solving. Delivered partially by teachers, FAST Track is incorporated into teaching throughout the day. A longitudinal study showed that it reduces aggression, increases prosocial behavior and increases academic engagement over sustained periods of time.
- Prevention is not effective at preventing all child psychopathology, and some severe problems are probably not preventable.

Study questions

1. What are the essential distinctions between prevention and treatment of psychological disorders?
2. What is the difference between primary and secondary prevention? Give examples, possibly hypothetical, of a primary prevention program and a secondary prevention program for the same disorder.
3. Why might a universal, primary prevention program be insufficient to prevent a targeted disorder?
4. Is a randomized trial the best way to evaluate a prevention program? Why or why not?
5. Define goal attainment scaling and state some of its advantages and disadvantages.

11 Psychological interventions with children and adolescents

Psychotherapy with children may or may not be conducted in a manner that resembles the widespread stereotype in which a person seeing a psychotherapist "opens up," reveals their feelings and inner conflicts and receives support from the therapist and insight about the causes of their difficulties. Many but certainly not all children have the capacity to undergo such a process, which of course depends on having the vocabulary needed to describe one's inner emotional life and to understand and make use of the therapist's input.

This chapter provides a global overview of psychological interventions in common use with children and adolescents. More information about the interventions used in the treatment of specific disorders appears in subsequent chapters. The chapter begins with an introduction to the major theories of psychotherapy. It continues with deliberation about the applicability of these approaches to the childhood and adolescent stages. Axline's non-directive play therapy is then introduced as a case example of a technique with an important place in the history of child psychopathology, followed by a section on contemporary evidence-based practice. The chapter continues with a section on the research basis of child and adolescent psychotherapy. The tool of meta-analysis is introduced at that point. The chapter concludes with some remarks about the emerging field of cybertherapy.

Theories of psychotherapy

Although there is considerable overlap among the various "schools" or approaches to psychotherapy, they are often classified as: (1) *psychodynamic*, which focuses on change in processes internal to the individual; (2) *humanistic/existential*, which often focuses on enhancing feelings of self-worth and experiencing acceptance as a person; and (3) *behavioral/cognitive*, focusing on change in behavior, sometimes by changing the thinking that is linked to maladaptive behavior. Table 11.2 contains a comparison of the major contemporary approaches to psychotherapy. A common element among most psychotherapies is their focus on a therapeutic alliance between the therapist and client. Given the great divergence among psychologists in their thinking about psychotherapy, it is important for psychologists and their clients, which include the parents of children in therapy, to agree on the purposes of therapy (Andersson and Cuijpers, 2009).

The term "psychological intervention" is used in the title of this chapter to encompass both the terms "psychotherapy" and "psychological treatment," each of which has specific connotations in the literature. Perhaps the most general of the many definitions of psychotherapy is "the treatment of mental or emotional problems by psychological means" (United States Office of Technology Assessment, 1980). Some contemporary users of this nomenclature have argued for a distinction between the terms *psychotherapy* and *psychological treatment* (Barlow, 2004; Andersson and Cuijpers, 2009). Psychotherapy represents a highly heterogeneous range of techniques that: (1) may or may not be validated by empirical research; and (2) may or may not have as their goal the alleviation of the symptoms of a mental health disorder; other goals may include self-discovery or personal development. Barlow (2004) argues that the term "psychological treatment" should be reserved for evidence-based interventions directed at a mental health disorder. In that sense, some but not all applications of psychotherapy can be considered a form of psychological treatment.

Developmental issues

Each of the major forms of therapy mentioned earlier (psychodynamic, humanistic/existential, behavioral/cognitive) was well developed for application to the problems of adults well before the basic principles on which the therapies were based were applied to children. Psychotherapy with children is fundamentally different from psychotherapy with adults because of its environmental embeddedness. As detailed by Weisz and Bearman (2010), the child may be the "patient" but the parents may well be the "clients." Parents usually initiate the process of therapy because children rarely present themselves to professionals asking for help with their psychological distress. Individual psychotherapy for the child may be part of the overall intervention plan but it is rarely the sole component. Even so, the parents may end up exerting themselves more than the child. Teachers also play important roles in children's lives; therefore, psychological treatment for children often involves work with them. Although the need to recognize and work from the child's perspective is increasingly acknowledged, this is not always easy to accomplish. In an interesting study by Yeh and Weisz (2001), there was only a 37 percent match between the problems listed by parents and children as reasons for their involvement with a mental health clinic.

Holmbeck, Devine and Bruno (2010) observe that if a 6-year-old and a 16-year-old are referred for the same problem, the treatment prescribed will likely not be the same in each case. However, despite the proliferation in research on child psychological treatment, surprisingly little is known about how to match treatment to the child's age or developmental level. Perhaps because therapy has not been adapted properly to the developmental level of younger children, it is often found that psychotherapy works somewhat better after the transition to early adolescence. This can be explained by the fact that the therapeutic approach most studied is cognitive-behavioral which, by its very nature, is related to the child's cognitive development. In order to profit optimally from cognitive-behavioral treatment, a child or adolescent must be capable of complex, symbolic abstract thinking. He/she must be capable of *metacognition* – thinking about one's own thinking processes. Implementation of any new behavior or way of relating to others requires the ability to plan and to anticipate the outcomes of new behaviors or new ways of relating to others. In Piagetian terms, these abilities relate to the emergence of formal operational thinking (Holmbeck et al., 2010).

Thus, cognitive development may be a *moderator* of the outcomes of psychotherapy, which means that the outcomes of therapy may be enhanced or weakened depending on the developmental level of the person in therapy. However, Holmbeck et al. also note that cognitive development may function as a *mediator* of the success of psychotherapy. In other words, the therapy may work because it helps accelerate the thinking skills of a child or adolescent who initially came to therapy with an immature level of cognitive development.

Finally, Holmbeck and colleagues mention one more way in which developmental issues are of fundamental importance to the psychological treatment, namely the parents' thinking about normal child development. These authors emphasize the importance of educating parents about the levels of emotional, cognitive and social development that are typical for children of the ages of their sons and daughters.

Dibs and a profession in search of itself

Laypersons around the world were offered a glimpse into the captivating process of child psychotherapy by Virginia Axline, whose 1964 book *Dibs: In Search of Self* (Axline, 1964) became a mass-market best seller. Dibs started therapy with Axline when he was 5 years old. He was brought to therapy because of his social isolation, difficulties in expressing his feelings, and sporadic outbursts of verbal and physical aggression. At times, he would lash out after being given an instruction by his teacher. A very likeable

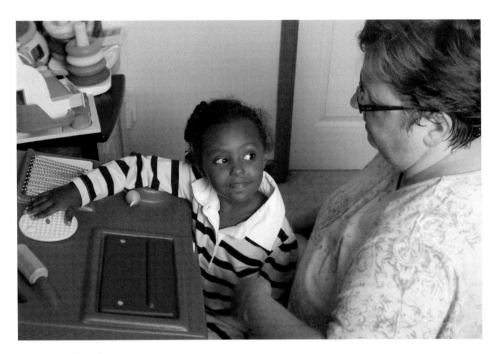

Figure 11.1 Play therapy.

boy in general, Dibs had an IQ well within the gifted range. However, he was quite sparing in his verbal communication with others. Because of his erratic behavior and withdrawal, Dibs' parents began to believe that he was crazy or schizophrenic. Before starting therapy with Dibs, Axline was invited to Dibs' school, where she confirmed the reports about Dibs' behavior through observation and discussions with the school staff. Difficult as school life was for Dibs, he would often engage in tantrums when it was time to go home.

Dibs participated in *play therapy*, in which play is used as a medium for self-expression and communication, recognizing the fact that verbal expression of problems may be outside the repertoire of many children's verbal skills and is an atypical experience for them. There were a total of eighteen sessions, which is shorter than many play-therapy interventions. From the start, Dibs related warmly and well to Axline and participated very willingly in therapy. Dibs' aloof mother could bring herself to do little more than bring Dibs to the play sessions. She

would not remain in the waiting room. Axline met Dibs' mother only twice, using these two meetings to provide the mother with the opportunity to express her inner feelings as well. Mom did express some remorse about the unhappy home environment she and her husband were providing for Dibs, which could be characterized as cold, somewhat harsh and devoid of emotional exchange. Axline listened empathically but offered no suggestions about other parenting strategies. Dibs' improvement in therapy was probably based in large part on the therapeutic relationship he developed with Axline. Using such toys as wooden soldiers, Dibs began to express his feelings about the emotionally cold and oppressive parenting he was receiving. Axline discovered his tendency to form strong opinions about things, to which he stuck with an arrogance uncommon for children his age. As time went on, Dibs began to explore the physical space of the play-therapy room. Dibs began to express himself, not only with Axline, but also with his parents. Although their involvement in therapy was minimal, the parents began to understand that Dibs' problems were largely a reflection of their own problems; they were saddened by this discovery. Dibs became less frozen in his approach to people and showed himself to be a spontaneous and creative boy.

Reflecting on the enduring message behind the Dibs story almost 50 years after it was first published, Jackson (2010) observes that the book serves as a megaphone to amplify Dibs' voice and make his feelings known. Jackson does not believe that Axline wrote the book to garner support for any specific school of psychotherapy. Her therapy with Dibs was vaguely psychoanalytic but not really rich in the interpretation of symbols or subconscious motives. Perhaps, however, the book is Axline's call to her profession to keep listening to the voice of children despite the then imminent effects of a behavioral movement in which emotions were dethroned from their central position in the understanding of psychopathology (Southam-Gerow and Kendall, 2002) and the effects of the systemic perspective (see Chapters 2 and 6) in which the child's voice can be obscured, if not obliterated, by a focus on the workings of a larger system. Research since Axline's time has confirmed, in general and across different forms of therapy, the importance of the therapeutic alliance in child psychotherapy (Karver et al., 2006). However, it has been confirmed (see meta-analysis by Dowell and Ogles, 2010) that child psychotherapy is greatly enhanced when the parents are extensively involved. It is unlikely that a contemporary child psychotherapist would allow the parents to drop their child off and not even remain in the therapist's waiting room or would refrain from giving advice to the parents of so needy a boy.

Research as a guide to practice in the psychological treatment of children

Research played very little role in the decisions taken by Axline about her care of Dibs and his family. This was not unusual at the time, or, to a much lesser extent, now: Many clinicians do not feel that

research results, especially those emanating from randomized clinical trials (discussed in Chapter 10) are relevant to decisions about their applications of psychotherapy (Persons and Silberschatz, 1998). However, in the years since Axline's work with Dibs, the move toward evidence-based psychological treatment has become a driving force behind many of the decisions taken in the psychological care of children, including any child psychotherapy that may be part of psychological treatment. Unfortunately, there has been much less research on child-centered psychotherapy, such as received by Dibs, than on other forms of psychotherapy, especially cognitive-behavioral psychotherapy. There are some exceptions. For example, Ray et al. (2013) conducted an interesting study with children in the first 3 years of primary school who were beginning to show emotional behavioral problems. The treatment group participated in a full course of child-centered play therapy whereas the control group received only an assessment using play techniques. Compared to the control group, the treatment group improved significantly in daily life functioning.

Emphasis on the empirical basis of psychological treatment is much more than a reflection of the empirical roots of the scientific discipline of psychology. In describing the forces behind the drive to catalogue and improve the empirical status of psychological treatments, Weisz and Kazdin (2010) recall that 50 years ago the field of psychotherapy was under siege. Mirroring similar pessimism about the effectiveness of psychotherapy with adults (e.g., Eysenck, 1952), several review papers reported that psychotherapy for children was ineffective, providing no more relief than membership in a control group (Levitt, 1957, 1963). In the intervening years, a number of task forces, notably those appointed by the American Psychological Association, have formalized standards for demonstrating that a particular treatment has empirical support. The general criteria that emerged from the deliberations of these task forces were summarized by Weisz and Kazdin (2010). These standards are essentially the same as those required for determining the empirical basis of medical treatments of any kind, which are described at the website of the CONSORT (Consolidated Standards for Reporting Trials) Group (www.consort-statement.org). There should be at least two studies on a particular treatment that demonstrate the standards expected. Ideally, the treatment should have been studied by at least one researcher who was not involved in the development of the treatment being evaluated. In these studies, the population should be clearly specified. The participants should be randomly assigned to treatment and control groups. Increasingly, the control condition receives the usual clinical care provided at a hospital or clinic rather than no treatment at all, which is usually not ethical in work with children already displaying symptoms of psychopathology. The standards also indicate that a procedures manual should be used to ensure that the treatment is implemented as prescribed. Furthermore, the effects of the treatment should be evaluated with multiple measures. If these measures involve ratings by parents or teachers, for example, the raters should be unaware of the treatment status (i.e., experimental or control) of the child they are rating. Finally, there should be a statistically significant difference at the termination of treatment between the experimental and control groups (Weisz and Kazdin, 2010). Not part of the formal guidelines but increasingly emphasized in the literature is the need for replication with children or adolescents from minority cultural backgrounds (Silverman and Hinshaw, 2008). Weisz and Kazdin (2010) emphasize that this is not a categorical system that separates empirically supported and unsupported interventions. Rather, it is a continuum, as described in Table 11.1. Thus, for some disorders, there may be several treatments that are considered well established. However, treatments that do not fully meet the standards are not totally dismissed.

Research on the effectiveness of the psychological treatment of children has flourished since the profession canonized its empirical heritage and advocated for it. Weisz and Kazdin (2010) estimate that, in comparison with the forty studies included

in the Levitt reviews, discussed earlier, that could have driven child psychological treatment into scientific oblivion in the 1950s and 1960s, there are now at least 2,000 relevant studies of the effectiveness of various interventions. This process has brought considerable legitimacy to clinical psychology in the minds of many, especially in establishing psychotherapy as a valid and effective method of providing healthcare. Indeed, the American Psychological Association's assertion that psychology is a health profession (Barlow, 2004) would have been considered very presumptuous without the empirical track record of the treatments that psychology can offer. Empirically supported treatments are now catalogued in the reports of various task forces, journal articles and websites (see, e.g., the special issue on evidence-based treatments of the *Journal of Clinical Child and Adolescent Psychology*, January, 2008). However, the gap between what researchers have found and what clinical psychologists do in their daily work remains wide, to the dismay of many.

The move toward evidence-based practice in psychotherapy has critics as well as advocates. Many of the critics are in agreement with the idea of validating psychotherapies scientifically but not with the way that this is being done by the task forces. Objections have been raised, first of all, to the mandatory use of procedures manuals. This does indeed ensure that the therapy being studied is the one that is prescribed and that different studies on the particular therapy are based on the same procedures. However, it has been noted that not all psychotherapies are easily manualized, especially those that are as complex as psychoanalysis. Wachtel (2010) noted that there is some empirical evidence that psychotherapy conducted without procedures manuals can be effective. The best evidence for this is probably the classic meta-analysis of the effects of adult psychotherapy by Smith, Glass and Miller (1980). Based on 475 original studies, that meta-analysis refuted the earlier detractors who claimed that psychotherapy was ineffective. The studies in the Smith et al. meta-analysis were conducted before

Table 11.1 **Categories of empirical support for therapeutic interventions**

Criteria 1: Well-Established Treatments

There must be at least two good group-design experiments, conducted in at least two independent research settings and by independent investigatory teams, demonstrating efficacy by showing the treatment to be:

a) statistically significantly superior to pill or psychological placebo or to another treatment

OR

b) equivalent (or not significantly different) to an already established treatment in experiments with statistical power being sufficient to detect moderate differences

AND

treatment manuals or logical equivalent were used for the treatment

conducted with a population, treated for specified problems, for whom inclusion criteria have been delineated in a reliable, valid manner

reliable and valid outcome assessment measures, at minimum tapping the problems targeted for change were used, and

appropriate data analyses

Criteria 2: Probably Efficacious Treatments

2.1 There must be at least two good experiments showing the treatment is superior (statistically significantly so) to a wait-list control group

OR

2.2 One or more good experiments meeting the Well-Established Treatment Criteria with the one exception of having been conducted in at least two independent research settings and by independent investigatory teams

Criterion 3: Possibly Efficacious Treatments

At least one "good" study showing the treatments to be efficacious in the absence of conflicting evidence

Criterion 4: Experimental Treatments

Treatment not yet tested in trials meeting task-force criteria for methodology

Source: Reprinted from The Second Special Issue on Evidence-Based Psychosocial Treatments for Children and Adolescents: A 10-year Update, Wendy K. Silverman and Stephen P. Hinshaw, *Journal of Clinical Child and Adolescent Psychology*, March 3, 2008, with kind permission of Taylor & Francis.

procedures manuals were in common use. Something of a compromise position was articulated by Kendall and Beidas (2007), who advocate for "flexibility within fidelity," that is, treatment manuals that are clear enough to be useful in documenting the accurate implementation of an intervention but that allow the intervention to be tailored in specified ways to the individual needs of the client and situation.

Critics have also objected to the requirement for participants in research on evidence-based psychotherapy to have a clear DSM diagnosis. Wachtel (2010) reminds those who set this requirement that most people coming to psychotherapy have more than one comorbid diagnosis. As well, many people come to psychotherapy with genuine problems that do not correspond to the formal criteria for diagnosis. Wachtel does not object to procedures manuals, DSM diagnosis and random assignment of participants to treatments when these methods are the best ones available for validating a particular procedure. In other cases, he argues, researchers should be studying the therapeutic processes that account for therapeutic change rather than the rote administration of a "canned" intervention.

Consistent with their reverence for data, some of the proponents of evidence-based practice have responded to such criticisms with data. An important example pertinent to the psychological treatment of children is a review article by Weisz, Jensen-Doss and Hawley (2006) showing that the treatments that have been endorsed as empirically supported are superior to "usual care." Usual-care conditions appear in psychotherapy research when it is unacceptable to deny clinical care to research participants who are displaying symptoms of a disorder, as in a no-treatment control group. The usual-care control group receives whatever treatment from clinicians to whom they would ordinarily be referred even if they were not participating in a study. The care received by a usual-care group is typically logged but not modified in any way because of the research. Thus, usual care is arguably the best representation in the scientific literature of the personalized clinician-designed care that many critics of evidence-based care advocate. Weisz, Jensen-Doss and Hawley (2006) compared usual-treatment groups with groups receiving treatments included in recognized lists of evidence-supported forms of therapy for children and youth. The therapies considered in the thirty-two studies they reviewed were aimed at a variety of problems including disruptive behavior disorders, depression and anxiety. On the whole, the therapies taken from the list of empirically supported treatments outperformed usual care. Although the difference between evidence-based and usual-care groups was not enormous immediately after therapy, the superiority of the evidence-based therapies increased somewhat at follow-up progress checks conducted several months later. Interestingly, among the thirty-two studies, those in which an explicit procedures manual was used for the evidence-based condition demonstrated only slightly greater effectiveness than

studies in which an evidence-based treatment was administered but without standard manuals. Another interesting finding is that in studies conducted by the developers of the particular treatment, the treatment was found to be more effective than when another researcher was replicating the treatment. This could be attributable to the original authors' experience and expertise or to some type of expectancy factor. In an interesting challenge to the interesting meta-analysis by Weisz and his colleagues, Spielmans, Gatlin and McFall (2010) published a recent meta-analysis in which they scrutinized the differences between the evidence-based treatments and "usual care" in great detail. Their results suggest that the superiority of the evidence-based treatments may be attributable to the fact that they are administered by personnel with greater training, more intensive supervision and more manageable workloads, not because of any fundamental feature of the treatments themselves. Thus, the meta-analytic data indicate substantial but not unlimited advantages of the empirically supported treatments over the routine treatments provided by mental health clinicians.

Confounding the arguments about current approaches to the identification of evidence-based treatments is the undeniable fact that treatments emanating from the behavioral and cognitive-behavioral traditions lend themselves best to manualization. Furthermore, the strong empirical foundations of these approaches inspire their advocates to conduct research on their success. As a result, there is simply much more research available on these approaches than any others, much of it showing that behavioral and cognitive-behavioral approaches are highly effective for many problems. However, Wachtel (2010) and other critics do not believe that they are involved in a fair fight. They argue that by writing such standards as manualization into the guidelines, proponents of behavioral approaches are, in the name of science, undermining theories of psychotherapy that differ from theirs.

Not surprisingly, the task forces that developed the guidelines for the identification of treatments that are

Table 11.2 **Comparison of major theories of psychotherapy**

Therapeutic Approach	Main Focus	Conception of the Problem	Solution Modality	Level of Therapist Input and Guidance
Psychodynamic	Interpersonal patterns and subconscious motivation	Inadequate or misdirected socialization	Resocialization by expert parent figure	Low to Medium
Humanistic/ Experiential	Emotions	Inability to express oneself; failure to achieve one's potential	Mobilization of client's internal resources	Low
Behavioral/ Cognitive	Observable behaviors and the thinking associated with them	Poor environmental conditioning	Diagnosing and correcting faulty thinking and reinforcement patterns by expert teacher	High

empirically supported offer no advice to practitioners who identify with the idea of empirical validation of therapies but not with the way this has been officially implemented. However, it seems logical for such disgruntled empiricists to accept the burden of evaluating in a careful way rather than assuming the success of their work with their clients. In its policy statement on evidence-based practice in psychology, the American Psychological Association (2005) has called for decisions regarding psychological treatment to be made in light of the relevant evidence base by trained clinicians who collaborate actively with the patient (or, by extension, the patient's parents). Hence, parents should know about the empirical status of treatments proposed for their children.

Meta-analysis: a tool for finding out what is known

An important part of identifying interventions that are empirically supported is summarizing the studies conducted on the intervention in question. As noted

earlier, solid empirical support is predicated on the results of a number of studies, including some conducted by researchers who were not involved in developing the original intervention. Although it might not seem to the uninitiated to be a great challenge to summarize the combined results of several studies, it in fact is. As psychological research has proliferated over time, it has become difficult to summarize the state of knowledge in a particular field. As chronicled by Light and Pillemer (1984) in a very readable primer on methods for the systematic review of scientific literature, politicians and policy-makers have expressed profound frustration over the failure of psychology and other scientific disciplines to provide a clear picture of what science has to say about a particular issue. It is rare in the social sciences for all studies on a given issue to yield consistent results. A science of literature review has emerged to provide the answers that simply cannot be reached by casual reading of individual studies one after another. If, say, twenty-four of twenty-nine studies on a particular form of therapy indicate that it is successful, should the results of the five naysayers be dismissed? Should they be dismissed even if they happen to be the five studies conducted with the largest, most representative sample sizes and the strongest measures of outcome? Should all twenty-nine studies be dismissed because their results are not consistent? As Light and Pillemer point out, the conclusions emerging from a perusal of the twenty-nine original studies is, first of all, time-consuming and inefficient. Secondly, without clear standards for what to look for in each study, the conclusion reached is likely to be highly subjective. Each reader is likely to pay most attention to studies and to features of studies that confirm his or her own biases. Thus, it is possible for reviewers of research in the same area to come up with diametric conclusions, even if their reviews are based on the same original studies, which they might not be. The standards for reviewing literature have become rigorous, enabling greater confidence in the results. "Vote count" reviews, such as reporting that twenty out of twenty-nine studies on a given issue yield significant findings, are no longer accepted as providing optimal information. In meta-analysis, the statistics reported in the original papers are amalgamated to yield a combined effect size. In many cases, the effect size is expressed in terms of standard deviation units. In the case of a treatment study, the effect size would be in essence an estimate based on the data from the studies included of how many standard deviations separated the treatment and control groups. Depending on the statistical adjustments performed on the data, there are several forms of effect sizes that are expressed in standard deviation units; the best known are Cohen's d, Glass' Δ and Hedges' g. In the case of Cohen's d, an effect size of .2 to .3 is considered small but may be significant both statistically and substantively depending on the nature of the data. A d of .5 indicates a medium effect, which is typical of many significant findings in the social sciences. Large effects begin at a d of about .8 (Cohen, 1992). Some meta-analysts prefer to express effect sizes in terms of the r statistic, which is the same as a Pearson product–moment correlation. It is common

practice nowadays to weight (i.e., multiply) the raw effect sizes from the original studies by the sample size in each study. The distribution of the effect sizes is also reported for good reason. In situations where there is little variation in the effect sizes pertaining to a particular treatment, the data want to tell a simple story about the basic success rate of the treatment. However, if there is considerable variation, unusual distribution, skew or outliers, the plot thickens (Borenstein et al., 2009; Cooper, 2010). It is important to look not only at the mean effect size but also at the distribution. If the distribution is not normal, there may be important information that can be discovered by inspecting, for example, any outliers or bimodal distributions. For example, it is possible (and, indeed, very common) that the studies showing the greatest effectiveness of a treatment were all conducted with adolescents rather than younger children.

Light and Pillemer (1984) provide a checklist useful to readers of a literature review (see Box 11.1). First of all, the reviewer should identify the precise purpose of the review. Is the reader looking for the "bottom line," for example the general success rate of a treatment, or is the reader more interested in detail about the specific ages, disorders or treatment settings in which the particular treatment works best? The reviewer should identify the procedure that was used to select the original studies, which should be not only clear but also unbiased. Ideally, the reviewer should have included studies that were not published in refereed scientific journals, which are known to be biased in favor of significant results. Non-significant findings can often be found in theses and papers presented at scientific conventions. The treatments included should be similar enough to warrant being combined. As well, the control groups in the original studies should be similar enough to be combined. For example, it may be deceptive to combine no-treatment controls with usual-care conditions.

If the early meta-analysts who were pilloried by Eysenck were guilty of combining "gold and garbage" to come up with a deceiving average effect size, this

Box 11.1 | **Checklist for evaluating reviews**

1. What is the precise purpose of the review?
2. How were the studies selected?
3. Is there publication bias?
4. Are treatments similar enough to combine?
5. Are control groups similar enough to combine?
6. What is the distribution of study outcomes?
7. Are outcomes related to research design?
8. Are outcomes related to characteristics of programs, participants and settings?
9. Is the unit of analysis similar across settings?
10. What are guidelines for future research?

Source: R. J. Light and D. P. Pillemer (1984) *Summing up: The science of reviewing research*. Cambridge, MA: Harvard University Press. By permission.

shortcoming has been more than remedied in recent meta-analytic practice. A meta-analysis should include some exploration of any statistical relation between effect size and research design. This can be accomplished, for example, by specifying the features that represent design quality and coding them, as on a 1 to 5 scale. It is often possible to analyze individually the influence of some important design features. For example, the report of the meta-analysis might contain a comparison of the effect sizes for studies conducted with rating scales that are statistically reliable and unreliable (or of unknown reliability). Other useful comparisons may include analyses conducted to determine whether treatment outcome is related to different program features, ways of administering the treatment, length of treatment, training of the therapists or the setting in which the treatment is conducted. A final element in Light and Pillemer's checklist concerns the outcome measures. If the outcome measures are not similar, differences among them in terms of responsiveness to the treatment being considered can be part of the story that the meta-analyst helps the researchers weave.

Meta-analysis and the rebuttal of the contention that psychotherapy is ineffective

Throughout this textbook, meta-analyses are cited rather than single studies whenever possible, especially in sections devoted to the outcome of treatments. This should hopefully provide an authoritative picture of the status of treatments for each disorder without burdening the reader with excessive detail about the original studies. The following paragraphs are devoted to several influential meta-analyses focusing on multiple disorders. These meta-analyses have shaped thinking about the general effectiveness or non-effectiveness of child psychotherapy.

As mentioned earlier, a classic meta-analysis of research on psychotherapy with adults (Smith et al., 1980) was used to counter earlier contentions that psychotherapy is ineffective. Not satisfied with the rebuttal, opponents dubbed the meta-analysis by Smith and his colleagues "an exercise in mega-silliness" (Eysenck, 1978). Eysenck's scorn was based largely on the combination of very heterogeneous studies, some of which betray exemplary research design while others do not. The lively debate that ensued led to improvements in meta-analytic procedures, which will be described later in this chapter. Additional meta-analyses of the adult literature followed. As well, several meta-analyses of child psychotherapy were offered in parallel to the adult reviews, starting with very influential papers by Casey and Berman (1985) and by Weisz et al. (1987). Both of these meta-analyses showed that child psychotherapy was, across disorders, age groups and outcome measures, quite successful, with mean effect sizes in the area of three-quarters of a standard deviation. Providing a most valuable international replication, a meta-analysis of German studies on child psychotherapy yielded essentially the same conclusion: Based on forty-seven comparisons between treatment and control groups in the German literature, Beelman and Schneider (2003) reported a mean effect size of 0.54. Weisz et al., whose meta-analysis was based on 150 outcome studies, demonstrated that behavioral treatments were more successful than other forms of psychotherapy. Encouragingly, they demonstrated that therapy was more effective for the specific form of psychopathology that was targeted in the individual studies than in improving other, more peripheral areas of functioning.

Several reviewers whose meta-analyses were published after the major papers discussed in the previous paragraph have provided important additional detail. Weiss and Weisz (1990) found that the apparent superiority of behavioral techniques could not be attributed to any superiority in the research methods used in the original studies documenting the success of behavioral methods. However, it has been consistently found that studies conducted with greater methodological rigor, behavioral or not, tend to have larger effect sizes than studies with more methodological flaws (Shirk and Russell, 1992). As mentioned earlier in this chapter as part of the critique of Axline's approach with the boy Dibs, Dowell and Ogles (2010), in a meta-analysis of forty-eight studies, showed that active parent participation in child psychotherapy significantly increases effectiveness. Also mentioned earlier, in support of Axline's emphasis on the therapeutic

relationship, is the meta-analysis of forty-nine studies by Karver et al. (2006), which indicated that a strong positive relationship was linked to effectiveness. In summary, meta-analysis has emerged as a tool that can be used judiciously not only to establish how effective psychological treatment of children is but also to discover which children respond best. The elusive search for the optimal match between therapy participants and treatments continues, with only some preliminary answers available now, thanks, to a considerable degree, to modern methods of synthesizing research findings across studies.

Technological innovations in the psychological treatment of children and adolescents

Just as an increasing number of young people are resorting to electronic communication in relationships with their peers, psychological intervention via electronic media is becoming widespread. Computer-assisted intervention is not usually designed with the aim of outperforming in-vivo psychological treatment with a therapist; its goal is usually to make psychological treatment more available to people in need of it or more efficient. Clearly, not all forms of psychological treatment lend themselves to computer-assisted delivery at the current stage of knowledge. However, as technology expands and improves, there are fewer modalities of human communication that cannot be, to some extent, conducted using some electronic tool. Hence, the possibilities for computer-assisted therapy are expanding at a very rapid rate.

There are two basic categories of *cybertherapy* or *computer-assisted therapy*, namely *telepsychology* and *virtual-reality therapy* (Botella et al., 2009). In *telepsychology*, the content of the intervention is delivered via the internet or another interactive modality such as a DVD. This modality works well, for example, in the delivery of cognitive-behavior therapy, which is typically delivered in a structured, sequenced manner, following a procedures manual (Anderson,

Jacobs and Rothbaum, 2004). The basic cognitive principles can be presented online using cartoons or vignettes. Computer technology can also be used to facilitate role-play practice of new ways of handling previously anxiety-provoking situations (Kendall et al., 2011). Telepsychology can also be used to train parents in ways of better handling their children's problems (Cefai, Smith and Pushak, 2010). Delivery of "real-time" therapy via videoconferencing, for example, is another form of therapy useful in helping people who do not have convenient access to a clinic or mental health professional in their communities. In *virtual-reality therapy*, the individual is placed in a computer-designed artificial environment that is made to simulate a real-life environment in which an individual is having difficulty functioning effectively. The computer program may vary the features of the environment to simulate different levels of the stimulus that is linked to discomfort or dysfunction.

Some of the subsequent chapters on the individual disorders contain descriptions of relevant interventions that are delivered electronically. The few examples presented here illustrate the range of disorders to which cybertherapy has been applied. First of all, teletherapy based on cognitive-behavioral principles has been applied widely to help children with internalizing disorders such as depression and anxiety (e.g., Cunningham et al., 2009; Kendall et al., 2010). Calear et al. (2009) applied cognitive-behavioral principles to a universal primary prevention program to combat childhood depression. Computer-based assessment of physiological processes related to emotional expression is the focus of a highly innovative intervention for children with autism spectrum disorder developed by Liu and colleagues (2008). Eating disorders were the targets of a web-based intervention for mothers and daughters implemented by Fang, Schinke and Cole (2010), which contained content directed at mother–daughter interaction as well as issues of nutrition and personal appearance.

The applications of virtual reality are as rich and diverse as the imaginations of the clinicians who take advantage of its potential. The best-known use of virtual reality in psychotherapy is in the graduated exposure of children and adults with anxieties and phobias to the stimuli that evoke their fears and anxieties, as discussed in Chapter 15. The anxieties treated range from social phobia (with virtual-reality studies conducted mostly with adults, e.g., Klinger et al., 2005) to school refusal (Gutierrez-Maldonado et al., 2009). Efforts continue to simulate a typical classroom to help children with attention deficit/hyperactivity disorder (ADHD), as in the Virtual Classroom developed by Rizzo et al. (2000). There has been some preliminary use of performance tasks in the virtual classroom to assess the response of children with ADHD to medication (Pollak et al., 2010). Baker, Parks-Savage and Rehfuss (2009) constructed a virtual environment to simulate children's social interactions in order to teach social skills to children who were disliked by their classmates. This approach could be extended to interventions for higher-functioning young people with autism spectrum disorder. Virtual environments have also been constructed to help teach and prompt empathy among children with autism spectrum disorder (Cheng et al., 2010). Finally, Wuang et al. (2011) demonstrated the successful use of Wii gaming technology to promote the visuo-spatial skills of children with Down's syndrome. It is important to remember many of these electronically facilitated interventions are still in their infancy. Probably none of them would qualify as well-established interventions according to the criteria discussed earlier in this chapter for empirically based treatments (e.g., Reger and Gahm, 2009).

It has been found that clinicians support electronically delivered psychotherapies to a limited extent, recognizing their appeal to young people and the ease of their dissemination. However, they often lament the lack of a therapeutic relationship, which, as discussed earlier, may be the hallmark of successful psychotherapy (Stallard, Richardson and Velleman, 2010). If the computer is not used for relational communication, there is no human therapeutic relationship. This would occur, for example, when accessing an online therapy program in which cartoons displaying cognitive-behavioral principles or facts about a disorder are displayed. However, as is evident in the email and text messages sent by young people, relationship communication nowadays can be electronic. Hence, it may not always be necessary for a child or family to be physically present in a therapist's office in order to have a therapeutic relationship. Furthermore, many of the successful computer-facilitated interventions include some personal contact with a therapist, as in the intervention by March, Spence and Donovan (2009) with children suffering from anxiety disorders.

Could Axline help a contemporary reincarnation of Dibs, a few years older than the Dibs she saw in play therapy, as a moderator of a chat room or monitor of a teletherapy intervention? The knee-jerk response is probably that she could not adapt to an approach that

she would find impersonal. However, a competent technophile could surely help demonstrate not only that relating online is possible but that the medium has many advantages, not the least of which is making it more likely that the therapist is available when the client most needs therapeutic input. The new technology can not only make therapy accessible to individuals in remote areas where no therapist is available, but it can also help engage some members of the vast population of ambivalent young people who need therapy by reducing the demands placed on them to present themselves at a given day and time in a clinic or therapist's office. Cybertherapy may seem less peculiar to young people accustomed to seeking answers to their questions and solutions to their problems online than to their parents. Hi-tech may also have more appeal to them than talking to wise but unfamiliar adults.

Summary

- Psychotherapy only sometimes consists of the child opening up to the therapist and, in turn, receiving insight. Some children lack the vocabulary for such a process. The three schools of psychotherapy are psychodynamic, focusing on changing internal processes; humanist/existential, focusing on enhancing feelings of self-worth and experiencing acceptance; and behavioral/cognitive, focusing on change in behavior and thinking. Most psychotherapists focus on the alliance between therapist and client. It is important for therapist and client to agree on the purpose of the therapy.
- "Psychological intervention" encompasses "psychotherapy," which may or may not be validated by research and may or may not aim to alleviate symptoms of a mental health disorder, and "psychological treatment," which, it has been said, should only apply to evidence-based interventions directed at mental health disorders.
- All of the schools of psychotherapy were developed for adults before being applied to

children. Children may be the patients, but adults are typically the clients, having presented the child for intervention. Psychotherapy will usually only be part of the process, with parents and teachers often involved. Though important, it can be difficult to understand the child's perspective.
- Little is known about matching treatment to the developmental level of younger children. Psychotherapy works somewhat better starting at early adolescence, when development brings metacognition and the ability to plan and anticipate the outcomes of one's own behaviors.
- Cognitive development may moderate the outcomes of therapy, but it can also be accelerated by therapy.
- Axline's *Dibs: In Search of Self* documented the boy Dibs' play psychotherapy. Despite his IQ in the gifted range, Dibs was socially isolated, had difficulty expressing feelings and had outbursts of verbal and physical aggression.
- Axline engaged Dibs in eighteen sessions of play therapy and met Dibs' mother twice, learning

of the cold environment, devoid of emotional exchange, Dibs lived in. Through a therapeutic relationship, Dibs expressed himself with toys, gradually learning to express himself to his parents, as well. His parents began to understand Dibs' problems reflected his environment. He became less frozen toward people, revealing his spontaneity and creativity.

- Axline's book was a call to therapists to continue to listen to children's emotions, despite the growing behavioral movement. Since then, the importance of the therapeutic alliance has been confirmed, but few contemporary therapists would allow as little parental involvement in the process.

- Many clinicians at Axline's time and to this day do not put much stock in research but the move toward evidence-based psychological treatment is a driving force behind many decisions taken now in the psychological care of children.

- About 50 years ago, there was great doubt about the effectiveness of psychotherapy. Several critics claimed it provided no more relief for children than leaving them untreated.

- Since the 1950s and 1960s, the number of empirical studies evaluating the effectiveness of treatments in child psychopathology has increased exponentially, lending considerable legitimacy to the field. However, there is still a large gap between what researchers have found and what clinical psychologists do in practice.

- Some critics object to the requirement of manuals for research, maintaining that some procedures are not easily manualized.

- Behavioral and cognitive-behavioral treatments tend to lend themselves best to manualization. These treatments are validated by more research than other approaches. Critics say the requirement of manualization in studies unfairly undermines treatments from outside these schools of thought.

- Standards have been established for reviewing literature, to reduce subjectivity and increase replicability in research reviews. In meta-analysis, the data from multiple studies are combined to provide a global index of the effects of interest.

- The reviewer should identify the purpose of the review, the method of selecting the original studies, which should include theses and other unpublished papers. The treatments and control groups involved should be similar enough to be compared.

- Meta-analysis should include exploration of the relation between effect size and research design, such as statistically reliable versus unreliable rating scales, or program features and delivery of treatment. If outcome measures are dissimilar, differences among them in responsiveness to treatments may be important.

- The 1980 meta-analysis of Smith et al. was used to counter contentions that psychoanalysis was ineffective, but was scorned by critic Eysenck. The debate led to improvement in meta-analysis, and more meta-analysis in both adult and child literatures. Influential meta-analyses from a number of sources demonstrated the effectiveness of child psychotherapy. Meta-analysis demonstrated that behavioral treatments and therapy targeted to specific forms of psychopathology were more effective than other treatments.

- Weiss and Weisz (1990) found that the superiority of behavioral techniques was not due to superior research methods, though it has been found that studies with greater methodological rigor tend to have larger effect sizes. Dowell and Ogles (2010) showed that parental involvement in psychotherapy improves results. Karver et al. (2006) show a link between a strong positive therapeutic relationship and success.

- Computer-assisted intervention is becoming more widespread, enabling more people to receive treatment. As computer technology expands, more treatments can be administered in that manner.

- There are two main types of cybertherapy. In telepsychology, the content of the intervention is delivered electronically. This works well in cognitive-behavioral therapy and can facilitate role-play practice, train parents in better ways of handling children's problems or deliver therapy to people in remote regions. Virtual-reality therapy simulates an environment in which the individual is having difficulty.

Study questions

1. What is the essential difference between psychoanalysis and humanistic/existential psychotherapy?
2. In what important ways is the work of psychotherapists who help children and adolescents different from the work of adult psychotherapists?
3. Should psychotherapists be required to use only techniques that have proven effective in evaluation research? Why or why not?
4. What is meta-analysis and how is meta-analysis useful in understanding how effective psychotherapy is?
5. What are some advantages and disadvantages of cybertherapy as opposed to in-vivo or in-person psychotherapy?

Part II High-incidence disorders

12 Disruptive, impulse control and conduct disorders

This chapter is devoted to conditions characterized by the violation of social norms and the disruption of orderly routines. The clinical diagnosis of disruptive behavior disorder evokes what has sometimes been seen as confusion between being bad and being sick. For instance, Heydon (2008) argues strongly for the "de-pathologizing" of behavior problems because considering them a disorder inevitably leads to blaming the child and his or her parents, absolving the community, school and society.

Beginning with this chapter, the chapters devoted to specific disorders are organized in similar sequence. This chapter begins with the important distinction between disruptive behavior disorders that are evident during childhood and those that first appear during adolescence; many experts consider these two separate disorders. The diagnostic criteria specified in the new DSM-5 and in the ICD are presented next. Considerable space is devoted to the possible causes of disruptive behavior disorders (including physiological, family, peer, media and neighborhood influences) and to the ways in which disruptive behavior disorders affect the functioning and well-being of children and adolescents. Information about the stability of disruptive behavior disorders and the prospects of recovery appear next. The chapter concludes with a descriptive summary of the major known treatments for disruptive behavior disorders and the evidence for their effectiveness.

Conceptual controversy: late-onset disruptive behavior disorders as a different disorder?

Recent findings differentiate among early-onset disruptive behavior disorder, with symptoms observable before age 10 years, and later-onset disruptive behavior disorders, with no noticeable signs until adolescence. Early onset is associated with a longer duration of oppositional defiant behaviors. Offset, or remission of oppositional defiant disorder (ODD) symptoms, usually occurs before 18 years of age. Seventy percent of all people who report having a history of ODD at any point in their lifetime indicated no symptoms after the age of 18 years. Research is increasingly indicating that early-onset (especially with remission during adolescence) and late-onset disruptive behavior disorders are separate in many ways, including especially their probable causes. For that reason, the disorder may be usefully subdivided according to age of onset. Looking at the relationship of ODD and compulsive disorder (CD) in a different way, ODD can be regarded as a disorder that is distinguished by its role as harbinger of other disorders. Although most of the participants in research differentiating early-onset and late-onset conduct problems have been boys there is some evidence that the distinction may also be useful in understanding and helping the relatively few girls who manifest conduct problems during childhood and adolescence (Brennan and Shaw, 2013).

Diagnostic criteria

DSM-5 considers several types of disruptive behavior disorder, including *oppositional defiant disorder* (ODD) and *conduct disorder* (CD), which were also disorders listed in DSM-IV. ODD usually appears earlier in life than CD, often before the child starts school. It consists of non-conformity to the basic rules of the home and school. CD, which is a frequent successor to ODD, involves more serious delinquency. CD, in turn, often leads to adult *anti-social personality disorder* (e.g., Burke, Loeber and Birmaher, 2002; see below). In the ICD-10 system, these two forms of disruptive behavior disorders are subtypes of a single disorder.

In DSM-5, ODD and CD are considered separate disorders, although, as mentioned already, it has been established beyond a doubt that CD is often preceded by ODD. Box 12.1 and 12.2 provide summaries of the changes in the diagnostic criteria in DSM-5. The ICD-10 also recognizes the interrelatedness of ODD and CD, but in a very different way. The symptoms it considers for the identification of disruptive behavior disorders are very similar to those

listed in the DSM-IV and DSM-5 (see Box 12.3). However, these symptoms are considered as indicative of the same disorder, called CD. The symptoms are divided into more severe and less severe. The ODD subtype of CD in ICD-10 is the less severe form; it can only be diagnosed if there are no more than two symptoms from the list of severe symptoms.

The difference between DSM-5 and ICD-10 may be more substantial than semantic. This is because the number of symptoms needed to meet the criteria for diagnosis is not the same in the two systems even though there is very little difference between the two in the symptoms listed or their descriptions. Any child who receives a DSM-5 diagnosis of ODD would be diagnosed using the ICD-10 criteria. However, the converse is not true: A number of children could be diagnosed as CD

| Box 12.1 | **Differences between DSM-IV and DSM-5 criteria for oppositional defiant disorder** |

- In both DSM-IV and DSM-5, oppositional defiant disorder is characterized by an angry mood and defiant behavior.
- In both DSM-IV and DSM-5, eight symptoms are listed. Examples of symptoms include losing one's temper, deliberately irritating others and blaming others for one's own mistakes. Four or more of the eight symptoms must be present.
- In DSM-5, the symptoms must be displayed toward at least one person who is not a sibling.
- In DSM-IV, there are no specific guidelines as to how often a symptom must occur. However, in DSM-5, precise guidelines have been added. For example, children under 5 are required to display the symptoms on more days than not for a minimum of 6 months. Additionally, in individuals aged 5 or older, symptoms must be present at least once a week for a minimum of 6 months.
- In DSM-IV, individuals diagnosed with conduct disorder cannot be diagnosed with oppositional defiant disorder. However, in DSM-5, this restriction has been removed.

Source: DSM-5 and DSM-IV-TR consulted June 28, 2013.

Box 12.2 | Differences between DSM-IV and DSM-5 criteria for conduct disorder

- In both DSM-IV and DSM-5, conduct disorder involves the violation of major rules and expectations.
- In both DSM-IV and DSM-5, the age of onset determines the code. If at least one of the listed conduct issues is present before age 10, the individual falls into the childhood-onset type. However, if no criteria are met before age 10, the individual is said to have the adolescent-onset type.
- Both versions list fifteen symptoms (conduct problems). Three or more must be observed within a period of at least 1 year. Examples of conduct problems include being physically cruel, destroying property and stealing.
- Both versions list the following specifiers: "mild," to be used if few conduct problems are observed and only minor harm is caused (e.g., lying); "moderate," to be used if the number of conduct issues and the amount of harm caused are above "mild" and below "severe" (e.g., vandalism); and "severe," to be used if many conduct problems are present or the conduct problems cause substantial harm (e.g., physical aggression).
- In DSM-5, an additional specifier, "with limited prosocial emotions," has been added. This specifier is used if the individual displays at least two of the following characteristics for at least 1 year: lack of guilt, lack of empathy, lack of concern about performance or shallow affect.

Source: DSM-5 and DSM-IV-TR consulted June 6, 2013.

Box 12.3 | ICD-10 diagnostic criteria for conduct disorders

Criterion list for all subcategories of conduct disorder

1. Unusually frequent or severe temper tantrums for developmental level
2. Often argues with adults
3. Often actively defies or refuses adults' requests or rules
4. Often, apparently deliberately, does things that annoy other people
5. Often blames others for one's own mistakes or misbehavior
6. Often touchy or easily annoyed by others
7. Often angry or resentful
8. Often spiteful or vindictive
9. Frequent and marked lying
10. Excessive fighting with other children, with frequent initiation of fights

11. Uses a weapon that can cause serious physical harm to others
12. Often stays out after dark without permission (beginning before age 13)
13. Physical cruelty to other people
14. Physical cruelty to animals
15. Deliberate destruction of others' property
16. Deliberate fire-setting with a risk or intention of causing serious damage
17. At least two episodes of stealing of objects of value from home
18. At least two episodes of stealing outside the home without confrontation with victim
19. Frequent truancy from school beginning before 13 years of age
20. Running away from home
21. Any episode of crime involving confrontation with a victim
22. Forcing another person into sexual activity against their wishes
23. Frequent bullying of others
24. Breaks into someone else's house, building or car

Categories
1. Conduct disorder confined to the family context
   a. Presence of three or more symptoms, of which at least three must be from items 9–24
   b. At least one of the symptoms from items 9–24 must have been present for at least 6 months
   c. Conduct disturbance is limited to the family context
2. Unsocialized conduct disorder
   a. Presence of three or more symptoms, of which at least three must be from items 9–24
   b. At least one of the symptoms from items 9–24 must have been present for at least 6 months
   c. Poor relationships with peer group as shown by isolation, rejection or unpopularity and by a lack of lasting close reciprocal friendships
3. Socialized conduct disorder
   a. Presence of three or more symptoms, of which at least three must be from items 9–24
   b. At least one of the symptoms from items 9–24 must have been present for at least 6 months
   c. Conduct disturbance includes settings outside the home or family context
   d. Peer relationships within normal limits
4. Oppositional defiant disorder
   a. Presence of four or more symptoms, of which no more than two from items 9–24
   b. The symptoms in A must be maladaptive and inconsistent with developmental level
   c. At least four of the symptoms must have been present for at least 6 months
5. Other conduct disorders
6. Conduct disorder unspecified

(ODD subtype) using the ICD-10 symptom who do not display enough symptoms to meet the DSM-5 minimum for these diagnoses. A few systematic studies indicate that the children in this "gap" may actually be quite needy (Rowe, Maughan, Costello and Angold, 2005; Sorensen, Mors and Thomsen, 2005).

Another important new feature in DSM-5 is a specifier to the diagnosis of conduct disorder based on callous-unemotional traits; the specifier is called "with limited prosocial emotions." Features associated with this specifier include not only callous and unemotional traits, which have been described in research, but also thrill-seeking, fearlessness and insensitivity to punishment. This specifier will hopefully assist clinicians in identifying this subgroup of children with CD who have been found to be especially difficult to treat. In particular, they do not appear to respond very well to behavioral techniques (these methods are discussed later in this chapter; Frick and Dickens, 2006). Unfortunately, this cluster of traits has been found to be fairly stable from late childhood to early adolescence and from adolescence to adulthood (e.g., Munoz and Frick, 2007; Loney et al., 2007), bolstering the argument for its inclusion in DSM-5. Research has also shown that *psychopathic traits* during the childhood years are more predictive of later anti-social behavior than other forms of CD (e.g., Loeber, Burke and Pardini, 2009; Thornton et al., 2013). Nevertheless, there is some concern that this specifier may harm some children who would be stigmatized by being labeled too early with a diagnosis that has many negative connotations (Pardini, Frick and Moffitt, 2010).

Perhaps the innovation with the widest impact will not be within the descriptions of ODD or CD but in the recognition that explosive, aggressive outbursts alternate in some people of all ages with periods of profound sadness. The DSM-5 diagnostic criteria for *intermittent explosive disorder* are displayed in Box 12.4. This addition could reduce what many have decried as an overdiagnosis of bipolar disorder by adding conceptual clarity and more precise diagnostic criteria. Hopefully, clinicians will be able to distinguish reliably among intermittent explosive disorder, oppositional defiant disorder, attention deficit disorder, bipolar illness and the new DSM-5 disorder of disruptive mood dysregulation disorder, which is discussed in Chapter 20.

DSM-5 also recognized the category of *anti-social personality disorder*, which is listed in the section on personality disorders as well as the section on disruptive, impulse-control and behavior disorders. The term *personality disorder* refers to problems caused by stable personality traits that are usually evident by early adulthood but that may be recognizable in adolescence. An anti-social personality is characterized by such traits as a chronic failure to conform to social norms, deceitfulness, irresponsibility and a disregard for the safety of others. Hopefully, research to come will confirm not only a satisfactory degree of reliability among diagnosticians on these categories, but also confirm that the different categories lead to effective and differential treatment. Finally, the DSM-5 section on disruptive, impulse control and conduct disorders includes the categories of *pyromania* (fire-setting) and *kleptomania* (the inability to resist the impulse to steal).

Prevalence

Disruptive behavior disorders are the most frequent reason for referrals of children and adolescents to mental health professionals in the United States (e.g., Dodge and Pettit, 2003). In the UK, the Office for National Statistics estimated in 1999 that 5.3 percent of children and adolescents displayed conduct problems severe enough to necessitate professional treatment (Office for National Statistics, 1999). Epidemiological studies indicate the prevalence

Box 12.4 | DSM-5 criteria for the diagnosis of intermittent explosive disorder

A. Recurrent behavioral outbursts representing a failure to control aggressive impulses as manifested by either of the following:

1. Verbal aggression (e.g., temper tantrums, tirades, verbal arguments or fights) or physical aggression toward property, animals or other individuals, occurring twice weekly, on average, for a period of 3 months. The physical aggression does not result in damage or destruction of property and does not result in physical injury to animals or other individuals.

2. Three behavioral outbursts involving damage or destruction of property and/or physical assault involving physical injury against animals or other individuals occurring within a 12-month period.

B. The magnitude of aggressiveness expressed during the recurrent outbursts is grossly out of proportion to the provocation or to any precipitating psychosocial stressors.

C. The recurrent aggressive outbursts are not premeditated (i.e., they are impulsive and/or anger-based) and are not committed to achieve some tangible objective (e.g., money, power, intimidation).

D. The recurrent aggressive outbursts cause either marked distress in the individual or impairment in occupational or interpersonal functioning, or are associated with financial or legal consequences.

E. The chronological age is at least 6 years (or equivalent developmental level).

F. The recurrent aggressive outbursts are not better explained by another mental disorder (e.g., major depressive disorder, bipolar disorder, disruptive mood dysregulation disorder, a psychotic disorder, anti-social personality disorder), and are not attributable to another medical condition (e.g., head trauma, Alzheimer's) or to the physical effects of a substance (e.g., a drug of abuse, a medication). For children ages 6–18, aggressive behavior that occurs as part of an adjustment disorder should not be considered for this diagnosis.

Note: This diagnosis can be made in addition to the diagnosis of attention deficit/hyperactivity disorder, conduct disorder, oppositional defiant disorder or autism spectrum disorder when recurrent aggressive outbursts are in excess of those usually seen in those disorders and warrant independent clinical attention.

Source: Reprinted with permission from the Diagnostic and Statistical Manual of Mental Disorders, Fifth Edition (copyright 2013). American Psychiatric Association.

rate for ODD at anywhere from 3 to 16 percent (Boylan et al., 2007).

Sex differences

Boys are two to four times more likely than girls to develop any form of conduct disorder (e.g., Dodge, Coie and Lynam, 2006; Earls and Mezzacappa, 2002). However, the ratio is even more imbalanced when one considers life-course-persistent conduct disorder, which is estimated to occur ten to fifteen times more frequently among boys than girls (e.g., Moffitt, 2006; Archer, 2004; Keenan and Shaw,

2003). Girls, of course, are not necessarily angels during the preschool years. Although they are usually not aggressive in physical ways, they are known to aggress in subtle non-physical ways such as spreading nasty rumors and getting other children to exclude the targets of their displeasure from playgroups (Crick, Casas and Mosher, 1997). Such *relational aggression* continues throughout the lifespan and is more typical among girls and women according to most studies (e.g., Crick et al., 2009). However, Chesney-Lind and Jones (2010) argue convincingly that, according to the most authoritative statistics available, physical violence by adolescent girls has in fact declined over the past few decades.

The sex differences in physical aggression and conduct disorder have been attributed to a wide variety of biological influences on anti-social behavior and violence, which range from the genetic to the neuropsychological and neurochemical, the hormonal and the obstetric (Eme, 2007; Raine, 2002; Rutter, Caspi and Moffitt, 2003). At the most basic level, sex chromosomes are the ultimate biological origin of all sex differences. There are many biological consequences of genetic sex differences. Hormones produced by gonads include androgens, estrogens and progestins (Collear and Hines, 1995), which have permanent effects on the neural system of the yet unborn child. There is a massive difference in the amount of testosterone to which members of each sex are exposed as a fetus, with prenatal output of testosterone peaking in males at Week 16. Relatively small amounts of testosterone circulate within the body of both sexes until puberty (Maccoby, 1998). However, at puberty, the male body has at least twenty times more circulating testosterone than the female body (Federman, 2006).

Taylor et al. (2000, 2002) propose that testosterone affects the individual's response to stress, making the classic "fight-or-flight" reaction more probable than the more nurturing tendency to "tend and befriend." Furthermore, testosterone may also act on the left-hemisphere language functions, perhaps reducing the likelihood of disputes being resolved using words and adaptive thinking such as problem-solving (Baron-Cohen, Knickmeyer and Belmonte, 2005; Baron-Cohen, Luctchmaya and Knickmeyer, 2004). The male disposition to perceive a situation as threatening may have to do with these left-hemisphere functions of language and cognition as well as with any inherent differences in the instinct to defend (Bettencourt and Miller, 1996; Knight et al., 2002). What proof is there that testosterone levels are associated with these factors or with aggression in general? Some of the most revealing evidence is from research showing that girls who are exposed to higher than normal levels of testosterone in the womb tend to engage later on in more rough-and-tumble play and more physical aggression than girls who had been exposed to typical levels of prenatal testosterone (Cohen-Bendahan, Van de Beek and Berenbaum, 2005; Eme, 2007; Hines, 2004). Just as the female brain may be better equipped to aggress verbally and to resolve disputes verbally, the prototypical male body is better equipped for physical aggression. The average man is taller by far than the average woman and has more muscle, a larger heart, 150 percent greater oxygen capacity, and stronger arms, chests and shoulders (Buss, 2004; Holden, 2004). The biological propensity to aggression by males is compounded by cultural and family influences in the socialization of the two sexes (Moffitt, 2006; Wood and Eagly, 2002).

Cultural differences in prevalence

There have been only a few cross-cultural studies on disruptive behavior disorders as a diagnosable condition. Most sources indicate that African-American youth in the United States display more of the symptoms of CD than their counterparts in other racial/ethnic groups, even in data based on their own self-report (e.g., Elliot, Huizinga and Menard, 1989). However, the data are not entirely consistent. Indeed, Vazsonyi and Chen (2010) found a higher rate of entry into delinquency among Hispanic-Americans than among African-Americans or members of the European-American majority. Interpretation of racial and ethnic differences in the actual arrest rates of young people is complicated by the possibility that racism could account for differential police action (Hawkins and Kempf-Leonard, 2005).

Although not specific to diagnosed disruptive behavior disorders, there has been considerable theorizing and some empirical research on the reasons why a culture might be characterized by high or low levels of childhood aggression. Pioneering research by Fry (1988) revealed dramatically different rates of both child and adult aggression in two otherwise similar Mexican villages quite close to each other, both inhabited by members of the Zapotec tribe. The results of this anthropological study strongly suggest that one of the obvious but nonetheless potent ways in which cultures shape the aggressiveness or non-aggressiveness of their children is by showing them more or less adult aggression. Bergeron and Schneider (2005) conducted a meta-analysis of data from thirty-six studies in which 185 comparisons of the aggression in pairs of countries were reported, with most of the samples consisting of children and adolescents. They found that aggression tended to be highest in more individualistic countries – countries where many citizens base their self-concepts on their identities as individuals and value individual prerogative – in comparison with more collectivistic countries, where the prevailing values emphasize belonging to groups. They also found that aggression was lowest in countries where value tended to be placed on moral engagement and on egalitarianism (which is by no means synonymous with individualism). In interpreting data on aggression from different societies, it is important to consider the methods used. For example, Weisz et al. (1988) compared the beliefs and expectations of parents in Thailand and the United States about children's aggression as well as their understanding of how aggressive they are. When questionnaires were used, Weisz and his colleagues found no significant difference in aggression between the two countries. However, direct observation of the children's play indicated dramatically higher rates of aggression in the United States.

Probable causes and concurrent impairment

The highly successful 1957 Broadway show (and subsequent film, in 1961) *West Side Story* provides less than subtle evidence of laypersons' beliefs about the causes of CD. In one of its crowd-pleasing musical numbers, members of a delinquent gang express their views on causes of conduct disorder to the local policemen, Officer Krupke. The delinquents declare in song that their mothers are all "junkies" and their fathers are all "drunks," and that they never got the love that every child should get. Their fathers beat their mothers and their mothers, in turn, beat them. So naturally they are all "punks." They then mock the social workers who try to get them to take respectable but low-paying jobs. Finally, they mock the judges, who might be inclined to be merciful because of their deprived childhoods. The song ends with a frank statement to Officer Krupke and the others involved in their cases: "deep down inside us we're no good!" Many professional researchers share this ambivalence about the formal diagnosis of oppositional defiant disorder and conduct disorder.

The biological basis of disruptive behavior disorders

Genetics[1]

Many authorities believe that children with disruptive behavior disorders inherit decreased baseline autonomic nervous system activity (Lahey et al., 1993; Raine, Venables and Williams, 1990). Accordingly, they require higher levels of stimulation in order to achieve optimal arousal. Among the evidence to support this are studies indicating a low resting heart rate among children with disruptive behavior disorders (e.g., Posthumus et al., 2009), which, although not evident in every study on the topic, is considered the most consistent biological marker of CD (see meta-analysis by Ortiz and Raine, 2004). According to *stimulation-seeking theory*, children and adolescents with

[1] Section written by Paul D. Hastings and Amanda Guyer.

disruptive behavior disorders may accomplish greater stimulation and arousal by engaging in sensation-seeking, high-risk activities. Another possibility, embodied in *fearlessness theory*, is that the low autonomic nervous system activity among children with disruptive behavior disorders results in a reduction in their fear of punishment (Cappadocia et al., 2009; Raine, 1993; Raine, Venables and Mednick, 1997).

Based mostly on twin studies, estimates of the heritability for externalizing disorders in general (i.e., the chances of inheriting ODD, CD and/or ADHD from parents with one or more of these disorders) range from around .50 (Gelhorn et al., 2005) to as high as .80. Heritability estimates for a specific externalizing disorder, such as ODD or CD, are still quite high, ranging from .35 to .60 (Hicks et al., 2004). Aggressive behavior itself is considered more hereditable than other aspects of delinquency such as theft (Eley, Lichtenstein and Moffitt, 2003). An explanation of heritability-index statistics and the methods used to derive them appears in Chapter 4, which contains several examples pertaining to conduct disorder.

Structural and functional neurophysiology

An important distinction has been drawn between aggression that is either *reactive* or *instrumental* in nature (Blair, 2010). Reactive aggression occurs in response to a trigger, something that proves to be frustrating or threatening to an individual, and is characterized by an attack (often angry) on what is thought to be the source of the trigger (e.g., a child hits a peer if he thinks the peer stepped on his foot). Instrumental aggression involves purposeful behaviors that are implemented with a goal in mind and that are not necessarily linked to emotions like anger (e.g., a child steals a peer's notebook so the peer cannot do her homework that night). Differentiating between these forms of aggression becomes important when considering the role of the biology because the neural systems engaged may differ based on the types of cognitions and behaviors involved.

Research conducted using animals has indicated that response to threats, such as in reactive aggression, is supported by a neural system involving the amygdala, hypothalamus and periaqueductal gray (Blair, 2010). The study of these basic neural systems involved in the threat response in animals can lead to an understanding of how these processes unfold in humans. In humans, the basic threat system response that accompanies reactive aggression is believed to be regulated by regions of the prefrontal cortex (PFC); specifically, the medial, orbital and inferior frontal areas. Brain regions that support goal-directed behaviors, such as the motor cortex and the caudate are thought to be involved in instrumental aggression or anti-social behavior. In addition, because engaging in anti-social behavior involves weighing the costs and benefits of making certain choices through one's behavior, it is believed that the amygdala and the orbitofrontal cortex (OFC) are integrally involved (Blair, 2007). As described in Chapter 5, the amygdala is important for learning and making a link between stimuli and certain outcomes whereas the OFC is critical for decision-making.

Effective prefrontal regulation inhibits reactive aggression. For example, when someone annoys you or gets in your way, appropriate social interaction would require that you inhibit or suppress an impulse to hit or push that person and instead generate a less confrontational behavior to manage the situation. Not surprisingly, adults with damage to the PFC display impairments in social awareness and decision-making and often have anti-social behavioral tendencies (Anderson et al., 1999; Blair and Cipolotti, 2000). Furthermore, damage to prefrontal regions that occurs early in development appears to be linked with dysfunctions in social cognition such as knowledge about appropriate social and moral expectations (Anderson et al., 1999). These findings fit well with the suggestion that dysfunction in neural regions involved in emotion regulation plays a role in anti-social behaviors.

Neuroimaging research in youth with anti-social behaviors or psychopathic tendencies is still in its infancy, but rapidly expanding. In boys with CD and psychopathic traits, increased gray matter volume has been noted (De Brito et al., 2009), which may signify delayed maturation of the PFC due to slow pruning of neurons or growth of myelin. Functional MRI studies have revealed some interesting findings as well. Several researchers have used tasks that involve emotional learning and decision-making such as emotional facial expression processing and moral reasoning. Results from studies conducted with adults displaying anti-social tendencies have shown consistently that activation of the amygdala and OFC is reduced in the diagnosed samples. In youth with CD, research also has revealed reduced amygdala activation in response to facial displays of negative affect (Marsh, Beauchaine and Williams, 2008; Sterzer et al., 2005).

In one fMRI study, boys with conduct disorder showed stronger activation in the amygdala, striatum and temporal poles while watching videos of people experiencing pain or not experiencing pain, either as an accident or on purpose by another person, than did boys in a control group without CD (Decety et al., 2009). Interestingly, the temporal poles project to the hypothalamus, which has a central role in autonomic regulation. The youth with CD also showed reduced co-activation of the amygdala and PFC, which suggests possible dysregulation of an arousal response to watching others in pain.

The role of the neurotransmitter system serotonin (5-HT) is discussed in Chapter 5. Children with disruptive behavior disorders are found in most studies to have lower serotonin levels than either typically developing children or children with internalizing disorders, such as anxiety or depression. Reduced serotonin leaves children with disruptive behavior disorders prone to impulsivity and less able than other children to regulate their emotions (Burke et al., 2002). In an interesting longitudinal study by Kruesi et al. (1992), serotonin levels were accurate predictors of aggressive behavior 2 years later. Cappadocia et al. (2009) emphasize the fact that dysfunctional serotonin levels are linked not only with aggression

but more specifically with emotion dysregulation, suggesting the validity and importance of emotion dysregulation theory.

Hormonal regulation and aggression

Among the most important accomplishments of recent research on the biological bases of aggression is the accumulation of evidence indicating changes in several related neuroendocrine systems that appear to be related to aggressive behavior in children. This evidence is discussed in greater detail in Chapter 5 and in a comprehensive review paper by Van Goozen, and colleagues (2007). As the reviewers point out, there are many more data about these processes in research conducted with adults. Transposition of the results of adult studies to inferences about children is very problematic because there are many differences between the ways that adult and child bodies work.

That crucial developmental difference applies most particularly to research on *androgens*, the hormones that stimulate the development of male characteristics. As detailed in the review by Van Goozen et al. (2007), elevated levels of the male hormone testosterone are clearly associated with aggressive behavior in laboratory animals and in adults. However, there is little convincing or consistent evidence of this effect in children below the age of puberty, except for the effects of prenatal exposure to testosterone discussed above.

Cortisol and disruptive behavior disorders

At first glance, it seems that studies of the relations between *hypothalamic-pituitary-adrenal (HPA) axis system* activity and disruptive behavior disorders lead to highly discrepant conclusions. Figure 12.1 illustrates the results of one of the studies on *cortisol* and disruptive behavior disorders. Some researchers have reported lower cortisol levels in children with disruptive behavior disorders than in other children (Hastings et al., 2009; Smider et al., 2002; Snoek et al., 2004); others have reported higher cortisol levels (McBurnett et al., 2005; Obradović et al., 2010) and some have reported that cortisol and aggressive

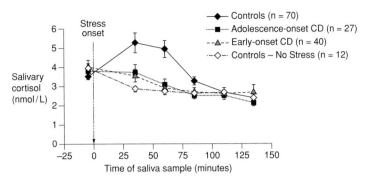

Figure 12.1 Adolescents with conduct disorder fail to show the normal HPA stress response of elevated cortisol levels in saliva after experiencing a stressful event.

or anti-social behaviors are not related to each other at all (Jansen et al., 1999; Spinrad et al., 2009). Although such inconsistency might lead one to abandon the idea that activity of the HPA axis makes any meaningful contribution to disruptive behavior disorders, a closer examination of the literature reveals two intriguing patterns. First, studies of older children and adolescents are somewhat more consistent than are studies of preschoolers and young children. This could suggest that the links between stress physiology and aggression strengthen with age. Second, studies of children and youths who have been diagnosed with clinical levels of disruptive behavior disorders are somewhat more consistent than are studies of aggressive children drawn from the general population, who typically show lower levels of aggressive and other anti-social behaviors. This might mean that there is something qualitatively distinct about the pathophysiology of children who show extreme anti-social tendencies.

With these caveats in mind, the overall nature of the relation between cortisol levels and disruptive behavior problems is that aggressive and disruptive children and youths have *lower* cortisol levels than children and youths without anti-social behavior problems. This is true both in terms of baseline diurnal cycles and acute responses to stressful events. The differences tend to be small, which might be one reason why they do not show up in all studies, but the differences are consistent enough to be of interest.

Lower baseline or diurnal (i.e., daytime) cortisol levels in children with disruptive behavior disorders have been shown by a smaller *cortisol awakening response* (CAR) (Freitag et al., 2009; Popma et al., 2007). Further, it seems that those anti-social children who do have low cortisol levels are worse off than others. Among boys with disruptive behavior problems, those who have particularly low baseline cortisol levels have the most severe problems (Van de Wiel et al., 2004) and their aggression is more stable and persistent over time (McBurnett et al., 2000).

Examinations of cortisol reactivity are even more striking. Stephanie van Goozen and her colleagues (Fairchild et al., 2008; Popma et al., 2006; Snoek et al., 2004; Van Goozen et al., 1998) have conducted several studies in which they compared adolescents with and without disruptive behavior disorders, looking at their acute cortisol reactivity in response to challenging tasks. The researchers used two tasks most often. The first, designed to evoke frustration, involves playing a competitive game against another youth (actually a pre-recorded video) who cheats and behaves in an antagonistic manner. The second, designed to evoke anxiety, involves public speaking (giving a speech to an audience). In these studies, youths with disruptive behavior disorders usually had equal or even higher cortisol levels before the tasks began compared to youths without problems. The participants with disruptive behavior disorders typically reported that they found the tasks to be just as annoying or unpleasant. However, youths with disruptive behavior disorders had lower cortisol levels 20 to 40 minutes after the challenging tasks were completed, meaning that they had smaller cortisol reactions to the provocations (Figure 12.1). Although they *said* that the tasks were aversive, the physiology of the youths with disruptive behavior disorders indicated that they did not react to the situations as stressful.

Research in this area may have important treatment implications: Boys with disruptive behavior disorders who show particularly weak cortisol reactivity to stress have been found to be less responsive to treatment programs than other youths with disruptive behavior disorders (Van de Wiel et al., 2004).

It is normal and adaptive to experience some physiological arousal when a potentially risky or challenging situation is encountered. In effect, that physiological reaction makes you "sit up and take notice" – you stop what you are doing, survey your surroundings for signs of danger and prepare to change your behavior in order to avoid being harmed. The subjective experience of that physiological response is likely to be a feeling of some anxiety or fear, or at least a sense of caution. In accord with the stimulation-seeking and fearlessness theories, some developmental scientists (Raine, 1997; Van Goozen et al., 2008) have proposed that children and youths with disruptive behavior disorders have strongly diminished stress response systems, or an underactive BIS (*behavioral inhibition system*), such that they experience fewer physiological cues to disengage from risky activities or withdraw from potentially deleterious situations.

Autonomic nervous system activity and disruptive behavior disorders

Children with disruptive behavior problems seem to have slow heart rates. In Ortiz and Rain's (2004) meta-analysis of forty studies on the relations between baseline heart rate and anti-social behavior, heart rate reactivity to various challenging and stressful tasks was considered in nine studies, involving almost 600 children. Their conclusions were striking: More disruptive and aggressive children had markedly slower baseline heart rates, and smaller increases in heart rate in response to laboratory tasks, than children without problems. Raine and colleagues found that children with slower heart rates when they were 3 years old exhibited more aggressive behavior when they were 11 years old.

Most studies of adolescents that have been completed since Ortiz and Raine published their meta-analysis have continued to support their conclusions, particularly with regard to heart rate reactivity. In a large group of young adolescents, lower resting heart rate was associated with having more externalizing problems, and predicted more aggressive and rule-breaking behavior in boys 5 years later (Dietrich et al., 2007; Sijtsema et al., 2010). Adolescents with a long history of delinquent behavior (early-onset disruptive behavior disorders) actually experienced decreased heart rates during a stressful gambling task, whereas those adolescents (later-onset disruptive behavior disorders) without problems and those who did not begin delinquent behavior until reaching adolescence had increasing heart rates (Bimmel et al., 2008). Finally, Hastings and colleagues (Hastings, Nuselovici et al., 2008) found that the heart rates of adolescent boys with externalizing problems were not related to their emotional arousal; their heart rates did not increase despite the fact that they reported feeling angry or scared while watching emotional films.

Given these consistent findings with adolescents, it is curious that the associations between disruptive behavior problems and cardiac arousal have not been as robust in studies of preschoolers (Crowell et al., 2006; Posthumus et al., 2009). This might suggest that maturational factors contribute to the patterns of reduced autonomic arousal seen in youths with disruptive behavior disorders. Furthermore, although studies of twins have shown that resting heart rate levels are largely determined by genetics (Boomsma et al., 1989), one twin study revealed that genetics made only a small contribution to the inverse relation between heart rate and anti-social behavior (Baker et al., 2009). Thus, despite the fact that early low heart rate predicts later disruptive and aggressive behavior (Raine, 1997; Raine, O'Brien et al., 1990), there is still room for debate about the underlying cause of this biological feature of aggressive, disruptive and delinquent development.

Regarding the parasympathetic nervous system (PNS), there is fairly consistent evidence that a weak physiological basis for emotion regulation, as reflected in lower *respiratory sinus arrhythmia* (RSA), characterizes youth with serious anti-social problems. Beauchaine's studies have shown that children and youths with disruptive behavior disorders have lower baseline RSA (Beauchaine, Hong and Marsh, 2008; Beauchaine et al., 2001) and do not experience the increase in RSA that accompanies sadness in children without problems (Marsh et al., 2008). In a play situation where higher RSA should support social engagement with peers, preschoolers with more externalizing problems showed RSA suppression (Hastings, Nuselovici et al., 2008). Conversely, using emotional and behavioral challenges that normally should induce some withdrawal of RSA in order to support orienting and attention, Calkins and her colleagues (Calkins et al., 2007; Calkins and Keane, 2004; Callicott et al., 2000) found that young children with externalizing problems show weaker vagal suppression than children without problems. Similarly, Katz (2007) found that young children with disruptive behavior problems who had been exposed to domestic violence actually showed *vagal augmentation*, or increased RSA, when they were deceived into thinking that a peer had provoked them. There have also been a few studies showing that RSA is associated with anti-social problems only for children living in troubled family circumstances, such as families with an alcoholic parent or high levels of marital conflict (El-Sheikh, 2001; El-Sheikh et al., 2009; Shannon et al., 2007). These are important reminders that any given biological

function does not operate in isolation; children's other regulatory systems and their socialization experiences are likely to shape the nature of the link between physiology and behavior. Overall, though, it seems clear that poor PNS regulation of cardiac arousal appears to distinguish children with disruptive behavior disorders from their peers without problems. They tend to have lower baseline RSA, they experience suppression of RSA in situations that do not call for it and they have weaker RSA suppression or even augmentation in response to tasks that require withdrawal of PNS influence.

Children and youth with disruptive behavior disorders also appear to show deficits in sympathetic nervous system (SNS) regulation (Beauchaine, 2012). Preschoolers, children and adolescents with disruptive behavior disorders have longer baseline pre-ejection period (PEP), or less PEP reactivity to challenging tasks (Beauchaine et al., 2001; Beauchaine, Neuhaus et al., 2008; Crowell et al., 2006). This is suggestive of weaker SNS influence over cardiac arousal, which could contribute to reduced heart rate reactivity to stress and challenges in disruptive and aggressive children. However, these effects for PEP have not been evident in all studies (Shannon et al., 2007; Willemen, Schuengel and Koot, 2009) and it remains to be seen whether further research confirms that children with disruptive behavior disorders have diminished SNS cardiac regulation.

There certainly is reason to expect that this will be the case, because disruptive behavior problems have also been associated with reduced activity on other measures of the SNS. More aggressive children have lower baseline and reactive *electrodermal activity* (EDA) and *electrodermal response* (EDR) (Lorber, 2004). For example, Van Bokhoven and colleagues (Van Bokhoven et al., 2005) found that aggressive children with lower baseline EDA were likely to still have high externalizing problems and diagnoses of disruptive behavior disorders years later, in their late adolescence. Similar to what has been reported for RSA, some researchers have found that lower EDA and EDR were associated with aggressive, disruptive and delinquent behavior only if other physiological or familial risk factors were present (El-Sheikh et al., 2008; El-Sheikh et al., 2009; Gordis et al., 2010). Remembering that measures of skin conductance are thought to reflect activity of the behavioral inhibition system (BIS), the fact that children and youths with disruptive behavior problems have weaker EDA and EDR suggests that they have less SNS arousal in response to punishment and avoidable dangers.

Cognitive dimensions of disruptive behavior disorders

Children with disruptive behavior disorders are known to display distinct patterns of thinking about themselves, about others and about what is right and wrong. One important way in which their thinking is maladaptive consists of *faulty attributions of intent*. In a social situation where the intentions of an individual are not really clear, children with disruptive behavior disorders are more likely than others to believe that another person intends to harm them (Dodge and Frame, 1982; Milich and Dodge, 1984). This is compounded by their problems in the area of *cue detection*: They tend more than non-aggressive children to reach a conclusion about a social situation based on very little information, often too little information for an accurate reading of the situation or the intentions of the people in it (Dodge and Newman, 1981; Milich and Dodge, 1984). Making matters even worse, once children with disruptive behavior disorders conclude that there is a problem, they have considerable difficulty thinking of solutions to it. They not only have trouble realizing that they have more than one solution available; they are also less likely than others to consider an amicable, non-aggressive solution (Rubin and Krasnor, 1986). Harboring the belief that aggression is a fully legitimate, perhaps wise and even necessary response may make it even more likely that these distorted beliefs will come to be reflected in anti-social behavior (Zelli et al.,

1999). The well-documented deficits in social information processing have inspired a number of promising interventions, which are discussed below.

Emotion dysregulation

The distorted cognitions of children who display problematic aggression are complemented by dysfunctions in the ways in which they come to experience particular emotions, in the circumstances in which they experience emotions, and in the ways they express their emotions (Cole et al., 2004; Keiley, 2002). As confirmed in a series of studies in which children with CD react to photographs depicting different facial expressions, children with CD appear to have difficulties feeling shame, fear and guilt in situations where most other children do (Eisenberg et al., 2001). Appropriate emotional responding in those situations would help them inhibit the impulse to act aggressively according to the research showing that such inappropriate emotional responses are correlated with problematic aggression (see meta-analysis by Card and Little, 2006; also observational research by Rubin et al., 2003). The physiological basis of emotion dysregulation is discussed in Chapter 5.

Family factors

Insecure child–parent attachment
Children with disruptive behavior disorders are often characterized by a history of insecure child–parent attachment. Importantly, this seems to apply to both child–mother and child–father attachment (DeKlyen, Speltz and Greenberg, 1998). The risk of CD or ODD is even higher when insecure attachment occurs in a home characterized by social adversity and maladaptive child-rearing practices (Greenberg et al., 2001). Research studying these attachment processes has succeeded in identifying specific patterns of insecure child–parent attachment that are most likely to predict aggressive behavior by children. According to an influential review by Lyons-Ruth, Alpern and Repacholi (1993),

disorganized or *controlling* attachment patterns tend to characterize the parenting of aggressive children. The disorganized attachment style is one of inconsistency. The child's responses to his/her caregiver may range from avoidant to overtly resistant; the child may appear confused or dazed. This may be because the parent's behavior may evoke both fear and reassurance in the child (Main and Hesse, 1990).

It is thought that these insecure attachment patterns between children and their early caregivers are reflected internally in subsequent insecure attachment organizations and in disturbed attachment bonds with romantic partners when they become adults. Anger, confusion and unresolved trauma are themes that recur in the narratives about adult attachment of adults who were known to have suffered from severe psychopathology as children; many of these adults had suffered another mental disorder in addition to conduct disorder (Allen, Hauser and Borman-Spurrell, 1996).

Inconsistent, ineffective and/or harsh parenting

Physical punishment may be both the cause and the effect of CD. Parents who are faced with defiance and non-compliance by their children may resort to physical methods more than others (e.g., Grusec and Lytton, 1988; Flynn, 1998). Although their desperation is understandable, harsh physical discipline has proven counterproductive. Children raised with high or moderate levels of physical discipline tend, on the whole, to engage in higher levels of anti-social behavior as adolescents than children of parents who used low levels of physical discipline or none at all (Farrington and Hawkins, 1991; Gershoff, 2002; Lansford et al., 2009). This is consistent with social-learning theory, according to which children who observe the use of aggression by a stronger person as a legitimate tactic for achieving compliance may subsequently use it on weaker individuals for exactly that purpose (e.g., Maccoby and Martin, 1983). It should be noted that sexual abuse as well as physical abuse has been implicated in the origin of CD (Nelson et al., 2002).

The effects of physical discipline have been found to vary according to culture, depending on whether it is perceived as part of the typical way of raising children by members of the culture. This may be because children may perceive physical correction as highly unfair and unreasonable in a culture where it is not seen as a sound way of raising children but might think otherwise if they believe that most other children are subject to the same modality of child-rearing (Grusec and Goodnow, 1994). Perhaps for that reason, harsh physical punishment, which is usually found to lead to greater child aggression in US research and in at least one influential German study (Engfer and Schneewind, 1982), seems not to work in this way for African-American children (Deater-Deckard et al., 1996; Lansford et al., 2004).

A more global perspective has been provided by Lansford et al. (2005), who worked with mothers of children 6 to 17 years old in India, Italy, Kenya, the Philippines and Thailand. Among other interesting findings, they discovered that mothers' use of physical discipline had much less to do with children's aggression in countries where the children perceived physical punishment as normative than in countries where there is less consensus that physical punishment is standard and legitimate.

Several types of individual differences, including gender, may moderate the effects of corporal punishment. For example, it has been suggested that corporal punishment short of physical abuse may be relatively normative in father–son relationships and perhaps less harmful in that context than in mother–son or father–daughter relationships in some communities (Nelson and Coyne, 2009). Some recent research has also revealed that certain genotypes (with risk conferred by a polymorphism of monoamine oxidizing gene monoamine oxidase A, or MAOA-uVNTR) interact with harsh parenting. In other words, genetic factors may leave some children more susceptible than others to the negative effects of physical discipline (Jaffee et al., 2005; Edwards et al., 2010); some other studies have failed to confirm this effect (see Young, Mufson and Davies, 2006).

"Coercive" processes in child–parent interaction

Seminal, now classic, work at the Oregon Social Learning Center has provided a fine-grained analysis of the child–parent interactions that escalate over time, with the child all too frequently ending up in trouble because of aggression and other forms of delinquency. The application of this work to parent training is described later in this chapter. Using precise observational data, researchers at the Oregon center apply social-learning theory (see Chapter 2) in conducting *micro-social analysis* of the ways children learn anti-social behavior by observing others and of the settings in which some children gradually become anti-social outside of the parents' easy reach. In addition to the analysis of behavior, the Oregon group has studied the cognitive and emotional processes that may lead the parent to get involved in a pointless and ineffective attempt at disciplining their children. In interpreting their child's behavior, for example, the parent of a child at early stages of risk may attribute a relatively minor incident of disobedience to the child being untrustworthy. They may believe that the child is deliberately trying to upset them. The parent becomes angry and aroused and may hit the child.

Coercive sequences in child–parent interaction often begin with something small that the parent could just as easily ignore. For example, the child may whine. The parent then starts to "natter" – to express displeasure or scold in a snide way that will simply irritate the child but not stop the whining. The child learns that whining leads to getting the parents' attention. The whining continues. The parents may continue to scold and eventually hit the child. In contrast, other parents might be more consistent in their discipline, either giving the whining child no attention at all or invoking a mild non-physical consequence that might stop the provocation.

Innocent as the whining may seem at first, Patterson labeled it, justifiably, a form of *coercion*, which may appear to be a very strong descriptor of a minor event if one forgets that such exchanges tend to escalate. All too often, the child learns to coerce the parent with increasingly maladaptive behavior that the increasingly overwhelmed and overstressed parent does not know how to manage (Patterson, 1982).

The Oregon group was among the first to discover that many parents indirectly and unintentionally contribute to their children becoming delinquent by allowing their children to roam the neighborhood without the parents knowing where they are or who they are associating with. This enables the children to learn to become delinquents from anti-social peers. Of course, parental monitoring can be overdone and might backfire in some situations. Furthermore, some parents may supervise their children more extensively because they see incipient delinquent behavior in their children; the delinquency is thus at least in part the cause of the monitoring, not vice versa (Laird et al., 2003).

Peer influences

Having the wrong friends

According to the *homophily principle* (e.g., Haselager et al., 1998), children (and adults) tend to befriend others who resemble them. Furthermore, once a friendship is formed and crystallized, the two friends tend to become even more similar over time, perhaps because of mutual influence (Kandel, 1978; Poulin et al., 2009). Accordingly, many children and adolescents with disruptive behavior disorders tend to have friends who are also aggressive. It is not surprising, therefore, that friendships with maladaptive peers are often cited as a cause of aggressive behavior. To the extent that such friends are actually to blame for problematic patterns of aggression, this would constitute an exception to the general rule that friendship offers important benefits to the developing child or adolescent, which were discussed in Chapter 7. Given the fact that aggressive children are usually shunned by most of their classmates (e.g., Greenman et al., 2009), one might think that aggressive children might not have any friends to be influenced by. This is often not the case: Aggressive children may not be accepted by the "mainstream" of their peer groups but tend to find friends among other aggressive groups, either one by one or by becoming part of a clique who share this common trait (Cairns et al., 1988; Mariano and Harton, 2005; Poulin et al., 1997; Poulin et al., 2009). In fact, their mutual propensity to aggression may be an important factor that influenced their attraction as friends (Bagwell, Newcomb, Bukowski, 1998).

Not surprisingly, research has revealed that having an aggressive friend leads to the maintenance of or increase in aggression (e.g., Adams, Bukowski and Bagwell, 2005; Snyder, Horsch and Childs, 1997). Vitaro, Boivin and Tremblay (2007) enumerate a number of theoretical models to explain how this might come about. They discuss, first of all, an *additive model*, in which the negative influence of an aggressive friend occurs independently of any risk factor within the individual or any other contextual risk factor. By contrast, an *interactive model* contains the assumption that the aggressive friend exacerbates pre-existing proclivities toward aggression within the individual, in more of a multiplicative rather than an additive model. In a *collateral model*, however, the friend does not influence aggression; it is the pre-existing proclivity toward aggression in the child or adolescent that results, coincidentally, in *both* the aggression and the selection of an aggressive friend. In something of a combination of these models, the *mediated model* is based on the belief that pre-existing proclivities toward aggression result in the selection of an aggressive friend and that the negative influence of the aggressive friend makes matters worse from that point on. At a more behavioral level, Dishion and his colleagues studied the conversations of aggressive children and their aggressive friends and found that they share *deviant talk*, in which deviant behavior is legitimized and encouraged by laughing or otherwise reinforcing the remarks of their friends. The term

cyclical attractor refers to the phenomenon in which two friends get stuck in talking about deviance, which becomes a predominant feature of their conversations. McDowell (1988) discovered a *matching law*, finding that aggressive boys tend to match the level and frequency of deviant talk to the level of their friends. Other than that, the conversations of aggressive boys and their friends may be quite immature. Dishion et al. (2004) followed dyads of boys who had begun participating in the Oregon Youth Study when they were 9–10 years old. Over the course of adolescence, the interactions of non-aggressive friends became organized and predictable. The interactions of aggressive boys with aggressive friends did not crystallize into a predictable pattern although deviant talk continued unabated. Probably making matters worse, the aggressive friends spent more of their free time in each other's company than the non-aggressive friends.

Media

Concern has been raised regarding the possible effects of violent television programming and, more recently, violent content in videogames. Researchers sometimes study this phenomenon in the laboratory. In such experimental studies, the participants observe violent media content in the laboratory and then participate in some situation, often a contrived one, in which their arousal, thoughts about aggression or aggressive intent are measured. Researchers using this method are able to accurately assess the amount and type of violence observed and, to the extent that their contrived situations represent real-life violence, the immediate effects of the stimuli. The disadvantage is, of course, the contrived nature of the experiment; the participants may not believe that the situation being simulated is real. Researchers using other methods, such as questionnaires or interviews, explore the extent to which violent media exposure occurs in the participants' daily lives. Such ecological validity, valuable as it is, may come at the expense of various forms of measurement error. Longitudinal research designs are being used in more recent research on the exposure to violent media contact, helping elucidate possible long-term effects.

According to a recent, authoritative meta-analysis by Anderson and colleagues (2010), there is no doubt that violent videogames are linked with violence by children. This effect is larger for the results of experimental studies than for other methodologies. Importantly, the studies reviewed by Anderson et al. include research reports from non-Western countries. Although the effects are larger in Western countries, violent videogames are nevertheless associated with problematic aggressive behavior by young people in non-Western societies. The authors speculate that youth in non-Western countries may tend to play these games in the company of their friends, which might attenuate the effects. Not all authorities find this evidence fully convincing, in part because the effects in many of the studies are not large in a statistical sense (Ferguson and Kilburn, 2010).

There is an enduring controversy as to whether violent media exposure has been proven to be a *cause* of violence by the viewers. Psychologists tend to be very cautious in making inferences of causation. Given the extensive correlational data, many major associations of mental health professionals believe that violent media exposure is almost surely a cause of aggression, just as many major medical associations believe that cigarette smoking is a cause of lung cancer. Strictly speaking, however, conclusive causal inferences cannot be made from correlational data, even with sophisticated statistical methods such as *structural equations modeling*, which do provide estimates of how likely a causal path is (Freedman, 1984).

Players of videogames interact psychologically with and thence *become* the protagonists in the games they play (Huntemann, 2000). Nevertheless, it is not yet clear that violent media exposure by itself has the power to create full-blown conduct disorder among masses of children with no particular genetic vulnerability to violence who have grown up in homes free of the modes of parenting that are known to contribute to aggression.

Neighborhoods at risk

Neighborhoods have distinct cultures (remembering that one definition of culture is "the collective programming of the mind which distinguishes the members of one category of people from another," Hofstede, 1984), just as countries and ethnic groups within countries do. Neighborhoods may also provide greater or lesser opportunities for associating with anti-social peers. A neighborhood can also increase or decrease the likelihood of isolated people, such as single mothers under financial stress, receiving support and counsel from others. Zalot et al. (2009) explored neighborhood factors that might increase the risk of the 11- to 16-year-old children of African-American single mothers developing comorbid conduct disorder in addition to the symptoms of attention deficit/hyperactivity disorder (ADHD). They used a variety of objective and subjective indices of neighborhood quality, including the mothers' ratings of their neighborhoods in terms of *social embeddedness* – the extent to which adults in the neighborhood interact socially and provide social support to each other; *sense of community* – including feelings of belongingness and trust; subjective satisfaction with the neighborhood; and perceptions of the crime rate. In general, these neighborhood factors were found to influence the likelihood of the children displaying comorbid conduct disorder. Direct exposure to violence in the community has been identified as a very potent risk factor for CD (e.g., McCabe et al., 2005).

Stability and prognosis

Obviously, the follow-up data currently available pertain to the diagnostic criteria in DSM-IV and older editions. Although, as noted earlier, DSM-5 has brought some important changes, these are not so drastic as to render the existing longitudinal data base irrelevant.

Most research indicates that ODD is quite stable. Its symptoms can be identified in preschoolers, although this is made difficult by the fact that a certain degree of oppositional behavior is common and very normal as part of the developmental stages that usually occur in early childhood (Egger and Angold, 2006; Tremblay et al., 2004). However, ODD in young children does not disappear with maturity as often as is sometimes thought; the disorder is associated with later pathology in a troublesome proportion of cases. It has been estimated, for example, that fully 50 percent of the preschool children who are diagnosed as having substantial conduct problems will be diagnosable with ODD 5 to 7 years later (Campbell, 1994).

ODD may not be very troublesome or persistent by itself (Loeber et al., 2009). However, as mentioned at the beginning of this chapter, an escalating spiral has been identified in which many children with ODD go on to develop CD. In fact, the risk of children with ODD developing CD is four times greater than the risk among children not previously diagnosed with either ODD or CD (Cohen and Flory, 1998). ODD has also been found to be a precursor of other mental health problems including depression and anxiety (Boylan et al., 2007; Nock et al., 2007) and ADHD (Nock et al., 2007). Nevertheless, it is important to remember that most children with ODD do not subsequently display the symptoms of CD (Loeber et al., 2000; Rowe et al., 2002).

Conduct disorder is a more serious condition than ODD, one that more clearly requires appropriate treatment. It is estimated that 2 to 16 percent of school-age boys and 1 to 9 percent of school-age girls display the full symptoms of CD (Loeber et al., 2000). CD is one of the most stable mental health disorders: It is estimated that 44 (Offord et al., 1992) to 88 (Lahey et al., 1995) percent of children diagnosed as having CD will still be diagnosable with CD several years later (Loeber et al., 2009). Boys diagnosed with CD between the ages of 7 and 12 years have been found to be at severe risk of developing anti-social personality disorders as adults (Burke et al., 2007; Lahey et al., 2005; Loeber et al., 2009). Besides coming into conflict with the law, many adolescents with CD drop out of school, engage in illegal substance abuse and become pregnant unintentionally (Bardone et al., 1996). The rates of mortality, physical illness and injury for adolescents with CD are higher than the corresponding statistics for non-diagnosed adolescents (Farrington, 1995; Kratzer and Hodgins, 1997; Loeber et al., 2009).

Loeber and colleagues (Kelley et al., 1997; Loeber et al., 1993, 1997, 1998) have identified three common pathways along which disruptive behavior patterns develop and escalate. The first is an *overt pathway*, with minor incidents of physical aggression leading to more serious physical aggression, with serious violence to follow. In contrast, there is also a *covert pathway*, marked by sneakier anti-social behaviors before age 15, leading to property damage and then to moderate to serious juvenile delinquency. Finally, children who begin on the *authority-conflict pathway* by exhibiting stubbornness and disobedience before age 12 may continue along those lines to more brazen acts of defiance to authority later on.

Adolescent-onset anti-social behavior continuing into adulthood is much more frequent than onset during childhood with anti-social behavior continuing throughout the lifespan (e.g., Fergusson and Horwood, 2002; Lahey et al., 2006). However, childhood onset has been associated with a more persistent, severe course of CD compared to adolescence onset (Lahey et al., 1998; Moffitt, 1993; Robins and Price, 1991). Childhood-onset CD is more closely related to adverse family conditions than is adolescent-onset CD, including family adversity and parental anti-social behavior. However, childhood-onset CD is also associated, to a certain extent, with neuropsychological deficit and low intellectual ability (Moffitt, 2003, 2006).

Adolescent-onset CD is associated with substance abuse and crime during adolescence or adulthood or both. However, adolescent-onset CD is not associated with as wide a range of negative adult outcomes in terms of education, work, health and family life as is childhood-onset CD (Odgers et al., 2007; Nagin, Farrington and Moffitt, 1995). Obviously, disruptive behavior disorder that persists over the lifespan is a more serious condition than disruptive behavior disorder that is contained to childhood and/or adolescence: It is estimated that individuals with life-course-persistent disruptive behavior disorders commit more than half of the crimes in the United States (Eme, 2007; Moffitt, 2005).

Prevention and treatment

Efforts at preventing childhood disruptive behavior disorders have redoubled in recent years. The best-known prevention program is Project FAST (Families and Schools Together) Track, developed and implemented at several sites across the United States. This program was discussed in Chapter 10.

Parent training

Working with parents seems logical in light of the many links between parenting and disruptive behavior disorders, discussed earlier in this chapter. It is imperative that the parents involved understand that their children's problems are not necessarily their fault but that their parenting is often the main causal element that can be changed.

Difficult as it may be to treat disruptive behavior disorders, several of the available interventions can be classified as either established or probably efficacious according to the standard guidelines for the classification of empirically based treatments endorsed by the American Psychological Association (see Chapter 11). The following summary is based on reviews by Farley et al. (2005) and by Eyberg et al. (2008) of the empirical status of treatments for children and adolescents, respectively.

The effectiveness of parent training for disruptive behavior disorders has been studied extensively and rigorously. Many of the relevant studies have been conducted with impressive methodological rigor, featuring random assignment of participants to treatment and control groups, clear specification of the intervention, verification that the intervention was delivered as planned, psychometrically sound

outcome measures, statistical correction in cases where a parent has dropped out of treatment, and long-term follow-up. A recent meta-analysis by Dretzke et al. (2009), in which the criteria for including an original study were very stringent, was based on fifty-seven separate studies. The results are unequivocal: Parent training consistently leads to systematic reduction in problematic child behavior, with improvements in parent-rated behavior ranging from about two-thirds of a standard deviation to almost three standard deviations. This estimate may be inflated because it is the parents themselves who are rating the behavior of their own children after having invested the time in a treatment program. Although fewer studies include independent outcome measures, these still indicate treatment effects that average at least half a standard deviation (Barlow and Stewart-Brown, 2000; Dretzke et al., 2009; Lundahl, Risser and Lovejoy, 2006; Reyno and McGrath, 2006). It has been estimated that 80 percent of children whose parents participated ended up better adjusted than the children of parents who did not participate. Importantly, two-thirds of the participating parents themselves ended up better adjusted than parents who did not participate (Serketich and Dumas, 1996). Impressive as these statistics are, they do reveal that there is a substantial minority yet to be reached.

These programs may be delivered to parents individually or in groups. Their content includes positive reinforcement for appropriate behavior, with a mild consequence if needed for misbehavior, such as removal for a few minutes to a time-out corner. Consistency is emphasized, as is carefully tracking progress with precise graphs and charts of the child's daily behavior. The best-known of these programs is Patterson and Guillion's (1971) Living with Children. An important innovation in parent training is the Triple P program developed by Matthew Sanders and his colleagues at the University of Queensland, Australia, described more fully in Chapter 6. The Oregon Social Learning Center, whose research was discussed earlier in this chapter, has led the field in developing empirically supported parent training interventions. Bank et al.

(1991) developed and evaluated a parent training program for youth with conduct disorder who had begun to get into trouble in the community. The parents participated individually in the program, each receiving an average of over 20 hours of direct contact with clinicians plus over 20 hours of telephone support, although there was no pre-specified time limit. The intervention focused on reinforcing prosocial behaviors and cooperation, providing negative consequences for risk behaviors and appropriately monitoring the youths' behavior at school and in the community. Written contracts negotiated individually between parents and children constitute an important part of the program. Parents learned how to monitor such behaviors as attending class, disobeying teachers, completing homework, associating with other youth who were in conflict with the law, staying out of the home after the set curfew and using illegal substances. For example, if a child had demonstrated a pattern of not attending school classes, daily telephone contact between parents and the school was set up. Instructions were given on how to discuss any behaviors that the parents could not directly observe and monitor. The parents were instructed to ask for receipts for any new items that were purchased. The clinicians taught the parents how to record these target behaviors on a daily basis on charts that could be reviewed regularly. Individualized systems of reinforcement and punishment were devised for each family, typically involving the gain or loss of free time or privileges. The children of families participating in the program, on the average, went on to commit significantly fewer delinquent acts than those in the community control group, who received whatever treatment was normally provided by the justice and mental health systems.

Unfortunately, not every parent who begins parent training participates fully and attends regularly; over one-fourth are known to drop out before the end of the program (Forehand et al., 1983). There has been extensive research to identify the "dropouts." Some parents feel uncomfortable with having their parenting observed as closely as is done in some parent training interventions (Forehand et al., 1983). As well, parents with stressful personal lives tend not to complete the program or benefit as fully as other parents (e.g., Friars and Mellor, 2009). Consequently, it may be useful to complement the behavior-management training with an intervention component designed to help the participating parents achieve better support or better management of their finances.

CASE STUDIES: Stewart Chris and their families receiving behavioral treatment

Stewart, a participant in the Incredible Years program

The case of Stewart, a participant in the Incredible Years program, is presented by Webster-Stratton and Reid (2011). Stewart was referred by his school psychologist because he was chronically aggressive and disobedient at school. His teacher and parents argued with each other about whether or not it was best for Stewart to remain in his school class or be transferred to a special facility. Stewart had no friends at school and talked about being the dumbest student in his class. At home, Stewart threw temper tantrums regularly, during which he insulted his parents, refused to follow their instructions and destroyed things. Stewart's parents tried to control his behavior by reasoning with him. At times, they would also send him to a time-out corner and withdraw privileges.

Stewart and his parents participated in the Incredible Years program for twenty-four weekly 2-hour sessions. The parent group was held at the same time as a therapeutic child play group for six children. In the parent group, Stewart's parents, Tim and Susan, expressed the long-term goal of improving their son's self-esteem. However, they realized that, in order to get there, Stewart would first have to learn to manage his behavior. One of the first suggestions made by the Incredible Years staff was that Stewart and his parents play together regularly and that, during playtime, Stewart was to be essentially free to decide what to do, giving him some sense of power when it was appropriate for him to be in charge.

Tim and Susan also learned emotion coaching. They taught Stewart the language to use to express his feelings and to use that language when he felt frustrated. They also taught and reinforced the social skills needed to cooperate with others, such as helping them and waiting for his turn. The Incredible Years staff worked hard to change Tim and Susan's habitual ways of dealing with Stewart's tantrums and insults. Tim and Susan had found it difficult to ignore Stewart's tantrums. In the program, they learned to coach Stewart to use calming words to cool himself down. Helped by role-play sessions in which the parent-group participants supported each other, they learned to use time-out appropriately when all else failed, following through consistently even on occasions when Stewart resisted for a long time. Their working together was facilitated by sessions at the parent group on communication and planning.

The improvement in Stewart's behavior at home did not alleviate the behavior problems at school. His teacher continued to request that he be transferred to another school. Tim and Susan had to struggle with Stewart in the mornings to get him to go to school. Relations between Stewart's parents and school staff were very strained. With some reluctance, Stewart's teacher agreed to attend the parenting clinic for four days of teacher training. The frustrated teacher was given a chance by the program staff to express her feelings about how Stewart's behavior was affecting the rest of the class. The staff also worked with the teacher on a positive behavior plan for Stewart. Stewart could earn breaks from schoolwork if he worked steadily and completed designated portions of the assigned work. Because of his attention problems, he was also allowed to move about the classroom at designated times. The therapists noticed that during his time in the "Dinosaur" group at the clinic (see next paragraph), Stewart enjoyed helping other children. Therefore, he was allowed to earn that privilege in the classroom as well. Finally, Stewart's school behavior plan included adult supervision of his recess play, with the provision for him to have normal recess play once his behavior improved.

Stewart first resisted participating in the Dinosaur social skills and problem-solving group, which reminded him of school. During the Dinosaur group sessions, the children are taught how to express their feelings, control their anger, solve social problems and use friendly talk to express their feelings. The group leaders learned to ignore his complaints and praise his sporadic attempts at joining in and cooperating. Stewart reacted very well to being given responsibilities. Soon, he was assigned the task of monitoring the friendly, positive behavior of another group member. This led to Stewart developing, for the first time, some friends. Mirroring the coaching provided by Tim and Susan, the group leaders helped Stewart stay calm and express his feelings. They modeled these social skills for him, sometimes with puppets.

In response to this intense, multimodal, and very well-coordinated treatment program, Stewart's behavior improved considerably. Nevertheless, progress was uneven. Incidents at home became very infrequent; Tim and Susan felt confident that they could handle whatever behavior problems Stewart would present. Progress at school continued somewhat but ongoing intensive coordination between the school, parents and the Incredible Years staff was necessary in order to maintain Stewart in his regular primary-school classroom.

Chris, who benefited from errorless behavior-management training

Ducharme, Di Padova and Ashworth (2010) present the case of Chris, age 7, to illustrate their use of errorless methods for managing children's behavior. Chris was referred to the psychologist by his school, which was a special school for children with special learning and behavioral needs. He had been diagnosed as having mild intellectual disability with mixed expressive-receptive language disorder. He also met the DSM-IV diagnostic criteria for attention-deficit/hyperactivity disorder, oppositional defiant disorder and conduct disorder. Since age 3, he has been treated with medications, both a psychostimulant for his attention problems and risperidone, an antipsychotic drug that is sometimes prescribed "off-label" (i.e., not for the purpose for which it received government approval) for his explosive outbursts. Chris was the youngest of three children, including an older sister who was in residential treatment because of aggressive behavior.

Chris' behavior was severely maladjusted and disruptive. At home, he hit his sisters, disobeyed his parents, destroyed furniture and walls, threw objects and urinated intentionally on the floor. He repeated frequently that he hated his mother. Unable to control him or to get him to go to his bedroom for a time-out period, Chris' parents had resorted to physically restraining him; this was the only way they could manage him. Although he did not comply with his teacher's instructions, his behavior at school was largely contained by the highly structured setting, with intensive individual attention and small classes with no more than ten pupils. However, he threatened to kill his camp counselor and was found with a knife in his possession the day after he made that threat.

Using modeling and role-play, the psychologist trained Chris' Mom to make effective requests. She learned to give directions in a brief, clear way, using a polite but firm tone, in the imperative mode.

During the baseline period, Mom kept track of Chris' compliance with such requests within the range of 10–40 seconds after they were made. In order to gauge subsequent practice, nothing was done during the baseline period to promote compliance other than improving the clarity of the requests. Indeed, Chris' problems continued unabated while the baseline data were being completed: He grasped a kitchen knife and threatened to kill his mother when she refused to serve him a second glass of juice.

The baseline data were used to classify the mother's requests into those with which Chris was more and less likely to comply. To achieve some degree of success as soon as possible, treatment began with Mom making high-probability requests and following them with copious praise and warm physical contact (kisses, hugs, pats) whenever Chris complied. Chris did not respond well to being touched, moving away and saying "leave me alone." Therefore, only praise was then used.

Even so, Chris resisted, telling his mother to "shut up." The therapist, who seemed to have developed a good rapport with Chris, had to praise Chris for accepting his mother's praise! Despite these setbacks, the detailed charts compiled by Mom and the therapists indicated some progress by the end of this initial phase.

It was apparent, however, that praise would not be sufficient. Therefore, tangible reinforcers, namely stickers and sports cards prized by schoolchildren, were introduced as an accompaniment to the praise. Mom distributed these inconsistently and Chris' compliance plummeted. When the therapist succeeded in getting Mom to be more consistent, Chris' compliance improved for a second time. Very gradually, the tangible reinforcers were faded out and Chris responded favorably to praise alone. In a parallel intervention at school, Chris' teacher was trained to deliver requests in the same way as his mother had learned to do; praise was used as a reinforcer. Rapid improvement ensued.

In implementing this successful, "errorless" intervention, many obstacles had to be overcome. Chris' mother was overwhelmed with the task of dealing with two problem children. She frequently canceled sessions because of stress. Tension in the family was another problem. The marital relationship was very strained, in no small part because of the tension created by the children's behavior. The impaired relationship between Chris and his Mom surely had a lot to do with his reluctance to accept positive reinforcement from her. Another complicating factor was the frequent adjustments of Chris' medication, which made it difficult to track the true effects of the behavioral intervention. Ducharme, Di Padova and Ashworth emphasize that sizeable treatment effects were achieved in this case, despite formidable obstacles, by using only positive methods.

Individual and group interventions for children – anger management

Anger is an emotion that is related to aggressive behavior. Inappropriate expression of anger is not only maladaptive in social situations but is also associated with heart disease and other health problems. Of course, children and youth with disruptive behavior disorders require help because of inappropriate management of anger by explosive outbursts and aggression. However, the alternative of totally repressing anger is not much more adaptive or healthy (see Kerr and Schneider, 2008 for a review). In a comprehensive anger-management intervention, the participants learn, first of all, to recognize the situations that may trigger their anger. They then learn to interpret these situations in as objective a way as is possible. Problem-solving is introduced to help consider alternatives to both holding one's

feelings in and explosive, aggressive outbursts. A skilled therapist can steer the participants toward the appropriate, assertive expression of their feelings. In typical anger-management programs, participants keep logs of their daily experiences with anger and the impulses to act on anger. They review these logs with their therapists, who assist them in evaluating their handling of the situations (Feindler, 2006). Anger-management interventions have an established though not totally consistent track record of reducing aggressive, disruptive behaviors (e.g., Lochman et al., 1989).

Social skills training

Some authors use the term *social skills* to refer to the overt behavioral skills that are needed for effective interpersonal interaction, others include underlying thinking skills (including social problem-solving, discussed earlier) and emotional processes, while yet others expand the scope to include virtually every ability needed to function successfully at school and in the community. Many social skills programs combine these components (e.g., Schneider and Byrne, 1987); social skills components are often combined as well with such behavior-modification techniques as token reinforcement for use of the skills learned (Bierman, Miller and Stabb, 1987; see also Cartledge and Milburn, 1994 for a comprehensive overview of social skills training techniques). Modeling methods are sometimes used to demonstrate the exact social skill that a trainee may lack. For example in Goldstein and Glick's (1998) *Aggression Replacement Training*, it might be established that a group participant is deficient in the skill of standing up for his rights. The leader would define the skill of doing so appropriately and assertively, break the skill down into steps that the participant could learn, demonstrate the skill, allow the participant to role-play it, and comment on the role-play.

Evaluative research does indicate that social skills training may be of some benefit for aggressive children and youth although these methods are probably more helpful to children with other types of psychopathology. Unfortunately, there is much less evidence of long-term effectiveness than there is of short-term effectiveness (see meta-analyses by Beelman, Pfingsten and Losel, 1994 and by Schneider, 1992). In many cases, the benefits of social skills training simply do not last or appear in settings other than the one in which the training was conducted. Gresham (1995) maintains that this is not surprising because, in his view, children with disruptive behavior disorders are not often deficient in social skills, meaning the knowledge of what to do and how to do it, but display marked deficiency in *social performance*. In any case, there has been something of a decline in social skills training for people with disruptive behavior disorders. These methods are, however, still useful in some situations, especially within multicomponent intervention packages such as FAST Track.

Catharsis: blowing off steam – or generating more steam?

It is often believed that vigorous physical activity, such as participating in fast-paced sports, will help children who are developing disruptive behavior disorders to channel their aggressive impulses onto targets other than other people. *Catharsis theory*, long since disproven by generations of researchers armed with punching bags and bobo dolls, maintains that venting one's anger on a target such as a punching bag will result in emotional release that will lead to dissipation of the anger. Doing nothing about one's anger, which is not healthy either, seems to be more helpful than hitting a punching bag (Bushman, 2002).

Participating in sport may, however, reduce disruptive behavior in young people under certain circumstances. Sports do of course have formal rules as well as informal behavioral norms. That reason has been offered for the *negative correlation* sometimes found between sport participation and delinquent behavior (e.g., Segrave and Hastad, 1982). Many coaches and masters of martial arts emphasize discipline and fairness. On the other hand, sports like hockey often entail a very explicit encouragement of aggression that could generalize. Not surprisingly, research on sport and aggression is highly inconclusive, with many studies indicating no relationship between sport participation and aggression or delinquency and yet others indicating that extensive involvement in sport might be linked with anti-social behavior (e.g., Begg et al., 1996).

In a recent Canadian study, Perron and colleagues (2012) found that the benefits or harmful effects of sports participation depend on the diagnostic status of the individual involved and whether or not he/she was previously a victim of bullying. Their data come from a longitudinal study of 918 children in Quebec, in which data were collected at four time points between age 6 and age 10 years. Among children who have not been victims and who show no signs of disruptive behavior disorders, those who are engaged regularly in sports are less likely than their non-active counterparts to develop disruptive behavior disorders at a later date. However, children who have been victimized or who already show signs of disruptive behavior disorders (and especially those who fit both of these descriptors) are *more likely* to develop disruptive behavior disorders if they have been active sports participants.

Drug therapy

At present, there appears to be no drug treatment that has been approved in any major jurisdiction for the treatment of disruptive behavior disorders. However, drugs are often prescribed for frequent comorbid conditions such as ADHD or anxiety (see Chapters 14 and 15). An international consensus statement prepared by experts in the field from several disciplines concluded that "pharmacological treatment of pure ODD should not be considered except in cases where aggression is a significant, persistent problem" (Kutcher et al., 2004). However, "off-label" prescriptions – prescriptions made by physicians for drugs to be used for reasons other than those for which they were developed – are quite common. In the case of disruptive behavior disorders, the antipsychotic drug risperidone is increasingly prescribed, although it is not approved for this purpose (Haas, Karcher and Pandina, 2008), generating extensive concern about side effects such as extreme weight gain (Panagiotopoulos et al., 2010).

Residential care, military-style "boot camps" and wilderness challenge experience

Adventure therapy is designed to help adolescents overcome their emotional and behavior problems by overcoming the challenges inherent in living in the wilderness. In doing so, the adolescents often need to develop a relationship of trust with fellow members of their adventure groups. Adventure-therapy programs are often characterized by close relationships with the counselors who teach the wilderness-survival skills. Outdoor-experience

programs have been found to enhance the self-concepts of young people in the general population (Hattie et al., 1997). When applied to children and youth with CD, however, the results are inconsistent. A meta-analysis by Wilson and Lipsey (2000) indicated highly inconsistent and generally non-significant results. However, this meta-analysis has been criticized for lumping together all therapies that are conducted outdoors, ranging from punitive military-style boot camps to developmentally sensitive outdoor experiences that advocates consider a more faithful interpretation of the underlying philosophy of adventure therapy. Gillis, Gass and Russell (2008) provide several examples of well-designed studies, featuring random assignment of participants and long-term follow-up, that illustrate the potential of the approach.

Conclusion and future directions

Over the past 50 years, psychology researchers have learned much about disruptive behavior disorders. Of all the disorders, this area has perhaps inspired the most impressive set of longitudinal studies that have successfully illuminated the developmental trajectories beginning with minor misbehavior and ending with a lifetime of crime. As part of this research effort, the family antecedents of disruptive behavior disorders have been traced. Less attention has been paid to the environment outside of the family although studies on peer, friend and neighborhood influence are increasing. Intervention research has produced some successful comprehensive, multimethod prevention and treatment programs, although these are not always as effective as their developers hoped they would be. Because of their efforts in conceptualizing and implementing the pioneer interventions it is now possible to revise somewhat the widespread belief that psychology can do little to alleviate CD.

At the same time, research in behavioral genetics has yielded a clear if somewhat worrisome tallying of the genetic transmission of problematic aggression.

Some researchers are beginning the productive process of delineating how environmental factors interact with genetic vulnerability. Research on the psychophysiology of disruptive behavior disorders has also yielded some important findings although more work, specifically with child samples, is sorely needed. Probably the most important avenue for productive research in the future is the integration of knowledge about the biology of disruptive behavior disorders with treatment efforts. This might take the form of greatly improved drug therapy, relaxation or biofeedback implemented in conjunction with interventions with families or, perhaps, peers and siblings.

At the same time, it is hopefully not too naïve to conclude with at least the hope that something can be done to correct the ways in which the broader social context may exacerbate disruptive behavior disorders. Perhaps social planners can help engineer urban communities that provide opportunities for more social interaction while reducing the violence observed by child residents. Perhaps some way can be found to reduce the level of violence depicted in the media and in videogames despite the fact that violent content may be healthy for the revenues of the companies that produce these products.

Summary

- There is some resistance to classifying as a mental disorder such behaviors as disobedience and fighting by children. It has been argued that the current system encourages practitioners to overlook the underlying causes of the behavior problems.
- Early-onset (especially with remission during adolescence) and late-onset disruptive behavior disorders are separate in many ways, including, especially, their probable causes.
- Oppositional defiant disorder (ODD) consists of non-conformity to the basic rules of the home and school.
- Conduct disorder (CD), a more extreme form of disruptive behavior disorder, often leads to adult anti-social personality disorder.
- In the ICD-10 system, these two forms of DBD are subtypes of a single disorder.
- It has been established beyond a doubt that CD is often preceded by ODD.
- New to DSM-5 is intermittent explosive disorder, which pertains to the inability to control the impulse to be aggressive far beyond a reaction that is in proportion to any provocation.

- It is also mentioned in DSM-5 that adolescents, especially, may receive a diagnosis of anti-social personality disorder based on a recurrent personality pattern of violating social norms.
- Epidemiological studies indicate the prevalence rate for ODD at anywhere from 3 to 16 percent.
- It is estimated that 2 to 16 percent of school-age boys and 1 to 9 percent of school-age girls display the full symptoms of CD.
- Boys are two to four times more likely than girls to develop any form of conduct disorder.
- Relational aggression, often observed in girls, is not considered in the DSM-5 diagnosis of ODD or CD.
- Most sources indicate that African-American youth in the United States display more of the symptoms of CD than their counterparts in other racial/ethnic groups, even in data based on their own self-report. However, the data are not entirely consistent.
- Many authorities believe that children with disruptive behavior disorder require higher levels of stimulation in order to achieve optimal arousal. In fact, this factor is considered the most consistent biological marker of CD.

- Heritability estimates for a specific externalizing disorder, such as ODD or CD, are quite high, ranging from .35 to .60.
- An important distinction has been drawn between aggression that is reactive and instrumental in nature. Reactive aggression occurs in response to a trigger. Instrumental aggression involves purposeful behaviors that are implemented with a goal in mind and that are not necessarily linked to emotions like anger.
- In humans, the basic threat system response that accompanies reactive aggression is believed to be regulated by regions of the prefrontal cortex.
- Brain regions that support goal-directed behaviors, such as the motor cortex and the caudate, are thought to be involved in instrumental aggression or anti-social behavior. It is believed that the amygdala and the orbitofrontal cortex (OFC) are also integrally involved.
- In boys with CD and psychopathic traits, increased gray matter volume has been noted, which may signify delayed maturation of the PFC due to slow pruning of neurons or growth of myelin.
- Children with DBD are found in most studies to have lower serotonin levels than either typically developing children or children with internalizing disorders, such as anxiety or depression.
- Changes in several related neuroendocrine systems appear to be related to aggressive behavior in children.
- Studies of the hypothalamic-pituitary-adrenal (HPA) axis system in older children and adolescents are somewhat more consistent than studies of preschoolers and young children. This could suggest that maturation is an issue, with the links between stress physiology and aggression strengthening with age.
- Studies of the HPA axis system in children and youths who have been diagnosed with clinical levels of DBD are somewhat more consistent than are studies of children drawn from the general population, who typically show lower levels of aggressive and other anti-social behaviors.
- Aggressive and disruptive children and youths have *lower* cortisol levels than children and youths without anti-social behavior problems.
- Children with DBD are known to display distinct patterns of thinking about themselves, about others and about what is right and wrong.
- In a social situation where the intentions of an individual are not clear, children with DBD are more likely than others to believe that another person intends to harm them.
- Children with DBD are often characterized by a history of insecure child–parent attachment.
- It is thought that these insecure attachment patterns between children and their early caregivers are reflected internally in subsequent insecure attachment organizations and in disturbed attachment bonds with romantic partners when they become adults.
- Most children with CD have been disciplined physically. Physical punishment may be both the cause and the effect of CD. Sexual abuse and physical abuse have been implicated in the origin of CD.
- Many parents indirectly and unintentionally contribute to their children becoming delinquent by allowing their children to roam the neighborhood without the parents knowing where they are or with whom they are associating.
- Many children and adolescents with DBD tend to have friends who are also aggressive.
- Violent videogames are linked with violence in children. However, these findings are correlational, so it cannot be conclusively determined that the violent videogames *cause* violent behavior.
- Most research indicates that ODD is quite stable. Its symptoms can be identified in preschoolers, although this is made difficult by the fact that a certain degree of oppositional behavior is common and very normal as part of the

developmental stages that usually occur in early childhood.

- CD is one of the most stable mental health disorders: It is estimated that 44 to 88 percent of children diagnosed as having CD will still be diagnosable as CD several years later.
- Although children with early ODD are at greater risk than others of developing CD later on, most children with ODD do not subsequently display the symptoms of CD.
- Boys diagnosed with CD between the ages of 7 and 12 years have been found to be at severe risk of developing anti-social personality disorders as adults.
- Adolescent-onset CD is not associated with as wide a range of negative adult outcomes in terms of education, work, health and family life as is childhood-onset CD.
- The best-known prevention program is Project Fast (Families and Schools Together) Track.
- Some worthwhile interventions have been developed for direct work with children and adolescents, often in conjunction with parent training.

- Parent training, either on its own or in conjunction with other intervention modalities, is at present the treatment of choice for young children with CD and ODD.
- Probably the most encouraging data about the effects of psychological interventions for children with DBD come from recent studies of interventions with several distinct components, typically implemented with parents, teachers and the children at risk themselves.
- Several prominent attachment theorists and researchers have attempted to improve child–parent attachment bonds in an effort to prevent or diminish conduct problems in children.
- Several researchers have recently begun combining interventions inspired by attachment theory with direct parent training in managing child behavior.
- Other interventions include anger-management programs and social skills training.
- The antipsychotic drug risperidone is increasingly prescribed, although it is not approved for the purpose of treating DBD.

Study questions

1. What important differences are there between early-onset and late-onset DBD?
2. In what different ways can parents cause or aggravate DBD?
3. How definite is the evidence that violent TV and other violent media content are an important cause of DBD? Explain your answer.
4. How treatable are DBD in childhood and adolescence? What is the most effective treatment?
5. How helpful is it likely to be to advise the parents or teachers of a boy showing signs of DBD that they should channel his energy by having him hit a punching bag or take up the sport of boxing?

13 Depression

Depressed mood has been called the "common cold" of modern society because it is so common. Some scholars object vehemently to that expression because it implies that depression is a minor problem (Allen, Gilbert and Semadar, 2004). Many psychoanalysts, especially in the mid-twentieth century, argued that depression was a defense mechanism that was a vital component of normal psychological development. They maintained that this defense mechanism appears only after the child discovers that all of his or her wishes will not be gratified and, thus, would not occur among children. They were wrong.

This chapter is devoted to the reasons why depression constitutes a major threat to the well-being of a very substantial portion of the child and adolescent population. The chapter opens with the interesting issue of whether depression often underlies other disorders, such as aggression, belying their outward appearance. As with the other chapters devoted to specific disorders, the diagnostic criteria appear before a discussion of the prevalence rates for the population as a whole, boys and girls, children and adolescents. Causes (physiological, familial and societal) are considered next, followed by a description of typical patterns of impairment, emphasizing cognitive and interpersonal factors. The stability of child and adolescent depression is discussed next. The final section is devoted to the major treatment modalities used to help children and adolescents facing the challenge of major depression.

Conceptual controversy: masked depression

Current clinical practice is to recognize and diagnose depression in children only when it clearly appears. However, the concept of *masked depression*, popular before the widespread adoption of DSM terminology, is occasionally used nowadays in writings about populations where showing one's weakness, lack of self-reliance or sadness is discouraged. These populations include boys and men (Addis, 2008; Rabinowitz and Cochrane, 2008) as well as African-Americans (Fuller, 1992). Aggressive and anti-social behaviors have been discussed most frequently as masked depression (e.g., Harper and Kelly, 1985). However, many other forms of psychopathology have sometimes been deemed to conceal underlying depressed feelings, including school refusal (Kolvin, Berney and Bhate, 1984) and body aches that could not be explained by physical ailments (Mascres and Strobel, 2000). Some longitudinal studies do indeed show that children and adolescents who were diagnosed as displaying "masked depression" in fact tend to proceed to overt depression in subsequent years (Christ et al., 1981; Strober, Green and Carlson, 1981). Although it was often maintained during the heyday of this concept that a well-trained, perceptive clinician should be able to detect the underlying depression (Carlson and Cantwell, 1980), the concept of masked depression waned with the increasing emphasis on clear diagnostic entities based on observable phenomena so that different clinicians seeing the same patient would come up with the same conclusion (see Chapter 3). Nevertheless, an important body of research reveals that early acting-out behavior can indeed lead to depression (Patterson and Capaldi, 1990). Over time, the professional community came to the grudging recognition that depression, not disguised as another condition, exists among children.

Diagnostic criteria

The DSM-5 criteria are numerous and very specific, which in principle should distinguish between the sad moments that occur in most people's lives and a condition that truly warrants professional attention. Boxes 13.1 and 13.2 contain a summary of the differences between the DSM-IV and DSM-5 criteria.

The ICD-10 allows for a lower threshold, with fewer symptoms required for diagnosis, as detailed in Boxes 13.3 and 13.4 (Andrews, Slade and Peters, 1999).

Prevalence

According to many sources, depression appears to be increasing among young people. Furthermore, the suicide rate among adolescents appears to have increased drastically over the past 50 years

---

Box 13.1 | **Differences between DSM-IV and DSM-5 criteria for major depressive episode**

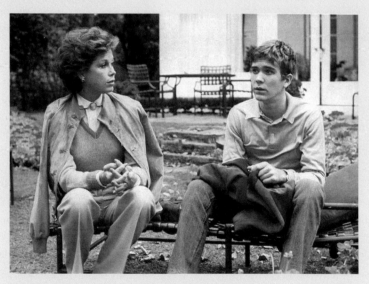

Figure Box 13.1 The film *Ordinary People* sensitized millions to the prevalence rate of major depression in young people.

- In both DSM-IV and DSM-5, the episode is characterized by a depressed mood and/or a loss of interest in pleasurable pursuits. Other symptoms may include unexpected changes in weight, irregular sleep patterns, psychomotor problems, fatigue, feelings of worthlessness, indecisiveness and suicidal ideation.
- In both DSM-IV and DSM-5, the individual must experience at least five of the symptoms for a period of at least 2 weeks.
- In both DSM-IV and DSM-5, it is noted that in children and adolescents, an irritable mood could be a symptom.

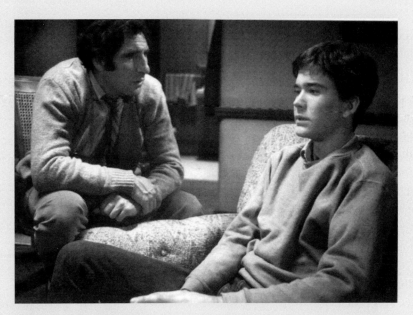

Figure Box 13.1 (*cont.*)

- In both versions, the individual must experience significant distress or difficulty.
- In both versions, the effects of a substance or treatment for depression cannot be the cause of the symptoms.
- In both versions, the symptoms cannot be caused by a medical condition.
- In DSM-IV, symptoms thought to be caused by the loss of a loved one are discounted. In DSM-5, this criterion has been removed. A lengthy footnote details factors to consider when attempting to distinguish grief from a major depressive episode. According to research, the loss of a loved one may not be substantially different from other stressors.
- In DSM-IV, the symptoms must fail to meet the requirements for a mixed episode (i.e., an episode during which criteria for both manic episode and major depressive episode are met). However, in DSM-5, the specifier "mixed features" has replaced the "mixed episode" criteria. The mixed features specifier is used if manic or hypomanic symptoms appear during the depressive episode. Additionally, an individual is still considered to have suffered a major depressive episode if the criteria for the "mixed features" specifier are met.
- A list of additional specifiers applicable to both major and persistent depressive disorders are included and explained in detail in DSM-5 (e.g., "with anxious distress," "with mood-congruent psychotic features").

Source: DSM-5 and DSM-IV-TR consulted June 28, 2013.

Box 13.2   Differences between DSM-IV and DSM-5 criteria for persistent depressive disorder

- In DSM-5, the name of the disorder has been changed from "dysthymia" to "persistent depressive disorder." This is due to the fact that dysthymia and major depression with chronic specifier have been merged; individuals receiving these two diagnoses seem to display similar features.
- In both DSM-IV and DSM-5, children and adolescents must frequently experience a depressed mood for a period of at least 1 year. Symptoms may include appetite issues, abnormal sleep patterns, low energy, low self-esteem, concentration problems and feelings of hopelessness.
- In both DSM-IV and DSM-5, the symptoms cannot occur solely in the context of a psychotic disorder.
- Both versions stipulate that the symptoms cannot be due to the effects of a substance or a medical condition.
- Both versions include the following specifiers: "early onset," to be used if the disorder presents before age 21, and "late onset," to be used if the disorder presents after age 21. Additionally, the most recent 2 years of the disorder should be noted, as well as any atypical features.
- In DSM-5, clinicians may also specify whether the disorder is in partial or full remission. A list of additional specifiers applicable to both major and persistent depressive disorders are included and explained in detail in DSM-5 (e.g., "with anxious distress," "with mood-congruent psychotic features").
- In DSM-5, there is also an option to specify whether the patient ever met criteria for major depressive disorder over the previous 2 years of persistent depressive disorder.
- In DSM-5, severity must be specified based on number of symptoms and degree of impairment.

Source: DSM-5 and DSM-IV-TR consulted June 6, 2013.

Box 13.3   ICD-10 Diagnostic criteria for depressive episode

Core symptoms:

- Depressed mood that is abnormal for the individual for most of the day and almost every day, largely uninfluenced by circumstances, for at least 2 weeks.
- Loss of interest and enjoyment in activities that are normally pleasurable.
- Reduced energy.

Additional symptoms:

- Loss of confidence and self-esteem.
- Unreasonable feelings of self-reproach or excessive and inappropriate guilt.
- Recurrent thoughts of death or suicide, or any suicidal behavior.
- Complaints or evidence of diminished ability to think or concentrate.
- Change in psychomotor activity, with agitation or retardation (either subjective or objective).
- Sleep disturbance.

General criteria for depressive episode:

A. Should last for at least 2 weeks.
B. No hypomanic or manic symptoms sufficient to meet the criteria for hypomanic or manic episode at any time in the individual's life.
C. Not attributable to psychoactive substance use or to any organic mental disorder.
D. To qualify for the somatic syndrome, *four* of the following symptoms should be present:
    1. marked loss of interest or pleasure in activities that are normally pleasurable;
    2. lack of emotional reactions to events or activities that normally produce an emotional response;
    3. waking in the morning 2 hours or more before the usual time;
    4. depression worse in the morning;
    5. objective evidence of marked psychomotor retardation or agitation;
    6. marked loss of appetite;
    7. weight loss;
    8. marked loss of libido.

   The distinction between mild, moderate and severe episodes is based on the number of *additional* symptoms.

Source: World Health Organization (1993). The ICD-10 Classification of Mental and Behavioural Disorders: Diagnostic Criteria for Research. Geneva, WHO.

Box 13.4 | ICD-10 diagnostic criteria for dysthymia

A. A period of at least 2 years of constant or constantly recurring depressed mood. Intervening periods of normal mood rarely last for longer than a few weeks and there are no episodes of hypomania.

B. None, or very few, of the individual episodes of depression within such a 2-year period are severe enough, or last long enough, to meet the criteria for recurrent mild depressive disorder.

C. During at least some of the periods of depression at least three of the following should be present:

1. a reduction in energy or activity;
2. insomnia;
3. loss of self-confidence or feelings of inadequacy;
4. difficulty concentrating;
5. often in tears;
6. loss of interest or enjoyment in sex and other pleasurable activities;
7. feeling of hopelessness or despair;
8. a perceived inability to cope with the routine responsibilities of everyday life;
9. pessimistic about the future or brooding over the past;
10. social withdrawal;
11. less talkative than normal.

Source: World Health Organization. (1993) The ICD-10 Classification of Mental and Behavioural Disorders: Diagnostic Criteria for Research. Geneva, WHO.

(Costello et al., 2006). Such statistics must always be interpreted with considerable caution for several reasons enumerated by Avenevoli et al. (2008). Prevalence rates may appear to be increasing only because parents, teachers and mental health professionals are becoming more aware of the problem.

The average concurrent prevalence rate in the twenty-eight epidemiological studies reviewed by Avenevoli and colleagues (2008) ranged from 1 to 2 percent among children and from 1 to 7 percent for adolescents. In their meta-analysis of twenty-eight studies involving a total of 60,000 observations of children, Costello et al. (2006) reported an average prevalence rate of 5.7 percent for adolescents and 2.8 percent for children. Thus, depression among children and adolescents is anything but non-existent. Although most children and adolescents will recover from their first bout with depression in a matter of months, 30–70 percent will have a relapse at some point in their lives. The risk of relapse is greater where there is a family history of depressive illness, another comorbid disorder or a stressful life event (Birmaher, Arbelaez and Brent, 2002).

Depressed children and adolescents often suffer from other mental health disorders at the same time. The highest comorbidity rate is with concurrent anxiety disorder, which can be diagnosed in 39 percent of depressed youth (Angold, Costello and Erklani, 1999). Many depressed children and youth can also be diagnosed as having conduct disorder (27.3% according to Angoldi et al., 1999) or attention deficit/hyperactivity disorder (with comorbidity reported in up to one-third of diagnosed children and youth; Faraone et al., 1998). These high comorbidity rates have important practical implications because multiple disorders have been associated with dramatically higher suicide rates than single disorders (e.g., Seligman and Ollendick, 1998).

Sex differences

Starting at puberty, adolescent girls suffer from depression far more extensively than adolescent boys – with most reviews indicating a prevalence rate for girls as twice that of boys starting at age 13 (Araya, et al., 2013; Hyde, 2005; Zahn-Waxler et al., 2008). The gender gap is documented so consistently that Hyde, Mezulis and Abramson (2008) maintain that it is the most robust statistical effect to be found in the psychopathology literature. Prior to adolescence, the prevalence rates are similar for boys and girls, with some studies even indicating a higher prevalence rate for boys. It is possible that the true differences between the prevalence rates for boys and girls are being exaggerated because girls are more willing than boys to acknowledge their depression and seek help for it (Hankin, Wetter and Cheely, 2008).

Sophisticated theoretical formulations have been proposed to explain why there is so strong a gender gap and why it becomes evident with the onset of adolescence. One possibility is the *gender-intensification hypothesis* (Hill and Lynch, 1983; Zahn-Waxler et al., 2008), according to which cultural expectations for conformity with traditional gender roles increase with the onset of adolescence, with girls expected to be dependent and self-effacing. Parents may unwittingly contribute to this by socializing their daughters to be dependent and to focus intensively on close relationships and the sharing of negative emotion (Brody and Hall, 1993; Eisenberg and Faves, 1994; Hankin et al., 2008). This occurs at the same developmental period during which hormonal changes are seen as increasing girls' needs for affiliation with others. Aggravating matters even further, affiliating with others during adolescence may be more complicated and stressful than in relating to peers as a child (Zahn-Waxler et al., 2008).

Girls tend to be more submissive in interpersonal relations than boys and tend to mull things over in their minds rather than come up with practical solutions that can be implemented with reasonable dispatch. The fact that girls and women are more oriented to interpersonal relationships than are boys and men may lead to the phenomenon of co-rumination, that is, not only brooding by oneself about a stressful event but joining together with a friend in brooding (Zahn-Waxler et al., 2008). Whether by co-rumination or not, girls are known to be more susceptible than boys to "depression contagion" or "catching" depression either from their mothers or close friends (Abela et al., 2006; Hankin, Wetter and Cheely, 2008; Prinstein et al., 2005).

The particular vulnerabilities of girls and women may also have a biological component (Hyde et al., 2008). One possibility is that the interactions between genetics and environmental stress are stronger in girls than in boys. As well, early puberty may constitute a stronger risk factor for girls than boys because puberty in boys leads to a strong, masculine appearance and demeanor whereas puberty in girls often leads to greater body mass, perhaps triggering depression through impaired body image. During puberty, a girl's estrogen balance may be disrupted, which may chemically trigger depression by disturbing serotonin processes.

Cultural differences

Cultural beliefs and stigma may result in keeping one's depression, or one's children's depression, a secret. Some maintain that members of different cultures experience depression in about the same way but differ in the extent to which they react to that feeling and in what they do about it (Furnham and Malik, 1994). However, cultural norms and prohibitions may actually be reflected in differences between cultures in the threshold at which people recognize themselves as being in a depressed state (Weisz and Eastman, 1995). As well, there may be cultural and gender issues in the environmental stressors than can trigger depression in a vulnerable individual.

Owning up to one's depression and seeking help for it, whether from a professional, a friend or a family member, can be seen as a confession of inadequacy. Although this can be a disincentive to seeking help in any culture, certain cultures are known to value and expect self-reliance more than others. For example, African-Americans, who have had to adapt to adverse circumstances, have developed an expectation, known as "John Henryism," that individuals fight hard and fight alone to overcome adversity. For that reason, African-Americans may not utilize mental health services for their depressed adolescents, even when they have the health insurance they need to do so (Breland-Noble, Bell and Nicolas, 2006). Being self-reliant and feeling that one is effective in resolving problems may, however, be a less important determinant of depression in highly collectivistic societies, such as East Asia, than in individualistic cultures such as the United States (Stewart et al., 2004). Owning up to being depressed may be particularly awkward for males in countries where there are sharp gender-role distinctions, which often include the expectation that males be self-reliant, as in Latin America (Lane and Addis, 2005). Any of these cultural factors may vary by social class within nations. Although the prevalence rates for young African Americans and Mexican-Americans appear to be higher than those for Anglo-Americans in some studies, this difference has been found to disappear once the lower socio-economic status of the ethnic minority groups is factored into the equation (Doi et al., 2001).

Being depressed or having a depressed child may bring shame (or the unwarranted fear that it will bring shame) to the family in some highly family-oriented cultures. For that reason, Chinese-Americans may be more likely to seek help for somatic problems than for emotional issues when they are depressed, reflecting at the same time Chinese teachings about the unity of mind and body (Kleinman, 1977). Rather than shaming themselves or their families, members of minority groups, such as black and Asian minorities in Great Britain, are thought to simply rely on their families to help with this form of mental illness rather than confiding in professionals (Furnham and Malik, 1994).

Probable causes and concurrent impairment

Physiological markers[1]

Individuals undergoing depression are known to be characterized by a number of distinct physiological markers. Modern methods including magnetic resonance imaging (MRI) and functional magnetic resonance imaging (fMRI) (see Chapter 5) have been used to demonstrate that there are differences between depressed and non-depressed children in the structures of several areas of the brain including, importantly, smaller frontal lobe volumes. The functions of the frontal lobe include planning to achieve goals and direct behavior based on emotion (Steingard et al., 1996; Nantel-Vivier and Pihl, 2008). In some of the fMRI studies, the children's brain functioning was studied as they observed photographs of facial expressions of fear. Thomas et al. (2001) found that depressed children displayed a blunted response in the amygdala. Other researchers have found a relatively low flow of blood in several regions of the brains of depressed adolescents, including left parietal lobe, anterior thalamus and right caudate nucleus (Kowatch et al., 1999).

With regard to neurochemical imbalances in depression, it is clear that serotonin, either by itself or in conjunction with other neurotransmitter systems, is linked to the onset of depression in adults; parallel studies with children and adolescents have yielded very inconsistent results (e.g., Frodl et al., 2010; Nantel-Vivier and Pihl, 2008).

Cortisol and depression

Hormonal factors may also be related to child and adolescent depression. The "stress hormone" cortisol, produced by the adrenal gland cortex, has been implicated. Many studies of hypothalamic-pituitary-adrenal (HPA) axis system functioning indicate that both *circadian* and *stress-reactive cortisol levels*

---

[1] Section written by Paul Hastings and Amanda Guyer.

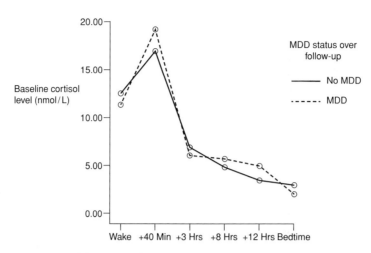

Figure 13.1 Adolescents with a stronger cortisol awakening response were more likely to be diagnosed with depression over the subsequent year.

are associated with depression. In adults, elevated baseline cortisol levels and high, flat diurnal slopes – that is, cortisol levels that do not decrease from morning to evening as much as would normally be expected – characterize as many as 50 percent of depressed individuals (Nestler et al., 2002). Prolonged exposure to elevated levels of circadian cortisol has physiological consequences that parallel depressive symptoms, including exhaustion and irritability (Gurguis et al., 1990). The degree to which cortisol levels are elevated is associated with the severity of depression (Pruessner et al., 2003), so the most depressed adults also typically have the highest cortisol levels. Recent research is identifying similar relations between cortisol and depression in children and adolescents, as well. Youths who report more negative affect (DeSantis et al., 2007) and adolescent girls with more internalizing problems (Klimes-Dougan et al., 2001b) have flatter diurnal cortisol slopes than youths without problems, who show more typical, negatively sloped patterns of cortisol production over the day. The cortisol awakening response (CAR) also is exaggerated in depressed adults (Vreeburg et al., 2009), young adults with depressed parents (Mannie, Harmer and Cowen, 2007) and preschool-aged boys with internalizing problems (Hatzinger et al., 2007).

The fact that parental depression predicts elevated cortisol in children before they show signs of clinical depression (Halligan et al., 2004; Mannie et al., 2007) suggests that chronically increased HPA activity might contribute to the emergence of depression. Two longitudinal studies of adolescents have shown that elevated cortisol predicts later depression symptoms (Goodyer, Herbert and Tamplin, 2003; Mathew et al., 2003). A recent study by Adam and her colleagues (Adam et al., 2010) went a step further by predicting which adolescents would develop full-blown clinical depression (major depressive disorder). They measured CAR and depression symptoms in 230 17-year-old youths, many of whom had high levels of *neuroticism*. Neuroticism is an aspect of personality that involves feeling high levels of negative emotions, and neurotic people tend to be more likely to develop depression (Kendler et al., 2004). Adam and her colleagues then contacted the young adults a year later, and again measured their symptoms of depression. Some of the young adults had experienced episodes of clinical depression in the intervening year. The participants who had highly elevated CAR a year earlier were three times more likely to have become depressed. Earlier high CAR predicted subsequent depression even after the researchers took account of experiences of stressful life events, and other factors that might have accounted for the finding.

Lopez-Duran and colleagues recently published a meta-analysis of studies on cortisol and pediatric depression (Lopez-Duran et al., 2009). They looked at seventeen studies of basal and diurnal cortisol levels in children and youths aged 4.76 to 15.8 years with diagnosed depression disorder. Aggregating across these studies, they concluded that depressed children and youths had significantly higher circulating cortisol levels than their non-depressed peers, across all times of the day. The difference between depressed and non-depressed peers was not large, but it was consistent, and it paralleled the patterns of high, flat curves identified in depressed adults. Lopez-Duran and colleagues also performed a meta-analysis of studies that had used the *dexamethasone suppression test (DST)*. Dexamethasone suppresses HPA activity, such that less cortisol is produced. They found that, across studies, depressed children and youths responded much less strongly to the DST than did children and youths without depression. Thus, their overactive HPA axis systems resisted the pharmacological agent and continued to produce an excess of cortisol.

If the circadian rhythm of HPA axis activity is dysregulated in depressed children and youths, what about cortisol reactivity to stressful events? Surprisingly, fewer investigators have examined this question. Three studies of depressed children (Luby et al., 2003; Luby et al., 2004; Rao et al., 2008) have produced inconsistent results, although this might be due to the difficulty of effectively eliciting cortisol elevations in preschoolers using laboratory stressors (Gunnar et al., 2009). There is a bit more evidence for increased cortisol reactivity being related to depression in adolescents, as youths with stronger cortisol reactivity to laboratory procedures designed to induce emotional stress are more likely to have depression (Rao et al., 2008) or internalizing problems (Klimes-Dougan et al., 2001b). Strikingly, one longitudinal study that followed youths for 10 years, from their adolescence into early adulthood, found that elevated cortisol reactivity to stress in

adolescence predicted whether depressed individuals had attempted to commit suicide in the subsequent 10 years (Mathew et al., 2003).

At least in adolescents, and possibly in children as well, depression and its associated problems appear to be linked with both increased diurnal HPA activity and increased reactivity to stressful events. Normally, elevated circulating cortisol would eventually cross the blood–brain barrier and signal the hypothalamus to end the cascade of hormones that result in cortisol secretion; perhaps this auto-regulatory feedback mechanism is impaired in depressed youths. Remember the adverse consequences of *hypercortisolism* on physical and mental health (see Chapter 5), and this should again call to mind the adage "too much of a good thing." The erosion of bodily resources that is incurred by chronically elevated cortisol levels might contribute to the lethargy, anhedonia (inability to enjoy things) and irritability that are typical of depressed youth.

Autonomic nervous system activity and depression

Given the lethargy and anhedonia that often characterize depressed youths, one might expect them to have relatively subdued autonomic states. However, there is little evidence that children with depression or at risk for developing depression differ from non-depressed children in their general levels of arousal, as reflected in such measures as baseline and reactive heart rate and blood pressure (Gump et al., 2009; Tonhajzerova et al., 2010).

This is not to say that depression has not been associated with any aspects of autonomic physiology. There is fairly robust evidence that depressed adults have low baseline *respiratory sinus arrhythmia (RSA)* and poor vagal regulation, reflecting weaker *parasympathetic nervous system (PNS)* control of cardiac activity (Rottenberg et al., 2007). Is this also true for pediatric depression? One team of researchers have found that higher RSA is weakly associated with adolescents' depression symptoms (Bosch et al., 2009; Greaves-Lord et al., 2007), but they seem to be the exception. Tiffany Field's studies have shown that infants with depressed mothers have poorer vagal regulation than infants of non-depressed mothers (Field et al., 1995). Children of depressed mothers have been found to show slower recovery of PNS activity after a disappointing experience (Forbes et al., 2006) and to have more symptoms of depression themselves if they showed weaker RSA responses to watching a sad film (Gentzler et al., 2009). Depressed adolescents also have lower RSA or heart rate variability than adolescents without depression problems (Shannon et al., 2007; Tonhajzerova et al., 2010). Overall, there is clear evidence that depressed children, and children at risk for depression, have relatively weak PNS activity, indicating that they are lacking in an important physiological basis for self-regulation of emotional states.

Fewer studies have examined how pediatric depression is related to measures of *sympathetic nervous system (SNS)* activity. Parental symptoms of depression have been found to predict children's internalizing problems only if children showed strong *electrodermal reactivity* to an emotional challenge (Cummings et al., 2007). Shannon and colleagues (Shannon et al., 2007) found that higher *pre-ejection period* reactivity, reflecting more SNS activity, was associated with more depression symptoms in adolescents, but only if their fathers engaged in high levels of anti-social behavior. Although the number of studies is yet small, there is at least some indication that increased SNS activity might be linked to children's risk for depression and related adjustment difficulties.

Summary

Theorists differ widely in the strength they assign to physiological factors as causal agents of depression. Depression may render the individual vulnerable to the stresses of life, meaning that physiology is, in essence, a partial cause of the disorder. However, as noted perceptively by Nantel-Vivier and Pihl (2008), stressful life events may also alter physiological processes. As well, psychotherapy may bring about an improvement in these processes (Purvis and Cross, 2007). Expanding further on the ways in which physiological vulnerability may interact with environmental stressors, Goodyer (2008) suggested two distinct functional frameworks depending on the area of the brain that is involved. In some cases, the neurologically based vulnerability evident early in life affects the child's ability for mood regulation, leaving him or her particularly susceptible to environmental stressors during adolescence. In other cases where other areas of the brain are involved, the physiological mechanisms affect thinking, motivation and behavior at any point in the lifespan at which negative life events are experienced. In summary, data available now provide some support for Nantel-Vivier and Pihl's bold, unambiguous and unqualified statement that "depression is a biological disease" (2008, p. 103). Biological it is, which by no means implies that depression is *only* a biological disease.

Family correlates of children's depressive disorder

Research has elucidated a number of diverse paths by which parents can influence the emergence of mood disorder in their children. All of these risk factors may be activated at times of family or personal crisis. This principle is the cornerstone of *diathesis-stress models* of depression, which can be applied to the interaction of any underlying vulnerability (cognitive, familial, etc.) – diathesis – with an immediate stressor in the environment – stress. For example, Abramson and his colleagues (e.g., Abramson, Alloy and Metalsky, 1988) proposed that people whose thinking patterns leave them vulnerable to dysphoric mood (as will be detailed later in this chapter) are more likely to suffer major depressive disorder at periods in which they are going through marked stress.

Parents' genetic contribution

Researchers working with adults have generally concluded that major depressive disorder among adults is family-based and heritable to a considerable extent (see review and meta-analysis by Sullivan, Neale and Kendler, 2000). Some authorities maintain that childhood depression is even more heavily determined by genetics than depression in adults. This belief is based, first of all, on the fact that depressed children are at very substantial risk of growing up to be depressed adults, as noted earlier. The fact that many of the relatives of children with depression suffer from depression as well provides additional evidence. However, in a systematic review of previous studies, Rice, Harold and Thapar (2002) located six follow-up studies in which children with depression were followed into adulthood. They also examined the results of four studies of the children of mothers with major depression. Taken together, these results indicate that the odds of having at least one relative who suffers from depression were about four times higher for the at-risk groups than for the normal control group. These odds provide some evidence for familial genetic transmission, but not necessarily greater transmission for childhood or adolescent depression than for depression among adults. Rice, Harold and Thapar also synthesized the results of ten twin studies (2002). There was considerable variation in the findings, which is not uncommon in twin studies. When parents filled out the questionnaire about their children's depression, there was moderate to high evidence of genetic transmission: Heritability estimates ranged from 30 to 80 percent, with all but one study indicating a heritability estimate above 50 percent. Ratings of depression by the children themselves suggested lower rates of heritability; the estimates ranged from 15 to 80 percent, but only one of six studies with self-report data indicated a heritability estimate over 50 percent. This difference in method may be attributable to *shared method bias* – the same conclusion emerging from a number of different measures obtained from the same informant – a methodological problem that can occur in any kind of research. When parents rate both their own and their children's adjustment, they may apply their own negative moods to all of their ratings, of themselves, their children and probably anyone else.

These twin studies have been complemented by only two adoption studies. In contrast with the twin studies, the two adoption studies in the data pool used in the meta-analysis indicated little correspondence between the parent-rated depression scores of biological and non-biological siblings, providing, obviously, no evidence of genetic transmission. Despite the inconsistent findings of the studies they summarized, Rice, Harold and Thapar concluded that there was significant support overall for the contention that childhood depression is partially determined genetically. Looking more closely at the data, they found that genetic influence appears to be most evident in the adolescent years. In middle childhood, however, environmental factors such as family adversity, harsh parenting and parental psychopathology appear to be more strongly determinant of children's depression. It has also been suggested that girls are more vulnerable than boys to the genetic transmission of depression and that the specific genes involved are not the same for males and females (Caspi et al., 2003). Greater susceptibility to genetic transmission by girls was confirmed in four of the six studies reviewed by Lau and Ely (2008), but two other studies indicated greater heritability for boys. Lau and Ely express the hope that molecular genetics will provide a clearer picture of the extent of the genetic origin of childhood depression than what the behavioral-genetic research has offered so far. However, the first few pioneering molecular genetic studies have not accomplished this; their results are somewhat inconclusive.

Given the recurrent evidence of small-to-moderate genetic influence, researchers have turned to the more challenging task of tracking the interactions between genetic and environmental influences. Working with a northern Italian sample, Nobile et al. (2009) detected a particularly high rate of parent-rated affective disorders (essentially symptoms of mood disorder) in children who were both members of single-parent families and were also determined to be genetically vulnerable according to DNA samples. Vulnerable gene composition has also been found to interact with child maltreatment in predicting the emergence of mood disorder in children (Kaufman et al. 2006). These gene–environment interactions and gene–environment correlations are of the magnitude that can be expected, according to the experts: Genetics probably does play a substantial causal role in childhood and adolescent depression, but works in complex interaction with powerful environmental factors.

Linking mothers' depression to children's depression

Probably the most consistent finding in the literature on children's depression is the fact that the children of mothers who are depressed themselves are at risk for depression. Based on many studies, it is estimated that 20 to 40 percent of the school-age or adolescent children of depressed mothers have experienced a depressive episode (Goodman and Tully, 2008). This rate is of course much higher than the incidence of depression in the general population. Before delving into the possible pathways by which mothers' depression might lead to mood disorder in children, it is worth remembering once more that this correlation, like any other correlation, does not indicate the direction of causation. Although, as discussed in Chapters 2 and 6, it is traditional (indeed, since biblical times) to infer that it is the parents that determine outcomes for their children, the opposite is not entirely inconceivable. Having a child with an inhibited temperament who is prone to be miserable could cause – or could exacerbate – a mother's negative mood. Some theorists postulate a bidirectional interactive process in which the child's negative mood escalates in counterpoint with negative parenting, with each element reciprocally contributing to the worsening of the other in a vicious cycle (e.g., Biglan, Lewin and Hops, 1990).

In any case, the fact that there is a significant correlation between mothers' and children's depression is not particularly informative by itself because there are many conceivable explanations for it, in other words, many ways in which

mothers' depression could be transmitted to their children, including, of course, their genetic bond. Prenatal experiences with mothers' depression may cause physiological changes associated with the regulation of emotion. Depression may affect the thinking, behavior and emotional expression that mothers direct at their children; this is considered in greater detail in the next section of this chapter. A mother's depression may also affect the quality of general family life, disrupting family harmony and marital satisfaction (Goodman and Gotlib, 1999). A mother's depression (or, indeed, a child's inhibited disposition) may affect the security of the child–parent attachment bond (Abela et al., 2009). Finally, a certain dysphoria can result from the observational learning that occurs when children observe and mimic the aspects of depression they observe their mothers displaying (Downey and Coyne, 1990).

Can't fathers also be depressed, and can't they also transmit depression to their children? Although some theorists believe that children are equally affected by depression in either parent, it has been demonstrated statistically that mothers' depression is more closely associated with children's depression than is fathers' depression (see, e.g., meta-analysis by Connell and Goodman, 2002). The most likely explanation for this is that mothers tend to be more involved in child-rearing activities on a daily basis than fathers. Therefore, children are more likely to be in direct contact with their mothers during depressed moods and be exposed more frequently to their mother's maladaptive behavior and thinking (Pleck, 1997). Another explanation is that depression may disrupt mothers' parenting more than fathers' parenting, with fathers tending to maintain a more stable, playful style of interaction with their children than mothers, even when they are depressed (Field, Hossain and Malphurs, 1999).

Insecure child–parent attachment and vulnerability to depression

Given the fact that the children of depressed mothers are at risk for becoming depressed themselves, researchers have taken up the challenge of finding out exactly why and how this occurs. One explanation that has been proposed is that depressed mothers are prone to insecure attachment bonds with their children (see Chapter 6 for an introduction to attachment theory) and that, in turn, these insecure attachment bonds lead to depression in the children. This may occur because as children develop self-awareness during the toddlerhood period, they develop their self-images that correspond to the way their mothers relate to them. If the toddler has experienced a positive, secure relationship with his or her mother, the corresponding self-image will be that of an emerging individual worthy of love. If, on the other hand, the early child–parent relationship has been one of rejection or insecurity, the child will develop a picture of himself or herself as unlovable (Bretherton, 1990). In a landmark longitudinal study, Toth et al., (2009) documented not only the fact that mothers' depression was associated with insecure infant–mother attachment, as was already known (see next paragraph), but also that the extent to which the children's representations of themselves at age 4 years were correlated with the mothers' depression depended on the insecurity of the attachment between them.

Considerable progress has been made in recent years in corroborating the broad premise that maternal depression leads to insecure child–parent attachment and thereby to depression in children. One important step has been determining exactly how insecure the attachment links between depressed mothers and their children are. Indeed, a significantly greater proportion of the relationships between depressed mothers and their children have been found to be insecure than the relationships between children and their non-depressed mothers. However, the results fluctuate considerably from study to study and the overall difference, although significant statistically, is not very large (see quantitative reviews by Atkinson, Niccols et al., 2000 and by Van IJzendoorn, Schuengel and Bakermans-Kranenburg, 1999).

Child-rearing and depression

Early research in this area, conducted primarily in the 1970s, focused on the feelings about parenting that were reported by depressed parents in questionnaires or interviews. The results are questionable from a methodological standpoint because of the inherent bias in reporting on one's own behavior, especially at an unhappy moment in life. Nevertheless, they do show quite poignantly how depression can pervade the child–parent relationship. The mothers reported that they were uninvolved with their children emotionally, profoundly dissatisfied in their role as parents and in life, and hostile and resentful (Lovejoy et al., 2000; Weissman, Paykel and Klerman, 1972).

Dissatisfied with the limitations of self-report methods, researchers began to favor direct observations of depressed mothers in interaction with their children. By 2000, enough observational studies had been conducted for there to be a comprehensive meta-analysis, by Lovejoy and colleagues (2000), who synthesized the findings of forty well-designed studies. This body of research has focused on both the lack of positive maternal behavior and on high rates of negative maternal behavior. The statistical results of the meta-analysis revealed that the negative behaviors were more linked with children's depression than was the lack of positive behavior, although both effects were statistically significant. Depressed mothers were found to be less responsive to the needs and emotions of their children than were other mothers. They do not communicate effectively with their children but impatiently issue directives and commands. They criticize frequently and appear hostile and irritated much of the time. There is also evidence that depressed mothers tend not to interact positively or playfully with their children as much as do other mothers.

That being established, the question remains as to how strong a causal role in the genesis of child depression is played by parental rejection or excessive parental control. McLeod, Weisz and Wood (2007) conducted a meta-analysis of forty-five studies on the associations between parenting and children's depression; the studies were not restricted to those focusing on depressed mothers. The meta-analysis revealed that the correlation between parenting and children's mood disorders was significant as expected, providing confirmation that the parenting behaviors measured are associated significantly with children's depression. However, the parenting measures explained only 8 percent of the variance in child outcome, a much smaller effect than is often suggested in the literature on parenting. This means that parenting should be considered as one of many possible causal agents. Some aspects of parenting were more predictive of children's depression than others. Parents' aversive behavior and the lack of parental warmth were found to be relatively strong predictors of outcome. Parental overinvolvement with the child's activities was a relatively weak predictor.

Maltreatment

Child abuse, be it physical, sexual or emotional, and neglect by parents or caregivers are known to lead to depression in children and adolescents (e.g., Cicchetti and Toth, 2005). Although child abuse is strongly linked with depression among both boys and girls, it has been established that girls are more vulnerable than boys to its effects (e.g., Fletcher, 2009a). Although it is not easy to establish the exact ways in which maltreatment leads to depression, one important theory that has been advanced is that maltreatment profoundly affects the child's sense of self and his or her ability to react to stressful life events (Molnar, Buka and Kessler, 2001). Children or adolescents who have been abused are thought to react emotionally to life stressors of a much lower magnitude than the level of stress that typically leads non-abused children to become depressed. This is sometimes called the kindling hypothesis and means that, as time goes on, less stress is required to trigger a depressive episode among children who have been victims of abuse or neglect. It is theorized that this

heightened sensitivity to stressors occurs because the experience of chronic abuse or neglect affects the physiological processes that trigger depression (Post, 1992), such as those discussed earlier in this chapter. A recent study by Harkness, Bruce and Lumley (2006), conducted with 103 depressed and non-depressed Canadian adolescents, provides research support for the contention that child abuse and/or neglect leaves individuals hypersensitive to stressful life events.

There has also been considerable exploration of the ways this specific vulnerability interacts with other possible influences that may cause depression and to possible protective factors that enable some victims of abuse and neglect to somehow avoid becoming depressed. The research questions examined have often been inspired by the concepts of *equifinality* – how and why individuals with different patterns of risk and protective factors end up with the same outcome – and *multifinality* – how and why individuals with the same patterns of risk and protective factors may end up with very different outcomes, that is, depression for some, other forms of psychopathology for others and no mental health problems for yet others (Cicchetti and Rogosch, 1996). In a ground-breaking recent study on the interaction between childhood maltreatment and genetic predisposition to depression, Cicchetti, Rogosch and Sturge-Apple found that among maltreated children and youth from low socio-economic status homes, only those who were found to be genetically at risk because of low monoamine oxidase A (MAOA) activity according to DNA samples developed depressive symptoms (2007).

Peer relations and depression

In the 1970s, at about the same time as cognitively based theories of depression began to achieve prominence, interpersonal theories were elaborated based on findings, obtained initially in work with adults, that the behaviors of depressed people are interwoven with identifiable patterns in the ways other people respond to them. The reactions of others may, in turn, perpetuate or aggravate the depressed state. In a ground-breaking study, Coyne (1976) randomly paired unacquainted adults, some of whom were found to be experiencing depressed mood. The participants in the study were instructed to speak to each other by telephone and try to become acquainted with the person they were speaking with. The depressed conversation partners left their listeners in a more negative mood than before the conversation. Although Coyne analyzed the taped conversations in many different ways, he was unable to pinpoint exactly what about the conversations might be linked to the increase in the negative affect of the listeners. Nevertheless, a highly unfortunate bidirectional process can reasonably be inferred in which this effect on others can be seen as both a cause and a result of the mood disorder. Potential companions tend, understandably, to avoid the person who engendered negative feelings. Their avoidance then confirms the expectations held by the depressed person that he or she is disliked and unwanted. In the process, the depressed person loses a potential source of social support that might act as a protective factor. Several research strategies have been used to confirm that this interpersonal process occurs between depressed children and their peers as it does with adults. The stigmatization of children with mood disorder was confirmed in a study by Walker and colleagues (2008), who presented vignettes depicting children or adolescents with depression, attention deficit/ hyperactive disorder or asthma to over 1,300 children and adolescents across the United States. Among the negative impressions of depressed children was the expectation that they would become violent.

Sociometric studies (i.e., those based on information from peers about their liking or disliking of other members of a social group – see Chapter 7) clearly indicate that depressed children and adolescents are not held in high esteem by their classmates and schoolmates (e.g., Hecht, Inderbitzen

and Bukowski, 1998; Kiesner, 2002; Nolan, Flynn and Garber, 2003; Oldehinkel, et al., 2007). As detailed in Chapter 7, children who are rejected in larger groups may still have a small circle of close friends. Unfortunately, children with depressive symptoms have been found to have relatively few friends (e.g., Schwartz et al., 2008). This may be because they deprive potential companions of the enjoyment of play interactions. In an observational study conducted by Rockhill et al. (2007), children with depressive symptoms were observed while playing a structured game with their self-reported best friends. The children with depressive symptoms and their friends said that they enjoyed the game less than did non-depressed children and their friends. In several other studies, depressed children have been found to display little interest in their peers and little inclination to be helpful or supportive to them (e.g., Rudolph and Clark, 2001). According to a number of studies, their interactions with friends and other children are characterized by constant requests for reassurance about their self-worth (see review by Joiner et al., 1999).

Victimization by bullies

Like maltreatment by parents, maltreatment by peers is a common pathway to depression among children and youth. Heart-rending reports of depression-related suicides by children and adolescents appear regularly in both the popular press and the professional literature. Correlations between victimization by peers and depression have emerged in a number of studies, such as a study conducted in the Netherlands by Van Hoof et al. (2008), one in New York by Klomek et al. (2007), an Irish study by Mills et al. (2004) and yet another study conducted in Italy by Baldry and Winkel (2004). However, in other research, including the New York study and a Finnish longitudinal study by Klomek and her colleagues (Brunstein Klomek et al., 2008), it emerges that the bullies may end up at least as depressed as the victims, if not more so. Furthermore, bully-victims, youngsters who are both bullies and victims at different times, often end up the most depressed of all. According to a Canadian study by Marini, Dane and Bosacki (2006), this is especially the case for indirect or relational bully-victims. In that study and a number of others, the researchers differentiated between direct bullying or direct victimization – which have to do with physical acts of aggression, direct extortion or threats to do either – and indirect or relational bullying or victimization – which involve the bully manipulating the victim's interpersonal relationships, for example by spreading rumors or excluding the victim from group activities or friendships. Tracking the results of a comprehensive anti-bullying program in the Netherlands, Vuijk and colleagues (2007) found evidence that direct victimization was linked to depression among boys whereas indirect victimization was implicated in the genesis of girls' depression.

As with the other possible causes of depression discussed in this chapter, victimization by child or adolescent peers probably interacts with other causal agents. Baldry and Winkel (2004) found that, although peer victimization was the strongest predictor of depression in their sample of Italian children, the risk increased if there was also abuse by parents. The possible interactions between peer bullying/victimization and other family risk factors, not to mention genetic risk, need to be scrutinized more fully in future research.

It has also been found that the bullying of adolescents of minority sexual orientation is a major contributing factor to depressive symptoms, especially in schools lacking in positive school climate (Birkett, Espelage and Koening, 2009). Moreover, young people who are questioning their sexual orientation but who do not identify as gay or lesbian are even more likely to react to peer bullying with depressive symptoms (Birkett et al., 2009). According to a large-scale epidemiological study by Roberts et al. (2013), the risk of bullying leading to depression is particularly high among young people who display gender non-conforming

behavior, regardless of their sexual orientation as adolescents or, later on, as young adults.

School effects

Given the centrality of school in the lives of children and adolescents, it seems unlikely that chronic unhappiness at school exerts no toll on pupils' well-being. Only a few studies have been conducted on this topic. Working with Australian young people 12 through 18 years old, Shochet and colleagues (2008) found, first of all, that school connectedness – meaning essentially a sense of membership and belonging in the school community – was related to self-reported depressive symptoms. Importantly, the study revealed only partial overlap between school alienation and insecurity of parent attachment. This suggests that alienation from school may occur and precipitate depression among many pupils who experience no difficulties in their relationships with parents. As with all other environmental correlates of depression, alienation from school may of course be either a cause or a result of the depression, or both.

Electronic communication and depression among young people

The advent of near-universal access to the internet in many countries has led to considerable reflection about the psychological implications of its use, including the possibility that it may increase the prevalence of depression. Indeed, the internet can be used to avoid interpersonal contact or to spend time aimlessly at games or information-seeking rather than to solve problems. However, the internet can also be used to establish and consolidate interpersonal relationships. Individuals who find it awkward to establish relationships in person may be more effective at doing so in the relatively anonymous environment of electronic communication, where the physical cues of awkwardness are often not involved (Schneider and Amichai-Hamburger, 2010). People undergoing stress or feeling depressed may be able to locate sympathetic, supportive people online where the potential network of contacts is almost infinite. Nevertheless, Kraut et al. (1998) argued that electronic communication is likely to increase depression because it usually involves substituting social interactions of lower quality for higher-quality interpersonal contact. Furthermore, the internet can be used for cyberbullying, which, like bullying in person, may conceivably lead to depression.

Although the possible benefits or harm of internet use have been studied in several countries, the results of studies to date are highly contradictory and confusing. According to the Youth Internet Safety Survey (2005), conducted by telephone in the United States, youth who reported depressive symptoms use the internet more frequently than others and use the internet more extensively to disclose personal information and feelings (Finkelhor, Mitchell and Wolak, 2011). In contrast, Gross (2004), who studied logs of instant messages sent by California high school students over a 4-day period, found no significant correlations between internet use and measures of psychological adjustment (depression, loneliness, social anxiety). Recent studies conducted in both the Netherlands and Korea (van der Eijnden et al., 2008; Yen et al., 2007) indicate that *compulsive* internet use is linked with depression, which does not mean of course that competent online social interaction has the same effect.

Some forms of psychotherapy for depression can be delivered online. The best-known online therapeutic program for depressed young people, known as MindGym, was developed in Australia. Some data indicate that these online interventions can be effective. Unfortunately, effectiveness is often compromised because the depressed children and adolescents often fail to log on as often as needed or go over the materials presented with sufficient attention (O'Kearney et al., 2009).

Cognitive roots of depression

The idea that maladaptive thinking may lead to depression can be traced in part to philosophers who

have delved into their own thoughts and thinking processes since ancient times, dating back at least to the times of the Stoic philosophers in ancient Greece, such as Cicero. Aristotle attributed misery to the inability of the individual to reconcile reason and faith. The eminent eighteenth-century German philosopher Immanuel Kant, one of the leading thinkers of the Enlightenment period, observed that mental illness developed out of failure to use "common sense" to correct "private sense." The leading interpersonal theorist in the field of mental health, Harry Stack Sullivan, introduced the concept of *parataxic distortion*, or the misreading of people with whom one shares close relationships, as a root of psychopathology. Subjective misinterpretation of interpersonal events and the behaviors it leads to constitute the cornerstone of contemporary cognitive-behavioral approaches. Cognitive-behavioral theory and therapy have evolved over the past 30 years to become the most influential theory of depression (Clark and Beck, 1999; Sullivan, 1953).

As part of the maturity of cognitive-behavioral approaches, there is now greater precision and detail in thinking about exactly how maladaptive thoughts might bring about depressed moods (see review by Abela and Hankin, 2008). One form of cognitive vulnerability is described by *hopelessness theory* (Abramson, Metalsky and Alloy, 1989), which subsumes three depressive thinking styles. First of all, the individual may believe that the causes of negative events are permanent and will be evident everywhere; there is therefore no escape from them. An individual may also believe that negative events have truly disastrous consequences, far worse than they actually are. The person may also feel that he or she is irreparably flawed, weakened by the negative events experienced in life. Making such inferences leads the individual to the belief that nothing can be done about the inevitable course of stressful events. Therefore, no effort is invested in coping with them.

Another approach to describing cognitive vulnerability, developed by the Canadian psychologist David Zuroff, is based on personality theory. Personality can be defined as a stable, organized set of characteristics or traits of an individual that influences the person's thinking, motivation and, especially, behavior across different situations (Ryckman, 2004). Zuroff delineated personality profiles that leave the individual vulnerable to depression. According to his theory, these include dependency, self-criticism and excessive need for approval (Zuroff, Mongrain and Santor, 2004). Similar to hopelessness theory in many ways, Beck's theory is based on the concept of *mental schema* (e.g., Beck and Alford, 2008). A schema is a stored body of knowledge that typically includes mental representations of oneself and of prior experiences. When faced with a new and potentially challenging situation, the individual activates schemata relevant to that experience. This activation influences how the individual understands the situation and, thence, how he or she reacts. In many cases, the individual interprets the situation as one that will lead to failure.

Response-styles theory, developed by Susan Nolen-Hoeksema (Nolen-Hoeksema, Girgus and Seligman, 1986) maintains that the way a person habitually responds to depressive symptoms determines the intensity and duration of the depressive episode. According to the theory, people may make things better by distracting themselves, avoiding thoughts that bring them to the stressful situation. They can make things worse by ruminating, that is, constantly mulling over the stressful situation, closing off other thoughts.

None of these refinements to cognitive-behavioral theory were developed to describe children's thinking. How well do these theories apply when transposed from the adult mind to the study of depression among children? Abela and Hankin's (2008) careful review includes twenty-seven prospective studies testing hopelessness theory with children or adolescents. Of these, twenty-three studies confirm either fully or partially the hypothesis that hopelessness predicts depression in the presence of a stressful life event. The data are strongest in confirming the predictive power of feeling that negative forces are stable and strong.

There is less evidence of risk associated with the belief that the individual who experiences the stressor suffers long-term damage from it. There have been five longitudinal studies conducted with children or adolescents on the predictive power of Beck's schema theory; all of these studies provide at least partial support for the theory. With regard to response-style theory, there are seven well-designed longitudinal studies providing evidence for the long-term harm associated with rumination. There is much less evidence that distraction helps protect a child or adolescent from depression. Compared to the other forms of cognitive vulnerability that have been proposed and investigated, support is more equivocal for personality vulnerability theory. Of the seven longitudinal studies focusing on self-critical personality styles, five indicate that such self-reproach is associated with subsequent depression. In contrast, only four of the eight longitudinal explorations show that a dependent personality style is linked with mood disorder. Thus, taken together, the evidence for the cognitive vulnerability theories is quite impressive.

Stability and prognosis

Although individual depressive episodes typically run their course over a period of months, depressed mood tends to pervade the ongoing life histories of children who suffer from this condition. For example, Fombonne et al. (2001a) interviewed 149 adults who had been seen as patients of the Children's Department of Maudsley Hospital in London 20 years earlier and who had been diagnosed as suffering from major depressive disorder. About two-thirds of the adults reported a major depressive episode during their adult years; about three-quarters reported some form of adult depression. Forty-four percent said that they had made at least one suicide attempt at some point, with more severe suicidality in the group that had been diagnosed as having both major depression and conduct disorder (Fombonne et al., 2001b). In a similar study conducted in New York City, adults who were seen at Columbia Presbyterian Hospital because of depression when they were children, 15 years earlier, were thirteen times more likely than children who had never been seen in a mental health clinic to have sought treatment as adults for a mental health problem (Goldstein et al., 2006; Zahn-Waxler et al., 2008).

Suicide is the most severe consequence of depression from adolescence on. Some form of suicidal event, but not death by suicide, was reported for 10 percent of the adolescents who participated in the influential Treatment of Depression Study (TADS), discussed in greater detail later in this chapter, during their 36 weeks of various forms of treatment (Vitiello et al., 2009). It has been found that fully one-third of the children and adolescents treated for depression in mental health clinics will make a suicide attempt by early adulthood (Kovacs, Golston and Gatsonis, 1993) and that 20 percent of those will make at least one further attempt (Harrington et al., 1994).

Prevention and treatment

Prevention of depression

Most prevention programs are based on the same cognitive-behavioral theory that underlies individual psychotherapy for depression. Thus, typical prevention programs feature classroom sessions in which the pupils might be taught how to identify and correct negative or irrational thoughts (e.g., Cardemil et al., 2007), how to generate creative, effective solutions to their interpersonal problems (e.g., Barrett et al., 2006) or how to relax (e.g., Hains and Ellman, 1994). Other content approaches include psychoeducation, which consists essentially of providing general information about depression and how to avoid it (e.g., Clarke et al., 1993). There have also been a few recent trials of prevention programs based on interpersonal psychotherapy with schoolchildren (e.g., Young, Mufson and Davies, 2006). These include a systematic comparison by Horowitz and colleagues (2007) of cognitive-

behavioral and interpersonal approaches, which showed that both were effective at the end of the intervention, although neither was at 6-month follow-up. Because most of the prevention programs are delivered in schools or recreational settings for children, relatively little attention has been paid to involving the family in preventive interventions. This might augment the effectiveness of the interventions delivered directly to the children and adolescents without compromising at all their brevity and preventive nature.

A recent and thorough meta-analysis by Stice and colleagues (2009) indicates that many of the prevention programs do in fact deliver what they promise: a significant if not enormous reduction in subsequent depression. These authors reviewed the results of forty-seven systematic trials of thirty-two different prevention programs. They reported an overall average effect size r of .15 for the difference in depressive symptoms between the beginning and the end of the interventions and of .11 for the difference between the start of intervention and the follow-up point. An effect size r of .15 corresponds to a difference of about 0.3 of a standard deviation unit between the average outcome for the group that received the preventive program and the control group. Applying the hypothetical method of calculating a binominal effect size display (see earlier discussion, p. 305), it can be estimated that a hypothetical 58 percent of prevention-group participants improved significantly compared with about 42 percent of control-group participants. Although this effect is not large, 41 percent of the programs reviewed succeeded in achieving significant reduction in depressive symptoms; 13 percent of the programs led to a significant reduction in future diagnosis of depressive disorder. Several characteristics distinguished programs with a higher success rate, most notably the characteristics of the participants. Preventive efforts directed at populations known to be at high risk for depression, such as populations with a high proportion of female participants, were more effective than universal or primary prevention programs, as might be expected. There was no difference in the effectiveness of programs based on different types of content, such as problem-solving, self-defeating cognition, social skills and psychoeducation. Although the overwhelming majority of the prevention programs were evaluated and conducted in the United States, Yu and Seligman (2002) introduced a school-based cognitive-behavioral prevention program to a relatively small sample of at-risk children in China, which achieved significant effects in terms of the children's depressive symptoms. Although cognitive-behavioral content has been used most often in direct efforts at preventing depression, other types of preventive interventions may also be useful. In addition to dedicated programs designed specifically to prevent depression, as reviewed by Stice and colleagues, preventive interventions that focus on the reduction of child maltreatment or of bullying in schools might also be effective.

Cognitive-behavioral therapy

Cognitive-behavioral psychotherapy aims at improving the various forms of distorted thinking that were discussed earlier in this chapter. Therapy can be delivered either individually or to groups. Part of its widespread appeal is its specific focus on cognition and on practical ways to implement change based on new beliefs. Typically, each session has a clear "agenda" and concludes with a homework assignment designed to help translate what has been discovered during the session into the client's real world. Cognitive-behavioral therapy is rarely a long-term endeavor: Reinecke and Ginsberg (2008) indicate that the therapist should strive to effect meaningful change in twelve to sixteen sessions.

All varieties of cognitive-behavioral therapy aim at providing the client with an understanding of the ways in which his or her thinking leads to feeling miserable, in the hope that the individual will recognize and interrupt such thoughts as they happen. However, cognitive-behavioral treatments differ in terms of how far they venture from their cognitive home base in seeking to change behavior. Meichenbaum (1977), a Canadian psychologist who pioneered in this field, aptly captures the difference by making the distinction between what he calls *cognitive-behavioral treatments*, which seek, essentially, to change behavior by changing cognition, and *cognitive-hyphen-behavioral treatments*, which work directly on both cognition and behavior. Adherents to Beck's traditional approach will pay primary attention to the correction of maladaptive schemata and beliefs. In contrast, Lewinsohn's approach to cognitive-behavioral therapy adds many complementary behavioral components such as relaxation training, direct instruction in social skills, and working on the client's schedule of pleasant activities (Reinecke and Ginsberg, 2008). Cognitive-hyphen-behavioral treatments for children often involve the parent in modifying the troubled child's environment or routine.

There is no doubt that cognitive-behavioral treatment of depression in childhood and adolescence is effective. Dozens of rigorous studies conducted with children and adolescents have been reviewed in a series of meta-analyses. The original meta-analyses appeared in the 1990s, and ended with the enthusiastic estimate of an effect size of about one standard deviation, meaning that there was, on the average, a difference between treatment and control groups of at least one standard deviation (Lewinsohn and Clarke, 1999; Reinecke, Ryan and Dubois, 1998). An effect of this statistical magnitude is considered large, indeed larger than most findings in the social sciences (Cohen, 1978). Another way of understanding this statistic is the binomial effect size display, a formula developed by Rosenthal (1991) to help explain the results of meta-analyses. According to that method, which is hypothetical (i.e., individual success rates are not calculated) it might be estimated that treatment is successful for 70–75 percent of the members of the treatment groups who received cognitive-behavioral therapy, whereas only 25–30 percent of the members of control groups would improve. Based on these very impressive data, many professionals began to consider cognitive-behavioral therapy as the preferred modality of treatment.

This is still true even though more recent studies have been based on increased expectations, leading to somewhat smaller effect size estimates in recent meta-analyses. Issues considered in more recent work include, especially, the long-term durability of the effects and, importantly, whether all of the participants were randomly assigned to the treatment or control groups. Applying very rigorous criteria to a meta-analysis, Weisz, McCarty and Valeri (2006) reported an average effect size of .34, much smaller than that indicated in previous meta-analytic reviews, but nevertheless significant and supportive of the efficacy of cognitive-behavioral therapy. Weisz, McCarty and Valeri also uncovered another substantial weakness in the studies they reviewed: Long-term outcome data were missing in many of the studies. The data from the few studies with long-term follow-up did not indicate effectiveness after, say, 1 year. This may be because, in most of the studies, there was no provision for seeing the client several months after the treatment was concluded for "booster" sessions, which is often recommended to maintain continuing effectiveness.

CASE STUDY: Lupita, challenged by depression and a troubled family

Jiménez Chafey, Bernal and Rosselló (2009) present a case study of a female adolescent in Puerto Rico who participated in psychotherapy for depression. At the time she came to the clinic, Lupita was living with both parents and a younger sibling. Although they remained together, Lupita's mother and father quarreled constantly and often separated for brief periods. Lupita's mother received regular care for depression and anxiety. Her father had been hospitalized for bipolar disorder. When she first came to the clinic, Lupita was attempting to transfer to a new school because of her low school marks and constant quarrels with her classmates. She cried often and felt sad. She always ate more than she should and had trouble sleeping. She felt irritable and anxious, and guilty because of the trouble she was bringing to her family.

Lupita participated in a twelve-session course of cognitive behavior therapy. During the first four sessions, the therapist focused on the influence of maladaptive thinking on Lupita's moods. Lupita learned strategies useful in "disputing" these thoughts when they came to her head. As homework, she completed a daily mood thermometer as well as a diary of positive and negative thoughts. The negative thoughts that Lupita needed to correct often pertained to being ugly, fat and overweight. Lupita also shared with her therapist her worries about not fitting in at her new school and not doing well there. She learned to challenge these negative expectations with language emphasizing the fact that the new school offered her a chance to start again with new teachers and new friends.

In sessions 5–8, the therapist concentrated on helping Lupita set specific goals for her life and move toward them. A time planner was added to her homework assignments. This middle phase of therapy included learning to stop thinking that she would make a fool of herself and was sure to be rejected by others. The final consolidation phase of therapy, covering sessions 9–12, was devoted to learning to communicate effectively with other people and to assert her wishes in an appropriate and effective way.

By the midpoint of her psychotherapy experience, Lupita's moods improved markedly. She even began to feel pretty at times. However, by the time the twelve sessions were finished, Lupita remained somewhat depressed. The perceptive therapist realized that not enough had been done to help Lupita deal with her family issues. In the back of her mind, Lupita always worried that her father would leave the home and perhaps divorce her mother. The therapist guided Lupita into realizing, first of all, that there was no clear evidence that her father in fact intended to leave. The therapist also helped Lupita to observe that many of her friends' parents were in fact divorced but they managed to adjust reasonably well to the divorce after an initial difficult period. At the end of therapy, the therapist strongly suggested to Lupita's mom that the parents seek marital counseling. After the additional four sessions, Lupita's symptoms abated considerably, to the point where she no longer met diagnostic criteria for major depression.

Jiménez Chafey, Bernal and Rosselló emphasize the cultural context of Lupita's difficulties. As discussed in Chapter 8 of this textbook, *familismo* is a core value of Latin American societies. They maintain that traditional manualized CBT may not be sufficient for Puerto Rican children because not enough attention is paid to the family situation. Therefore, they have added a standard, manualized family intervention to the CBT manual they use in Puerto Rico.

Other forms of psychotherapy

The established efficacy of cognitive-behavior therapy derives in part from the fact that its proponents are empirically oriented and have conducted many well-designed studies of its effects. Other forms of therapy are beginning to receive greater attention in both practice and evaluative research. Spielmans, Pasek and McFall (2007) published the best review of high-quality controlled studies in which different forms of therapy were implemented with depressed children and youth. Their review is based on twenty-three studies of "bona fide therapy" (i.e., therapy based on an established theoretical model and established, documented methods) and twelve studies on placebo attention groups (i.e., where the participants received the same amount of therapist attention but the group leader did not conduct therapy but perhaps engaged in general discussion. Bona fide therapies (CBT, interpersonal, parent training, behavior therapy, social skills training) were much more effective than the placebo groups. The review

indicates only *one* systematic comparison between CBT and another bona fide therapy (interpersonal); both were effective and the difference was not significant. Interpersonal psychotherapy, like cognitive-behavioral therapy, is a time-limited, focused procedure. It focuses on the interpersonal relationships of the depressed individual at the time of the onset of a depressive episode (Mufson, Pollack et al., 2004). Thus, future research may well indicate that other forms of therapy are as effective as CBT. In any case, given the research showing the effectiveness of several forms of psychotherapy, it is important for clinicians to favor proven methods over unproven ones.

Pharmacotherapy

Since the 1950s, knowledge about the physiological processes implicated in mood disorder has been applied to the development of pharmacological interventions to help alleviate its symptoms. Like all other types of treatment, pharmacological treatment of depression was first developed for adults, then extended downward to see if the same drugs would be effective for children and adolescents. The effectiveness of psychotropic medication is typically evaluated using a rigorous research design known as the randomized clinical trial, which usually involves randomly assigning participants to receive either the medication or a placebo tablet. Ideally, the trial should be double-blind, meaning that neither the child taking the medication nor anyone who is rating changes in the child's behavior knows whether the child is receiving active medication or not. The randomized clinical trial must be conducted with a large enough sample to detect statistically any difference between active medication and placebo, both of which may well work. Special considerations apply when conducting randomized clinical trials with children. In some situations, it may be considered unethical to prescribe placebo medication to a child in need of care. On the other hand, it is important to know and understand the size of the placebo effect. Adolescents, and, even more so, children, are known to exhibit substantial responses to placebos, especially in the treatment of depression (Cohen, D. et al., 2008). Although the minds of children and adolescents are surely capable of the experience of melancholy, perhaps skepticism about medical treatments is not likely to emerge until later on in life, leading to high expectations for any treatment prescribed.

It is important to note that there are different families of psychotropic medications used to treat depression, each acting in different ways. Tricyclic antidepressants have been available since the 1950s; they work on two neurotransmitter systems, the noradrenergic and the serotonergic (Fombonne and Zinck, 2008). It has become evident that tricyclic antidepressants are less than optimal for children with major depression because their effectiveness rate tends not to be much higher than that of placebo tablets and because there are substantial side effects, including increased heart rate and blood pressure, vertigo and sedation, which have resulted in sudden deaths of a small number of children (Biederman, 1991; Fombonne and Zinck, 2008).

In the past 25 years, a family of more advanced "second generation" antidepressants known as selective serotonin reuptake inhibitors or SSRIs has largely replaced the "first generation." SSRIs work mainly by interfering with the transporter system that reuptakes serotonin from the synaptic cleft into the presynaptic neuron, reducing depression by increasing the levels of serotonin in the synapse. The complex formulations of SSRIs lead to other potentially beneficial but secondary physiological changes. Therefore, there may be individual differences in response to different drugs within the SSRI family. They also vary in terms of how quickly they take effect and how long their effectiveness lasts (Fombonne and Zinck, 2008; Stahl, 2000). The SSRI most used for child and adolescent depression is fluoxetine. The use of SSRIs to treat child and adolescent depression reached three million prescriptions in the United States by the year 2002 (Hampton, 2004). However, careful scrutiny of the results of randomized clinical trials led to the discovery that for some reason there is a small but significant increase (2%) in suicidal ideation in a small number of young people taking SSRIs. This led to warnings about SSRIs for young people in both the United States and the UK, with special caution against using SSRIs as the sole intervention. As a result, the practice decreased in both countries, as the data on suicidality undergo continued careful scrutiny and as new medications are being developed. In the United States, prescriptions for antidepressants to young people dropped by 58 percent. Referrals to physicians for child and adolescent decreased rapidly and, among those who were referred, three times as many received treatment(s) other than antidepressants compared with the period before the warnings (Libby et al., 2007). Perera et al. (2007) tracked the recommendations made in a South London mental health clinic for depressed children and adolescents from 2003 through 2006. The number of cases not receiving any psychological therapy while on medication dropped from 43 percent the year before the warning about suicidal ideation to 14 percent the

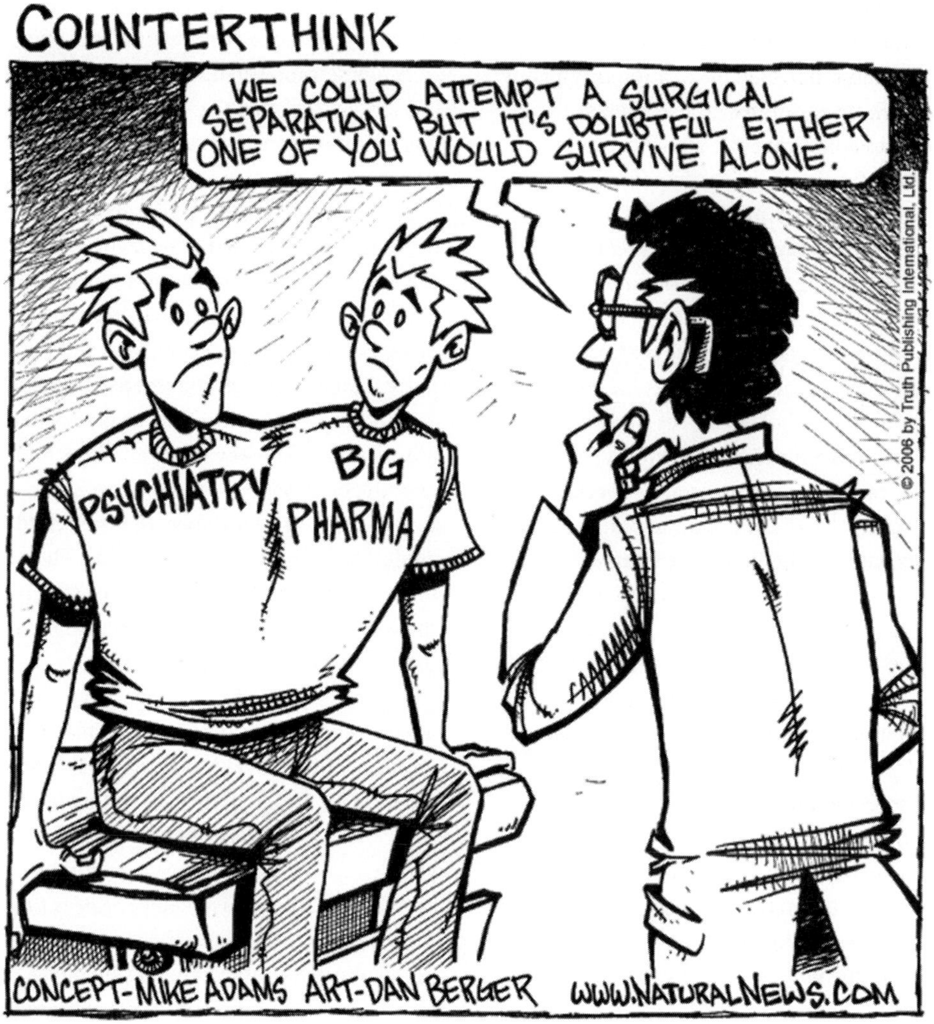

Figure 13.2 The use of medication to treat adolescent depression is controversial.

year after (although not to zero, as recommended in the national guidelines).

As with the other treatments, there are problems with assuming that children will react to medications in the same ways as adults do. As mentioned earlier, children and adolescents tend to respond substantially to placebo medications. As well, it is known that the bodies of children and adolescents may not respond physiologically to antidepressant drugs in the same ways as the bodies of adults do.

The limited data on these differences consist largely of data on differences between young and mature animals. The neurotransmitter systems of young people are not fully mature and may not function like those of adults until they are fully developed (Bylund and Reed, 2007).

Concerns about the undesirable side effects of conventional antidepressants have motivated some users to seek natural, homeopathic alternatives. The most widely used homeopathic medicine in the treatment of depression is St. John's wort, which is the most frequently prescribed medication for adolescent depression in Germany. St. John's wort may be somewhat helpful in the treatment of mild or moderate depression. However, there are only very limited data confirming its effectiveness and, natural though it is, problems do arise when it is taken at the same time as a number of other medications (Seelinger and Mannel, 2007).

Combining pharmacological interventions with psychotherapy

Interest in combining pharmacology and psychotherapy arose in part from concerns about the safety of SSRIs and other antidepressants. Furthermore, it may be unwise to maintain young people on medication for periods of several years; relapses may well occur when the medication is discontinued.

Research to evaluate a combination of two therapies that have each been proven effective must be designed carefully. Sample size must be large enough to detect the difference between the success of the combined treatment and its components. Of course, both long-term and short-term effects must be measured. It may be useful to include outcomes other than relapse, such as improvement in interpersonal functioning or academic performance. Because one of the possible benefits of combined treatments is that improvement may be generated with lower dosages of medication, dosage issues must receive attention. Timing is another issue because medication may work faster than psychotherapy. If psychotherapy is delayed until the medication has shown its effects, the child or parents may be poorly motivated to participate in psychotherapy, not realizing that it may prevent relapse down the road.

The best-known and most systematic study in which pharmacotherapy, cognitive-behavioral psychotherapy and their combination were compared with placebo medication is the Treatment for Depressed Adolescents (TADS) study, conducted in the United States with 327 young people 12 through 17 years old. The initial results, after 12 of the 36 weeks of treatment, indicated that the combined treatment was superior to medication alone, although the difference was not large (73 percent versus 62 percent). Unlike the results of many previous studies, cognitive-behavioral therapy was not significantly more effective than placebo. However, suicidal ideas were more common among participants treated with fluoxetine alone. Longer-term results differed considerably from the initial findings, indicating clear advantages for the combined group in terms of lower relapse rate, fewer suicidal thoughts and improved social and academic functioning. By the end of the 36-week treatment, the psychotherapy group demonstrated improvements similar to those of the other treatment conditions; the delayed effect may be because of time needed to fully implement the "menu" format used to individualize the psychotherapy (Curry, 2009; Kennard et al., 2009).

Implementing the combination treatment is a challenge in clinical care as well as research. It is easiest for physicians to prescribe medication; it is easiest for psychologists to conduct psychotherapy. Combining these therapies entails a level of coordination between professionals of different disciplines that is often elusive.

Prescriptive physical exercise

Depressed people withdraw from interpersonal contact and reduce their physical activity. Lack of exercise may be not only a result of depression, but also a partial cause or, at the least, a factor in sustaining the depressed state and making things worse. Therefore, physical exercise may also be a useful treatment. In a careful review of the research, Mead et al. (2008) conclude that prescriptive exercise is definitely superior to no treatment. Several studies also indicate that prescriptive exercise may be about as effective as short-term psychotherapy. There are many methodological problems with the studies on prescriptive exercise, including, most importantly, a lack of long-term follow-up. This may be particularly important in this case because many people, depressed or not, who do not exercise regularly are known to abandon their exercise regimens after their initial enthusiasm has waned. In addition, little is known about the possible benefits of combining prescriptive exercise with the other treatments discussed in this chapter.

Conclusions and future directions

Depression during childhood and adolescence has emerged in the past 30 years as both a very widespread and a very treatable condition. Given its prevalence, both primary and secondary prevention programs appear to be a cost-effective way of reducing the suffering it causes. Nevertheless, not every child at risk will improve because of preventive efforts alone. Therefore, it is important for mental health professionals to find ways of delivering effective and cost-effective treatments where diagnosable depressive conditions emerge. Societal efforts to remove the stigma from those who seek those treatments may literally save the lives of some young people.

Summary

- Only recently has the professional community recognized the existence of childhood depression, or, as early mental health practitioners called it, *melancholia*.
- The concept of masked depression is no longer used as frequently as it was before the requirements for objective criteria in diagnosis appeared in the DSM system. Masked depression is non-apparent depression that may show up as aggression, anti-social attitude, school refusal or body aches with no physical basis. These may be common among boys and men, and among certain groups such as African-Americans who are not encouraged to display negative feelings.
- Prevalence rates of depression appear to be rising, perhaps because of increased awareness of the problem. Concurrent prevalence rates (i.e., depression at a single point in time) range from 1 to 2 percent for children and 1 to 7 percent for adolescents. Cumulative prevalence rates (i.e., depression at least once in one's life up to the present moment) range from 1 percent and up for children under 9 and 4–24 percent for adolescents. Attention Deficit Hyperactivity Disorder (ADHD) and, especially, anxiety disorder are often comorbid with depression.
- Starting at puberty, girls appear to be more likely to have depression than boys. However this may be due to girls being more willing to discuss their depression while boys do not report it.
- Gender differences may result from increased dysphoric mood stemming from negative body image among girls. Other explanations include the fact that girls are required to become increasingly self-denying and deferent at the onset of puberty, and may experience high levels of anxiety at puberty.
- Girls are more prone to depression contagion, co-rumination and displeasing body images than are boys. These may be based on biological and hormonal changes affected by disruptions in serotonin levels, which lead to the depressive symptoms.
- Members of certain cultural groups may not report on their depression due to their group's self-reliance values (e.g., African-Americans or Latin-Americans) or due to a cultural fear of bringing shame to the family (e.g., Chinese-Americans).
- MRI and fMRI technology has allowed scientists to discover that depressed children have smaller frontal lobe volumes than non-depressed children. The frontal lobe is involved in directing behavior based on emotion and on goal-planning.
- Poor functioning of the amygdala, left parietal lobe, anterior thalamus and right

caudate nucleus, as well as increased levels of serotonin and cortisol, have been implicated in depression.

- Consistently elevated cortisol levels (signifying high hypothalamic-pituitary-adrenal or HPA activity) are a meaningful predictor of subsequent depression.

- Depressed children and youths are dexamethasone-resistant, meaning that they are resistant to the chemicals meant to suppress HPA activity. Therefore cortisol levels may be elevated in depressed children.

- The only evidence to show a link between autonomic nervous system (ANS) activity and depression pertains to depressed adults, who have weaker parasympathetic nervous system (PNS) control of heart activity than non-depressed adults.

- Infants, young children of depressed mothers and depressed adolescents also show weak PNS activity. Higher electrodermal (EDA) and pre-ejection period (PEP) reactivity signaling higher sympathetic nervous system (SNS) activity is associated with depression and poor adjustment symptoms in adolescents.

- Physiologically, depression may affect one's ability to regulate emotions in general or to respond appropriately during particularly stressful events. Physiological factors interact with environmental factors in the emergence of depression.

- Depression has a moderate heritable component. This vulnerability is thought to interact with environmental stressors to bring on depression. More twin studies than adoption studies have indicated a genetic basis for depression.

- Family adversity is another strong contributor to depression.

- In some cases, genetic predispositions to depression may only be activated when combined with environmental risk factors such as low socio-economic status (SES), single-parenthood or a mother's emotional distress and punitive disciplinary style.

- A child's shyness, behavioral inhibition, low self-esteem, neurotic personality and expression of negative emotion may be proximal personality features linked with depression. A mother may cause her child to be depressed, but the child may also make the mother more depressed, or both.

- Prenatal experience may interact with genetic contributions to depression.

- An insecure attachment between caregiver and infant may put the child at risk for developing depression.

- Research shows that depressed mothers harbor personal dissatisfaction and hostility, which can affect their relationships with their children.

- Parental depression accounts for only 8 percent of the variance in child depression in one meta-analysis. Fathers' depression has not been studied widely but the effect is smaller than those of maternal depression. Strong parental criticism and lack of warmth contribute to child depression more than parental overinvolvement.

- Negative parenting may interact with other factors leading to child depression including the child's inhibited temperament, stressful life events and low SES.

- The effects of controlling parents may be greater in children from cultures that do not place high value on filial piety.

- Girls may be more prone to depression following child abuse than boys, with both genders being more sensitive to stressors as the abuse continues over time.

- The effect of low SES and abuse may only have an effect where children have low monoamine oxidase A (MAOA) demonstrating the importance of studying the interactions of environmental and biological factors.

- Depressed children may depress other people they know, leading to a vicious cycle of dejection causing increased depression, causing further dejection, etc . . .

- Depressed children have little inclination to be helpful or supportive to their friends, resulting in having fewer of them, and in having friends who do not optimally enjoy activities with them.

- Being bullied or even being a bully has been linked with depression.
- The internet has been seen as exacerbating depression but also as a buffer against depression because it can help one overcome awkwardness and make more friends.
- Online psychotherapy for depression can be effective if used properly.
- Different but related theories of depression maintain that thoughts of hopelessness, as well as seeing negative events as permanent, global and characteristic of one's self, lead to depression (hopelessness theory).
- The personality theory of depression maintains that dependency, self-criticism and need for approval lead to depression. Mental schema theory states that maladaptive schemata (mental representations of oneself, or of events) lead to depression. Response-style theory avers that how one habitually responds to depressive symptoms affects the duration and intensity of the episode.
- Childhood depression often leads to adult depression. Suicide is the most severe consequence of depression.

- Prevention programs are often based on cognitive-behavioral theory. Primary prevention programs have been successful, with one meta-analysis reporting a moderate effect size for depressive outcomes.
- Other programs such as interpersonal therapy show immediate but not always long-term success.
- Cognitive-behavior therapy is to be distinguished from cognitive-hyphen-behavior therapy, which includes addressing maladaptive thoughts as well as changing behavior directly (e.g., via relaxation and social skills training) to help alleviate depression.
- The placebo effects of drugs prescribed for depression are large.
- Antidepressants include tricyclic antidepressants (not optimal for children), and SSRIs (with substantial individual differences in effectiveness). Pharmacological treatments have different effects on children than they do on adults and should thus be administered with caution. The Treatment for Depressed Adolescents (TADS) study showed that combining psychotherapy with pharmacology was superior to psychotherapy alone in the long term. Prescriptive physical activity is about as effective as short-term psychotherapy.

Study questions

1. Name several different reasons that can explain the difference between depression among girls and boys.
2. In what ways can the differences among the core features of different cultures relate to differences in the prevalence of major depression among members of the cultures?
3. What are some symptoms of depression that could very possibly be related to high levels of cortisol?
4. What are some reasons why mothers' depression might be more strongly related than fathers' depression to the depression of sons and daughters in intact families?
5. According to response-styles theory, what is a major way used by individuals experiencing depressed feelings to unwittingly make their depression worse?

14 Attention deficit/hyperactivity disorder

No other childhood disorder is as controversial as is Attention Deficit/Hyperactivity Disorder (ADHD). Some consider this condition an epidemic that is responsible for the underachievement at school and at work of a substantial segment of the population, whereas others regard it as a fabrication of the pharmaceutical industry. The "epidemic" is sometimes attributed to a mismatch between society's demands for focused attention and what some see as the inherent tendency of many children, especially boys, to wander and explore.

The first published medical report of attention deficit with hyperactivity did not appear until the beginning of the twentieth century. However, a poem written by German physician Heinrich Hoffman in 1844 appears to have been part of the collective memory of several generations of members of the medical profession from that point on (Thome and Jacobs, 2004):

"Let me see if Philip can
Be a little gentleman;
Let me see if he is able
To sit still for once at the table."
Thus Papa bade Phil behave;
And Mama looked very grave.
But Fidgety Phil,
He won't sit still;
He wriggles,
And giggles,
And then, I declare,
Swings backwards and forwards,
And tilts up his chair,
Just like any rocking horse–
"Philip! I am getting cross!"
See the naughty, restless child
Growing still more rude and wild,

Till his chair falls over quite.
Philip screams with all his might,
Catches at the cloth, but then
That makes matters worse again.
Down upon the ground they fall,
Glasses, plates, knives, forks and all.
How Mama did fret and frown,
When she saw them tumbling down!
And Papa made such a face!
Philip is in sad disgrace…

The poem goes on to describe horrific consequences, including capital punishment, for Philip's mischief (Thome and Jacobs, 2004). In the very early 1900s, such disorders as ADHD were considered "defects of moral control" (Still, 1902, cited by Mayes and Rafalovich, 2007).

Moral development issues are totally absent from contemporary thinking about ADHD. However, Philip's problems in sitting still remain one of the major features of the disorder as it is now conceptualized. The following brief section is devoted to the debate between those who consider excess movement the core symptom and the many who focus more extensively on inattention. A more heated controversy is mentioned next, namely whether the disorder exists at all or is being fabricated to suit the interests of drug companies and school authorities. Diagnostic criteria follow, together with consideration of a very typical feature – impairment of peer relations – which, although not a diagnostic criterion is a universal feature. Information about the prevalence of ADHD follows, emphasizing age, sex and cultural differences. A section on the possible causes and correlates of ADHD appears next before information about possible causes and typical consequences. The controversial issue of how to treat ADHD is the subject of the final section of the chapter.

A disorder of attention or a disorder of movement?

As currently conceived, the broad syndrome of ADHD is characterized in terms of observable behavior by inattention and/or hyperactivity (excessive movement). However, many authorities would prefer to define it in terms of the cognitive or neurological dysfunctions that are associated with it, such as the executive functions of the brain, which will be discussed later in this chapter (e.g., Brassett-Harknett and Butler, 2007; Swanson et al., 1998). The prevailing consensus is that ADHD cannot be defined on the basis of underlying cause or causes. That is mostly because the causes, which may be identifiable in *groups* of children already known to have ADHD, may not be identifiable in each individual case.

As will be discussed later, the current conception of ADHD involves subtypes distinguished by the relative strength of each of the primary symptoms, inattention and hyperactivity, in the behaviors of individual children. Hyperactivity and impulsive behavior were assigned greater emphasis in the years following the identification of the disorder as early as 1902 (Still, 1902, as cited by Rapport et al., 2009). A major conceptual shift occurred once the seminal Canadian research by Virginia Douglas in the 1970s demonstrated marked attention problems in many of the children who had been diagnosed as hyperactive (Douglas, 1972). Starting with DSM-III in 1980, attention problems moved to the forefront; excessive movement is no longer needed in order to diagnose ADHD. Some of the impetus for this may derive from the long tradition of studying the processes of attention in the discipline of psychology, dating back to the work of one of the founding fathers of the profession in the nineteenth century, William James,

who wrote an essay entitled *Stream of Thought* that contains reflections on the focusing of interest and attention (James, 1981)

Conceptual controversy: a real disorder or a fabrication of the drug companies?

Based on the higher rates of identification in North America than in most other countries (Timimi, 2005), some have argued that ADHD is a cultural product of the Western societies (Anderson, 1996; Timimi and Taylor, 2004). Societal pressures on parents result in competing demands to control unruly children but to limit the range of acceptable child-rearing methods that can be used to control maladaptive behavior. According to Timimi et al. (2002), this "cultural anxiety" has led to the deflection of the focus of attention away from societal problems to the individual child, fostering the popularity of the diagnostic category of ADHD and of psychostimulant medications far beyond the "true" need (see also Carey, 2002; DeGrandpre, 1999; Diller, 1998). Some have gone as far as to contend that the construct of ADHD is a fabrication of the pharmaceutical industry (Baughman, 2006). Needless to say, the unsubstantiated "cultural perspective" on ADHD is considered a misrepresentation of basic facts by the professional authors of an international consensus statement on ADHD (Barkley, 2004).

Diagnostic criteria

The debate about the best diagnostic criteria includes heated discussions about the age at which the condition should first be diagnosed. Probably the most important change in the DSM-5 criteria, summarized in Box 14.1, is increased recognition of the different manifestations of ADHD at different ages. The criteria mention that some sign should usually be evident by age 12, without restricting diagnosis to a particular age range.

Box 14.1 Differences between DSM-IV and DSM-5 criteria for attention deficit/hyperactivity disorder

- In both DSM-IV and DSM-5, the symptoms are divided into two categories: inattention and hyperactivity/impulsivity. The individual must display at least six of the symptoms in one of the categories for a minimum of 6 months. However, an individual might display various symptoms in both categories.
- Examples of inattention include failing to attend to details, having a hard time focusing and appearing to not listen. Examples of hyperactivity/impulsivity include being fidgety, restless and loud.
- In both DSM-IV and DSM-5, the symptoms must cause significant impairment.
- In DSM-IV, the symptoms must cause *impairment* in two or more settings. In DSM-5, however, the symptoms must be *apparent* in two or more settings.
- In DSM-IV, the symptoms must be present before the age of 7. In DSM-5, this age criterion has been raised to 12.
- In DSM-IV, three types are listed: "combined type," to be used if the inattention and hyperactivity/impulsivity criteria are satisfied for the past 6 months; "predominantly inattentive type," to be used if the inattention criterion is met, but the hyperactivity/impulsivity criterion has not been met for the past 6 months; and "predominantly hyperactive-impulsive type," to be used if the hyperactivity/impulsivity criterion is satisfied, but the inattention criterion has not been met for the past 6 months.
- In DSM-5, the current presentation (not type) must be specified. The three types listed in DSM-IV are retained as presentations in DSM-5.
- In DSM-5, additional specifiers have been added. The "in partial remission" specifier is to be applied if the full criteria are no longer met, yet the symptoms still result in impairment. The current severity must also be specified (i.e., mild, moderate or severe), based on number of symptoms and degree of impairment.

Source: DSM-5 and DSM-IV-TR consulted May 6, 2013.

This contrasts with the implication in DSM-IV that there is a single disorder that, if present, surely has to be evident by age 7 (Barkley, 2010). These changes mean that DSM-5 has opened the door for more children to be diagnosed with ADHD than ever before. Indeed, as discussed later in this chapter, there is increasing awareness, on the one hand, of adolescent and adult ADHD, as well as, on the other hand, of ADHD in preschoolers.

In fact, the American Academy of Pediatrics revised its practice guidelines in October 2011 to allow for the use of medication in the treatment of hyperactive preschoolers as young as 4 years (http://pediatrics.aappublications.org/content/early/2011/10/14/peds.2011-2654.full.pdf). The nomenclature "hyperkinetic disorder" is used in ICD-10, as detailed in Box 14.2. However, over time, the DSM and ICD criteria are becoming

Box 14.2 | ICD-10 Diagnostic criteria for hyperkinetic disorders

A. Demonstrable abnormality of attention, activity and impulsivity at home, for the age and developmental level of the child, as evidenced by 1, 2 and 3:
1. at least three of the following attention problems:
   a. short duration of spontaneous activities;
   b. often leaving play activities unfinished;
   c. overfrequent changes between activities.
   d. undue lack of persistence at tasks set by adults;
   e. unduly high distractibility during study, e.g., homework or reading assignment;
2. plus at least three of the following activity problems:
   a. very often runs about or climbs excessively in situations where it is inappropriate; seems unable to remain still;
   b. markedly excessive fidgeting and wriggling during spontaneous activities;
   c. markedly excessive activity in situations expecting relative stillness (e.g., mealtimes, travel, visiting, church);
   d. often leaves seat in classroom or other situations when remaining seated is expected;
   e. often has difficulty playing quietly;
3. plus at least one of the following impulsivity problems:
   a. often has difficulty awaiting turns in games or group situations;
   b. often interrupts or intrudes on others (e.g., butts in to others' conversations or games).
   c. often blurts out answers to questions before questions have been completed.
B. Demonstrable abnormality of attention and activity at school or nursery (if applicable), for the age and developmental level of the child, as evidenced by both 1 and 2:
1. at least two of the following attention problems:
   a. undue lack of persistence at tasks;
   b. unduly high distractibility, i.e., often orienting toward extrinsic stimuli;
   c. overfrequent changes between activities when choice is allowed;
   d. excessively short duration of play activities.
2. and by at least three of the following activity problems:
   a. continuous (or almost continuous) and excessive motor restlessness (running, jumping, etc.) in situations allowing free activity;
   b. markedly excessive fidgeting and wriggling in structured situations;
   c. excessive levels of off-task activity during tasks;
   d. unduly often out of seat when required to be sitting;
   e. often has difficulty playing quietly.

C. Directly observed abnormality of attention or activity. This must be excessive for the child's age and developmental level. The evidence may be any of the following:
   1. direct observation of the criteria in A or B above, i.e., not solely the report of parent or teacher;
   2. observation of abnormal levels of motor activity, or off-task behavior or lack of persistence in activities, in a setting outside home or school (e.g., clinic or laboratory);
   3. significant impairment of performance on psychometric tests of attention.
D. Does not meet criteria for pervasive developmental disorder, mania, depressive or anxiety disorder.
E. Onset before age of 7 years.
F. Duration of at least 6 months.
G. IQ above 50.

Source: World Health Organization (1993). *The ICD-10 Classification of Mental and Behavioral Disorders: Diagnostic Criteria for Research*. Geneva, WHO.

more similar, as is the case for most disorders (see Chapter 3).

Is ADHD really a single disorder?

Many experts believe that ADHD consists of more than a single disorder. DSM-5 identifies different presentations of ADHD, retreating from the previous DSM-IV position that there are different subtypes. Nigg (2006) offers useful medical analogies to describe the relationship of the various manifestations or subtypes of ADHD to the main disorder. He suggests that inattention or hyperactivity are the final symptoms of some underlying condition; thus, they are analogous to the current medical understanding of a fever. Regarding the underlying disease entity, there are many different forms of cancer that bear some general resemblance to each other but differ markedly in their causes, the bodily functions they disrupt and their seriousness; the various forms of ADHD are similar in many ways.

Among the many controversies pertaining to ADHD is the lingering doubt that the condition as currently delineated is really one single disorder. The delineation of different presentations in DSM-5 implies, of course: (1) that different people demonstrate different clusters of symptoms but (2) that the subtypes nonetheless are part of a single disease entity. Several alternative propositions are, however, very tenable. From a developmental perspective, many individuals are hyperactive early in life but demonstrate mostly symptoms of impulsivity by the time they reach adolescence; most school-aged children diagnosed as ADHD display both types of problem behaviors. Thus, what are now considered different forms or presentations of ADHD might in fact be representations of developmental stages within many if not most individuals. On the other hand, if the presentations really differentiate individuals, it may not necessarily make sense to consider them parts of the same disorder.

There is even some evidence that the different underlying symptoms and presentations may differ in the ways they are affected by genetics. In an influential meta-analysis of twin and adoption studies, Nikolas and Burt (2010) found that both inattention and hyperactivity were highly heritable, with genetic factors accounting for a hefty 71 percent of the variance in inattention and 73 percent of the variance in hyperactivity. The genetic effects on symptoms of hyperactivity appear to be *additive*. In other words, the degree to which a child demonstrates hyperactivity depends on the sum of genetic influences from both biological parents across genetic loci. This is analogous to physical height: How tall a child grows is a function of the sum of genetic markers for tallness inherited from the child's mother and father. In contrast, inattention seems to reflect the interaction rather than the sum of the genetic markers, just as the color of an offspring's eyes depends on the interaction of the eye-color alleles passed on by each parent, some being dominant over others, and not on the total number of eye-color alleles the child receives.

Impaired peer relations as a marker of ADHD

The diagnostic criteria fail to convey very fully how constant the troublesome interactions between children with ADHD and those around them are. Pelham and Fabiano (2008) estimate that children with ADHD have one negative interaction per minute with their parents (from data reported by Danforth et al., 2006), two negative exchanges per minute with teachers or peers at school (based on data reported by Abikoff et al., 1993), plus 0.7 per minute with peers outside of school (based on Pelham and Bender, 1982). Added together, this makes well over a million negative interpersonal interactions per year, not counting sleep time!

CASE STUDY: Sally, whose relations with family members and peers are impaired by ADHD

The case of Sally, described by Schwartzberg (2000), illustrates some of these negative peer interactions and their consequences. Schwartzberg begins the case study with a description of a typical interaction between Sally and her father. When Michael Howard came home from work he found his 7-year-old daughter Sally and her friend riding their bikes full speed around the driveway. Sally bounded over to Michael and energetically greeted him by leaping into his arms. She then pulled away from her father and ran wide circles around the driveway loudly ordering her friend to get off her bike. While inside the house, Michael heard a screaming match erupt between the two young girls before Sally's friend finally stormed off. Before Michael could mention the incident to his wife Karen, Sally flew into the kitchen, clambered up onto the counter and just as quickly tumbled down to the floor in a shower of coupons and receipts. Later during dinner, Sally threw a temper tantrum after her mother refused her requests for chocolate milk. After several minutes of screaming and crying Michael gave in and poured a glass of chocolate milk in an attempt to calm Sally down, but the tantrum was already in full swing and lasted until Sally finally fell asleep for the night. Both parents were exhausted, and Karen particularly irritated with what she saw as Michael yet again undermining her authority and giving in too easily to Sally's demands.

Michael and Karen were also very concerned about a letter that arrived earlier that week from Sally's teacher requesting a meeting to discuss their daughter's behavior and academic problems.

They had been receiving similar notes since Sally started preschool. Even as early as infancy, Sally seemed irritable and difficult to soothe. Sally's parents felt that, compared to her peers, she required more extreme discipline measures, was more accident-prone and a poor judge of her own limitations. When Michael and Karen met with Sally's teacher, she described Sally's classroom-specific problem behaviors: "She jumps out of her seat and runs to the window to look at anything that catches her eye . . . she blurts out answers for other children or before she hears the whole question . . . she's frequently talking when she should be working and that just disrupts the entire class . . . she acts very bossy with other children . . . " The teacher recommended a psychological evaluation to identify any underlying problems. She also stressed the negative long-term effects that Sally's academic and social failures could have on her self-esteem. Michael and Karen agreed to a referral to the school psychologist.

The school psychologist took a multimodal approach to Sally's evaluation, gathering information from several sources and contexts and using a selection of measures before reaching a conclusion. A rating scale was completed by Sally's parents and teacher to compare her behavior at school and home to established norms. Sally's behavior was also directly observed by the psychologist in the classroom and during individual sessions. Sally completed a battery of psychological tests to measure intellect, academic achievement and emotional and psychological functioning. Collateral information was also obtained about Sally's behavior from her grandparents and her medical history from her pediatrician. All information confirmed the diagnosis of ADHD.

Sally's treatment involved three components. First she was placed on a trial run of methylphenidate. After a month of no noticeable progress the dosage was increased and her behavior in the classroom and during interactions with peers gradually improved. Sally herself remarked that she found it easier to concentrate on homework and play sports when on the medication. Second, a classroom-based intervention was developed which involved moving Sally's desk away from distracting stimuli, clearly posting and reviewing the daily schedule and classroom rules and preparing for transition periods with a gentle warning. A token system was also implemented which reduced the incidence of Sally's disruptive behavior in the classroom. Finally, Sally's parents received training on ADHD-management strategies which emphasized the importance of consistency and predictability within the home. As Michael and Karen's confidence in their parenting skills grew and Sally's behavior continued to improve, positive interactions became more frequent in their household and the family began to enjoy each other's company.

Studies have shown without exception that peers dislike children with ADHD (see review by Mrug, Hoza and Gerdes, 2001). Laboratory studies have shown that it takes no more than 30 seconds and a few quick social interactions for other children to reject a peer with ADHD as a prospective friend or companion. Other children find them disruptive, unpleasant and socially unskilled (e.g., Milich and Landau, 1982). An intensive longitudinal study of the friendships of children with ADHD, featuring direct observation of the interactions of the friends, revealed that children with ADHD tend to be insensitive to the wishes of their friends and may compromise their friendships by breaking the rules of games they enjoy (Normand et al., 2011).

CASE STUDY: Jeff, a boy with ADHD and learning disabilities adjusting to a new blended family

Jeff, age 13, was brought to the psychologist (Barry Schneider, author of this textbook) by his parents, who were alarmed about the low grades on his report card from the prominent private school he attended. Jeff's family had moved extensively since he started school due to Jeff's father's career as a foreign-relations officer with the government. During his preschool years, Jeff attended a very child-centered preschool with a very favorable staff–student ratio. Jeff reportedly thrived in that environment in which he was encouraged to interact with play materials and use them in highly creative ways. The family's first overseas posting occurred soon after Jeff started formal schooling. At the small international school he attended, Jeff managed to keep up with his classmates, although his mathematics grades were always weaker than his marks in other subjects. Jeff has always been an outstanding athlete, excelling especially in basketball and volleyball. Socially, he has always had a wide circle of friends, many of whom participate in sports with him. Recently, however, a subtle pattern of behavior problems has emerged. Jeff's younger brother, Robert, reported to their Mom that Jeff had been bullying and teasing several of the younger, weaker pupils at his school. His math teacher suspected Jeff of cheating on an exam. Jeff forged his mother's signature on several letters from the school concerning his effort, achievement and behavior.

Recently, there have been many problems in Jeff's parents' marriage. The parents argue constantly whenever they are together and by phone. Jeff's mother constantly reproaches his father for leaving her alone with four children for months at a time. Jeff has always been closer to his father than to his mother. His mother has begun to have difficulty getting Jeff to comply with her instructions at home. Until the current year, Jeff's academic marks were generally average at best. However, in their ratings of Jeff's behavior, some of the teachers remarked that Jeff was often daydreaming.

After interviewing the family and gathering comprehensive information about Jeff's developmental, school and family history, the psychologist began his contacts with Jeff with some informal conversation and picture drawing in order to establish rapport. Jeff was fully cooperative and friendly. He answered all questions readily although without much elaboration. The psychologist then asked Jeff to write paragraphs about the best and worst days of his life. His best day was a day at the beach alone with his father. His worst day was when his mother left the house briefly after a family fight. The psychologist noted that Jeff's handwriting was a bit immature and that his writing was full of grammar, punctuation and spelling problems. The content was clear but Jeff elaborated little about the two events and did not indicate any emotional reaction to them.

The psychologist continued with a standard battery of IQ and achievement tests. Results indicated average intelligence overall but some weakness in short-term memory. Jeff's achievement scores were very variable. Jeff often missed the right answer in mathematics problems by only digits. Jeff's scores in reading words and passages were quite high but he did poorly in spelling, mathematics and written expression, with scores 1 to 3 years below the average for pupils at his level.

The psychologist's assessment included standardized rating scales completed by both parents and by several of Jeff's teachers, using the Conners-3 scales. In both the parent and teacher ratings, the highest scores (meaning more problems) were on the Inattention scale. On that scale, Jeff's scores were well in the clinical range, in the top 1 percent of scores usually obtained about children his age. Somewhat lower scores, at just about the boundary of the clinical range, were evident in the teacher ratings for Learning Problems as well. The psychologist concluded from all information available that Jeff's outgoing ways and athletic prowess had concealed an underlying attention deficit. The fact that he was inattentive but not hyperactive made this problem even more difficult to detect. As with many children who have attention problems, Jeff was also displaying learning and behavior problems.

The psychologist's first step in helping Jeff and his family was *psychoeducation* – explaining the nature of these conditions. The psychologist met with the school to provide suggestions about handling bullying. He was also able to set up a "daily report card" in which the teachers quickly provided feedback each day to Jeff's mother on his effort and behavior; Jeff could earn special privileges for cooperating. At his mother's insistence, Jeff was not referred to a psychiatrist for an opinion on the need for psychostimulant medication. Three months later, however, Jeff's father persuaded his mother to do this. Jeff did well on the medication. He also benefited from training in study skills. The psychologist advised Jeff's parents on how to manage his behavior consistently and positively. He also referred the parents for marriage counseling. Jeff's schoolwork improved and there were no further reports of bullying or sneaky behavior.

Prevalence

In estimating the prevalence of ADHD, it is imperative to discount prevalence estimates that are based exclusively on ratings by a single informant. Relying solely on teacher ratings or solely on parent ratings could lead to the shocking conclusion that as many as one child in five or six has ADHD (e.g., Gadow et al., 2000; Nigg, 2006; Nolan, Gadow and Sprafkin, 2001; Wolraich et al., 1996). Fortunately, much lower prevalence rates emerge when the full diagnostic criteria are used, including the provision that the disorder must in fact interfere with some aspect of the child's functioning (Gordon et al., 2005). The DSM-IV (American Psychiatric Association, 2000, p. 90) indicated the typical prevalence rate, based obviously on DSM-IV diagnostic criteria, as 3–7 percent of school-age children. That prevalence rate is consistent with most other reputable estimates

(e.g., Scahill and Schwab-Stone, 2000). Data are not yet available on prevalence rates calculated with DSM-5 criteria. However, the more liberal criteria suggest that the rates will be higher.

Many adults remember their school days as a time when no children were diagnosed as having ADHD, leading logically to the question of whether the disorder itself is actually increasing in frequency. Unfortunately, any increase across time is virtually impossible to document scientifically, in part because awareness of the disorder, which has surely increased, increases the likelihood of its being diagnosed. However, it is not inconceivable that there has been some kind of change in the school environment that has resulted in an increasing mismatch between its demands and the capabilities of a specific group of children to focus their attention. Furthermore, the possibility that there has been an increase in some form of environmental contaminant or some change in the typical child's diet cannot be ruled out (Nigg, 2006).

The statistics on the prevalence of ADHD include the vast majority of children who have not only ADHD but also some other debilitating comorbid disorder. It comes as no surprise that many children with ADHD are also aggressive and defiant; 30–50 percent also meet the diagnostic criteria for oppositional defiant disorder or conduct disorder. It is typically reported that at least a third of children diagnosed as having ADHD are also suffering from major depression; comorbidity with anxiety disorders is also substantial. At least one-fourth of children with ADHD display concurrent dyslexia or learning disorders using very conservative diagnostic criteria for the diagnosis of the learning problems; other estimates would suggest that the majority of children with ADHD experience substantial academic problems (Spencer, Biederman and Mick, 2007). Many children with intellectual disabilities have attention problems. A recent study by Neece et al. (2013) indicates that it is probably useful and valid for researchers and clinicians to be more sensitive to the comorbidity of ADHD and intellectual disability.

ADHD as a lifelong debilitating condition

It was once believed that ADHD is a disorder that affects only school-age children. However, it is now known that ADHD can affect people throughout the lifespan: At least 70 percent of children with ADHD continue to display symptoms of the disorder as adolescents (August, Braswell and Thura, 1998; Barkley et al., 1990; Brassett-Harknett and Butler, 2007). This does not mean, however, that they display exactly the same symptoms: Hyperactivity tends to decline with maturity whereas problems of inattention tend to persist (e.g., Hart et al., 1995). In a comprehensive, longitudinal analysis, Langberg, Epstein, Altaye et al. (2008) reported a decline coinciding with the onset of adolescence in the major core symptoms of ADHD: inattention, hyperactivity and impulsivity, according to both parent and teacher ratings. However, many of the behavior

problems associated with childhood ADHD continue into adolescence, especially conduct problems, juvenile delinquency and substance abuse (e.g., Barkley et al., 1990; Molina and Pelham, 2003). In a recently reported longitudinal study, Kuriyan et al. (2013) traced a long-term link between the diagnosis of ADHD during school years and subsequent difficulty finding and maintaining employment. The risk was even higher for people who presented disciplinary problems in school in addition to the diagnosis of ADHD.

ADHD: a boys' disorder?

The overwhelming majority of children (at least two-thirds; Biederman, 2005; Brassett-Harknett and Butler, 2007) referred for treatment because of inattention or hyperactivity are boys. The reasons for these sex differences are the subject of heated controversy. The sociological literature contains some scathing diatribes against the diagnosis of ADHD, which the authors see as societal repression of the natural temperaments of boys and men. The most scornful is probably a chapter in a 2006 anthology by Rosenfeld and Faircloth about various aspects of what they call the medicalization of men's bodies. Hart, Grand and Riley (2006) maintain that the construct of ADHD is an expression of middle-class anxiety about the socialization of boys in the face of the demands for docility in schools and in the workplace. Reflecting on the escalating rates of boys in the United States being diagnosed with ADHD, psychiatrist and anthropologist Melvin Konner commented in a 1994 *New York Times* article that Tom Sawyer and Huckleberry Finn would today be diagnosed as having ADHD and treated with psychostimulant medication. The columnist concluded with the contention that "now, if a guy cannot at the very least manage to finish college, the surging, indifferent Mississippi of the world's economy is likely to take his little raft and break it into bits" (Angier, 1994).

Many articles in the popular press emphasize differences between boys' and girls' brains and the effects of these differences on learning and school behavior. There is only limited and somewhat inconsistent research evidence of such differences. Several researchers have found differences between girls and boys with ADHD in the size of the splenum of the corpus callossum, which facilitates communication between the left and right hemispheres of the brain (Hutchinson, Mathias and Banich, 2008; Valera et al., 2006). There is preliminary evidence of sex differences in the EEG (electroencephalogram) patterns of boys and girls with ADHD (Barry et al., 2006). An initial investigation using proton magnetic resonance spectroscopy, a non-invasive modern neuroimaging technique, to explore the right frontal lobes of children with and without ADHD, suggested sex differences that may be very important. Nevertheless, these potentially consequential sex differences in brain structure do not appear to result in any difference between the executive functions of boys and girls with ADHD (Rucklidge, 2006; Seidman et al., 2005; Weyandt, 2005).

Although many more boys are diagnosed with ADHD than girls, it has become clear that ADHD among girls has long-lasting and profound consequences. In the first longitudinal study in which girls with ADHD and a suitable control group were followed into adulthood, Biederman et al. (2010) worked with ninety-six girls with ADHD and sixty-one girls without the disorder, all between 6 and 18 years at the start of the disorder. Eleven years later, the girls with ADHD were far more likely than the controls to display a variety of negative mental health problems, including depression, anxiety, eating disorder, substance abuse and anti-social behavior. Using multiple methods, including teacher ratings, direct observation of classroom behavior and standardized tests of academic achievement, Dupaul et al. (2006) found that US girls with ADHD were at least as likely as boys with ADHD to experience marked problems at school. Adolescent girls with ADHD are *more* likely than their male counterparts to experience comorbid depression and anxiety (Lahey et al., 2007). Similarly, in a large-scale Canadian study, adolescent girls with

ADHD were found to have higher rates of comorbid anxiety and depression; in that study, boys tended to display higher rates of comorbid aggression (Romano et al., 2005).

ADHD: An artifact of Western culture?

The extent of cross-national and cross-cultural variation in ADHD is not clear. Most epidemiological studies and large intervention studies on ADHD have been conducted in North America, leading some researchers to question the generalizability and the meaningfulness of these studies for non-North American settings. Systematic reviews (Faraone et al., 2003; Polanczyk et al., 2007; Skounti, Philalithis and Galanakis, 2007) also confirm wide variations in the estimates of the prevalence of ADHD among children and adolescents in different countries. These estimates range from 0.9 to 20 percent. The discrepancies have led some authors to speculate about different reasons for such apparently divergent findings. Large-scale multisite cross-cultural studies confirm that when a uniform set of rigorous, standardized diagnostic criteria is used by skilled clinicians across clinics in Africa, Australia, Europe and North America, ADHD prevalence rates are very similar (Buitelaar et al., 2006; Polanczyk et al., 2007).

Working in Cuba, where medical knowledge is high but where medication for ADHD is very scarce, Schneider et al. (2011) found that ADHD was indeed diagnosed, although perhaps not as often as in countries where the diagnosis leads to specific treatment. Cuban children with ADHD were more likely to be referred for psychiatric help – the only way of receiving medication – if they also displayed comorbid behavior problems and came from families under stress. Taken together, all evidence indicates that ADHD diagnostic criteria identify a similar frequency of an underlying construct in different locations, independent of local judgments. Nevertheless, even if cultures do not vary in the prevalence of ADHD, they still can vary in terms of their tolerance for inattention and hyperactivity and in the social sanctions inflicted on children with the disorder (Rohde et al., 2005).

Stability and prognosis

The World Health Organization World Mental Health Survey initiative (Lara et al., 2009) was designed to determine the continuity of ADHD from childhood to adulthood in ten countries. This influential study involved a total of 43,772 participants from ten countries, including seven developed countries (United States, Belgium, France, Germany, Italy, Netherlands and Spain) and three developing countries (Colombia, Lebanon and Mexico). Averaged across countries, 50 percent of the childhood cases of ADHD were found to meet full criteria for ADHD in adulthood; the stability rate ranged from 33 to 84 percent across the countries.

This sobering picture of the stability of ADHD over the lifespan is compounded by parallel data illustrating the impact of the disorder on functioning in adolescence and adulthood. Barkley and colleagues (2006) followed a group of young adults in Wisconsin who had been rigorously diagnosed as hyperactive 13 years prior to the follow-up; the researchers also followed an undiagnosed community control group for the same period. Members of the hyperactive group discontinued their schooling at an earlier age than did the controls, often without completing their school programs to graduation. They also had poorer school results and repeated school years more often. The hyperactive group had fewer friends than did the controls and reported lower self-esteem. Because many of the control-group participants were in university at the time of follow-up, a greater proportion of the hyperactive children were working. However, they were dismissed from jobs more frequently than were the control participants and received lower performance evaluations by their employers. In another 10-year follow-up study, Biederman, Monuteaux and their colleagues (2006) examined the lifetime prevalence of major mental health problems among young adults with chronic ADHD. ADHD subjects had significantly higher rates than their non-diagnosed counterparts of anxiety disorders, several types of phobia, major depression, bipolar disorder and alcohol and drug dependence.

Probable causes and concurrent impairment

Throughout the century-long history of ADHD, leaders in research on ADHD have argued vehemently for better recognition of its biological roots and the other disorders that often occur with it. Efforts for the recognition of the role of the brain in mental health have been described as a crusade against "brainlessness" (Eisenberg, 1986, 2007). Eisenberg, an influential Harvard psychiatrist in the field for over 50 years until his death in 2009, noted that the idea of neuropsychological origin appealed to many parents who believed that the diagnosis *proved* that they were not responsible for their children's many problems. Most scientists today concur with the view that ADHD is predominantly caused by neuropsychological factors although, as scientists, they still experience difficulty regarding the available evidence as conclusive proof. The most difficult notion to accept is the inference of brain damage without any clear evidence, at least in the individual case, of damage to the brain (Eisenberg, 2007; Taylor, 2009). This may change over time with the ongoing improvement of techniques for the direct examination of brain-wave patterns. One method using electroencephalogram (EEG) technology was introduced in the United States in 2013 (Leichti et al., 2013) but many experts remain skeptical about the value of this diagnostic procedure.

Many theories have emerged over the years about how children with ADHD come to have their damaged, dysfunctional or different brains. Neurologists Strauss and Werner (1942) proposed that congenital brain damage could be inferred from behavioral symptoms. Some contemporaries shied away from the implications of the term "brain damage" by substituting the term "brain dysfunction," thereby not implying that any damage had actually occurred. Backing off a bit further, many writers added the adjective "minimal," implying, perhaps, that the damage is so small that it cannot be detected. The terms *minimal brain damage*, *minimal brain dysfunction*, *minimal cerebral damage* and *minimal cerebral dysfunction* were used widely in the 1950s and 1960s, over the objections of critics who already knew that there was no clear scientific validity for the idea (Birch, 1964; Eisenberg, 2007). Reflecting on this development, Eisenberg (1986) observed that psychiatry had drifted from brainlessness to mindlessness.

Although evidence of many neurological deficits among children with ADHD has accumulated, some emerging facts have diminished somewhat the fervor that accompanied the earlier quest for a single overarching neurological explanation of ADHD. Most important is the recognition that the behaviors corresponding to atypical brain structure or atypical brain function are highly variable, making it impossible to diagnose brain damage in any meaningful way from observable behavior (Taylor, 2009).

Nigg (2006) argues that it is highly unlikely that a single pathway accounts for ADHD in all its forms but that different causal paths may eventually be identified for different manifestations of ADHD. This means not only that the different subtypes of ADHD may have different causes (see section "Is ADHD really a single disorder?"), but also that the causes of a child's problem may depend on the comorbid conditions that accompany his or her attention deficit disorder – whether, for instance, the individual also has an anxiety disorder, oppositional defiant disorder, etc. (Castellanos and Tannock, 2002; Nigg, 2006; Nigg, Goldsmith and Sachek, 2004). As shown in Table 14.1, it is possible to trace different pathways from different types of child temperament to ADHD and to delineate the developmental stages that are most relevant to these pathways.

Neurobiological characteristics of ADHD[1]

Much of the work on ADHD has focused on understanding ADHD in relation to specific cognitive and behavioral processes including response inhibition, working memory and different types of attention processes (e.g., sustained attention, selective attention, executive attention) (Durston, 2008; Epstein et al., 2009). A deficit in response inhibition, or a weak ability to deliberately respond to a non-target stimulus and not respond to a target stimulus, is one of the most robust and consistent findings across children, adolescents and adults with ADHD (Willcutt et al., 2005).

Brain regions engaged during response inhibition tasks include prefrontal regions, such as the dorsolateral prefrontal cortex (DLPFC). In general, children and adolescents (and adults) with ADHD show less frontal lobe activation than individuals without ADHD; this pattern of reduced activation emerges across the orbital, inferior, middle and superior frontal areas. The hypothesis underlying this relatively consistent finding is that input from frontal regions is required in order to control inhibitions (Garavan et al., 2002), and the reduced input associated with ADHD results in their undercontrolled behaviors. Youths and adults with ADHD also consistently show reduced activation of the caudate region of the striatum during response inhibition tasks (Durston et al., 2006; Epstein et al., 2007; Pliszka et al., 2006; Rubia et al., 1999; Vaidya et al., 1998). Based on these findings, researchers have concluded that the fronto-striatal network is under-recruited in ADHD patients during response inhibition or suppression of a prepotent tendency (Booth et al., 2005; Durston et al., 2006; Pliszka et al., 2006), and that this pattern does not seem to vary by age (Epstein et al., 2007).

Children with ADHD also show working memory deficits relative to healthy control children (Willcutt et al., 2005). To date, neuroimaging studies of

[1] Section written by Paul Hastings and Amanda Guyer.

Table 14.1 **Nigg's model of temperament, development and clinical presentation of ADHD**

ADHD pathway	Key develop-mental period	Developmental sequence and speculative temperamental precursors	Clinical presentation
1. Primary ADHD with secondary Conduct Disorder (CD)	Toddlerhood/preschool	Weak regulatory control at 1–2 years; secondary breakdown in ability to dampen negative affect; disrupted socialization a key moderator	Impaired executive functioning; mild deficits in affect regulation; secondary ODD or CD in some cases
2. Primary ADHD with little or no comorbidity	Infancy	Extreme positive approach at 6–18 months, with permissive socialization	"Normal" neuropsychological profile; little or no clinical comorbidity; altered delay–reward gradient
3. Secondary ADHD with primary socialized CD	Infancy	Extreme negative approach at 6–12 months disrupts later regulation development; thus secondary executive deficits	Mild executive function deficits; notable hostility and poor affect regulation; ODD, then CD
4. Secondary ADHD with primary unsocialized CD	Infancy	Extreme low anxiety (low negative withdrawal) disrupts later consolidation of regulation	Low arousal, low heart rate; aggressive conduct problems; risk for later psychopathology
5. Primary ADHD with anxiety	Infancy/toddlerhood	Weak regulatory control at 1–2 years, with low hostility but high negative withdrawal (anxiety)	Executive deficits, with notable anxiety or anxiety disorder
6. Primary or secondary ADHD	Infancy	Cognitive regulation is disrupted in relation to high anxiety/intrusive thoughts; high scores on anxiety	Inattentive on CPT but OK on executive tasks; high anxiety, maybe "anxious impulsivity"; overarousal

Source: Nigg, J. T., Goldsmith, H. H. and Sachek, J. (2004). Temperament and attention deficit hyperactivity disorder: The development of a multiple pathway model. *Journal of Clinical Child and Adolescent Psychology*, *33*, 49. Reprinted by permission of the publisher (Taylor & Francis Group, www.informaworld.com).

working memory and ADHD have been conducted only in adult samples. In a PET imaging study, adults with ADHD show less activation in frontal, temporal and occipital areas (Schweitzer et al., 2004) and greater activation in midbrain, striatal, cerebellum and middle frontal gyrus during these kinds of working memory tasks.

With regard to attention, several kinds of tasks have been used to see how the brain responds during different attention processes in individuals with ADHD. Effective control of attention during performance on attention tasks is supported by neural input from the prefrontal and parietal cortices. Neuroimaging studies indicate an overall pattern of underactivation of the fronto-parietal-striatal regions in individuals with ADHD when performing attention tasks (Bush, Valera and Seidman, 2005; Durston et al., 2003). In part, the striatal underactivation findings converge with other work that indicates anomalies in the transmission of dopamine (Ernst et al., 1998). Research on the structure and function of the brain also shows smaller volumes and atypical function of the cerebellum in association with ADHD (Schweitzer et al., 2000; Schweitzer et al., 2004).

Overall, the neural pathways most prominently altered in ADHD are the fronto-striatal-cerebellar, fronto-parietal-thalamic and fronto-cingulate circuits. A common denominator across these three networks is the frontal cortex. Perturbations in these regions could stem from the structure (e.g., reduced size), connectivity (e.g., inter- or intraregional communication) or neurochemical make-up (e.g., dopamine neurotransmission) of the circuits. Indeed, studies of individuals with ADHD suggest that, relative to people without the disorder, ADHD is associated with smaller frontal lobes (Valera et al., 2007), thinning of the cortex (Shaw et al., 2006) and a developmental lag in cortical gray matter thickness (Shaw et al., 2007).

Frequently mentioned in this literature are the *executive functions* of the brain (Boonstra et al., 2005; Willcutt et al., 2005; Barkley et al., 2006; Biederman et al., 2008). The concept of executive functions refers to a set of brain processes that control a person's ability to plan, make decisions, solve problems, respond to a novel situation or react to a dangerous or difficult situation (Norman and Shallice, 2000). Table 14.2 summarizes the major behavioral consequences of impaired executive functioning in children with ADHD.

Cortisol and ADHD

Although some studies suggest that children with ADHD have lower cortisol levels than children without ADHD (Klimes-Dougan et al., 2001a; Randazzo et al., 2008; Reynolds, Lane and Gennings, 2010), other studies have shown the opposite

(Sondeijker et al., 2007; White and Mulligan, 2005). At least two issues complicate the picture. First, children with ADHD have notoriously high rates of comorbid disorders, meaning that it is quite common for children with ADHD to also have other psychological difficulties (Connor et al., 2003). In fact, disruptive behavior disorders (DBDs) and anxiety disorders are fairly common in children with ADHD and these two types of problems have opposite relations with cortisol levels. It is possible that the unrecognized presence of comorbid problems has obscured some efforts to understand the associations between ADHD and hypothalamic-pituitary-adrenal (HPA) axis system activity. There is research that suggests that if children *just* have ADHD, *without* comorbid disruptive behavior problems, then their HPA responses to stress and challenge are not any different than those of children without ADHD (Snoek et al., 2004).

The second issue is that ADHD itself is a multifaceted disorder. Children might be primarily hyperactive and impulsive, primarily inattentive and unfocused, or both. It is possible that there are physiological differences between children that correspond to the different subtypes of ADHD they manifest, including differences in HPA activity. For example, some studies suggest that children with combined hyperactive and inattentive symptoms have lower than normal cortisol reactivity to stress, even if they do not have comorbid DBDs (Hastings et al., 2009; Van West et al., 2009). This contrasts with the argument from some researchers that it is the presence of comorbid DBDs that contributes to lower cortisol reactivity in children with ADHD (van Goozen et al., 2007).

Given the studies that currently exist, it would be premature to draw any strong conclusions about how – or even whether – cortisol levels might play a role in ADHD. There are certainly other aspects of neurophysiological functioning that distinguish children with ADHD from their peers without problems. That might also be true for HPA axis activity, but more research will need to be

Table 14.2 **Major behavioral consequences of impaired executive functioning in children with ADHD**

Executive function	Example of resulting impairment
1. Organize, prioritize and activate	Trouble getting started
	Difficulty organizing work
	Misunderstand directions
2. Focus, shift and sustain attention	Lose focus when trying to listen
	Forget what has been read and need to re-read
	Easily distracted
3. Regulate alertness, effort and processing speed	Excessive daytime drowsiness
	Quickly lose interest in task
	Effort fades quickly
	Difficulty completing a task on time
	Slow processing speed
	Inconsistent productivity
4. Manage frustration and modulate emotion	Very easily irritated
	Often sad, worried, unhappy
	Fussy about getting things perfect
	Feelings hurt easily
	Overly sensitive to criticism
5. Working memory and accessing recall	Forget to do a planned task
	Forget intended words or actions
	Difficulty recalling learned material
	Difficulty following sequential directions
	Lose track of belongings
	Quickly lose thoughts that were put on hold
6. Monitor and regulate action	Find it hard to sit still or be quiet
	Rush things, slap-dash
	Often interrupt, blurt things out

Source: Reprinted from *Clinical Psychology Review*, *27*, Brassett-Harknett, A., and Butler, N., Attention-deficit/hyperactivity disorder: An overview of the etiology and a review of the literature relating to the correlates and lifecourse outcomes for men and women, pp. 188–210, 2007, with permission from Elsevier.

done before we can make that determination with confidence.

Autonomic nervous system activity and ADHD

Researchers have speculated that ADHD would be associated with reduced *electrodermal activity* (EDA) and *electrodermal response* (EDR), because a weak *behavioral inhibition system* (BIS) was thought to contribute to the impulsivity that characterizes this disorder (Daugherty, Quay and Ramos, 1993). Fowles (1988) argued that stronger EDA reflected stronger BIS influence. Studies have been equivocal (Zahn, Schooler and Murphy, 1986). Many have, indeed, found that children and youth with ADHD have reduced EDA and less frequent EDR (Beauchaine et al., 2001; Iaboni, Douglas and Ditto, 1997; Snoek et al., 2004). But a number of studies have failed to find differences between children with and without ADHD (Pliszka et al., 1993; Satterfield et al., 1984; Zahn, Rapoport and Thompson, 1980), and one has even found that girls with ADHD have higher EDA and more EDR (Hermens et al., 2005).

Although there have been fewer studies of cardiac activity in children with ADHD (Shibagaki and Furuya, 1997), a slightly more consistent pattern exists. There is little evidence that children with and without ADHD differ in baseline heart rate, but several researchers have found that children with ADHD have relatively smaller heart rate reactivity (Iaboni et al., 1997; Jennings et al., 1997; Sroufe et al., 1973). Still, there are divergent findings, as other researchers have found that they have slightly stronger reactivity (Snoek et al., 2004; Zahn, Little and Wender, 1978). Interestingly, one study has suggested that patterns of heart rate reactivity might differ across the subtypes of ADHD. Boys with only inattention problems did not differ from boys without ADHD, but boys with hyperactivity problems showed reduced heart rate reactivity (Dykman, Ackerman and Oglesby, 1992).

There have been even fewer studies of the contributions of the *parasympathetic nervous system* (PNS) and *sympathetic nervous system* (SNS) to cardiac activity, as measured through *respiratory sinus arrhythmia* (RSA) and *pre-ejection period* (PEP)

respectively, in children with ADHD. Beauchaine and colleagues (Beauchaine et al., 2001) did not find that male adolescents with ADHD differed from adolescents without ADHD on baseline or reactive measures of RSA and PEP. Bubier and Drabick (2008) also reported that ADHD symptoms were not related to children's RSA, but more hyperactive children had reduced PEP reactivity to emotional films, suggestive of decreased SNS influence. Utendale (2005) found that boys with the hyperactive-impulsive subtype of ADHD showed very strong RSA suppression in anticipation of having their blood drawn in a hospital clinic. Working with a sample of children who had relatively few problems, El-Sheikh and colleagues (El-Sheikh and Whitson, 2006) reported that combined patterns of RSA and *skin conductance level* (SCL) reactivity predicted that children would have more ADHD-related problems when their parents had high rates of marital conflict. But both RSA withdrawal with low SCL reactivity (or *coinhibition* of the PNS and SNS), and RSA augmentation with high SCL reactivity (or *coactivation*), were associated with more problems.

Overall, the research on the autonomic physiology of children with ADHD has not produced an altogether clear set of findings. They might experience relatively low autonomic reactivity to events, but there is some evidence that they do not. They might have different patterns of PNS and SNS activity than children without ADHD, particularly reduced SNS, but this cannot be stated with complete certainty. It is possible that the heterogeneity of ADHD – the fact that the disorder encompasses three subtypes, and is so often accompanied by other emotional and behavioral problems – has confounded efforts to find consistent patterns of autonomic physiology. ADHD is a disorder with many faces; under those faces might beat many different hearts.

Genetics and ADHD

Whatever the exact brain mechanisms linked to ADHD may be, there is little doubt that ADHD is in large part transmitted genetically. This is confirmed beyond doubt by an array of family, twin and adoption studies (e.g., Banerjee, Middleton and Faraone, 2007; Faraone and Doyle, 2000; Thapar, Langley et al., 2007; Wallis, Russell and Muenke, 2008). Reviewing the research on the genetic basis for ADHD, Brassett-Harknett and Butler (2007) conclude that heritability estimates in the original studies they perused ranged from .50 to .98. Accordingly, ADHD is considered one of the most genetically influenced of all mental disorders (Faraone et al., 2005). The concordance rates for monozygotic twins are very high, ranging from .80 to .98. Thus, of all the causal factors that have been identified and proposed, scientific evidence is the strongest for the genetic pathway, which does not of course exclude non-genetic causes. Much less is known about the exact mechanism or mechanisms by which genetic transmission occurs. A number of different genes have been linked with ADHD but research remains quite inconclusive in that regard (Brassett-Harknett and Butler, 2007; Faraone and Doyle, 2000; Segman et al., 2002). Thus, the consensus of experts is that ADHD is in large part genetically determined; there is no consensus as to *how* it is genetically determined.

Family factors

If there is one principle that unites all major contemporary authorities on ADHD and almost all scholars who have studied the condition over the past century, it is the emphatic refutation of the idea that ADHD results from deficiencies in the family environment. Nevertheless, family dysfunction and family stress are no doubt important consequences of ADHD and important exacerbating factors. Furthermore, even if bad parenting is not the cause of ADHD, as most research suggests, equipping the parents of children with ADHD with truly optimal parenting skills may be an important part of the treatment, remembering that certain irrefutable causes, such as genetics, are not very amenable to treatment.

Thus, it should be noted that correlations between family problems and ADHD symptoms are only helpful in understanding the patterns of family interactions typical of the families of children with ADHD, not for helping decide whether the aspect of family functioning in question is the cause or the effect of the child's ADHD. In any case, the risk for ADHD has been found to increase as a function of the number of indicators of adversity in the child's background: family history of ADHD, comorbid psychopathology, adverse home or community environment (Biederman, 2005). Most experts agree that the biological factors inherent in the child interact with environmental factors in producing the symptoms observed in each child. It is unlikely that genetics account completely for children's ADHD because the concordance rates between monozygotic twins do not approach 100 percent (Faraone and Biederman, 2000; Kuntsi and Stevenson, 2000; Johnston and Mash, 2001). It is possible that a very healthy family environment may act to a certain degree as a protective factor against children predisposed to ADHD. This is unlikely to be demonstrated conclusively because such families rarely are participants in research on the disorder (Johnston and Mash, 2001).

Whatever the role of families in the emergence of ADHD, the family environments of children with ADHD have been found to be more stressful and conflict-ridden than the families of undiagnosed children (Brown and Pacini, 1989; DuPaul et al., 2001; Gadow et al., 2000; Johnston and Mash, 2001). The parents of children with ADHD are known to use negative methods of child discipline more than others and to be more negative in their exchanges with their children (Barkley, Karlsson and Pollard, 1985; DuPaul et al., 2001; Johnston and Mash, 2001). Negative parenting emerges more saliently as a distinguishing feature of the families of preschool children with ADHD than in studies conducted with school-age populations (Mash and Johnston, 1982). Such negativity, again, could be the cause or result of ADHD, or both, or a factor that exacerbates other causes. In many but not all studies, the parents of children with ADHD report relatively low levels of satisfaction with their marriages (Befera and Barkley, 1985; Johnston and Mash, 2001; Murphy and Barkley, 1996; Shelton et al., 1998). Often, the negative parenting is compounded by other family problems such as poverty and maternal depression (Campbell, 1994; Campbell and Ewing, 1990; Johnston and Mash, 2001). In several studies, family functioning has been found to improve after children are placed on medication (Barkley, 1988, 1989; Johnston and Mash, 2001; Schachar et al., 1987).

Prevention and treatment

Pharmacological treatment

Of the most common psychological disorders of children, ADHD is the one most closely associated with treatment by means of psychotropic medication. The usefulness of medication for ADHD was discovered by accident, in the Bradley Home, a prestigious private treatment center in Rhode Island for children with emotional problems, in the 1930s. Believing that the children's problems were caused by abnormalities in the structures of their central nervous systems, psychiatrists performed brain surgery, specifically a spinal tap, on the children. The children developed headaches after the surgery, which the psychiatrist Charles Bradley tried to relieve with the amphetamine Benzadrine. The Benzadrine did nothing for their headaches but Bradley observed that the young patients improved both their work habits and behavior once they returned to school after surgery. Therefore, Bradley decided to try Benzadrine on another group of disturbed children who had not undergone brain surgery and it worked. Bradley considered the beneficial calming effect of a stimulant medication as paradoxical. A theory-based explanation for the "paradoxical" effect emerged soon after by other researchers working at the Bradley Home. Maurice Laufer and Eric Denhoff (1957, cited by Mayes and Rafalovich, 2007) proposed that the cortex of the brain could become overwhelmed by more stimuli than it could manage. They hypothesized that the amphetamines in some way altered the functions of the diencephalon, a small part of the brain that functions in essence as a traffic director that sorts and directs impulses coming from the brain's sensory receptors.

The researchers at the Bradley Home, as biologically oriented as they were and enthusiastic as they were with their discoveries, did not advocate widespread medication at the expense of all other interventions (Mayes and Rafalovich, 2007). Psychotropic drugs were used infrequently with children through the 1950s. The 1960s brought marked improvements to both the medicines and the methods used to evaluate their usefulness. The Geigy pharmaceutical company developed the stimulant *methylphenidate*, better known by its trade name of Ritalin, a drug as effective as its predecessors but without substantial side effects in most cases. Federal regulatory authorities in the United States introduced procedures by which the developers of new psychotropic drugs request approval for their dissemination. New standards were developed for the research required to demonstrate the effectiveness of new drugs. Previously, the impressions of the prescribing physician were quite acceptable in scientific circles. *Randomized clinical trials* with *double-blind* assignment to treatment and placebo groups became the gold standard, as they have remained until the present day. The effects of the medications are rated, daily if possible, by parents and/or teachers who do not know if the child is on the medication or the placebo on the day the ratings are being filled out. Not even the prescribing physician knows: Another individual not involved in the study or the treatment will have placed the medicine and placebo tablets into envelopes labeled with the dates that the contents should be taken by the child. Only once the daily ratings have been completed does that individual reveal the roster of dates and the nature of the tablets taken by the child on each day.

The road to the current widespread use of psychotropic medication for children's ADHD was by no means a smooth one. By the end of the 1960s, only 0.002 percent of children across the United States were actually on stimulant medication. Nevertheless, newspaper reports in 1970 indicated that 5–10 percent of the children in the public schools of Omaha, Nebraska were on the medication, which was urged upon their parents by school authorities. This was in fact an error; it was 5–10 percent of the children diagnosed with special behavior and learning needs, a figure that was unusual at the time but not in US schools today. Furthermore, the schools had made no provision for the supervision of the administration of the medication during the school day. This was necessary because unlike current successors such as Biphentin, which provide for the slow time release over 24 hours of essentially the same product, Ritalin washes out of the body after a few hours and the medication must be repeated. Journalists and some sociologists issued widely read condemnations of the "medicalization" of what should be considered normal aspects of child behavior, decrying the collusion among teachers who were in essence performing the diagnosis, physicians who dispensed the medication readily and the pharmaceutical firms who profited from the entire enterprise. In the politically charged 1970s, when many educated people challenged authority in general, the diagnosis of ADHD leading summarily to the prescription of Ritalin was dubbed "the chemical straightjacket," one of the most nefarious mechanisms of social repression. Hyperactivity was dismissed as a myth created as part of this conspiracy (Conrad, 1975; Schrag and Divoky, 1975). The negative impressions left in the media resulted in tightening of the federal legal restrictions on the provision of stimulants for children (Conners, 2000; Mayes and Rafalovich, 2007). Going even further, Ritalin was withdrawn from the market for a period of time in Sweden and the UK (Bramble, 2003).

The furore abated and restrictions on the prescription of Ritalin were eased. Prescriptions for Ritalin mushroomed, reaching about 9.3 percent of the child population in the West Coast of the USA in the years 1999 to 2001 (Jick, Kaye and Black, 2004). Since then, prescriptions for children have leveled off to approximately 5 percent of children of elementary-school age in the USA, with much lower rates, approximately 0.3 percent, for children under 6 years old (Zuveka, Vitiello and Norquist, 2006). Recent years have seen the introduction of several types of improved drugs. One of these is Adderall, essentially an improved version in the same family as Benzadrine, the amphetamine used by Bradley in the 1930s, but with far fewer side effects. An important advantage of Adderall over Ritalin is that Adderall can be taken once a day, eliminating the need for in-school administration, which can be stigmatizing and create logistic and liability problems for the schools. In parallel, a longer-lasting second generation methylphenidate drug similar in chemical composition to Ritalin, named Concerta, appeared, also eliminating the need for administration during the day. Within a few years after its introduction in 2000, Concerta had almost completely replaced Ritalin in common medical practice in the United States. Finally, an antidepressant – Strattera – was shown to have some effect on ADHD. Strattera is typically used with the group of children who do not respond well to drugs in the stimulant family (Swanson and Volkow, 2009).

The widespread prescription of stimulant medication for ADHD together with the awareness that ADHD may continue into adolescence and adulthood has led to some concern about the implications of children and adolescents being on stimulant medication for extended periods of time. This of course is not generally considered in the trials conducted by pharmaceutical companies eager to demonstrate the effects that will lead most readily to approval of their products. Indeed, those companies have been accused not only of failing to explore long-term effects but of concealing data that indicate that the drugs are not as effective as other studies indicate. Professional regulation is now making that practice less blatant (Eisenberg, 2007).

Nevertheless, despite a number of follow-up studies of limited scientific rigor (reviewed by Satterfield et al., 2007), there are few well-designed studies at this point of the long-term effects of medication, with at least one study showing somewhat mixed success in measures administered at 1-year follow-up (Coghill, Rhodes and Matthews, 2007). Aside from the possibility that the drugs may simply not maintain their effectiveness, there have been warnings raised about their effects on children's physical growth (Jensen et al., 2007; Swanson et al., 2006; Swanson et al., 2007) and about whether they might provoke, in a small number of cases, cardiovascular adverse events (Kollins and March, 2007). Some concerns have been expressed that the widespread use of psychostimulants may lead to drug abuse (Volkow and Swanson, 2003), with other results suggesting that appropriate medication might actually lead to *less* drug abuse (Wilens, 2003). Recent review articles suggest that there is no evidence of any positive or negative correlation between being medicated for ADHD and abusing drugs of any kind. However, some of the drugs seem to find their way to young people for whom they have not been prescribed (Swanson and Volkow, 2009).

Although psychostimulant medication is frequently associated with the United States, it is by now accepted in most parts of the world, even in such countries as the UK where there was once considerable opposition to it. However, there are important cross-national differences in the way it is used. First of all, as discussed earlier, the ICD-10 criteria used in most European countries effectively reduce the number of children diagnosed as having ADHD because those criteria specify problem behaviors in more than one setting, for example both home and school. Furthermore, many physicians in the UK prescribe medication only when psychosocial approaches have proven insufficient whereas routine prescription of medication as the first intervention is very common in the United States (Taylor, 2009). Schlachter (2008) attributes this difference to a more psychosocial conception of ADHD in the UK

compared with a more medical model that prevails in the United States and in Australia.

Psychological therapies for children with ADHD

The prevailing psychological therapies for children with ADHD can be categorized as: (1) behavioral family intervention; (2) cognitive and cognitive-behavioral intervention; (3) social skills training; and (4) behavior modification at school.

Behavioral family intervention

Parent training is derived from the behavioral principles that emerged during the refinement of behavior modification during the 1960s and 1970s. These principles can be imparted either in groups of parents or individually, often during visits to the parents' homes. The parents are taught, first of all, to consistently deliver some kind of *positive reinforcement*, immediately, consistently and for well-defined forms of appropriate behavior. It is important for them to use positive reinforcement several times more frequently than punishment. In the event of negative behavior by the child, a brief, non-physical, immediate consequence, such as spending a few minutes in a time-out corner where little attention or enjoyable activities are available, is applied immediately. Most importantly, parents are trained to be specific, systematic and consistent. As the intervention is delivered, the parents learn to measure the child's behavior specifically and systematically in order to gauge progress.

The many studies on the effects of behavior-management training for the parents of children with ADHD and comorbid conditions have been systematically reviewed a number of times (see, e.g., Baer and Nietzel, 1991; Chronis, Jones and Raggi, 2006; Corcoran and Dattalo, 2006; DuPaul and Eckert, 1997; Fabiano et al., 2009; Lundahl, Risser and Lovejoy, 2006; Pelham and Fabiano, 2008; Purdie, Hattie and Carroll, 2002; Serketich and Dumas, 1996; Stage and Quiroz, 1997; Van der Oord et al., 2008). The review articles, even those featuring statistical meta-analyses, provide diametrically different conclusions but most of these articles indicate effects that are at least moderate (e.g., Van der Oord et al., 2008). According to Fabiano et al. (2009), the effect size for studies using the "gold standard" of evaluation methodology, the randomized clinical trial averages out to 0.83 of a standard deviation, which is moderate and which does indicate effectiveness. Similar statistics have emerged in a number of the previous meta-analyses listed above. However, most of the previous meta-analyses did not include *within-subjects designs*, including *single-subject designs*. In this research strategy, the child's behavior is measured, usually by means of direct observation, at a number of consecutive time points. The intervention is introduced during the interval between some of the time points; its impact is judged according to the change in the child's behavior. In the more rigorous studies, the intervention is removed briefly afterwards to demonstrate its connection with the behavior change assuming, of course, that it is ethical to do so and that the behavioral improvement in question is something that can be reversed. Fabiano et al.'s (2009) meta-analysis indicates that the average effect sizes for these within-subjects designs is several times greater than that of studies evaluating behavioral intervention using between-groups designs. While the effectiveness estimates are used in the heated exchanges between advocates of behavioral techniques and pharmacotherapy, the meaningful questions of whether the two might be best combined, or whether each is useful when and where the other is not, are beginning to be examined, especially in the ongoing analyses of the MTA study results (see below).

Cognitive and cognitive-behavioral intervention: an uphill battle?

It is the fervent wish of many parents and teachers to find out how to *teach* children with ADHD the basic thinking and concentration skills they lack. Techniques for teaching these skills have indeed been developed. However, Hinshaw (2006) pointed out an important distinction between cognitive-behavioral

interventions for children with ADHD and cognitive-behavioral interventions for such conditions as depression and anxiety. As detailed in Chapter 13, the depressed or anxious child usually displays some form of cognitive *distortion*, such as seeing the world as a very gloomy place. In contrast, the cognitive-behavioral therapist working with a child with ADHD is dealing with a cognitive *deficiency*, a chronic deficiency of some kind in the way the child processes information. This means that cognitive-behavioral interventions may, on the one hand, be particularly appropriate in dealing with some of the core deficits in ADHD. At the same time, it also means that they may be particularly difficult to implement successfully. Barkley (2007), however, offers a totally converse argument, insisting that these interventions lack conceptual foundation because we now know that the cognitive and behavioral deficits that are part of ADHD did not arise from deficits in social-learning or social-modeling processes that these interventions seek to correct.

In any case, some cognitive and cognitive-behavioral therapists have taken up the challenge of tackling ADHD, and not without some success. In their useful review of this limited literature, Toplak et al. (2008) separate cognitive from cognitive-behavioral interventions. Cognitive interventions, which feature direct exposure to cognitive stimuli, involve attempts to train such thinking processes as fixation, attention or working memory. Cognitive-behavioral techniques, in Toplak's review, include, for example, teaching children to monitor their own thinking processes in order to correct errors as well as training in systematic problem-solving, a classical cognitive-behavioral technique. Evaluations of cognitive-behavioral interventions are plagued with methodological problems, including administering the cognitive-behavioral interventions to children already on medication, making it impossible to establish which therapy might account for any treatment gains. As well, random assignment to treatment and control groups was conducted only in some of the studies. Thus, the results are difficult to interpret. Furthermore, the findings are mixed: Effect sizes vary enormously, with changes reported only in cognitive processes but not attention or behavior in many of the studies.

The review by Toplak et al. is somewhat more optimistic with regard to direct cognitive training, although they were able to locate only six original studies on the topic. Thus, research has yet to demonstrate the usefulness of cognitive or cognitive-behavioral techniques in the treatment of childhood ADHD in any convincing way. This does not necessarily mean that these methods should be totally dismissed, as many practitioners and researchers have done.

Social skills training

As noted earlier, one of the primary manifestations of ADHD is impaired peer relations. Social skills training is a popular intervention designed to improve peer relations. Although children with ADHD do lack social skills, the conceptual basis for applying social skills training to children with ADHD is somewhat uncertain. In common with children displaying other externalizing disorders, such as oppositional defiant disorder (which is highly comorbid with ADHD), children with ADHD may not really be lacking in the social skills themselves, if one understands the word "skill" to mean the mental knowledge of what should be done in a social situation (see Schneider, 1993a for a discussion of this terminology). In contrast, children with ADHD may lack whatever is needed – motivation, judgment, understanding of the situation at hand, freedom from anxiety, positive expectations or self-confidence – to actually use skills they know (Gresham, 1997; Wheeler and Carlson, 1994). If that is the case, the kind of social skills training that focuses on teaching the abstract skills alone may not be very applicable.

Several different varieties of social skills training have been attempted with children with ADHD. In virtually all of the interventions, a combination of social skills training approaches has been used. In almost all interventions, the skills to be learned are modeled, either in demonstrations by the therapists or on video. These skills include making

conversation, listening, sharing, making requests in an assertive way, making compliments where justified in an appropriate manner and handling criticism. The demonstrations are usually followed by practice by the participants by means of role-play. Many of the interventions also include cognitive components, such as problem-solving, mobilizing thought to achieve self-control, learning to appreciate the perspective of the other person in a social situation and maintaining perspective when faced with anger-provoking situations (Abikoff et al., 2004; Antshel and Remer, 2003; Miranda and Presentacion, 2000; Pfiffner and McBurnett, 1997; see review article by De Boo and Prins, 2007). Often, some measure is added to help promote maintenance of the skill learning and transfer of the learning to new settings. These include daily report cards and arranging for teachers and/or parents to provide systematic positive reinforcement when they see the newly acquired behaviors (Abikoff et al., 2004; Abikoff, 2009; Pfiffner and McBurnett, 1997).

De Boo and Prins (2007) provide a careful, detailed review of the results of these studies and their research designs. They conclude that four studies, including three featuring random assignment of participants to either social skills training or a control condition (Antshel and Remer, 2003; Miranda and Presentacion, 2000; Pfiffner and McBurnett, 1997) demonstrate beneficial effects of social skills training at the end of the intervention. However, Abikoff et al. (2004) found no incremental benefit of social skills training over and above the gains achieved by medication alone. Unfortunately, no follow-up measures are reported in the De Boo and Prins review. De Boo and Prins argue that this data base enables social skills training to be considered an effective experimental intervention for ADHD pending further study. Aberson, Shure and Goldstein (2007), in an editorial in the *Journal of Attention Disorders*, maintain that social problem-solving training may eventually prove beneficial for children with ADHD. Nevertheless, the community of ADHD researchers remains largely unconvinced (e.g., Pelham and Fabbiano, 2008). Barkley (2007) maintains that social skills training may even have negative effects in some cases, perhaps because of stigma and/or because in some studies aggressive children are grouped together for social skills training, leading unwittingly to the cross-fertilization of anti-social attitudes.

Direct, contingent reinforcement of appropriate behavior in the classroom

Probably the most effective and most practical intervention focusing on classroom behavior management is the daily report card, where the child is given some form of reward at home for achieving his/her behavioral goals at school on the particular day. The goals are set up to provide some degree of challenge for the child, which is often increased as the intervention continues (Chronis et al., 2001; Fabiano and Pelham, 2003; McCain and Kelley, 1993). The literature contains at least twenty-two studies documenting the effects of direct contingent reinforcement of appropriate social behavior by children with ADHD (Wells et al., 2000). A meta-analysis indicates effectiveness approaching 1.5 standard deviation units, which is very impressive. Not surprisingly, the greatest gain has been reported in measures of behavior as opposed to measures of academic achievement (DuPaul and Eckert, 1997).

Another format in which direct contingent reinforcement has been provided with considerable success to children with ADHD is the special therapeutic summer camp. William Pelham and his colleagues have operated such a summer camp in the United States for a generation, providing at the same time treatment, evaluative research and training for future psychologists. During the 8-week program, a token or point system as well as systematic praise by the staff are used to reinforce appropriate social skills. Complementing the contingency-management program are parent training, training in social problem-solving as well as coaching in both academic and sport skills (e.g., Pelham and Hoza, 1996).

Despite these clear successes, contingency-management approaches are not without their drawbacks. The most formidable obstacle is ensuring that the teacher is in agreement with the program and willing to carry it out, which is not always the case even though it can be argued that the results in terms of improved behavior represent a very good return on the teacher's time investment. As with all other known interventions for children with ADHD, there is no reason to believe that the benefits of contingency management will continue if and when the contingency management is discontinued.

Treatment modalities compared – the MTA study

The treatments discussed in the preceding sections differ in terms of their theoretical roots and the professional identities and values of those who are likely to implement them. Nevertheless, there is no reason in theory why they cannot be combined. Furthermore, for all the therapies discussed, the evaluation research is lacking in many important ways. Perhaps the most important gap is in the examination of the long-term effects of all of the treatments.

The comprehensive MTA study in the United States was designed to provide the best answers to questions about the long-term impact of the major modalities of treatment, together and in combination. The participants were 579 children at six sites across the United States. They were all diagnosed at the beginning of the study as having ADHD, with both inattention and hyperactivity. They were randomly assigned to several treatment groups, with treatments spaced over 14 months according to a set protocol. One group, medication-only, received medication that was "titrated" (adjusted to determine the optimal dose for each individual), and monitored monthly at a clinic. The multicomponent behavior-therapy condition consisted of twenty-seven sessions of parent-group training supplemented by an 8-week summer treatment program and 12 weeks of classroom behavior modification, which included a half-time teacher's aide and ten teacher consultation sessions. The combination condition involved both the medication and the multicomponent behavior therapy. These treatment conditions were compared with a usual-treatment condition, in which the participants received no special treatment from the MTA staff but continued with whatever treatment or treatments they were already receiving in the community (MTA Cooperative Group, 1999a, 1999b).

At the end of the 14 months of treatment, all groups had improved. However, participants in the medication and combined-treatment conditions showed the greatest improvement in the core symptoms of ADHD and in comorbid symptoms of oppositional defiant disorder. In some other areas, the combined-treatment group displayed better outcomes than the behavior-modification and control groups, especially in terms of comorbid depression and anxiety, school achievement and parent–child relations. There were even some important gains for the medication-only group in terms of peer relations (MTA Cooperative Group, 1999a, 1999b). These results, obtained at the end of treatment, raised considerable doubt as to the additional benefit accrued with the behavior-management procedures. That condition did lead to important incremental gains in some areas of functioning but not in the core symptoms of the disorder, and only at gargantuan additional cost in terms of time and money.

However, even by the first follow-up at 10 months, about half of the advantage initially displayed by the medication and combination conditions over the other groups had dissipated (MTA Cooperative Group, 2004). By the next follow-up, at 36 months after treatment, the treatment groups no longer differed in terms of either the symptoms of ADHD or comorbid oppositional defiant disorder. Molina and eighteen co-authors (Molina et al., 2009) presented the results of the follow-up data collected after 8 years, when the participants were adolescents 13 to 18 years old. Many of the participants in the original medication treatment had stopped taking their medication. Nevertheless, even when this was taken into account, there were virtually no significant differences among the original treatment groups. Sadly, however, most

of the participants were still exhibiting many types of maladjustment.

Thus, the MTA study provides by far the most authoritative, long-term picture of what can be expected of the major treatments in current use for childhood ADHD. The message delivered most clearly by the MTA results is that things are by no means clear. The predictors of long-term effectiveness do not necessarily correspond to results for short-term effectiveness. More research is still needed to determine whether the combination of the major modalities of treatment brings any incremental gain over interventions based on a single modality. Another sobering conclusion of the MTA study is that ADHD (to which the MTA study was restricted) is a handicapping condition with long-term effects that we have only begun to learn to treat.

The MTA study was conceived at a time when ADHD in adolescence and adulthood was only beginning to be considered and when ADHD in girls was usually relegated to footnotes. Future efforts at clarifying and expanding the work will hopefully consider both age and sex effects in response (Pelham and Fabiano, 2008), which could conceivably occur for all of the interventions, pharmacological and psychosocial.

Neural-based interventions

Given the consensus that ADHD is related in some way to brain abnormalities or dysfunctions, should not the brain be the locus of therapeutic intervention? As mentioned earlier, neurosurgery was attempted, without success, as early as the 1930s. Perhaps the recent technological advances in neuroimagery will eventually result in renewed interest in some form of surgical intervention. In the meantime, many practitioners have embraced neurofeedback techniques, in which behavioral methods are used to train children with ADHD to become aware of and modify abnormal EEG patterns (Butnik, 2005). As reviewed by Toplak et al. (2008), studies conducted to establish the effectiveness of neurofeedback are mostly of very poor quality. The most frequent flaw is the failure to control for the effects of medication; most of the participants in the studies are already on medication and remain so. Another problem is that the outcome measures are not robust indices of focused attention in real-life settings but often the scores of neuropsychological tests or laboratory procedures. Therefore, Toplak et al. conclude that there is little research support for neurofeedback.

Other researchers have been developing interventions addressed at the executive-function deficits of children with ADHD. The best-known of these efforts is the Cogmed program, whose purpose is to enhance working memory. Preliminary findings do indicate some degree of success, at least in improving working memory (Gibson et al., 2009). Further research is needed to confirm that Cogmed or similar interventions have their place as a direct intervention with children diagnosed as having ADHD.

Diet

The contention that ADHD results from poor nutrition resonates with the instincts of many mothers and caregivers. That is in fact one reason that makes it difficult to study the effects of special diets: The fervent beliefs and expectations of parents generate a strong placebo effect that may mask the true effects of the diet or the lack of such effects. The most elaborate theory linking poor nutrition to ADHD was developed by Dr. Benjamin Feingold (1975a), stating that food additives such as chemical preservatives and artificial colors were the cause of hyperactivity and learning disabilities. Feingold (1975b) reported that 40 to 70 percent of children with ADHD who were placed on a diet free of such additives demonstrated significant reduction in ADHD symptoms. Because most packaged foods contain preservatives, this diet requires extensive commitment by parents. The same media that lambasted the spread of Ritalin in the 1970s extolled the virtues of the Feingold diet. Of course, the scientific community would only accept these

findings if they were replicated by independent researchers with careful controls for placebo effects, for example, obtaining ratings from informants other than parents who did not know when the participants were on the diet. More rigorous yet, *challenge studies* involve placing children who appear to respond to the diet on a "control" diet that looks like the foods permitted in the Feingold diet but actually contained some substances that are prohibited. A meticulous meta-analysis by Kavale and Forness (1983) showed that the more rigorous the research design, the smaller the apparent effects of the diet. Kavale and Forness concluded that, overall, the true effects of the diet are trivial, with 55 percent of subjects in the control groups displaying gains equivalent to those of the experimental (diet) group.

Sugar and other sweets have sometimes been associated with ADHD in the popular press as well. In a study by Milich and Pelham (1986), children who had consumed no soft drinks overnight were given soft drinks with either sugar or an artificial sugar substitute the day after; there were no differences in the observed behaviors of the two groups. Nevertheless, many parents and professionals are not prepared to dismiss the issue. There may well be a subgroup of children who display ADHD-like symptoms because of allergies to some food substances. Clinical psychologist Vincent Monastra (2004), in a book on parenting children with ADHD published by the American Psychological Association, presents a very balanced view when introducing his chapter on nutrition:

In this chapter, I want to focus on the dietary habits of your child and how they relate to attention, impulsivity, and hyperactivity. Why? Is it because I think that ADHD is caused by inadequate nutrition? No, that's not the reason, although there is evidence that children who have deficiencies of iron, zinc, and magnesium will show symptoms of inattention, impulsivity, and hyperactivity. Is it because I think that food allergies cause ADHD? Again, the answer is no, although there are well-controlled studies that indicate that symptoms that mimic ADHD can be caused by allergic reactions to foods like wheat, corn, soy, eggs, milk, and certain food dyes and additives. There are several reasons why it is important for you to understand how foods contribute to a person's ability to attend, inhibit impulsive behaviors, analyze information, regulate emotional responses, and solve problems. Our selection of foods will determine whether we have the capacity to manufacture the essential neurotransmitters necessary for brain functions. What we eat will determine whether we will have the materials necessary to manufacture the enzymes, cells, and tissues essential for life functions. In addition, should we mistakenly eat foods that cause allergic reactions, our ability to attend, think, and control our emotions will be compromised. Because of this, I routinely request that all of my patients be screened for common food allergies prior to initiating medication for ADHD or making specific dietary recommendations to address nutritional deficiencies.

Conclusions and future directions

How likely is it that neuropsychologists will soon pinpoint the exact cause of ADHD? Very possibly, the complexities of the brain may become better understood although research may not lead to a single form of brain dysfunction that triggers inattention and hyperactivity. More important, though, is the challenge of linking treatment more directly to the brain dysfunctions that may be discovered. Perhaps the new technology will enable direct examination of the workings of interventions, including, but not necessarily limited to, pharmacological interventions.

The current awareness of the possible biases of research on the treatment of ADHD will hopefully lead to a clearer picture of the effects of the various interventions, less fettered by disciplinary allegiance and commercial interests. As part of that process, the appropriate coordination of pharmacological and psychosocial therapies will hopefully emerge.

Summary

- ADHD consists of two primary symptoms, inattention and/or hyperactivity (i.e., excessive movement).
- Some critics argue that ADHD is a result of societal pressures on parents to control their unruly children or that the pharmaceutical industry is responsible for the construct of ADHD.
- DSM-5 presumes that the disorder has to be evident by age 12. There is evidence of adolescent and adult ADHD, as well as ADHD in preschoolers as young as 4 years.
- The counterpart disorder in the ICD-10 is hyperkinetic disorder.
- There is much debate about the different presentations of ADHD (i.e., hyperactive, impulsive or both) and whether they represent entirely different disorders or can be considered part of the single disorder ADHD.
- Genetics play a role in the symptoms of ADHD, with both inattention and hyperactivity being highly heritable.
- Children with ADHD have many negative interpersonal interactions throughout the day with their parents, teachers and peers at school, and peers outside of school. These impaired peer relations have been as reliable as the core symptoms of ADHD (inattention and hyperactivity) at statistically differentiating children with and without ADHD.
- Although difficult to document scientifically, the frequency of ADHD diagnoses may be increasing, most likely due to awareness of the disorder.

Environmental and dietary factors cannot be ruled out as explanations for the increase.

- ADHD can continue throughout an individual's life, although the symptoms often shift from those of hyperactivity to those of inattention.
- The majority of children diagnosed with ADHD are male. Many point to demands placed by schools on boys that are inconsistent with their natural temperaments.
- Research on girls with ADHD has revealed that, compared to their male counterparts, they are more likely to experience comorbid depression and anxiety, whereas boys often experience comorbid aggression. ADHD in girls has also been related to eating disorders, substance use disorders and anti-social behavior later in life.
- There is some discrepancy in the prevalence of ADHD among various countries. However, when rigorous, standardized testing is done, these differences are often minimal.
- Childhood ADHD often persists into adolescence, and, to some extent, into adulthood.
- Individuals with ADHD are more likely than others to discontinue their schooling at an earlier age, to demonstrate poor school results and to repeat school years. They have fewer friends and lower reported self-esteem, and often have comorbid anxiety disorders, mood disorders and substance use disorders.
- Although it is assumed that ADHD is of neurobiological origin, it is awkward to conclude that brain damage exists when no damage to the brain is apparent. In previous years, the terms "brain/cerebral dysfunction" were used to avoid implying physical damage.
- Many contemporary scientists believe that there is not a single pathway accounting for ADHD in all its forms.
- Cognitive and behavioral processes related to children with ADHD include response inhibition, working memory problems and impairment of different types of attention processes.
- Response inhibition (i.e., the ability to suppress actions one would make in response to a stimulus

that is not relevant to the context or situation at hand) is affected in people with ADHD throughout their lives. It is linked to the fronto-striatal network of the brain.

- Working memory deficits can also be found in people with ADHD, linked to reduced activation in the frontal, temporal and occipital areas, and a greater activation in midbrain, striatal, cerebellum and middle frontal gyrus regions.
- Underactivation of the fronto-parietal-striatal regions in individuals with ADHD is seen during attention tasks. The frontal lobe is implicated in these dysfunctions. A smaller frontal lobe, thinner cortex and developmental delay in gray cortical matter thickness are associated with ADHD.
- Conflicting results exist regarding the cortisol levels in children with ADHD. This may be because some comorbid disorders, such as disruptive behavior disorder and anxiety disorders, have opposite relations with cortisol levels.
- The autonomic nervous system may be associated with ADHD, although research has been inconsistent with respect to electrodermal activity and electrodermal response processes in children with the disorder. Relatedly, some data indicate that boys with ADHD, especially, have lower heart rate reactivity than is typical of boys the same age.
- There are some additional distinguishing features of the cardiac activity in children with ADHD, including differences in baseline or reactive measures of respiratory sinus arrhythmia and pre-ejection periods. This varies among different presentations of ADHD. The inconclusive evidence with regard to the autonomic physiology linked with ADHD may be due to the heterogeneity of the disorder.
- ADHD is in large part genetically determined; however, the exact genetic route is not known well. In fact, it is considered one of the most genetically influenced of all mental disorders.
- Parenting and deficiencies in the family environment, although very often present, are not

viewed as causes for ADHD in children. However, equipping the parents with optimal child-rearing skills constitutes a very effective form of treatment.

- The parents of a child with ADHD are more likely than others to act negatively toward their children and use negative methods of child discipline. These parents report low levels of satisfaction with their marriages. The negative parenting is often compounded by other family problems such as poverty and maternal depression.

- ADHD is one of the psychological disorders of children most closely associated with treatment by means of psychotropic medication. Amphetamines, methylphenidate (Ritalin), Biphentin, Adderall, Concerta and Strattera have all been used in the treatment of ADHD, some with more benefits and fewer side effects than others.

- Some concerns have been expressed regarding pharmaceutical companies not exploring the long-term effects of drugs they develop. There are some cross-national differences in the use of pharmacological treatment.

- Psychological therapies used for children with ADHD include: behavioral family intervention (e.g., encouraging positive reinforcement and brief, non-physical punishments), behavior modification at school (using the daily report card approach), cognitive-behavioral interventions with children (training thinking processes such as fixation, attention and working memory) and social skills training (improving peer relations by teaching listening, sharing, appreciation, etc.).

- The MTA study is the largest investigation of the major treatments of ADHD in children and their relative benefits. Initial findings favored medication over behavioral treatment. However, the benefits of medication were much less evident in longer-term follow-up data.

- Neural-based interventions are designed to help children with ADHD become aware of and modify abnormal EEG patterns, using neurofeedback techniques. However, due to the fact that current research has not controlled for the effects of medication, very little support exists for neurofeedback. Other neural-based interventions, such as Cogmed, show some degree of success at improving working memory, but this gain has not been directly linked to the core symptoms of ADHD.

- Diet has been a concern for parents. Some studies have shown a significant reduction in ADHD symptoms when food additives were eliminated from the child's diet. However, many researchers point to the expectations of the mothers or caregivers as generating a strong placebo effect.

- Academic interventions, such as tutoring, may be a useful treatment or adjunct treatment for children with ADHD.

Study questions

1. How suitable are teacher ratings as the main component of the assessment of possible ADHD?
2. What are some important differences between the typical symptoms of ADHD in children, adolescents and adults?
3. How accurate is the contention that ADHD is caused by brain damage?
4. What are the "executive functions" that are typically impaired among children and adolescents with ADHD?
5. How important is it for children with ADHD to follow a specific prescribed diet?

15 Anxiety disorders

Anxiety is characterized by distress or uneasiness regarding danger, real or perceived, or concern about an upcoming stressful event. According to a classic theory proposed by Alpert and Haber (1960), anxiety is often facilitative and helpful. It can lead to trying harder at a pursuit in which one wants to do well. Anxiety can also serve a protective function by steering children and adults away from situations in which they will experience danger or so much failure and disappointment that they will lose enthusiasm for whatever endeavor is involved. Anxiety becomes debilitative when it begins to interfere with successful functioning in family, school and work settings. Indeed, fears are a very integral and usually constructive part of the normal development of children. It is useful to conceptualize *fear* or *panic* as pertaining primarily to an imminent threat or danger, whereas anxiety refers to worrying about a real, imagined or exaggerated threat that will occur in the future (Craske, 1999). Throughout childhood, children worry about getting sick, failing in school and looking foolish (e.g., Ollendick, Matson and Helsel, 1985). This makes it difficult to notice that some children experience anxiety on a chronic basis at levels well above the norm for their ages. In fact, problematic anxiety is very common among children and adolescents. However, anxious children and adolescents, who rarely disrupt the routines of families and schools, often remain unnoticed. Even the mental health community has only developed awareness of the extent of the anxiety problems of young people in the past 30 years or so. Although some anxiety problems begin in early childhood, anxiety disorders at that stage are only beginning to receive the attention of researchers and practitioners. Conditions that interfere substantially with the daily lives of school-age children and adolescents remain relatively understudied compared to other psychological problems that are very prevalent in the population at large.

This chapter begins with a delineation of the distinct forms of anxiety disorder. The basic notion of considering anxiety a disorder is discussed next, including the possible advantages and problems inherent in doing so. Diagnostic criteria and information about the prevalence of anxiety disorders among children and adolescents are presented next. In the section on prevalence, particular emphasis is placed on sex differences, culture and gender diversity. Details about the physiological, family, societal and peer-group factors in the emergence of anxiety disorder are considered next, followed by a brief section on stability and prognosis. The chapter ends on a happy note with descriptions of treatments for children's and adolescents' anxiety disorder, several of which are quite successful.

Distinct types of anxiety disorders

Anxiety disorder, like disruptive behavior disorder, is an umbrella term that includes a number of distinct disorders, some of which are more prevalent among children and adolescents than others. *Separation anxiety disorder* refers to excessive distress about separating from one's caregiver. In *social anxiety* or *social phobia*, the feared situation is social contact, especially with an unfamiliar individual or one who might evaluate an individual negatively. *Specific phobia* involves an excessive fear of a specific situation, such as one in which a snake may be encountered; fear of high places is another example. *Panic disorder*, rarely diagnosed in children, involves repeated, short episodes of intense anxiety that appear suddenly and unpredictably, often accompanied by strong physical symptoms and a fear of a disastrous outcome. *Agoraphobia*, the fear of crowds, is also more common among adults than children, but may be related to *school refusal* or *school phobia* in childhood. Agoraphobia often involves panic attacks and therefore is often considered a condition very close to panic disorder (Beesdo, Knappe and Pine, 2009; Beidel and Alfano, 2011). *Generalized anxiety disorder* refers to frequent worry or fear that occurs in a wide range of situations. Two additional conditions are considered anxiety disorders in DSM-5 but not in ICD-10. *Obsessive-compulsive disorder* (OCD) consists of unwanted thoughts or impulses that may be accompanied by repeated ritualistic behaviors, such as constant washing of the hands. As is the case for the other anxiety disorders usually diagnosed at this point only with adults, there is an increasing awareness that there are some cases of OCD in children. *Selective mutism* involves not speaking in some social situations, such as those at school, where speaking is expected. Onset often occurs before the child is 5 years old (American Psychiatric Association, 2000). Opposition to adult authority may be a feature of some cases of selective mutism. A new category, pragmatic (social) communication disorder appears in DSM-5 for the first time. Hopefully, diagnosticians will be able to distinguish reliably between this form of language/communication disorder and such anxiety disorders as social anxiety and selective mutism.

School refusal, referred to in many older writings as school phobia, is a complex and heterogeneous phenomenon that is sometimes associated with anxiety disorders. Although this phenomenon is rarely characterized by a specific phobia directed at the school itself, it may be a manifestation of separation anxiety, social anxiety or generalized anxiety (Kearney, 2008). School refusal is the subject of Chapter 22.

Conceptual controversy: turning ordinary shyness into an illness?

There has been relatively little challenge to the notion that anxiety disorders, like other diagnosable conditions, reside within the individual and that the increase in their diagnosis in recent years is attributable to increased awareness of the problem. However, the notion of diagnosing social anxiety or social phobia on an individual basis has not escaped the wrath of some social critics. They attribute this practice to the pressures of a mass society to conform to its social norms. They regard the individual diagnosis as a means of marginalizing people who are simply not sociable (Wakefield, Horwitz and Schmitz, 2005). Thus, just as the diagnosis of ADHD is seen by some as a way to suppress behaviors that might disrupt order, anxiety disorder is seen as a way to suppress non-conformity and non-participation. Shared with ADHD in these criticisms is the contention that the "medicalization" of what has always been seen as a common personal characteristic emerged at about the same time as prescription medications were developed to treat them (e.g., Lane, 2007).

Diagnostic criteria

In recent years, it has been increasingly recognized that children can and do suffer from anxiety disorders. Indeed, the retrospective reports of adults suffering from anxiety disorders frequently indicate the belief that the problem started in childhood, even though it was not recognized (Beesdo et al., 2009; Kessler et al., 2005). The DSM-III, introduced in 1980, represented a gigantic forward leap with the designation of a separate category entitled "anxiety

---

Box 15.1 | Differences between DSM-IV and DSM-5 criteria for social anxiety disorder (social phobia)

- In both DSM-IV and DSM-5, the disorder is defined in terms of a marked fear of social situations in which a person will be evaluated or scrutinized.
- In both DSM-IV and DSM-5, it is stipulated that these social situations must almost always provoke fear or anxiety.
- In both DSM-IV and DSM-5, it is specified that the fear or anxiety must be out of proportion to any actual threat that is posed by the situation. However, in DSM-5, it is noted that an individual's socio-cultural context must be taken into account when determining what qualifies as excessive.
- Both versions recognize that children may express their social anxiety in distinct ways, such as by crying or tantruming.
- Both versions exclude the diagnosis of social anxiety/phobia if the problems are caused primarily by a medical condition or another overriding psychological condition, such as substance abuse.
- In both DSM-IV and DSM-5, children must experience symptoms for a minimum of 6 months.
- In DSM-IV, the specifier "generalized" is included to be used if most social situations cause the individual anxiety; this specifier has not been retained in DSM-5.
- In DSM-5, the "performance only" specifier has been added, to be used if the anxiety occurs only in relation to public speaking or performance.

Source: DSM-5 and DSM-IV-TR consulted June 26, 2013.

---

disorders of childhood." This was not retained in DSM-IV or DSM5, whose developers substituted the recognition that some forms of anxiety disorder occur across the lifespan. The descriptions and diagnostic criteria of the other anxiety disorders contain a few modifications to be used when a problem of a child or adolescent is diagnosed. Many experts consider these modifications as minimal, insufficient and, in some cases, of limited scientific validity (Beesdo et al., 2009). Despite these criticisms, little significant change appeared with the release of DSM-5. The most substantial recognition that the anxiety disorder manifests itself in distinct ways during childhood is in the case of social anxiety disorder/social phobia. The

diagnostic criteria for children's anxiety disorders in ICD-10 are very similar to those in DSM, except for the fact that more conditions are considered anxiety disorders in ICD-10, as mentioned earlier. Boxes 15.1, 15.2 and 15.3 summarize the changes between DSM-IV and DSM-5 criteria for social anxiety disorder, generalized anxiety disorder and separation anxiety disorder. Compared to other disorders, relatively little has been changed. Although there are no specific diagnostic criteria for anxiety disorders in adolescents in either the ICD or DSM systems, many anxiety conditions, especially social anxiety disorder (social phobia), do emerge at that stage, when peer relations increase in importance.

Box 15.2   Differences between DSM-IV and DSM-5 criteria for generalized anxiety disorder

- There are no substantive differences between the DSM-IV and DSM-5 criteria.
- In both DSM-IV and DSM-5, the disorder is characterized by excessive worry and anxiety about various activities in an individual's life.
- In both DSM-IV and DSM-5, it is noted that the generalized anxiety should not fall exclusively within the confines of another anxiety disorder that is more specific, a somatoform disorder, a mood disorder, a psychotic disorder or an autism spectrum disorder.
- Both versions exclude the diagnosis of generalized anxiety disorder if the symptoms are caused primarily by a drug or general medical condition.
- In both versions, the child must experience one or more of the listed symptoms. Examples of symptoms include restlessness, fatigue and trouble sleeping.
- In both versions, the worry must be present on most days for at least 6 months.

Source: DSM-5 and DSM-IV-TR consulted June 6, 2013.

Box 15.3   Differences between DSM-IV and DSM-5 criteria for separation anxiety disorder

- In both DSM-IV and DSM-5, the individual must experience a fear of being separated from home or from attachment figures.
- In both DSM-IV and DSM-5, eight symptoms are listed. Three or more of the listed symptoms must be present. Examples of symptoms include distress when the individual is separated from the home or an attachment figure; worry about something happening to an attachment figure; intense fear of being alone; refusal to attend school; nightmares that possess a separation theme; fear of sleeping apart from an attachment figure; and physical symptoms like headaches or nausea.
- In both versions, the disturbance must last for at least 1 month.
- Both versions note that the disturbance should not occur solely in the context of a psychotic disorder or an autism spectrum disorder. Both versions also note that the disturbance should not be better described by another anxiety disorder.
- In DSM-IV, the specifier "early onset" is included to be used if the disorder is present before the age of 6. However, this specifier has not been retained in DSM-5.

Source: DSM-5 and DSM-IV-TR consulted June 28, 2013.

CASE STUDY: Andrea, social anxiety hidden behind a punk self-presentation

Andrea, age 14, was referred to the psychologist (Schneider, author of this book) by her parents, who were concerned that she was spending hours alone in her room, listening to music through her earphones. Andrea was spending virtually all of her waking hours, except for school and mealtimes, alone in her room. She had developed a particular interest, which the parents called an obsession, with post-hardcore punk music. Andrea's room was decorated with photos of her favorite band, the Omegas. Punk-theme tattoos covered most of her body. Her parents did not agree with the tattooing, which was done when Andrea's mother was out of town visiting Andrea's ailing grandmother. To her mother's dismay, Andrea insists on wearing t-shirts adorned with the names of punk-rock groups.

Andrea's mother insisted on speaking to the psychologist alone for the first session. She was having considerable difficulty getting Andrea to agree to see the psychologist. She expected Andrea to say very little. She and Dad accompanied Andrea for the second session. Mom works part-time as a bookkeeper for a pharmacy; Dad is an accountant who works long hours for a large company. Mom was soft-spoken and matter-of-fact in her conversation, expressing little emotion. She reported that she secretly checked Andrea's room for drugs while Andrea was at school but fortunately found none. Mom and Dad were both very concerned about doing the right thing and about the negative image Andrea was projecting to neighbors and relatives. They also very sincerely wanted Andrea to be happy, which she is not. Mom has tried to discuss Andrea's problems with her, but Andrea denies having any. Andrea's relationships with her Dad and younger brother are even more distant. Andrea's brother, David, is reported to be friendly, outgoing and successful in school.

To his surprise, Andrea was quite friendly during her first session with the psychologist. She said that she loved her parents deep inside but found them too conventional for her taste. She complained that they were constantly trying to change her into someone else, someone that she did not want to be. The psychologist asked her what kind of person she really wanted to be. Andrea was evasive, giving the impression that she did not really know. After a moment of reflection, Andrea said that she wanted to express herself freely, unlike most of the people she knows who are trying to show off. She said that both her school program – in visual arts, to capitalize on her talents in drawing and painting – and the punk music derived from her need to express herself freely.

The psychologist ventured that most young people interested in punk music are trying to express their resentment and need to rebel. Surprising the psychologist once more, Andrea said that she did not really resent anyone or anybody but just wanted to be left alone. She said that the interest in post-hardcore punk came from her friend Beverly, who was her only friend. When questioned, Andrea revealed that she only saw Beverly about once every 3 weeks and exchanged text messages with her about once a week. Their relationship did not appear very close.

The psychologist asked Andrea about her contacts with the rest of her fellow students in the art program. Andrea said that she had few such contacts. She disparagingly called most of them conventional people who dressed in identical fashion sportswear and penny loafers. However, Andrea admitted that it would be nice to at least have a friendly conversation with someone at school once in a while. When asked whether she was lonely, Andrea immediately responded "yes."

The psychologist proceeded to inquire about the efforts Andrea had made to establish at least harmonious relations with her schoolmates. Andrea had made none. She felt that any such approaches would surely be rebuffed. No one would want to associate with anyone whose interests were so different from theirs.

The psychologist began to suspect that Andrea's hardcore punk image was really a shield against facing her inner social anxieties. He asked Andrea to complete a standard questionnaire about the symptoms of social phobia as well as other questionnaires about depression and peer relations. Andrea's score fell within the clinical range for social phobia. She was also somewhat depressed and, not surprisingly, reported difficulties in peer relations.

The psychologist helped Andrea work through a standard, multicomponent intervention for young people with social phobia. Before he could begin the intervention, though, he had to engage Andrea in several discussions to determine what she really wanted: to be on friendly terms with others without giving up her individuality. Once there was agreement on the objectives, Andrea proceeded well through the components of the intervention. She learned to suspend judgment about other people until she had gotten to know them a bit. She also learned to stop her somewhat automatic thinking that no one would like to befriend her. She learned systematic relaxation techniques, especially deep breathing.

The most difficult component of the intervention was graduated exposure. Andrea had to first do no more than say hello to some of her classmates. She did that with little difficulty. However, the next step involved a more extended conversation about a neutral topic, such as which teachers they found the most irritating. Andrea's stomach fluttered and she did not accomplish this until encouraged by the psychologist for several weeks to continue. Eventually, Andrea was able to make conversation at school. She no longer sat alone at lunch and was invited to some after-school events at the homes of her schoolmates.

By the time of her termination of therapy, Andrea was feeling less lonely and more confident. She had not changed her hardcore punk appearance. As advised by the psychologist, Andrea's parents made more sincere attempts at relating with Andrea in different ways. They did their best to support her and share her experiences rather than instruct her on how she should lead her life.

Prevalence

An authoritative estimate of the lifetime prevalence of *any* anxiety disorder is about 15–20 percent. The most frequent anxiety disorders among children and adolescents are separation anxiety, with prevalence rates estimated at about 3–8 percent, social phobia, which affects about 7 percent of the child and adolescent population, and specific phobias, with a prevalence rate of about 10 percent. The prevalence rate for generalized anxiety disorder in children and adolescents is thought to be about 4 percent. Agoraphobia and panic disorder affect fewer than 1 percent of children, although as many as 3 percent of adolescents reportedly suffer from panic disorder and 3–4 percent experience agoraphobia (Beesdo et al., 2009; Beidel and Turner, 2005; Bowen, Offord and Boyle, 1990). Complementing the statistics on the lifetime prevalence of anxiety disorder are epidemiological results about the number of children and adolescents who meet the diagnostic criteria for anxiety disorders at any specific moment in time, which is estimated at between 2.5 and 5 percent (Costello, Compton et al., 2003; Rapee, Schniering and Hudson, 2009). There is considerable comorbidity among the different forms of anxiety disorder, with anywhere from 40 to 60 percent of children and adolescents who display one anxiety disorder also displaying diagnosable symptoms of another anxiety disorder (Rapee et al., 2009).

Most children and adolescents with anxiety disorders also display symptoms that correspond to the diagnostic criteria for other forms of psychopathology. The most common comorbid condition is depression, with comorbidity rates reported in different studies ranging from 16 to 62 percent (Beidel and Alfano, 2011; Brady and Kendall, 1992). One possibility that could explain this comorbidity is that chronic, crippling anxiety leads over time to depression (Anderson and Hope, 2008; Chorpita and Daleiden, 2002). In Clark and Wilson's (1999) *tripartite model* (see review by Anderson and Hope, 2008), *negative affect* is seen as the common component that links the two disorders. Separating them is, first of all, *positive affect*, which is pervasively low only in people suffering from depression, who feel tired and sluggish whereas people with anxiety disorders generally do not. Another distinguishing feature of the two disorders is *physiological hyperarousal*, which includes somatic tension, shortness of breath, etc. Physiological hyperarousal is particularly noticeable in panic disorder but perhaps less extensively in other anxiety disorders. In another version of the tripartite model, it is fear rather than physiological hyperarousal that differentiates between anxiety and depression (Anderson and Hope, 2008; Chorpita et al., 1998).

Comorbidity between anxiety disorders and externalizing disorders such as attention deficit/ hyperactivity disorder or oppositional defiant

disorder is also substantial, ranging across studies from about 17 to 34 percent, with higher comorbidity typical in older child samples (Beidel and Alfano, 2011; Stavrakaki et al., 1987). There are conflicting findings about the links between different forms of anxiety and substance abuse. Whether or not young people with anxiety problems engage in risky addictive behavior may depend on the expectation that their peers will approve or disapprove of their substance abuse (Zehe et al., 2013).

Developmental issues

The typical age of onset differs among the various forms of anxiety disorder. Specific phobia and separation anxiety, which are the most closely linked with the developmental experiences of the childhood years, often appear for the first time during childhood and often decrease with the onset of adolescence (Beesdo et al., 2009; Kessler et al., 2005; Rapee et al., 2009). Social phobia may appear in young children, usually from about age 7 years, but is more typical from middle childhood onwards, with some but not all studies indicating an increase during adolescence (Canino et al., 2004; Kearney, 2005; Rapee et al., 2009). Generalized anxiety disorder can appear at any age within the childhood and adolescent years (Beesdo et al., 2009; Kessler et al., 2005; Rapee et al., 2009).

Sex differences

The overwhelming majority of studies indicate that girls with anxiety disorders of all types outnumber boys considerably, by a ratio of 2:1 or higher in most studies. The greater risk for females also occurs for depression, as noted in Chapter 13. However, unlike the case of depression, girls and women are at higher risk for anxiety disorders at all ages, whereas in depression the male:female ratio depends on the age of the sample (Costello, Compton et al., 2003; Rapee et al., 2009). Explanations for the gender difference range from differences in hormones to fear by girls and women of maltreatment by men to society's greater acceptance of negative emotions and the behaviors used to express them by males (Harmon, Langsley and Ginsberg, 2006). Kearney (2005) speculates that boys may be less likely than girls to discuss their anxiety with others. On the other hand, he notes that boys may be referred for professional help more readily than girls because anxiety is more inconsistent with society's normative expectations for boys' behavior. It should be noted that in certain culture-specific manifestations of anxiety, such as *taijin kyofusho*, discussed later, the prevalence is actually higher among males than among females (Suzuki et al., 2003), even though Japanese girls, like girls elsewhere, have been found to report more anxiety symptoms in general than Japanese boys, consistent with the worldwide pattern (Ishikawa, Sato and Sasagawa, 2009).

Sexual orientation

Gay and bisexual adolescents have been found to experience higher levels of social anxiety, in particular, than their peers of majority sexual orientation according to a study by Safren and Pantalone (2006). These researchers identify a lack of social support as a cause of this. Other possible explanations for this are many, including restricted social contacts due to negative attitudes by their peers, the stress of attempting to initiate satisfactory social relationships while concealing their sexual orientation, the effects of being teased, bullied and/ or abused and the lack of adult and peer role models. More research directed specifically at this population is needed. Such research may eventually elucidate useful directions for prevention and treatment.

Cultural differences

There are important cultural differences in demands for outgoing, social behavior as opposed to valuing of shyness and modesty. Perhaps for that reason, some studies conducted with adults have confirmed higher rates of social anxiety among East Asians than among people from English-speaking countries

(Heinrichs et al., 2006). In some collective cultures, such as those of East Asia, individuals are profoundly concerned about "face," that is, about their own reputation or the reputation of their family. This can be a source of stress by itself, and one that appears to be represented in high rates of social anxiety among adults in East Asian cultures.

Cultural differences interact with developmental differences. The core values of a culture may affect the parenting that children receive but the values themselves may not be completely inculcated until adolescence or adulthood. This may apply to the concern for face and the proneness to shame that are common among East Asians. Perhaps developmental issues explain the fact that, unlike data pertaining to adults, highly variable results have been reported in studies of the self-reported anxiety of children in Japan and China. Some reports indicate higher anxiety among East Asian samples of elementary-school children than among European-Americans (e.g., Ollendick et al., 1996), with other reports indicating the opposite (Essau et al., 2004; Iwawaki et al., 1967). Of course, these results may be affected by the willingness of children to divulge their anxiety in self-report questionnaires, which may itself be affected by culture.

Some culture-specific patterns of anxiety and social withdrawal have been reported in Japan most extensively but also in other East Asian countries. These are discussed most extensively in the adult literature although they are not limited to adults, as discussed by Miyaki and Yamazaki (1995). *Taijin kyofusho* (e.g., Ono et al., 2001) is characterized by an extreme fear of embarrassment. One form of the disorder, perhaps the best known, is characterized by a marked fear of conveying an offensive body odor. Other forms involve fear of making eye contact and fear of offending by blushing (Suzuki et al., 2003). Another condition, known as *hikikomori* (Teo and Gaw, 2010) involves social withdrawal to the extent of becoming a recluse, spending months in parents' homes and refusing to attend school or see other people. Only in some cases is *hikikomori* associated with anxiety.

Ataques de nervios (literally "nerve attacks") are a specifically Latin American constellation of symptoms including panic, troubled thinking and somatic symptoms. The people affected and those around them believe that the individual has suffered some kind of attack, probably because of stress. They experience problems in breathing, numbness, shaking and shouting. They may fall to the ground or strike out at others (Lewis-Fernandez et al., 2002). In some ways, *ataques de nervios* resemble panic attacks. However, its symptoms are often broader than those of panic attacks. Latin Americans use the term to refer to a wide range of mental health problems. Almost all the literature on *ataques de nervios* pertains to adults (Varela and Hensley-Maloney, 2009). However, a recent study of children and adolescents in Puerto Rico and Hispanic neighborhoods of New York City revealed that 4 to 5 percent of the children were identified as having had an *ataque* (Lopez et al., 2009).

Probable causes and concurrent impairment

Genetics

The heterogeneity of the phenotypes in anxiety disorder and in the genetic complexity underlying the diverse phenotypes constitutes a formidable challenge (Smoller, Block and Young, 2009). Nevertheless, some clear evidence of genetic causation is available. First-degree relatives of a person with an anxiety disorder are four to six times more likely to have the specific or generalized anxiety disorder that affects their relatives than the general population incidence of the particular disorder (Hettema, Neale and Kendler, 2001). As well, there is a considerable risk of a first-degree relative having any form of anxiety disorder, not necessarily the specific anxiety disorder that affects the family member (Smoller, Gardner-Schuster and Misiaszek, 2008). Twin studies, which provide more direct evidence of heritability, indicate a concordance rate of 12–26 percent for monozygotic twins, compared

with 4–15 percent for dizygotic twins (Hettema et al., 2001). These data have been used to estimate the heritability of anxiety disorders, yielding heritability estimates that range from 20 to 40 percent, similar to those for depression but lower than of a number of other mental health disorders (e.g., Hettema et al., 2005; Scherrer et al., 2000; Smoller et al., 2009).

That being established, the more formidable task is identifying the genes that are involved. This is difficult because, in contrast with some disorders that often result from a mutation of a single gene, anxiety disorders result from the complex interactions of the workings of several genes. To date, researchers have identified several chromosomal regions, although with inconsistent results that vary from study to study as well as different findings for the different types of anxiety disorders. It is possible that many more genes are involved than have been studied to date. Smoller and colleagues (2009) believe that further progress will depend not only on improved technology but also on greater clarity in the subtyping and diagnosis of anxiety disorders.

Temperament

Another way of looking at the possible genetic roots of children's anxiety problems is to consider the genetic transmission of temperament rather than the genetic transmission of diagnosable disorder. *Behavioral inhibition* is characterized by the consistent display of fearfulness and withdrawal, especially in unfamiliar situations. Approximately 10–15 percent of young children are classified as behaviorally inhibited in most research. They are often timid, quiet, speaking little and smiling infrequently; they often cling to their mothers. The heritability of behavioral inhibition is estimated at .50 to .70 (Hirshfeld-Becker, 2010; Kagan, Reznick and Snidman, 1988). Early behavioral inhibition has been linked to the emergence of social phobia in particular but sometimes to other anxiety disorders as well. For example, in a longitudinal study by Schwartz, Snidman and Kagan (1999), it was found that 34 percent of the participants who were inhibited

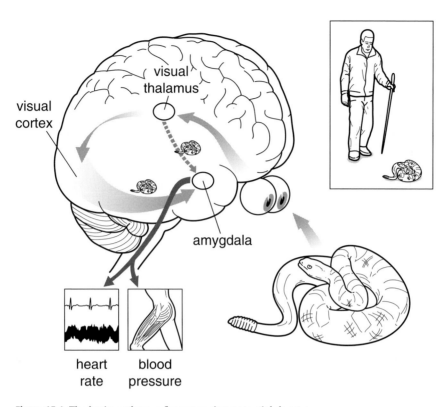

Figure 15.1 The brain pathways for processing potential danger.

as toddlers went on to develop social phobia at age 13 compared to 9 percent of toddlers who were not inhibited during their early childhood years. These and many similar findings about temperament have led to questions about the fundamental relationship between temperament and psychopathology: Is psychopathology merely the upper extreme of the distribution of temperament, or are psychopathology and temperament separate but related constructs (Rapee and Coplan, 2010)?

Psychobiology[1]

Considerable animal and neuroimaging work delineates the engagement of a neural "fear-circuitry" that processes and responds to danger and threat in one's surroundings (LeDoux, 1994)

[1] Section written by Paul Hastings and Amanda Guyer.

(see Figure 15.1). This neural circuitry centers on the amygdala, which is located in the medial temporal lobe, but also includes the ventral prefrontal cortex (vPFC), and the anterior congulate cortex. The amygdala particularly aids in processing information about salient emotional stimuli (LeDoux, 1994), including those positive or negative in valence (Breiter et al., 1996; Morris et al., 1996; Yang et al., 2002).

Much work on the brain and anxiety focuses on how individuals attend and respond to threatening stimuli and factors that modulate those responses. Two frequently used task paradigms in this kind of research measure emotional face processing and attention orienting. These kinds of tasks have been especially useful in studies of children, in part because they use pictures rather than words. With regard to emotional face processing, when individuals view fearful faces (which convey that

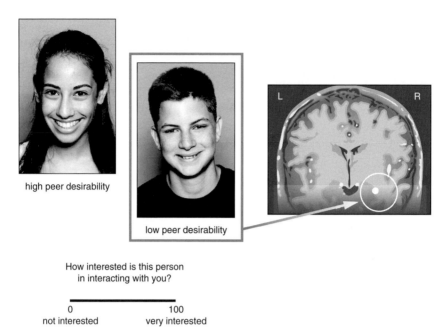

high peer desirability

low peer desirability

How interested is this person
in interacting with you?

0   100
not interested   very interested

Figure 15.2 Socially anxious children show a heightened amygdala response to peer evaluation.

there is danger in one's surroundings), the amygdala appears to be particularly responsive (Adolphs et al., 1995; Whalen et al., 1998). This has been supported by several fMRI studies that indicate fearful facial expressions, more than neutral or other emotional expressions, engage the amygdala (Breiter et al., 1996; Morris et al., 1996; Whalen et al., 2001). Further evidence comes from lesion studies, which show that adults who have amygdala lesions have difficulty recognizing fearful faces, but not other facial emotions (Adolphs et al., 2005; Adolphs et al., 1999).

In adolescents with anxiety disorders, higher levels of amygdala activity occur in response to fearful faces as compared to adolescents with no psychiatric disorders (Thomas et al., 2001). Similarly, adolescents with high social anxiety symptoms show greater amygdala response to fearful faces (Killgore and Yurgelun-Todd, 2005). Another study of adolescents with anxiety disorders also found more amygdala response to fearful faces but particularly when the anxious adolescents were thinking about

how afraid they felt while looking at those faces (McClure et al., 2007). Additional work has used a type of face viewing task that simulates potential peer evaluation, a prominent threat to individuals with social anxiety (Guyer et al., 2008). In this study, socially anxious adolescents had greater amygdala activity while they were waiting to be told whether unknown peers would accept or reject them for a social interaction. Across these studies, the documentation of abnormal amygdala function suggests that anxious adolescents are readily influenced by threatening cues, which engages the overinvolvement of amygdala; in turn, this set of processes may compromise emotion regulation and perpetuate chronic, extreme anxiety.

Anxiety involves hypervigilance and enhanced attention to threat; hence, several paradigms have been designed to measure how anxious individuals orient their attention to threat stimuli (Bar-Haim, Dan et al., 2007; Mogg and Bradley, 1998; Pine, Guyer and Leibenluft, 2008). Attention bias to threat is considered to be greater if it takes an individual longer to draw attention away from a threat cue, such as an angry face, in order to respond to a target stimulus. Behavioral studies have shown that adults with high anxiety levels orient toward threat whereas those with low anxiety levels orient away from threat (Mogg and Bradley, 1998; Mogg, Millar and Bradley, 2000; Monk et al., 2004). Children and adolescents with anxiety disorders also show biases toward threat stimuli, such as angry faces (Dalgleish et al., 2003; Taghavi et al., 1999). Neuroimaging research has further shown that adolescents with anxiety disorders show more amygdala activity to threat stimuli than adolescents who are psychiatrically healthy. Such higher levels of amygdala activations are positively associated with greater attention bias as measured by response time (Monk et al., 2008).

Based on EEG, electroencephalographic asymmetry has been found in children with behavioral inhibition and anxiety, who show relatively greater activation of the right frontal lobe than is evident in the left frontal lobe (Perez-Edgar and Fox, 2005). Measuring frontal EEG asymmetry is often considered as a way to quantify the neurobiological roots for the motivational systems of approach and withdrawal behavior. Specifically, the left frontal region directs approach emotions and behaviors to desired stimuli and the right frontal region guides withdrawal behaviors from perceived aversive stimuli. Thus, EEG activity asymmetries have been examined to understand how children differ in the degree to which they approach or withdraw from stimuli. Behavioral inhibition also is thought to be accompanied by increased amygdala response to novel, feared stimuli. In the first longitudinal neuroimaging study of young adults who were characterized as behaviorally inhibited or uninhibited in early childhood, greater amygdala activation was found in response to unfamiliar faces (Schwartz et al., 2003). A similar pattern of heightened amygdala response to fearful faces has been found in adolescents who were behaviorally inhibited across childhood (Perez-Edgar et al., 2007). Thus, young children with a temperamental profile of behavioral inhibition appear to develop the patterns of exaggerated

amygdala response to potentially threatening stimuli (unfamiliar and frightened faces) that are characteristic of adults with anxiety disorders.

Some of the strongest evidence for the importance of emotion regulation in adolescent anxiety problems comes from studies of the prefrontal cortex (PFC). Hyperactivity of the PFC in anxiety disorders may be interpreted as the failure to inhibit inappropriate responses (Thayer and Lane, 2000). Three studies on adolescent anxiety disorders have shown that, in addition to enhanced amygdala response, the ventral prefrontal cortex (vPFC) also shows heightened activity in response to threat stimuli (Guyer et al., 2008; McClure et al., 2007; Monk et al., 2008). Input from vPFC regions is thought to come online during longer durations of threat processing, as opposed to the immediate, rapid response period when the amygdala acts as a fast threat detector. Recruitment of the vPFC further along in sequence of reacting to threat may serve the purpose of regulating the amygdala and associated emotions and behaviors. As such, the vPFC may play a role by stepping in at different time points to help regulate emotional responses via cognitive functions to inhibit behaviors or thoughts, or updating rules or goals. Several researchers have examined whether children's anxiety problems are related to diurnal cortisol levels. The time of day seems to matter. Some researchers have suggested that shy preschoolers (Schmidt et al., 1997) and anxious adolescent girls (Schiefelbein and Susman, 2006) have high cortisol levels in the morning, but many studies have shown that children's anxiety problems are not associated with cortisol awakening response (CAR) or morning cortisol levels (Freitag et al., 2009; Greaves-Lord et al., 2009; Hastings et al., 2009). Things look different later in the day according to several studies indicating higher afternoon cortisol levels among socially wary preschoolers (Essex et al., 2010; Smider et al., 2002). Similarly, Forbes and her colleagues (Forbes et al., 2006) reported that children and youths with diagnosed anxiety disorders had higher cortisol levels in the 2 hours preceding sleep than did children and youths with depression or without psychiatric diagnoses. Overall, then, these studies suggest that anxious children and youths *might* have more active HPA axis systems, especially in the latter part of the diurnal cycle.

It is more certain that anxious children have unusually strong cortisol reactivity to stressful events (Gunnar, 2001). These include normal, everyday challenging events, like spending time in daycare or preschool (Gunnar et al., 2010; Watamura et al., 2003), and more creative stressful events that researchers have used to elicit acute cortisol responses in children. Working with children and youths referred to a clinic for their emotional and behavioral problems, Douglas Granger and his colleagues (Granger et al., 1996; Granger et al., 1994) had children and their parents discuss and attempt to resolve an issue of intense conflict in the parent–child relationship. Children who showed stronger cortisol reactivity to the conflict discussion had more social difficulties related to anxiety and withdrawal from others, and when seen again 6 months later, more internalizing problems and symptoms of anxiety disorders. Public speaking is quite stressful for many people, and adolescents required to give a speech in front of an audience have been found to show larger increases in cortisol levels if they have more anxiety symptoms (Klimes-Dougan et al., 2001). Similarly, most children don't like getting needles, but preschoolers with more internalizing problems (Kestler and Lewis, 2009) and boys with anxiety disorders (Hastings et al., 2009) show particularly strong cortisol reactivity to inoculations and blood-draw procedures.

Despite a wealth of information illustrating that anxious adults show exaggerated physiological reactivity to various challenges and stressful events, there have not been as many investigations of the autonomic parameters of anxiety disorders in children and youth (Merikangas et al., 1999). Deborah Biedel and Samuel Turner have conducted a number of psychophysiological studies comparing children with and without anxiety problems, or comparing children with parents who do or do not have anxiety disorders. Although anxious children

do (Beidel, 1991; Turner, Beidel and Epstein, 1991; Turner, Beidel and Roberson-Nay, 2005). Children and adolescents with anxiety or internalizing problems either do not differ (Bimmel et al., 2008; Hastings, Zahn-Waxler and Usher, 2007; Pine et al., 1998), or they have faster (Beidel, 1991; Dietrich et al., 2007; Olsson et al., 2008) baseline heart rates than children without problems. More consistently, studies show that having anxiety or internalizing problems is associated with greater heart rate and blood pressure reactivity to challenges like public speaking, taking tests and seeing frightening stimuli (Hastings et al., 2007; Pine et al., 1998; Weems et al., 2005). Interestingly, anxious children also are able to monitor the speed of their heart rates more accurately than children without anxiety problems (Eley et al., 2007; Eley et al., 2004), suggesting they might be more highly attuned to their bodily cues of arousal and distress.

Does the heightened cardiac arousal of anxious children stem from strong sympathetic nervous system (SNS) activity, weak parasympathetic nervous system (PNS) regulation or some combination of the two? Unfortunately, there is little research on cardiac pre-ejection pulse (PEP) in children with anxiety problems. Indirect measures of SNS influence suggest that the cardiac activity of anxious adolescents is affected more by the SNS, compared to youths without anxiety problems (Mezzacappa et al., 1997). Jerome Kagan (Kagan, Reznick and Gibbons, 1989) has argued that temperamentally inhibited children have stronger SNS activity than others. Correspondingly, faster PEP (reflecting greater SNS activity) has been found to characterize young children who have extremely fearful responses to strangers (Buss et al., 2004), and also fearful adolescents (Gunnar et al., 2009).

More research has confirmed that respiratory sinus arrhythmia (RSA), the marker of PNS influence over cardiac arousal via the vagus nerve, is associated with anxiety and internalizing problems. Some studies have indicated that children with anxiety and internalizing problems have low baseline RSA or less heart rate variability (Greaves-Lord et al.,

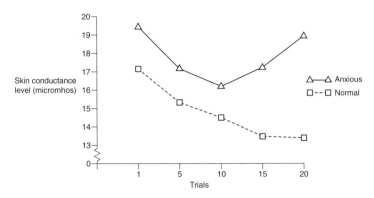

Figure 15.3 Children with anxiety disorders react to a picture of a snake with increasing skin conductance levels.

2007; Pine et al., 1998), but more studies have shown that low baseline RSA increases the risk for anxiety problems if other factors are present, such as poor parenting or troubled families (Bosch et al., 2009; El-Sheikh, 2005; El-Sheikh, Harger and Whitson, 2001; Hastings, Sullivan et al., 2008). If lower RSA reflects less parasympathetic contribution to effective emotional self-regulation, than it makes sense that poorly regulated children would be at greater risk for manifesting anxious adjustment when they are raised in maladaptive conditions. Changes in RSA in response to a variety of tasks or challenges also have been associated with children's anxiety and internalizing problems, both directly (Boyce et al., 2001; Gazelle and Druhen, 2009; Hastings, Nuselovici et al., 2008), and in the presence of other risk factors (El-Sheikh, 2001; El-Sheikh et al., 2009; El-Sheikh and Whitson, 2006). Although findings are mixed, there is evidence that the pattern of RSA change that characterizes anxious children is one of exaggerated withdrawal of PNS activity. This is logical because stronger RSA suppression is thought to support the kinds of defensive and avoidant behaviors that are associated with the fight-or-flight response. When anxious children experience stress, their PNS withdraws its calming influence, their heart rates accelerate and they become physiologically prepared to take flight.

Finally, some studies have identified associations between children's anxiety and internalizing problems and the other two indicators of sympathetic nervous system activity, electrodermal activity (EDA) and salivary alpha-amylase (sAA). More non-specific electrodermal response, and greater electrodermal response and electrodermal activity reactivity to frightening stimuli, have been found to characterize children with anxiety problems or children with anxious parents (Figure 15.3) (El-Sheikh and Harger, 2001; Turner et al., 1991; Turner et al., 2005; Weems et al., 2005). This would suggest that increased SNS activity, as well as decreased parasympathetic nervous system activity, contribute to anxious children's autonomic arousal. Mona El-Sheikh and her colleagues (El-Sheikh et al., 2008) have found that children with higher EDA or more sAA have more internalizing problems when they also have stronger hypothalamic-pituitary-adrenal (axis system) (HPA) reactivity, as shown by elevated cortisol levels (Figure 15.4). Multiple physiological systems probably are working in combination to affect children's emotions and behaviors. Anxious children seem prone to an experience of globally heightened reactivity when they are faced with intimidating challenges.

Parenting

Children's anxiety, even if not caused initially by any aspect of family life, generates parental behaviors that may lead to greater anxiety (Wood et al., 2003).

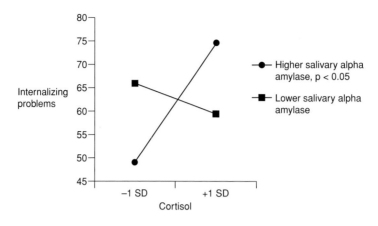

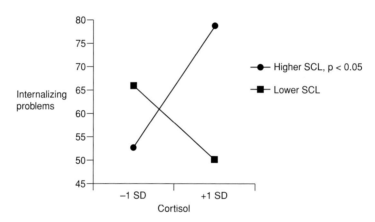

Figure 15.4 Children with high salivary alpha-amylase or skin conductance levels (both are sympathetic indices) and high cortisol levels (HPA axis) have the most internalizing disorders.

Recent progress in theory-building and research has led to the specification of different parenting styles that are linked with children's anxiety disorders. Based on the two dimensions of parental warmth and parental control, these styles can be dichotomized as either models of *affectionless control* or *affectionate control*. Control becomes a central issue because of the belief of many experts that anxiety disorders arise when children feel that they have no control over their lives or social situations. Some overcontrolling parents dominate in ways that are devoid of warmth and affection (Chorpita and Barlow, 1998; DiBartolo and Helt, 2007). Others, often because they perceive their inhibited children as vulnerable and fragile, are equally controlling and overprotective but in ways that convey affection and even overindulgence. They deny their children age-appropriate opportunities to explore the social world and learn social skills, making it even more difficult for the children to overcome their difficulties (Rubin and Mills, 1991).

Although the parents of anxious children are often anxious themselves, it should not be assumed that it is the parents' anxiety that leads to overcontrol and/or lack of warmth. In a meta-analysis of twenty-three studies conducted with 1,305 parent–child dyads, Van der Bruggen, Stams and Bögels (2008) found no significant links between parental anxiety and overcontrol of their children. However, the links between the children's anxiety and the parents' control were significant. Among the participants in a recent observational study by Van der Bruggen, Bögels and Van Zeilst (2010), fathers' anxiety was in fact associated with *lower* levels of parental control. Interestingly, mothers with both very high and very low levels of anxiety controlled their children more than did mothers with moderate levels of anxiety. These preliminary findings provide a reminder that moderate levels of anxiety can be facilitative. More revealing, however, was the finding that the child's anxiety predicted overcontrol by parents more strongly and consistently.

Attachment and anxiety

Manassis (2001) elaborated on the specific ways in which maladaptive attachment patterns might be linked to anxiety disorders. She speculated that different insecure attachment styles would be associated with the different forms of anxiety disorders. She suggested, first of all, that separation anxiety disorder would be linked with ambivalent attachment, in which the child alternates between seeking contact with the caregiver, exhibiting distress when the caregiver becomes unavailable and displaying anger afterwards. Manassis proposed that, in this situation, the caregivers become frustrated with the children's inconsistent attempts at relating, which only worsens the situation. In contrast, she speculated that children involved in avoidant attachment relationships with their caregivers, displaying low levels of contact as well as low levels of distress, might develop a pattern of limiting social contacts that leads to social phobia. Disorganized attachment patterns, which are characterized by a lack of a coherent pattern of attachment relations, sometimes accompanied by the child developing a concern about the caregiver's adequacy and well-being, might be associated with social phobia accompanied by separation anxiety according to Manassis' theory.

Several studies conducted with school-age children have confirmed that secure child–parent attachment is generally linked with lower levels of both social anxiety and separation anxiety (Bar-Haim, Dan et al., 2007; Bohlin, Hagekull and Rydell, 2000; Brumariu and Kerns, 2008; Moss et al., 2006). Summarizing the results of forty-six original studies conducted with almost 9,000 participants, Colonnesi and her colleagues (2011) found that anxiety was moderately correlated with insecure attachment. Many anxious children were found to display ambivalent attachment patterns (see Chapter 6).

The father's role

As reported in the section on genetics earlier in this chapter, children are more likely to develop anxiety disorders if they have relatives with anxiety disorders. Although research results are not entirely consistent, this increased risk appears to apply to both fathers and mothers, especially in the case of social phobia (Bögels and Phares, 2008). Observational studies suggest that fathers of anxious children are highly controlling, provide little useful guidance and may not engage in playful interactions with their children. This was demonstrated graphically in a study by Greco and Morris (2002), in which the fathers of anxious young children were frequently observed to physically grab the origami materials from the hands of their children and to take over from their children the task of assembling the paper figure. Perhaps because of this type of fathering, highly anxious children indicated in a study by Perry and Millimet (1977) that they got along better with their mothers than with their fathers. Based on the results of the few studies available, Bögels and Phares (2008) propose that the parenting provided by fathers is more affected by their own anxiety, especially social anxiety, than is the parenting provided by mothers. These authors report some new data suggesting that this transmission of anxiety from parent to child is more likely in sons than in daughters. In another recent study, McShane and Hastings (2009) found that fathers' supportiveness in relating to their preschool children was correlated with lower levels of anxiety among daughters but not sons.

Peer relations

Rubin and his colleagues describe a spiral in which children who are initially shy during early childhood are rejected by their peers because of their non-participation in group activities and atypical behaviors. This rejection is then mirrored in a negative self-concept, which increases the child's anxiety and social withdrawal. Withdrawal from social participation also restricts the natural, developmental unfolding of the social-cognitive and social skills needed for competent social relationships because these skills are learned and practiced in social interactions. In many but not all cases, the spiral ends with anxiety disorder and/or depression (Rubin, Coplan and Bowker, 2009). One of the possible determinants of progression along this spiral is whether the withdrawn, inhibited child's parents grant autonomy to the child or overcontrol and overprotect, as will be discussed shortly (Rubin, Burgess and Hastings, 2002).

Studies on the peer reputation of anxious children and adolescents confirm, first of all, that they are often disliked by their peers (Degnan, Almas and Fox, 2010; Gazelle and Ladd, 2003; Greco and Morris, 2005; Inderbitzen, Walters and Bukowski, 1997; Verduin and Kendall, 2008; Vernberg et al., 1992). An observational study by Spence, Donovan and Brechman-Toussaint (1999) revealed that children diagnosed with social phobia receive relatively few positive responses from their school peers. Peers also make negative remarks about them (Waas and Graczyk, 1999). They are victimized at school by bullies. This victimization may be both the result of their anxiety in social situations, which marks them as targets, and the cause of further anxiety (Siegel, La Greca and Harrison, 2009; Storch, et al., 2005). There is some evidence that the experience of being bullied not only increases anxiety but that, by increasing anxiety, the bullying affects cortisol levels in the brain (Carney et al., 2010). Friendships may provide some support that buffers the consequences of being disliked by most members of the peer group (Erath et al., 2010).

However, studies about the quality of the friendships of socially anxious children and youth have indicated inconsistent findings as to exactly how supportive and intimate the friendships actually are (Rubin et al., 2006; Fordham and Stevenson-Hinde, 1999; Schneider, 1999). This is important for future researchers to resolve because research has shown that anxious children who have friendships of good quality respond better to psychotherapy than other anxious children (Baker and Hudson, 2013).

Researchers have invested considerable effort in attempts to determine exactly what brings about the scorn and rejection of anxious children and youth by their peers. Raters who view videotapes of the speech or social interactions of anxious children and adolescents can easily distinguish them from videotapes of participants without anxiety. The anxious speakers are often rated as awkward in their body language, speech and facial expressions (e.g., Miers, Blöte and Westenberg, 2010). Schneider and his colleagues conducted a series of studies on the friendships of anxious children. When observed in interaction with their friends during games and negotiations about the sharing of desired objects, anxious children were found to be quiet and unassuming, reluctant to engage in friendly competition or to compare their artwork with that of their friends (Schneider, 1999, 2009). Related to these deficits in social interactions with even close friends may be a less mature understanding of the basic concept of friendship than is prevalent among age-mates. In written compositions about their expectations of their best friends, socially withdrawn and anxious children wrote that they expected their friends to satisfy their own psychological needs more often than did other study participants, who were more likely to recognize the reciprocal nature of friendship (Schneider and Tessier, 2007).

Stability and prognosis

Research findings about the stability of child and adolescent anxiety disorders vary considerably.

Important in understanding the data is the distinction between *homotypic continuity* and *heterotypic continuity* – whether the child or adolescent has the same exact form of anxiety disorder at follow-up or any form of anxiety disorder or psychopathology. In studies focusing on homotypic continuity at two specific time points, the stability rate may be no higher than 15 or 20 percent. Specific phobia in particular may disappear with the onset of adolescence (Beidel and Alfano, 2011). However, other than children with specific phobia, it is very likely that a person who has suffered from an anxiety disorder during childhood or adolescence is very likely to suffer from some type of anxiety disorder and/or depression during a substantial part of adolescence or adulthood, with full remission occurring in fewer than one-third of cases according to most studies (Beesdo et al., 2009; Bittner et al., 2007; Rapee, Schniering and Hudson, 2009).

Much less is known about the long-term prognosis for children and adolescents with anxiety disorders than for children with most other forms of psychopathology that are very common. The main reason for this gap in knowledge is that recognition has only come recently that children's anxiety disorders are a widespread and debilitating problem. Therefore, not many longitudinal studies of children with anxiety problems were launched a few generations ago. However, with time, it is increasingly recognized that early anxiety often leads to social exclusion and to later depression (Gazelle and Ladd, 2003; Gazelle, Workman and Allan, 2010).

Anxiety disorders also affect school participation, academic achievement and, indeed, enrolment in school. Ameringen, Mancini and Farvolden (2003) conducted a study with adult patients admitted to the psychiatry department of a hospital in Hamilton, Ontario, Canada. Of the 201 whose primary diagnosis was anxiety disorder, 49 percent reported leaving school prematurely. Of these, 24 percent cited anxiety as the reason for leaving school.

Prevention and treatment

Primary prevention

Because almost everyone experiences anxiety to some degree, the content of the cognitive-behavioral interventions described in the next section may be useful to the general population of children and adolescents, not just to those who are at risk of developing anxiety disorders. Recognizing this, several Australian researchers have adapted the content of the Coping Cat program, described in the subsequent section on therapy, for use as a primary prevention technique. The prevention program has been delivered mostly in schools, either by psychologists or by schoolteachers; evening sessions are held for parents. Evaluations of the program indicate that program participants who were at risk of developing anxiety disorders were less likely to develop full-blown disorder than were members of the control groups (Barret and Turner, 2001; Lowry-Webster, Barrett and Dadds, 2001). Other school-based prevention programs have been conducted in interventions ranging from two sessions to a full school year. In a comprehensive meta-analysis of the benefits of twenty school-based prevention and early-intervention programs, Neil and Christensen (2009) reported that three-fourths of the programs were successful in reducing the anxiety of children and adolescents significantly. Unfortunately, very few of the researchers gathered long-term follow-up data to assess the maintenance of the effects of the prevention programs. Despite this shortcoming, it is reasonable to conclude that primary and early secondary prevention of anxiety constitutes a worthwhile investment.

Cognitive-behavior therapy

Cognitive-behavioral methods are the most widely used form of treatment for children and adolescents and, to date, the most successful. Most cognitive-behavioral interventions are specified in procedures manuals that have facilitated the evaluation of their effectiveness. The exact ways of delivering cognitive-behavioral therapy (CBT) and the content of the interventions that are considered cognitive-behavioral vary considerably.

The pioneering cognitive-behavioral intervention for children and youth with anxiety disorders was introduced by Phillip Kendall of Temple University in Philadelphia in 1994 (Kendall, 1994). The Coping Cat program consists of four basic components: (1) recognizing anxiety and its physical manifestations (sometimes called *psychoeducation*); (2) learning to recognize and label the emotions that arise in situations that provoke anxiety; (3) learning to cope, for example by using self-talk to assess situations objectively, determining the best ways of dealing with them and learning how to relax while under stress; and (4) learning to praise oneself for making progress. Different versions of the program have been developed for children from 8 to 13 years old and adolescents 14 to 17 years old. In order to prepare the participants for venturing out into situations they find anxiety-provoking, they prepare an *exposure hierarchy* in which they start by listing situations that provoke only slight anxiety, placing highly anxiety-provoking situations at the peak of the hierarchy. Relaxation and guided visual imagery prepare the child or adolescent for gradual exposure to the situations that provoke anxiety. "Homework assignments" are designed to help transfer what is learned to the participants' daily lives. Typical assignments include the practice of new skills or the observation of specific situations (Hudson and Kendall, 2002). During the final sessions of the 16-week program, the therapist encourages the participant to begin attempting the situations in the hierarchy, starting with those at the bottom of the list, which are those at which the child or adolescent is most likely to succeed at first. In complementary parent sessions, the parents learn about the content of their child's treatment and how they can help (Kendall, 1994; Kendall and Hedtke, 2006).

The evidence for the effectiveness of this and similar programs is impressive. Based on a thorough review of thirty-two studies known for their methodological rigor, Silverman, Pina and Viswesvaran (2008) concluded that both individual and group cognitive-behavioral therapy could be rated as "probably efficacious" according to the standards specified for evidence-based treatments (see Chapter 11). There appears to be no systematic difference between the effectiveness of group and individual administration. Cartwright-Hatton et al. (2004) estimated that an average of about 57 percent of children in treatment groups improved at the end of treatment to the point that their problems were no longer diagnosable as anxiety disorders, compared with the spontaneous recovery of about 30 percent of the participants in control groups. Follow-up of treatment participants for as long as 7 years after the end of therapy indicates very satisfactory maintenance of the improvement for many children with anxiety disorders (Kendall, Safford, Flannery-Schroeder and Webb, 2004). This does not mean, however, that a miracle cure has taken place and that all anxiety is gone forever. Many former participants do experience some degree of anxiety, often not enough for them to be diagnosed again as having an anxiety disorder but enough to seek some "booster" help (Hudson, 2005). Furthermore, children and adolescents with social anxiety do not seem to respond as well as young people with other forms of anxiety disorder at 7-year follow-up. Kerns et al. (2013) speculate that, in order to achieve long-term success with children with social anxiety, social skills training may have to be added to the cognitive elements of CBT.

Most of the studies confirming the effectiveness of CBT involve comparisons of active treatment with children and adolescents on a waiting list. In an important methodological advance, Hudson et al. (2009) compared cognitive-behavioral treatment with a control condition in which the participants received an equivalent amount of support and attention from their therapists. The responses of the control-group participants to an expectancy questionnaire indicated that they found the treatment credible and expected to improve. The results showed that the cognitive-behavioral intervention was clearly superior.

CASE STUDY: Bruce, an 8-year-old with social anxiety and selective mutism

Reuther and colleagues (2011) present an interesting case study of an 8-year-old with both social anxiety and selective mutism who was helped by CBT. Bruce, who lives with both his parents and several siblings, came for treatment with his mother. At the time he started treatment, Bruce would speak only to members of his immediate family but not to his teachers, schoolfriends, classmates or grandparents. He would only speak to his parents and siblings while they were in their own home. Bruce had previously seen a psychiatrist, who prescribed Prozac, an antidepressant in the SSRI class of medications. During the weeks during which he was on Prozac, Bruce managed to utter one short phrase on a single occasion, the first time he ever spoke in school. Bruce seemed to get along well with his classmates despite his refusal to speak. In fact, they often spoke for him.

The clinic at which Bruce was treated used a variety of methods to assess Bruce's difficulties, including a standardized assessment interview designed for the diagnosis of anxiety disorders, the Anxiety Disorders Interview for Children: DSM-IV Parent version (ADIS-IV; Silverman and Albano, 1996). At the beginning of the individual assessment sessions, Bruce was frozen and totally unresponsive. However, as contact continued, Bruce began to point with his fingers to respond. This enabled the diagnosticians to establish on the basis of at least receptive language that an intellectual disability was highly unlikely. Bruce would not speak with his family members during a family assessment session at which a therapist was present but did speak in a session that the therapist observed through a one-way mirror. The diagnoses of social phobia and selective mutism were clearly indicated by all sources of information available to the diagnostic team.

A standard CBT protocol was supplemented by a number of preliminary sessions designed to increase communication between Bruce and his therapists. At the same time, the therapist encouraged the family to stop accommodating Bruce's non-communication by speaking for him in social situations. During the first four sessions, Bruce played a game with his family members at the clinic, with the therapist progressively joining in, first from outside the room, then from the edge of the room until, at last, the therapist could join the game as a full-fledged participant. Small prizes were offered as reinforcers at the end of each session for Bruce's cooperation with the therapist's integration into the communication. After four sessions, Bruce made eye contact with the therapist and met the goal of saying at least three words to the therapist at least three times during a session.

From this point on, the standard CBT procedures could be implemented, including psychoeducation about the nature of anxiety, construction of an anxiety hierarchy, graduated exposure to situations of increasing anxiety as indicated in the hierarchy, and social skills training. Bruce's family were present for the first few CBT sessions, but this was faded out subsequently. Progress outside the therapy sessions was tracked as well. Bruce's verbal interactions with adults and peers at school were tracked; he earned special privileges, such as a pizza meal or movie, for increasing his interactions each week. For the last few of the twenty-one CBT sessions, Bruce was able to check in with the clinic receptionist when he arrived each time. Bruce was talking regularly to both teachers and peers at school. At follow-up visits at 1 month and 6 months, it was determined that the treatment gains had been maintained and that Bruce's behavior no longer corresponded with the diagnoses of selective mutism or social phobia.

Alternatives to CBT

Research support for psychotherapies other than CBT in the treatment of anxiety disorders among children and adolescents is extremely limited. Other approaches have indeed been tried, such as brief psychoanalytic therapy in which the core goals are insight, self-expression through play and the experience of a close therapeutic relationship (Warren and Messer, 1999). School-based humanistic counseling has been shown to be effective for early adolescents suffering from "emotional distress," many of whom may have suffered from anxiety problems, according to a preliminary randomized trial conducted in Strathclyde, Scotland (Cooper et al., 2010). However, because of their very limited basis in research, approaches other than CBT cannot be considered science-based at this point, especially in light of the substantial data from CBT studies indicating that children's and adolescents' anxiety problems can be treated successfully in psychotherapy.

New technology for delivering CBT

Although the relationship with a therapist is often considered fundamental in psychotherapy, it is important to remember that many relationships in contemporary society, including therapeutic relationships are developed and maintained at least partially online. Furthermore, geography and life circumstances may preclude personal on-site participation in individual or group CBT at treatment sites. Kendall et al. (2011) emphasize the distinction between *computer-based therapy*, in which the entire therapy would be delivered through a website or CD, and *computer-assisted therapy*, in which some of the content is delivered using electronic means. However, there is still a therapist known to the treatment participant. Contact between the therapist and the treatment participant might be partially by email, chat or telephone, reflecting the realities of communication for many children and adolescents. Several studies have demonstrated the viability of computer-assisted therapy for children

and adolescents with anxiety disorders (e.g., March et al., 2009).

Virtual-reality therapy is an exciting new technique in which the person seeking treatment is brought to a space in which an environment that has generated anxiety is simulated visually and auditorily. The anxiety-inducing elements of the environment can be increased or decreased in intensity or proximity by the software that generates the environment, as shown in Figure 15.5a and b. These techniques have been used successfully in the treatment of adults' anxiety disorders but are only beginning to be used with children and adolescents. So far, most of the applications have been to specific phobia or school refusal. However, the technique has the potential to facilitate the exposure component of CBT for other anxiety problems including social phobia (Bouchard, 2011).

Family treatment

Although it is believed by many professionals that parent involvement is crucial in the treatment of anxiety disorders as in most forms of child psychopathology, there is no clear, consistent empirical evidence for that contention (Rapee et al., 2009; Silverman et al., 2008). Wood and his colleagues (2006) developed the Building Confidence program directed at enhancing child–parent communication and age-appropriate granting of autonomy, reducing problematic overcontrol and intrusiveness by the participating parents. The participants were the parents of children and early adolescents with anxiety disorders, 6 to 13 years old. The children whose parents participated in the Building Confidence program improved more than the children in a control group that received traditional child-focused CBT. In working with young children who have anxiety problems, intervention with the parents alone may be optimal. A recent study with waiting-list control by Cartwright-Hatton and his colleagues (2011) was conducted with the parents of children from 2.5 to 9 years old. The results demonstrated that an intervention focus

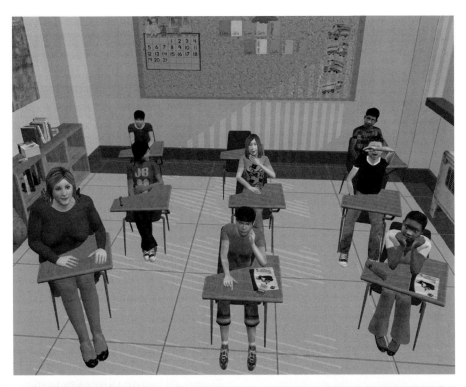

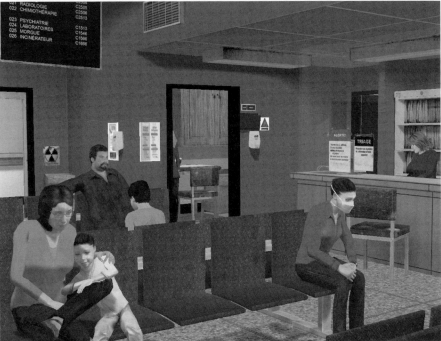

Figure 15.5a and b Images used in the treatment of social and generalized anxiety at the Virtual Reality Laboratory at the Université du Québec en Outaouis.

on parent–child communication and appropriate discipline resulted in substantial improvement in the child's symptoms. Similar success was reported by Rapee and his colleagues (2005), who conducted a six-session parent-group intervention with parents (mostly mothers) of 3- to 5-year-olds showing early signs of problematic anxiety.

Pharmacotherapy

Several different types of medication are known to relieve anxiety in children and adolescents as well as the adults for whom the medications were first developed and tested. A specific class of medications developed for anxiety problems, benzodiazepines, does exist. The most common of the benzodiazepines is Valium (diazepam). Although the benzodiazepines do bring short-term relief, there are many problems in using this type of medication, starting with the fact that its effectiveness lasts only a few hours. More importantly, side effects include addiction as well as building up a tolerance to the medication, leading to the need for higher doses (Pine and Klein, 2010). However, and probably because of the many similarities between anxiety and mood disorders, discussed earlier in this chapter, the SSRIs (serotonin reuptake inhibitors), developed for the treatment of depression, are effective in reducing anxiety disorders as well; the SSRIs have fewer side effects than the other medications available. In a number of studies, therapy with SSRIs has been proven more effective than placebo medication. However, the effects of children and adolescents taking SSRIs on a long-term basis are not known (Rynn et al., 2011). Furthermore, there have been some warnings from government regulatory agencies that in a very small number of cases, children and adolescents who take SSRIs may experience agitation and increased suicidal thoughts (Pine and Klein, 2010). Therefore, it is probably prudent to use SSRIs in only certain specific cases where it is clear that CBT alone will not bring improvement and even then under regular professional supervision. Several studies have yielded inconsistent evidence that the combination of CBT and pharmacotherapy will lead to any greater effectiveness than either of these therapies by themselves (Beidel and Alfano, 2011; Rynn et al., 2011). Therefore, at the current state of knowledge, there is no basis for complementing CBT with pharmacotherapy in general. This situation may change with new research and the appearance of new medications, and with research based on larger sample sizes and valid, multiple measures of outcome (Beidel and Alfano, 2011).

Conclusions and future directions

Although the current data base pertaining to the anxiety disorders of children and adolescents is not small, most experts in the field believe that awareness of these problems is just beginning. Most cases of child and adolescent anxiety disorder probably remain unnoticed and untreated. If one adds the probable cases of anxiety-related school refusal (see Chapter 22) to the number of undiagnosed cases of anxiety disorders that have formal diagnostic status at present, the total surely reaches a very substantial part of the total population of children and adolescents.

The familiar tone of the scenarios in the major CBT intervention packages may leave the impression that the treatment of anxiety disorders is easy; it is not. Interaction styles rooted in individual temperament and exacerbated by parental overcontrol and isolation from peer interaction do not change without considerable effort. Existing interventions have, fortunately, a solid track record of success. Most experts believe that the interventions still need fine tuning in order to achieve optimal effectiveness.

Thus, the field of anxiety disorders in children and adolescents may not benefit from any sudden, revolutionary development in research and treatment in the next few years. However, by continuing along the trajectory of the past 30 years or so, during which the magnitude of the problem has entered into widespread awareness, much further progress may well be made.

Summary

- Anxiety is best thought of as fear of a real, imagined or exaggerated future event, as opposed to fear or panic pertaining to a primarily imminent threat or danger.
- There are many different forms of anxiety disorder including separation anxiety disorder (separation from one's caregiver), social anxiety (fear of social contact) and obsessive-compulsive disorder (OCD).
- Selective mutism is defined as not speaking in certain social situations, such as at school.
- Some social critics believe that anxiety disorder diagnoses are a means of suppressing children who are not sociable.
- The estimated lifetime prevalence of anxiety disorders is 15–20 percent. Some consider anxiety disorders the most prevalent childhood psychopathology around.
- Most children and adolescents with one specific anxiety disorder will have another anxiety disorder. Depression is comorbid with anxiety disorders 16–62 percent of the time.
- Clark and Wilson's tripartite model attributes the link between depression and anxiety mainly to negative affect, but also to low positive affect.
- Girls are at greater risk for anxiety disorders than boys across cultures. This could be due to real causes such as hormonal causes in girls, fear of maltreatment by men or, alternatively, simply because it is more socially acceptable for girls to have anxiety (e.g., in English-speaking cultures).
- Gay and lesbian adolescents are at greater risk for anxiety as well. This may be because of homophobic bullying, social isolation alienation and lack of social support.
- Studies conducted with East Asian adults suggest that a focus on reputation and the avoidance of shame leads to higher rates of anxiety than in English-speaking cultures. Studies conducted with East Asian children and children of Anglo-European origin have yielded less consistent results.

- Social phobias in certain cultures are particularly debilitating. Because being nice, outgoing and sociable is a core value in Latin America, social anxiety may be particularly debilitating there.
- Concordance rates from twin studies for diagnosed anxiety disorders are 12–26 percent for monozygotic (MZ) twins, compared with 4–15 percent of dizygotic (DZ) twins. The genetic heritability estimate for anxiety disorders ranges from 20 to 40 percent.
- Among preschool children, 10–15 percent are found to be behaviorally inhibited.
- The heritability estimate for behavioral inhibition is .50 to .70.
- fMRi and structured observation task studies performed with child and adolescent participants as well as brain lesion observations of adults and animal lesion studies implicate abnormal amygdala function as a psychobiological cause behind anxiety.
- Children with high anxiety are more likely than those with low anxiety to orient toward threatening stimuli such as angry faces. Children with post-traumatic stress disorder (PTSD), however, often orient their gaze away from threat.
- In studies of children displaying high levels of anxiety, behaviorally inhibited children showed strong amygdala activation in response to fearful faces.
- The ventral prefrontal cortex (vPFC), responsible for inhibiting inappropriately lengthy anxiety responses to stimuli, is also overactive in anxious adolescents.
- For some, but not all anxiety disorders, anxious children and youths display more active hypothalamic-pituitary-adrenal (cortisol) reactivity in the latter parts of the day.
- Children with anxiety display elevated cortisol responses in conflict situations with their parents, public speaking engagements and at the advent of getting hospital needles.

- Across studies, children and adolescents with anxiety do not always differ in baseline heart rate and blood pressure compared with children and adolescents with less anxiety. Children and youth with anxiety, however, consistently show greater heart rate and blood pressure specifically in response to fearful situations like public speaking.

- Sympathetic nervous system (SNS) activity in adults is associated with anxiety. More anxious children experience lower parasympathetic nervous system (PNS) activity than do less anxious children, especially when other environmental factors are involved such as poor parenting or troubled family circumstances.

- Traditional socialization theory avers that negative parenting practices exacerbate children's anxiety symptoms.

- Fathers' anxiety predicts low levels of parental control, while mothers both high and low in anxiety demonstrate high levels of parental control. Either affectionate or affectionless overcontrol by parents can exacerbate anxiety symptoms in children.

- Manassis' theory suggests that separation anxiety disorder is linked with ambivalent attachment between child and caregiver; social anxiety is linked with avoidant attachment; and social phobia together with separation anxiety disorder is linked with disorganized attachment (no coherent attachment pattern).

- Large-sample research confirms that anxiety is moderately correlated with insecure and ambivalent attachment; secure attachment is associated with lower levels of social anxiety and separation anxiety.

- Children's anxiety is linked to overcontrol in fathers' parenting, with preliminary research showing this is especially the case with boys. Many children with anxiety disorders get along better with their mothers than with their fathers.

- Anxious children often enter a vicious cycle in which their anxiety leads to social exclusion, which in turn damages their self-concept, which in turn increases their anxiety, leading to more social exclusion, etc…

- Anxious children are more likely than non-anxious children to be disliked by peers and victimized in bullies. Negative behaviors of peers of an anxious child may be provoked by the seeming awkwardness, unfriendliness and social immaturity of the anxious children.

- One study revealed that in a sample of 201 adult psychiatric patients, 49 percent reported having left school prematurely, and 24 percent of these reported anxiety as the direct cause.

- The stability rate of anxiety disorder from childhood to adulthood is no more than 15–20 percent when based on homotypic continuity (continuity of the same form of anxiety disorder). Continuity rates are higher for heterotypic continuity of anxiety disorder (continuity of *any* kind of anxiety disorder).

- While longitudinal studies on the continuity of anxiety disorders are scarce, researchers have established to some degree that early anxiety leads to later social exclusion and depression.

- Participants in a primary prevention program based on Coping Cat have been shown to be less likely to develop full-blown anxiety than child members of a control group.

- Kendall's cognitive-behavioral therapy (CBT) interventions, including Coping Cat, treat anxiety in children by educating them about anxiety, helping them label their anxious emotions, teaching them coping strategies for anxiety and encouraging them to praise themselves for progress in dealing with their symptoms.

- While not always successful, CBT is considered efficacious according to the standards specified for evidence-based treatments.

- Alternatives to CBT (e.g., psychoanalytic therapy, humanistic therapy) have not been scientifically validated for treating anxiety disorders.

- CBT can be delivered using computer-based methods where therapy is delivered entirely over the internet or via CD. Computer-assisted therapy is delivered in part by computer with some interaction with a live therapist.

- Virtual-reality therapy is a form of computer technology that helps children overcome phobias with graduated, therapist-controlled exposure to simulated anxiety-provoking stimuli.
- Family treatment has not been consistently validated as critical in individual CBT therapy for children. However, some research shows that adding a family component to child treatment results in significant improvements in the reduction of anxiety symptoms.
- Benzodiazepines (e.g., Valium) have been used to treat anxiety, but their effects last only hours and bring unwanted side effects such as addiction. Selective serotonin reuptake inhibitors (SSRIs) bring fewer side effects than benzodiazepines in anxiety treatments. However, SSRIs may elevate suicidal ideas slightly. Many authorities suggest that they only be prescribed to children and adolescents if psychotherapy fails.
- Only a few studies have shown the greater effectiveness of the combination of CBT and pharmacotherapy on anxiety disorders over either form of therapy alone.
- Advances in the pharmacotherapy of anxiety disorders will be made when specific forms of anxiety disorder are considered one at a time, as opposed to as all anxiety disorders combined. Their evaluation would be facilitated by experimentation with large samples and diverse measures of participant outcomes.

Study questions

1. What forms of anxiety disorder cannot be formally diagnosed among children?
2. What are some possible reasons for the higher rates of anxiety disorder among adolescents of minority sexual orientation?
3. What features of East Asian society may relate to anxiety disorders in those populations, including some of the anxiety conditions that are specific to East Asian culture?
4. What lessons can be learned about anxiety disorder from psychophysiological studies of human response to threat?
5. What is the most effective form of treatment for anxiety disorders in childhood and adolescence?

Part III | Developmental disorders

Intellectual disability

Terminology and stigmatization, intended and unintended

The title of this chapter, intellectual disability, is the new name for this disorder in DSM-5. It was known as *mental retardation* in DSM-IV. The change reflects contemporary usage by experts on intellectual disability, who consider the previous term, "mental retardation," as highly stigmatizing. The term and its derivative "retard" have come to be used as pejorative, as is the case for the previous terms "feeble-minded," "idiot," "imbecile" and "moron," which were used by psychologists and physicians without any intent to offend several decades ago (Schalock et al., 2007; Switzky and Greenspan, 2006). There is nothing inherently pejorative in the term "mental retardation," which in itself signifies no more than that the individual's intellectual development is delayed in comparison to the development of other people; this is indeed true for this segment of the population. Certainly, the professionals who used that term in their research and clinical writing intended no other meaning, including, for example, those who contributed articles to what was called until very recently the *American Journal on Mental Retardation*. However, as language evolved, the word "retard" came to be used pejoratively in daily speech. A recent survey of over 1,000 US youth ranging in age from 8 to 18 years revealed that 92 percent of respondents had heard the "r-word" used in a negative way. Only about a third of these respondents were fully aware of its meaning (Siperstein, Pociask and Collins, 2010). Although the same word seems not to be used as extensively as an epithet in the UK, *BBC News Magazine* reported in 2008 that other pejorative words are

(Rohrer, 2008). Hopefully, the new term "intellectual disability" will not acquire a pejorative connotation over time, perhaps because of its grammatical structure and inherent meaning.

Schalock et al. (2007) elaborate on the implications of the terms *disability* and *intellectual disability*. They note that construct of "disability" implies the interaction between a person and his or her social context. Hence, disability does not reside entirely within the individual; "disability" refers to the limitations of the individual that restrict his or her ability to function in society. Thus, part of the thrust toward revising the terminology reflects the contemporary emphasis on the social context of psychopathology in general, on the interactions between person and environment. Schalock and his colleagues believe that the new term is one around which persons with developmental disabilities will be better able to unite in crystalizing a "disability identity" that will facilitate political action to promote the interests of the group. The American Association on Intellectual and Developmental Disabilities (formerly the American Association on Mental Retardation) has adopted the following definition: "Intellectual disability is characterized by significant limitations both in intellectual functioning and in adaptive behavior as expressed in conceptual, social and practical adaptive skills; this disability originates before age 18" (Luckasson et al., 2002).

At the same time as it permits an emphasis on person–environment interaction, the new term "intellectual disability" reflects the widespread desire of many theorists and professionals to distance themselves from the former reification of the concept of IQ (see Chapter 2). In the heyday of IQ testing, culminating in the 1950s, it was possible to diagnose intellectual disability solely on the basis of low IQ scores. Beginning in 1959, formal diagnostic criteria were modified somewhat to specify that low IQ had to be manifest in a deficiency in *adaptive* behavior, thus moving closer to the current emphasis on the person with disabilities in social context. Reflecting the best thinking of the time at which it was introduced, this was the basis for the diagnosis of mental retardation in DSM-IV. Finally, the term "intellectual disability" is notable for the absence of any connotation of disease or physical abnormality (Schalock et al., 2007). For all these reasons, a consensus in favor of the term "intellectual disability" (or "disabilities") has emerged and is used in DSM-5. It should be noted that the term "learning disability" is sometimes used in the UK to refer to intellectual disabilities. In most other English-speaking countries and in this textbook, the term "learning disability" is used to refer to conditions otherwise known as specific learning disorder or dyslexia – see Chapter 18. In DSM-5, intellectual disability is part of the broad category of neurodevelopmental disorders, pertaining to conditions that are usually evident very early in a person's life, usually before the start of schooling. Included among the neurodevelopmental disorders in DSM-5 are intellectual disability, communication disorders (e.g., language and speech disorders), autism spectrum disorders, attention deficit/hyperactivity disorder, specific language disorder and motor disorders. The communication disorders listed in DSM-5 include a new diagnostic category called social (pragmatic) communication disorder, which was introduced in this textbook in Chapter 15, in which the new disorder is compared with social anxiety disorder. The term "mental retardation" remains in ICD-10 but is sure to be replaced by "intellectual disability" once ICD-11 appears in a few years.

Important as terminology and language are, the impending change in nomenclature is not likely by itself to totally eliminate either the stigma attached to people with intellectual disabilities or inattention to many of their needs. As introduced in Chapter 2, there has been a trend over the past several centuries to demarcate firmly the distinction between intellectual disorder and other forms of psychopathology. This was embodied in the separation in DSM of Axes I and II, which began with DSM-III but which has been eliminated. The distinction between the axes was introduced for the most benevolent of reasons, namely to ensure that clinicians do not overlook important underlying and enduring conditions. However, intellectual disability was separated from most other psychological disorders that are usually first seen in childhood. This continued the practice that started several centuries ago of separating people with intellectual disabilities from other people suffering from the clinical syndromes. As noted by historian Jonathan Andrews (1998), who specializes in the study of the history of ideas about mental illness, this separation is based on the assumption that intellectual disability is incurable, reflecting accurately the fact that contemporary science includes no technique that can change a person with an intellectual disability into a person without one. For that reason, "idiots" were excluded from British insane asylums like Bethlem beginning at the end of the seventeenth century. Although they were deemed untreatable at the time, people with intellectual disability were also deemed to be harmless and free of evil intent, even as they were thought to be incapable of rational thinking. These ideas were expressed by Shakespeare in *Hamlet*, in which he wrote about "a tale told by an idiot . . . full of sound and fury, signifying nothing." Andrews (1998) comments that these ideas, benevolent as they may have been, have served throughout the ages to obscure the fact that people with intellectual disabilities can indeed be taught many things. As will be discussed later in this chapter, they can also experience many forms of mental suffering aside from intellectual disability that psychologists can help alleviate.

Box 16.1 | **Differences between DSM-IV and DSM-5 criteria for intellectual disability (intellectual developmental disorder)**

- In DSM-5, the name of the disorder has been changed from "mental retardation" to "intellectual disability (intellectual developmental disorder)."
- In both DSM-IV and DSM-5, the disorder is characterized by general impairments in intellectual ability.
- In both DSM-IV and DSM-5, the individual must score 70 or lower on an IQ test, or approximately in the lowest 1 percent. However, in DSM-5, there is an emphasis on ensuring that the test is culturally appropriate.
- In both versions, the disorder must first appear relatively early in life. In DSM-IV, this is defined as prior to age 18, but in DSM-5, this is defined as during the period of development.
- DSM-5 emphasizes that there must have been significant impairment in an important area of daily life.

Source: DSM-5 and DSM-IV-TR consulted June 6, 2013.

Table 16.1 **Typical features of different levels of intellectual disability**

Level	Identifiable Organic Cause	Intellectual Functioning and Language Proficiency	Self-care	Social Functioning
Mild	Usually none identifiable	• Usually acquire language, but with some delay • Many have difficulty with abstraction and synthesis • Usually require special educational programming and profit from it • Usually capable of reading and writing but with difficulty	• Function independently in eating, washing, dressing, bowel and bladder control. May achieve independent functioning later than most children	• May achieve age-typical social relationships in settings in which little academic achievement is required • May have difficulty in social interactions requiring advanced coping skills or functioning in more than one culture • Same range of social maladaptation as in typical populations

Table 16.1 **(cont.)**

Moderate	Usually	• Language develops slowly and remains immature, with some able to participate in uncomplicated conversations	• Self-care and motor skills develop slowly but most become fully active and mobile • Many require supervision throughout their lifetimes	• Many are able to establish social contact and converse but not at the level of typically developing populations
		• Some master rudimentary reading, writing and counting • Often have very different abilities in different domains (language, memory, visuo-spatial, motoric)		
Severe/ Profound	Almost always	• Marked impairment of language and thinking abilities • Some able to master rudimentary vocabulary and/or non-verbal communication	• Marked impairment of motor skills • Limited mobility • Many are incontinent • Most require constant supervision throughout their lifetimes	• Most have very limited capacities for social interaction but many may be able to learn eye contact, basic greetings, motor skills to help with some household tasks

Source: ICD-10 Guide for Mental Retardation, World Health Organization, Geneva, 1996.

Conceptual controversy: should intellectual disability be considered a form of psychopathology?

Rarely raised these days is the question of whether intellectual disability should be considered a form of psychopathology at all. However, it has been argued that intellectual disability by itself constitutes nothing more than the lower end of the population distribution of cognitive skills and adaptive behavior and is not necessarily pathological. From that perspective, only the large number of individuals who have an emotional or behavioral disorder as well as intellectual and adaptive skills well below the norm should be considered among the population of people with mental illness (Bebko and Weiss, 2005).

This chapter continues with information about the epidemiology of intellectual disability, including information about diagnostic criteria, prevalence and comorbid conditions. Included in the section on epidemiology is information about the most common syndromes in intellectual disability and their causes. Peer, family and cultural factors are considered next. A variety of interventions are discussed subsequently. The chapter closes with a discussion of the ever-increasing efforts to facilitate participation by children and adolescents with intellectual disability in community life to the greatest extent possible.

Diagnosis, prevalence and major causal syndromes

An important advance in DSM-5 is that equal or even greater weight is now assigned to adaptive functioning as opposed to IQ scores, which featured more prominently in the DSM-IV criteria. Adaptive functioning refers to the age-appropriate basic skills required in daily life, including the skills needed to care for one's body and belongings, protect oneself from danger, follow rules, learn in school or engage in paid work, relate to others, make decisions, maintain one's health, communicate successfully and use means of transportation. Adaptive behavior is typically assessed by obtaining information in an interview or questionnaire from people in the child's environment, such as parents, teachers and caregivers. The DSM-5 criteria include both deficit in intellectual functions, which can often be measured with intelligence tests, and deficit in adaptive functioning. Importantly, however, it is the individual's adaptive functioning that determines whether his or her intellectual disability is to be considered mild, moderate, severe or profound. This decision is justified by the fact that it is the level of adaptive functioning, rather than the IQ score, that determines how much support and care the person needs.

Many authorities regard intellectual disability of moderate, severe and profound degrees as very distinct from mild intellectual disability, almost to the point of delineating two separate disorders. The ICD-10 guide comments that the functioning of people with mild intellectual disability (mental retardation) is more similar to that of people with typical intellectual development than to the functioning of people with more pronounced intellectual disabilities. An organic cause can only be identified in some cases. Their self-care skills are typically delayed, but they can function well if given proper support. If given proper instruction, they may master rudimentary elements of reading as needed for basic community interaction. As adults, they can perform useful work under supervision, often in sheltered workshops (World Health Organization, 1996). Many young people with

moderate to severe intellectual disability have been able to learn to communicate with sign language at a level higher than they could achieve with verbal expression (e.g., Dalrymple and Feldman, 1992).

In contrast, individuals with severe and profound intellectual disability often are impaired in their motor functions and are likely to require assistance with basic self-care throughout their lives. In most cases, damage or atypical development of the central nervous system can be identified (World Health Organization, 1996).

The definitions and diagnostic criteria for intellectual disability in DSM-5 and ICD-10 are deceivingly simple. The population of children and adults with intellectual disabilities are in fact a far more heterogeneous group than the diagnostic categories suggest. This can be attributed chiefly to the fact that causal etiology has been eliminated from these diagnostic systems, as discussed in Chapter 3. However, in the case of intellectual disability, many of the physical and behavioral features of the pathology are more closely identified with known symptom patterns than is true for most other disorders.

Prevalence

Estimates of the prevalence of intellectual disability among children and adolescents depend heavily on the cut-offs specified for both adaptive behavior and IQ. Prevalence data based on DSM-5 criteria are not yet available. However, prevalence studies that are not based on any version of DSM can be used as a guide. There are consequences of different cut-off points that have been debated widely, as reviewed by MacMillan, Siperstein and Leffert (2006). The controversy pertains to cases of mild intellectual disability. As noted by Siperstein and his colleagues, these are the cases that are likely to pose any challenge to clinicians contemplating diagnoses. They also represent the majority of children who are diagnosed with intellectual disability, as many as 80 percent. Unlike children with more severe intellectual deficits, which are usually obvious to most observers, they often have no physical anomalies. By the time they reach school age, children with mild intellectual disability may require no particular assistance with personal hygiene, self-care or locomotion. There is often no known medical reason for their intellectual disabilities. Furthermore, their intellectual challenges may be apparent only in the school setting. A disproportion of children diagnosed as having mild intellectual disability come from poor families, often of minority cultural origin, in which the parents have limited formal education. For these reasons, the diagnosis of mild intellectual disability can be seen as stigmatizing and unwarranted. This issue calls into question the very purposes of diagnosis and classification as discussed in Chapter 3. Children with mild intellectual disability might be better off not being diagnosed unless diagnosis provides access to substantial special services, which may or may not happen. MacMillan, Siperstein and Leffert note that that in recent years, there has been a tendency, especially among educational authorities, to avoid the category of mild intellectual disability in the identification of pupils requiring special services (MacMillan, Siperstein and Leffert, 2006). As the number of pupils diagnosed as having intellectual disability has decreased, there has been a concomitant increase in the number of pupils diagnosed as having learning disabilities (in the North American use of the term, with reference to such conditions as specific learning disorders – see Chapter 18). These authors question the benefit of this misdiagnosis. They offer several suggestions for improvement. First of all, they suggest that there be a separate diagnostic category for children with mild intellectual disabilities, as was common in diagnostic schemes that were used up to the past few decades. Second, they suggest that consideration be given to replacing IQ measures with more specific measures of social cognition that focus on specific cognitive abilities that relate directly to successful functioning inside and outside of school. Finally, they argue for refinement of the measurement and definition of adaptive behavior, to include specific behaviors inherent in adapting to the social demands of both teachers and peers.

Incidence estimates of intellectual disability vary considerably. If IQ were the only identification criterion, as it usually was until the 1990s, it can be estimated that 2.28 percent of the population would have IQs falling below two standard deviations below the mean. However, the addition of the adaptive behavior criterion reduces the incidence considerably, perhaps to 1 percent (Yu and Atkinson, 1993). A recent authoritative meta-analysis of fifty-two incidence studies conducted in many countries around the world reported an overall incidence rate of 10.37 per 1,000 members of the population, although studies conducted exclusively with child and adolescent samples tended to report higher incidence rates, averaging 18.3 per 1,000 people. Most but not all studies of both children and adults indicated a higher incidence rate for males. Incidence is higher in low-income countries than more prosperous ones; it is also higher in rural areas and urban slum areas than in more prosperous urban areas (Maulik et al., 2011).

Einfeld and Emerson (2010) comment on several factors that may increase or decrease the prevalence of intellectual disability over time. An increase may occur because more mothers are having children at later ages than in previous years. Older mothers are at greater risk of having a child with an intellectual disability than younger mothers. Contemporary Western women may choose to wait before having a child in order to pursue higher education or establish themselves in careers that were not easily accessible to women in previous eras. On the other hand, prenatal screening for Down's syndrome and improved medical care before and during pregnancy may reduce the incidence over time.

The most common syndromes associated with intellectual disability and their causes

Down's syndrome accounts for the largest proportion of intellectual disabilities. It affects about 1 in 800 babies and is more likely to occur when the mother is over 35 years old at the time of the baby's birth. It is a genetic disorder but not one that is usually inherited. It occurs because of a biological error that causes there to be, at the time of conception, forty-seven chromosomes instead of the usual forty-six. The extra chromosome interferes with the development of the brain, thus causing intellectual disability. People with Down's syndrome are often recognizable by their facial features, including slanted eyes and flat bridge of the nose. Although some may be considered stubborn by temperament, many people with Down's syndrome relate well socially despite their intellectual challenges (World Health Organization, *Mental Health and Substance Abuse*, n.d.).

Fragile X syndrome is the most common form of intellectual disability than can be inherited. It occurs when there is a change in the FMR1 gene of the X chromosome, hence its name. That chromosome is responsible for the generation of a protein that affects brain development. Only some children born with Fragile X turn out to have an intellectual deficiency. This occurs quite often in boys, about 80 percent of the time, but only occasionally in girls. Other children with Fragile X may develop learning disabilities, autism or attention deficit disorder. Fragile X syndrome manifests itself socially and behaviorally in many different ways. Some children with Fragile X do well socially whereas others display marked social anxiety. Yet others face the same challenges in relating to others as do children with autism spectrum disorders and/or attention deficit disorder (Hagerman and Hagerman, 2002).

Prader-Willi syndrome is another condition present at birth. It occurs in approximately one live birth out of 10,000 to 20,000. The syndrome is caused by a gene change that occurs randomly, meaning that the syndrome often emerges in children with no family history of the disorder. In most cases, the child is born without part of the material in the father's chromosome 15. There are also some children with Prader-Willi syndrome with two copies of the mother's chromosome 15. These children typically go through two developmental phases: At first, they fail to grow and thrive but from about age 2 years onwards they tend to overeat and gain weight. People with Prader-Willi syndrome are often recognized by physical signs of the disorder, including almond-shaped eyes, narrow bifrontal skull and small limbs. Males often

have undescended testicles. In addition to intellectual challenges, some children with Prader-Willi syndrome experience problems of psychosocial adjustment ranging from anxiety to attention problems to compulsive biting of the skin (Chen et al., 2007).

Comorbidities

Progress has been made in recent years toward recognizing the fact that children and adults with intellectual disabilities can also exhibit the same forms of psychopathology as people without intellectual disability. These include disruptive behaviors, attention deficit, psychosis, depression and anxiety. The term *dual diagnosis* is used for the simultaneous diagnosis of intellectual disability and another form of psychopathology, in most cases an emotional or behavioral disorder. The responsibilities of helping professionals in providing care to children with dual diagnoses are beginning to be recognized and understood. Prior to this advance, any other problems suffered by people with intellectual disabilities were usually considered just a manifestation of their low intelligence (Hodapp and Dykens, 1991). This resulted, all too often, in inadequate attention to the emotional or behavioral problems. Institutions specializing in disruptive behavior disorders, for example, may specify a minimum IQ for children as part of their admissions criteria.

Although these conditions may no longer be seen as artifacts of intellectual disability or additional manifestations of the syndromes that caused it, the fact that the comorbid condition co-occurs with intellectual disabilities poses additional challenges for clinicians charged with assessment and treatment (Wallander, Dekker and Koot, 2003). These challenges include, first of all, conducting diagnostic procedures using language that can be understood by the children. This is paralleled of course by difficulties in interpreting the responses of children with limited cognitive development. Perhaps for that reason, many responses are wrongly interpreted as hallucinations, resulting in an overdiagnosis of comorbid psychotic condition. Rating scales completed by adults who are familiar with the child's behavior may be particularly useful in situations of possible dual diagnosis. In diagnosing a behavior disorder or emotional problem that might be considered comorbid, the developmental level of the child must be considered. For example, a 12-year-old who has developed in most areas to the level of a typically developing 2-year-old might be expected to have the tantrums that are typical of 2-year-olds (Einfeld and Emerson, 2010).

Although it is now recognized that children with intellectual disability are subject to the full range of comorbid psychopathologies as are other children, the sad reality is that they are subject to more of them, perhaps because of genetic or environmental factors that may or may not be intrinsically related to intellectual disability (Bebko and Weiss, 2005). However, some theorists have suggested that intellectual disability has a *pathoplastic effect* – that it acts to compound the severity of some comorbid conditions (Einfield and Emerson, 2010; Smiley and Cooper, 2003). Whatever the causes of the comorbid conditions, it has been estimated that anywhere from 15 to 60 percent of people with developmental disabilities also suffer from another type of psychiatric disorder, with an average across studies of 37.5 percent, which is much higher than the rate of psychiatric disturbance in the population at large (Yu and Atkinson, 1993).

CASE STUDY: Mark, facing the dual challenges of self-injurious behavior and intellectual disability

Stein, Blum and Lukasik (2005) present an interesting case study that illustrates how intellectual disability can interact with, and sometimes complicate, another mental health problem. Mark, 7 years old, has an intellectual disability in the severe range. He also displays recurrent self-injury, more at home than at school. He hits his face with his fist and bangs his head against the wall, floor and table, causing some bruising. The behaviors occur at all times of the day and in a wide variety of situations. For example, he might be watching television or playing with a toy and suddenly starts banging his head. These behaviors have occurred intermittently over the several years prior to Mark's first appointment at the mental health clinic. However, in the 6 months prior to the appointment, the problematic behaviors have become more frequent and intense. Mark's parents report that these self-injurious behaviors often occur for no apparent reason, but also at times when he is unable to do something. Mark's parents attempted to manage his behavior with verbal reprimands, which had no effect at all.

Self-injurious behavior is frequent among children with autism spectrum disorders (see next chapter) but there are no other signs of autism in Mark's behavior, nor any signs of a seizure disorder. Mark eats and sleeps well. He has a working vocabulary of about twenty words. Mark goes to school, where he attends a special class of eight students, taught by a teacher and two assistants. Mark lives with both his parents and two younger siblings. Mark's mother has been somewhat depressed since the birth of her younger son, now 5 years old.

Stein's article about Mark's case includes the opinions of a consulting pediatrician and child psychologist. Dr. Blum, the pediatrician, urges a thorough medical and dental examination to ensure that Mark is not suffering some kind of pain that he cannot describe. If medical problems are ruled out, Dr. Blum suggests that Mark's self-injurious behavior is a way of getting attention. Dr. Lukasik, the psychologist, also suggests exploration of the possibility of comorbid attention deficit/ hyperactivity disorder. She urges careful examination of the situations that seem to provoke Mark's behavior, leading, hopefully, to some direction as to better ways of expressing himself, choosing activities he likes while avoiding others, and getting attention. Bloggers who commented on the case by internet urge exploration of possible anxiety or depression, although they recognize that these conditions are difficult to diagnose because of Mark's limited range of expression. Other bloggers suggest exploring the possible effects of family factors, including Mom's depression. Other comments suggest further exploration of possible underlying medical conditions, including migraine headaches and ear infections. Thus, Mark's intellectual disability, manifest especially in his difficulties in communicating verbally, makes it extremely difficult to understand and treat his behavior problems. The professionals contributing to the blog suggest a wide range of treatments, from trials on several different medications to training in the use of sign language to let others know when he is frustrated. One particularly sensitive blogger also suggested that respite care be arranged so that Mark's parents might have some time for themselves and a break from the challenges of parenting their son.

Peer relations of children with intellectual disabilities

The basic innate need for interpersonal contact applies to all persons, including those with intellectual disabilities. Peer acceptance has become a particularly pressing need since the advent of the mainstreaming movement because rejection by peers can torpedo the successful integration of pupils with intellectual disability into school settings where they might be able to manage otherwise. In fact, many authorities believe that social integration is the most important benefit of mainstreaming (see below) both to children with intellectual disabilities and to the peers who come into contact with them (e.g., Haring, 1991). Therefore, most of the recent research has focused on relationships between children with and without disabilities. However, relationships among, and friendships between, children with intellectual disabilities remain an important source of human social contact, especially for children who are not attending regular schools. As noted in Chapter 7 and emphasized by Haring for persons with intellectual disabilities, a social network of any individual

consists of relationships of varying degrees of closeness and depth. Accordingly, acceptance by classmates who may not be close friends is important in establishing a climate of acceptance, whereas close friendships have particular psychological and developmental significance.

Research on the overall peer acceptance of children and adolescents with intellectual disabilities in unequivocal: The hoped-for social integration of pupils with disabilities in US schools, discussed later in this chapter, has simply not happened. In studies conducted as late as 2006, it has been found that children and adolescents with intellectual disabilities are three times as likely to be rejected by their school peers as are other pupils. Only 10 percent of pupils indicate that they have even a single friend with an intellectual disability (Siperstein and Parker, 2008). Similar research in other countries yields the same conclusion, such as a well-designed study conducted in the Netherlands by Geurts et al. (1987). Solish, Minnes and Kupferschmidt (2003) found that about half of the Canadian children with developmental disabilities whose caregivers participated in their survey had no friends at all. Part of the problem may be that children with intellectual disabilities fail to make social contact with other children at play (e.g., Bebko et al., 1998; Guralnick and Groom, 1987; Jenkins, Odom and Speltz, 1989); instead they tend to play alone. This is unfortunate because it has been shown that children with intellectual disabilities who do make social contact are more likely than other children with intellectual disabilities to be included in activities with peers (Siperstein and Leffert, 1997). The peer rejection of children with intellectual disabilities at school appears to recur in recreational, social and leisure activities according to a recent Canadian study by Solish, Perry and Minnes (2010).

Webster and Carter (2007) reviewed the friendships of children with intellectual disabilities as well as other forms of developmental disability. They note that these friendships might appear to be quite different from friendships between typically developing children. In some cases, the friends may share the decision-making and power in the relationship. In other instances, however, the typically developing friend may assume the role of helper or tutor (Murray-Seegert, 1989). This can bring some degree of satisfaction to both friends. Therefore, the apparently unequal balance of power does not necessarily mean that the principle of equity in friendship (see Chapter 7) is not at work (Schneider, Wiener and Murphy, 1994). A longitudinal perspective on the relationships, which is very rare in research, may be particularly illuminating in this regard because there are some anecdotal accounts of friendships that began with the typically developing child helping a friend with disabilities. Over the course of time, however, the balance of power and, perhaps, of satisfaction in the relationship, may become more equal (Salisbury and Palombaro, 1998; Webster and Carter, 2007).

In their review, Webster and Carter (2007) highlighted some of the methodological limitations of the few studies conducted on the friendships of children and adolescents with intellectual disabilities. Some of the problems are no different from the methodological shortcomings in research on the friendships between children with any type of psychopathology or no psychopathology at all.

The most frequent problem is making an inference about friendship, which is a dyadic phenomenon (see Chapter 7) on the basis of information provided by only one of the friends. Other methods of studying friendship, such as direct observation of the interactions of the two friends, have been used in only a few studies conducted with participants who have intellectual disabilities. These few results indicate that the friendships of children and adolescents with intellectual disabilities are less intimate than the friendships of peers without disabilities, as was reported in a study using a participant-observation methodology by Zetlin and Murtaugh (1988). Perhaps because of the lack of intimacy, the friendships of participants with disabilities were also found to be less stable than the friendships of other participants. A more recent interview study by Matheson, Olsen and Weisner (2007) revealed that adolescents with mild intellectual disabilities tended to conceive of friendships in terms of immediate companionship rather than closeness, intimacy or support. This thinking could be either a result or a cause of their lack of friendships.

Much of the social life of adolescents in contemporary Western societies is conducted at least partially by electronic communication. Many adolescents with mild intellectual disabilities are capable of using cell phones and email. Even when educated in segregated special schools, they may communicate electronically with adolescents in other settings. Unfortunately, this subjects a substantial number of them to cyberbullying, as detailed in a recent Dutch study by Didden and his colleagues (2009).

Family and cultural factors

Families play a substantial role in determining how close children with intellectual disabilities come to developing to the highest level possible within the limits of their potential in as natural an environment as possible. For many families, having a child with an intellectual disability is, at least at first, a source of profound sadness and grief. Some may turn to science for an explanation of what has happened and attempt to determine how likely they are to have other natural children with intellectual disabilities (Statham et al., 2011). Others may seek support through religion (O'Hara and Bouras, 2007). This may either strengthen their faith or lead them to question their beliefs. Indeed, in many cases, a substantial number of families of children with intellectual disabilities eventually come to believe that the birth of their children was a positive event that strengthened them in a number of ways (Dura-Vila, Dein and Hodes, 2010). Sometimes personal characteristics of the parents serve them well in adjusting to the situation. Parents are more likely to adjust well if they believe either that they are in control of the situation or that it is attributable to fate. Less adaptive beliefs include perceiving themselves inadequate to handle the situation or thinking that they are at fault in some way for their child's disability (Green, 2004). Individual child factors also contribute to the parents' coping or lack of it. As noted earlier, the age of the mother at the time of the child's birth is correlated with the likelihood of the child having Down's syndrome. Hence, parents, especially older parents, live with the stress of wondering who will care for their children once they are unable to do so. Importantly it is not usually the intellectual deficiency by itself that leads to families feeling or being unable to cope, but the more challenging behaviors that often accompany intellectual disabilities (Einfeld and Emerson, 2010; Magaña et al., 2006). On the other hand, the endearing features of many children with intellectual disabilities, such as those with Down's syndrome, are surely a factor that promotes their own adjustment and that of their families.

The financial hardship for families caring for children with intellectual disabilities can be substantial. Longitudinal methods are imperative for studying this economic strain because, as noted earlier, mild intellectual disability is associated with lower socio-economic status in general. Emerson

et al. (2010) followed the families of a large sample of children with intellectual disabilities in the UK for 1 year, comparing changes in their financial status with similar data from UK families whose children did not have intellectual disabilities. The families supporting children with disabilities were far more likely than the others to be poor from the start of the data collection or to become poor over the year. The families of children with disabilities were also less likely to escape from poverty. A specific precipitating event, such as a worsening of the child's behavior or change in the parents' ability to offer care, was identifiable in many of the families whose economic status declined markedly.

Important cultural differences in the reactions of families have been reported. In some cultures, having a child with an intellectual disability brings shame upon the family. People of different cultures and religions interpret the arrival of a child with intellectual disability differently. In some societies, parents may see it as a punishment for something they have done, as a way of testing them or as a special blessing. This may result from different interpretations of the same precept in the same religion, such as the Hindu belief in fate. The belief that the intellectual disability can be cured in some way is also more frequent in some non-Western cultures than in the majority Western culture (Dura-Vila, Dein and Hodes, 2010).

As discussed in Chapter 8, many non-Western cultures are highly oriented toward the extended family. Grandparents and other relatives tend to be, as would be expected, important sources of practical and social support for parents of children with intellectual disabilities. At the same time, their presence can instil a heightened sense of responsibility and ambivalence about depending so heavily on relatives. Perhaps for that reason, the support provided by relatives may be accompanied by greater rather than lesser distress (Blacher and Baker, 2007). Lin et al. (2013) conducted a qualitative study of the experiences of fourteen families of girls with Rett syndrome in several parts of China. Rett syndrome, which mostly affects females, is a genetic disorder that usually results in severe intellectual impairment together with impaired gait and limited hand dexterity. Some children with Rett syndrome acquire spoken language to some degree but most communicate by varying their eye gazes. Most of the parents interviewed felt helpless and desperate. They lacked adequate information about their daughters' disabilities. They were profoundly concerned about their daughters' futures. Compounding these difficulties is the stigma they face from both inside and outside their families. For instance, unlike most grandparents in China who willingly help take care of their grandchildren, many of the grandparents of the girls with Rett syndrome refused to become involved. The interviewed mothers felt that people on the street stared with disdain on them and on their daughters.

A positive outlook does not necessarily translate into optimal parenting. Many parents of children with intellectual disabilities are known to over-restrict and overprotect their children, which may interfere with optimal development (Dura-Vila, Dein and Hodes, 2010). Fortunately, there is much that helping professionals can do to assist parents of children with learning disabilities. Among the helpful services is respite care for the child for brief periods of time and support groups for the parents. However, probably the most helpful service is training in handling problem behaviors positively and effectively (see review by Hastings and Beck, 2004). Some reports indicate that it is common for fathers to avoid the challenges of parenting a child with intellectual disability, even when the mother is employed. This has become a matter of concern, with some authorities suggesting special interventions to increase "mindfulness" with regard to the fathering role (MacDonald and Hastings, 2010).

Interventions for children and adolescents with intellectual disability

Intellectual stimulation

It is important to bear in mind that the IQs of people with mild intellectual disability tend to be correlated with the IQs of their natural parents but that this is not the case for people with moderate, severe or profound degrees of intellectual disability (Einfeld and Emerson, 2010). Thus, one of the major causes of mild intellectual disability (and, once more, not other forms of intellectual disability) may be insufficient intellectual stimulation. This has also been noted in the case of children raised in very unstimulating institutions (Kephart, 1940), which was one of the reasons why orphanages have been closed in many countries.

Given the specter of large numbers of children being diagnosed as having intellectual disability without evident cause other than lack of stimulation, many daring educators and prevention scientists have attempted to change things with programs aimed at teaching cognitive skills. These efforts reached a crescendo in the 1970s and 1980s. Perhaps the boldest effort was sponsored by the government of Venezuela as an attempt to improve the literacy rate, which at the time was only 15 percent. In 1979, Luis Alberto Machado was appointed that country's Minister of Intelligence and was assigned the task of disseminating interventions to improve the thinking skills of the country's poor. His ideology is summed up in the title of his book *The Right to be Intelligent* (Machado, 1980). Thinking exercises were disseminated to masses of children in the schools of the poorest parts of the country. One of the advisors to the project was Israeli psychologist Reuven Feuerstein, who developed thinking exercises for underprivileged immigrant children to that country. Feuerstein's philosophy is also captured by the title of one of his books: *Don't Accept Me as I Am: Helping "Retarded" People to Excel* (Feuerstein, Rand and Rynders, 1997). An important part of Feuerstein's thinking is the abandonment of "static" approaches to the assessment of intelligence and replacing them with "dynamic" assessment. In other words, rather than asking questions to which the answers depend on previous instruction, Feuerstein advocates assessment by means of trial teaching. If the child is capable of learning what is taught during the dynamic assessment session, this is considered the true index of the child's ability. Feuerstein's program has been implemented with different populations around the world. Although children may benefit from these exercises, many members of the scientific community remain largely unconvinced of their long-term general benefits and even less convinced that the program can prevent or reverse intellectual disability (e.g., Forsyth, 2004). A somewhat similar consensus has emerged about the results of some US programs in which mothers in communities of low socio-economic status are coached and encouraged in providing more cognitive stimulation to their children. One of the best-known of these programs was developed by psychologist David Weikart, with increasing IQ specified as one of the primary objectives. The participating children were followed for many years. It was found that their life achievements were enhanced, which has led to the Perry Preschool project being largely considered a success. However, once more, there was no effect on IQ (Locurto, 1991; Schweinhart and Weikart, 1989).

Social skills training

The mainstreaming movement, discussed later in this chapter, aims at including as many pupils with intellectual disability as possible in regular schools. This philosophy has spurred interest in the systematic, direct and specific teaching of social skills to children and adolescents with mild intellectual disability. It has been argued that such training may make the difference between being self-sufficient and being chronically dependent on others in school, community and work settings (Sukhodolksy and Butter, 2007). It might be argued that social skills training is not particularly relevant in several other areas of psychopathology because the children involved already know the skills but do not use them for one reason or another (see Chapter 12). However, in the case of intellectual disabilities, there is a very substantial possibility that the skill knowledge is lacking and that social skills training thus constitutes a central modality of intervention.

Vaughn and her colleagues (2003) prepared a thorough review of research on social skills interventions for children with disabilities, including intellectual disabilities. The original studies reviewed pertained to a wide range of social skills training techniques. In many studies, appropriate social behavior is prompted as the child interacts with peers. Reinforcement of appropriate target behavior is often used. Other interventions involve play materials. In some cases, adults become involved in children's play at first and then reduce their involvement (Jenkins, Odom and Speltz, 1989). Yet other interventions are based on the modeling of the desired behaviors (Odom and McEvoy, 1988). Many of the studies were conducted with diverse populations, including children with a range of disabilities, developmental or otherwise; these are somewhat difficult to interpret. However, three studies devoted specifically to intellectual disability are listed, all of which demonstrated positive results for the social skills interventions. A dissertation by Bradley (1987, cited in Vaughn et al., 2003) focused on sharing. During five 10-minute sessions, a teacher prompted and praised sharing behaviors. Jenkins, Odom and Speltz (1989) reported positive results for a ten-session intervention in which children participated in structured play. Finally, LeBlanc and Matson (1995) demonstrated the effectiveness of a social skills intervention that involved modeling by puppets and by peers, followed by systematic reinforcement of the behaviors targeted.

Peer-mediated interventions

There have been some successful interventions in which classroom peers have volunteered as mediators in interventions for children with intellectual disability. For example, McMahon and her colleagues (1996) asked typically developing classmates to instruct elementary-school children with intellectual disability in the skills needed to play common board games. The intervention led to an increase in some types of social interaction between classmates with and without intellectual disability.

Box 16.2 | **Nirje's eight planks of normalization**

Plank 1. Individuals should follow the normal rhythm of the day.

Plank 2. Individuals should follow a normal routine of life.

Plank 3. Individuals should follow the normal rhythm of the year.

Plank 4. Individuals should participate in the normal developmental experiences of the life cycle.

Plank 5. The right of individuals to make choices should be valued.

Plank 6. Individuals should be entitled to experience normal sexual pleasure.

Plank 7. Individuals should participate in normal productive work and receive appropriate compensation for the work they do.

Plank 8. Individuals should enjoy living, learning and recreational facilities similar to those enjoyed by other members of the community.

Source: Based on Nirje, B. (1969). The normalization principle and its human management implications. In R. Kugel and W. Wolfensberger (Eds.), Changing patterns in residential services for the mentally retarded (pp. 181–95). Washington, DC: President's Committee on Mental Retardation, and Perske, R. (2004). Nirje's eight planks. *Mental Retardation*, *42*, 147–50.

Participation in school and community life

The tradition, as old as the history of institutions, of sending children and adults with intellectual disabilities to institutions, special classes and special schools, has been seriously questioned in the past 40 years. In many countries, that tradition is dead or dying. The ideology that led to its demise is called *normalization*. The term is somewhat misleading because its dictionary definition implies that the people involved will be made "normal"; in fact the intent is that they be made as "normal" as possible (Perske, 2004). The philosophy of normalization was nurtured by the close contact between pioneering theorists in Scandinavia, led by Bengt Nirje (1969), and in the United States led by Wolf Wolfensberger (e.g., Wolfensberger and Tullman, 1982).

Nirje's principles are contained in eight "planks," summarized by Perske (2004) (see Box 16.2). The first is that people, regardless of their disability, should have a normal routine of day. In other words, they should dress, eat, sleep, etc., at the same times as most people. They should also have normal connections to physical space, meaning that, as is usual for most people, home, school and work should not occur in the same physical setting. Plank Three refers to a normal cycle of holidays, which should be special for people with disabilities as for most other people. They should also be allowed to transition into the different spaces normally provided to people at different stages of the life cycle, such as close, family spaces for infants, spaces with extensive social contact for adolescents and, ideally, supportive spaces for old age. Plank Five specifies that individuals should have the freedom to make choices about their lives to the greatest extent possible. They should also have the opportunity for romantic and sexual relations. They should have the opportunity to participate in the economy as far as possible, earning money and learning how it is used. Finally, they should live, learn and engage in recreation in places and ways that are as similar as possible to those used by most people.

Wolfensberger's position about normalization is summarized by the definition he proposed: Normalization implies, as much as possible, the use of culturally valued means in order to establish and/or maintain valued social roles for people (Wolfensberger and Tullman, 1982). He elaborated on this general position in a number of ways. First of all, he observed that differentness by itself need not be viewed as deviant until it becomes evaluated negatively by others. Their devaluation of defined groups of people will, in his view, cause those people to be treated badly. Maltreatment will also be aggravated by devaluing with inappropriate language and labels. For example, a school class for children with intellectual disabilities should not be given the name of a type of animal, like the "lions" or the "turtles," lest they be treated like animals. Their activities should be referred to as activities, not as "therapy," for example "work therapy," "reading therapy." Wolfensberger postulated that if a group of people is perceived as deviant, they will begin to behave in deviant ways.

Wolfenberger argued that psychologists should advocate for persons with intellectual disabilities, first of all, by attempting to change the perceptions and values of the community as a whole. Part of this can be achieved by normalizing the means by which professional services are delivered. For example, counseling provided to the families of children with intellectual disabilities and behavior problems should resemble as far as possible counseling provided to other families whose children demonstrate behavior problems. Providers of service must strive to be aware of the largely unconscious processes that are linked with devaluing groups of people. They should do everything in their power to make it possible for children and adults with intellectual disabilities to relate to others in normal and positive roles, such as those of neighbor, pupil, teacher, friend, guide or tenant. Importantly, Wolfensberger emphasized that it is more likely that a group will be stigmatized if it is congregated in large numbers. He remarked that

a single person walking with a limp is unlikely to be noticed on a street but if six people walk together on a street, all with limps, it will attract attention. This principle applies especially to the size of institutions (Wolfensberger and Tullman, 1982).

The reasons behind the thrust toward normalization can be understood in light of some of the failures of large institutions. Although, as in Scandinavia and Germany, attractive, progressive institutions were sources of pride, there were other types of institutions. One of the worst actually led to a rebellion that was the subject of a book by D'Antonio (2004). The book documents the systematic physical, sexual and verbal abuse suffered by children who were sent to Fernald State School in Massachusetts after being diagnosed as mentally retarded, usually on the basis of a single IQ test. Such was the fate of 8-year-old Fred Boyce, who was sent to the school in 1949. Staff members would call the residents "retards" or "morons." If they talked during meals, an attendant would tear a piece of bread, throw it to the floor and force the offenders to push it across the floor with their noses. Eventually, some of the boys, including several who did not really have intellectual disabilities, began to rebel. Some began to insist that they did not belong at Fernald and that some mistake was made. Repeat IQ testing, administered after persistent complaints, sometimes revealed no indication at all of intellectual disability, leading to the release of some residents. Others ran away. By the 1970s, several former residents began legal action against the school and were awarded compensation for the abuse they suffered. It emerged that the residents had been involved without their consent in research about the effects of radioactive oatmeal conducted by scientists at Harvard University and the Massachusetts Institute of Technology in nearby Boston. Legal procedures also forced improvement in conditions at the school.

The principles espoused by Nirje and by Wolfensberger began to be reflected in laws about the schooling and institutional placement of children with intellectual disabilities beginning in Scandinavia in the 1950s, accompanied by heated debate. In Denmark and Sweden, especially, this was seen as a continuation of a social commitment to citizens in difficulty that was a century old at the time. Prior to the advent of the normalization movement (also referred to as the *mainstreaming movement*, especially as applied to schools), this social commitment was translated into the establishment of separate schools and institutions for children with intellectual disability, which were considered exemplary and were a matter of national pride (Ericsson, 1985). In the United States, the landmark Education for All Handicapped Children Act or, as it is more commonly known, Public Law 94–142, was passed in 1975. The law includes a requirement that pupils with disabilities had to be educated within publicly funded government school systems and, importantly, that they had to be educated in the *least restrictive setting* possible (US Department of Education, 2007). This means that it became illegal to educate a child in a special, segregated school for children with disabilities if the child is capable of being educated in a regular neighborhood school. Elaborate procedures were established to document that these provisions were followed. As a result, many special schools and special classes were eliminated, changing drastically the nature of the duties assigned to regular school teachers. European countries vary widely in their endorsement and implementation of the philosophy of mainstreaming. In the UK, there is little consistency in the practices of local authorities. It is reported that just under half the pupils with intellectual disabilities in the UK attend regular local schools (Einfeld and Emerson, 2010). Special schools remain very much the norm in Germany, a country that has pioneered high-quality programming for children with intellectual disability for over a century (Opp, 2007). In contrast, one of the most radical shifts in policy in any country was Italy's "psychiatric revolution" of the late 1970s (Dosen, 1994). This "revolution" brought about in a very short time the closure of virtually all special schools. Manetti, Schneider and Siperstein (2001) studied the experiences of children in a school

in Genoa who were provided the opportunity of volunteering to help in a special unit for children with severe intellectual disabilities at their schools. The volunteers seemed to benefit in several ways from the experience, demonstrating positive attitudes about intellectual disability in general. However, the six pupils with mild intellectual disabilities who were enrolled in regular classes in the school were still rejected socially by their classmates.

In short, many of the hopes of initial proponents of mainstreaming remain unfulfilled. Siperstein and Parker (2008) note that the mainstreaming movement was designed to bring about physical integration, instructional integration and social integration. Physical integration – the placement of children with intellectual disability in regular-school classrooms, has largely been achieved. It is very difficult to determine whether instructional integration – providing academic instruction to children with intellectual disabilities through reasonable modification of regular-class teaching – has been achieved. However, with regard to social integration, there is no doubt. As discussed in the section on peer relations earlier in this chapter, dozens of studies clearly demonstrate that children with intellectual disabilities tend to be rejected by their typically developing peers. This is by no means limited to the United States: Schoolchildren in countries as diverse as Zambia (Nabuzoka and Ronning, 1997) and the UK (Furnham and Gibbs, 1984), like their American counterparts, have been found to reject their classmates with intellectual disabilities.

It is abundantly clear that physical integration by itself does not necessarily bring about social integration; interaction between children with intellectual disability and their classroom peers who do not have disabilities must be systematically encouraged (e.g., Jenkins, Odom and Speltz, 1989). This need not be difficult to do. This social interaction has been successfully stimulated in many ways, including peer tutoring, matching children with intellectual disabilities and other pupils who serve as "buddies," active encouragement of interaction by the teacher and many others (see review by Siperstein,

Norins and Mohler, 2006). Some data suggest that pupils with intellectual disabilities are more likely to be included in small-group academic activities at school than when the lesson is directed at large classes (Carter et al., 2008). Interaction during sport activities has been fostered by *inclusive sports* programming, which is characterized by non-competitive interaction in a supportive atmosphere (Siperstein, Glick and Parker, 2009).

It is also important to note that, despite the fact that the mainstreaming movement has not achieved all it hoped to, there is no reason to believe that children with intellectual disabilities are better off socially in segregated special classes or schools. Webster and Carter's (2007) review includes three studies in which mainstreamed and segregated schools are compared in terms of the likelihood of pupils with intellectual disabilities having friends. The results are inconclusive, with one study leading to the conclusion that friendship is more likely in self-contained facilities (Cuckle and Wilson, 2002), compared with two others reporting the opposite (Buysse, Goldman and Skinner, 2002; Fryxell and Kennedy, 1995).

Present and future roles for child-clinical psychologists

Unfortunately, there is no treatment that a mental health professional can offer that will result in the elimination of an intellectual disability. However, as time passes and efforts increase, new ways of helping children with intellectual disability emerge.

Mainstreaming must be recognized as a reality in an ever-increasing number of places around the world. At the same time, it must be acknowledged that mainstreaming only works where there is active effort at making it work, using established interventions together with innovative new ones. The challenge of making mainstreaming work whenever possible provides many new roles for the psychologist. The traditional role of diagnostician remains. However, as IQ is increasingly supplemented by other variables in diagnosis, such as adaptive behavior, the psychologist is increasingly liberated from the stereotypical role of testing technician. Precision is still required in IQ testing, which has become very sophisticated methodologically. The same sophistication is required but elusive in the assessment of adaptive behavior and comorbid conditions. Beyond diagnosis, the psychologist can play a fundamental role in conceptualizing, delivering, supervising and, importantly, evaluating interventions for children, schools and families. Moving far beyond the role as pawn whose IQ tests were once used to send children to institutions like the Fernald School in Massachusetts, the psychologist can become, aside from a clinician, an advocate for children and adolescents with intellectual disability. However, families will remain in most cases the main advocates for children with intellectual disability. Consequently, perhaps the major role and opportunity for psychologists is in supporting the parents of children with intellectual disabilities and helping them apply the scientific principles of behavior management.

Summary

- The term, "intellectual disability," which appears in DSM-5, implies a more integrated concept of psychopathology than the previous term, "mental retardation," which has come to be used in pejorative ways. Intellectual disability is determined by both measured IQ and adaptive functioning. Adaptive functioning refers to the skills needed for daily living and communication.
- Intellectual disability has varying levels, differentiated primarily by levels of adaptive functioning.

- People with mild intellectual disability often have no signs of cerebral or physical impairment and are capable of caring for themselves and forming interpersonal relationships that are rewarding.
- Moderate intellectual disability is associated with greater limitations in the ability to care for oneself and is often linked to an organic cause.
- Severe intellectual disability has clearly defined roots in damage to or dysfunction of the central nervous system. Individuals with severe intellectual disability have marked impairments in their motor functions and capacities for self-care.
- Incidence estimates vary considerably. Children and adult males, people from low-income countries and people from rural areas have a higher incidence than their counterparts in other places.
- Down's syndrome, a non-inherited genetic disorder featuring one extra chromosome at the time of conception, accounts for the largest proportion of these cases. This forty-seventh chromosome interferes with brain functioning, causing intellectual disability and noticeable facial differences.
- Fragile X syndrome, an inherited change in the FMR1 gene of the X chromosome that may ultimately cause an intellectual disability, causes learning, social and/or behavioral problems for the child.
- Prader-Willi syndrome, randomly present at birth due to a lack of genetic material from the father's chromosome 15, is observed to cause physical differences, intellectual difficulties and often psychosocial maladjustment (e.g., anxiety, attention problems).
- Sometimes a dual diagnosis is needed, where the child has another form of psychopathology along with the intellectual disability, most often an emotional or behavioral disorder.
- Theorists have suggested that intellectual disability has a pathoplastic effect, i.e., it acts to compound the severity of its comorbid conditions. Professionals are becoming more

attentive than previously to the needs of people with dual diagnoses.
- Proper social integration into peer groups and classroom settings is paramount in enabling children with intellectual disabilities to benefit from the highest level of social exchange they are capable of. However, children with intellectual disabilities are more likely to be rejected by their school peers than those without an intellectual disability.
- An important methodological flaw in both this domain and child psychopathology in general is the fact that some studies have obtained information about the dyadic phenomenon of friendship from only one of the friends. Accordingly, knowledge about friendships in which one of the friends has an intellectual disability is very limited.
- Financial hardship is a problem that may occur within families caring for children with intellectual disabilities. Often, such families are more likely to be poor from the start or become poor over 1 year, precipitated commonly by a worsening of the child's behavior or a change in the parents' ability to offer care.
- In some cultures, having a child with intellectual disability is seen as a punishment. In others, it is seen as a blessing. Importantly, members some non-Western cultures believe intellectual disabilities can be cured in some way, a belief that is less common in many Western cultures. The presence of extended family members often contributes to the parents' distress; in others, family members may play a supportive role.
- Several interventions have been found to be somewhat successful for children and adolescents with intellectual disabilities, notably intellectual stimulation and social skills training (particularly for those with mild intellectual disability), and peer-mediated interventions (delivered by typically developing classmates).
- Normalization refers to the idea that people should be regarded as normal no matter what their disability or ability may be. For example,

they should be allowed the freedom to make their own age-appropriate choices and thus be treated similarly to other children or adolescents of the same developmental stage. This also means referring to children with special needs using appropriate terminology rather than stigmatizing labels; educating and helping them in ways that are as similar as possible to the services received by other children; and helping them in the community to the extent possible.

- The normalization movement, also known as the mainstreaming movement, has led to policy changes intended to educate and help as many children with intellectual disabilities in their home schools and communities, or, if necessary, in special settings that are as small as possible and as similar as possible to normal community settings.

Study questions

1. What are the major reasons for the changes in the name of the disorder in DSM-5 to "intellectual disability" and for the changes in the diagnostic criteria?
2. What causes Down's syndrome?
3. What type of parenting is typical in families of children and adolescents with intellectual disability? Is this type of parenting helpful?
4. What measures are probably necessary for the mainstreaming movement to achieve its main goals?
5. Given that psychological interventions cannot eliminate intellectual disability, how can psychologists facilitate the development and progress of children and adolescents with this disorder?

17 Autism spectrum disorders

Of the major psychological disorders that affect children and adolescents, autism is probably the one that remains the most shrouded in mystery. Is there any meaning to the stereotyped movements and idiosyncratic verbalizations of children with autism? Is their avoidance of social contact caused by any aspect of their environment? Is there a reason why the prevalence of autism seems to be increasing? And, most importantly, can children with autism be helped, and, if they can, how?

This chapter begins with a capsule historical sketch in which the emergence of the contemporary concept of autism is traced. Diagnostic criteria are presented next, including a discussion of the recent elimination of the category of Asperger's syndrome in DSM-5. The apparent increase in the prevalence of autism in recent years is discussed next, together with controversial recent data about the stability of the disorder. The likely causes and features of the disorder are the focus in the following section, which includes both causal factors that are endorsed by contemporary research and some of those that are interesting museum pieces. Early signs of autism spectrum disorder are also presented in the section on causes and correlates. The chapter closes with the increasingly optimistic (or, better said, increasingly less pessimistic) story of the treatments that have been developed and evaluated.

Emergence of the contemporary concept of autism

The idiosyncratic, puzzling behaviors displayed by autistic children and adults have inspired a number of intriguing theories about the origin of the disorder, few of which have withstood the test of time. Some sources report that the first account of the condition, not yet named, was in 1747, when certain personal traits of Scottish landowner Hugh Blair, such as his tactlessness, unusual gaze, obsessive and repetitive behavior and odd mannerisms were discussed during his divorce proceedings. Blair collected feathers and sticks for no apparent reason. People at the time called the condition "silent madness" (Frith, 2003; Wolff, 2004). Many contemporary authorities believe that the "wild boy of Aveyron," who was found in the woods in France in 1798 when he was probably 11 or 12 years old, had autism. However, the fact that the boy grew up in social isolation would be atypical for the disorder as it is now known; autistic-like behaviors resulting from such isolation are often called "quasi-autistic" (Wing, 1997; Frith, 2003). Although not yet labeled as such, the first case reported in the medical literature is probably the 13-year-old whose case is described in a chapter called "The Insanity of Early Life" in Henry Maudsley's (see Chapter 2) 1879 textbook *The Physiology and Pathology of the Mind* (Wolff, 2004).

Autism was formally identified as a syndrome in the seminal work of Leo Kanner in the 1940s (Kanner, 1943). The symptoms he described included extreme aloneness and abnormal speech with echolalia (meaningless repetition of words). He noted the inappropriate use of pronouns in the children's speech and their inability to move beyond the very literal meaning of words and sentences. He observed their monotonous, repetitive behavior. Kanner emphasized that the condition was usually present from the beginning of life. He believed it to be quite rare. He insisted that the condition be recognized as distinct rather than a form of schizophrenia or psychosis. Kanner emphasized the lack of warmth in their parents. Rutter's influential research in the 1960s validated the syndrome. Importantly, Rutter's work suggested a strong genetic basis for the disorder (e.g., Rutter, 2001). Lorna Wing, a British psychiatrist who became interested in autism because of her daughter's condition, is credited with introducing the idea that autism is not a single syndrome but can be best described as a spectrum of disorders. She included Asperger's syndrome (Wolff, 2004), a term that was eliminated in 2013 with the release of DSM-5, as will be discussed later in this chapter.

Diagnostic criteria

According to current knowledge and diagnostic practice, the autism spectrum disorders are conceptualized as somewhat heterogeneous but grouped together on the basis of a neurologically based deficit in social communication and social interaction. However, in the years since the disorder was first identified by Kanner in 1943, ideas about the core deficit underlying autism have shifted repeatedly. The history of ideas about the core deficit in autism once included the belief that it was a disorder caused by a deficit in the mechanisms governing the child's ability to receive emotional contact. This deficiency, it was thought, could be remediated by intensive psychotherapy that would "re-charge [the] low affective battery" (Deslauriers and Carlson, 1969). The specifics of this approach have long since been discarded although it remains clear that children with autism do have a dysfunction in the basic understanding and expression of emotion (Losh and Capps, 2006).

A core deficit in receptive language was once believed to be the core deficit in autism. This belief was tempered when it was shown in longitudinal research that some children with autism improved their language skills over time but still displayed pronounced deficits in relating socially to others (Cantwell et al., 1989). However, with the exception of some higher-functioning individuals, most children with autism display language patterns that can be described as both delayed and deviant. Their intonation is often idiosyncratic. Their language is not coordinated with that of the persons around them. They often confuse pronouns. For example, in making a request, they might ask if *you* want a glass of water when they themselves are the ones who want a drink. This pronoun confusion, originally notice by Kanner (1943) may reflect confusion about the identities of self and others. Some children with autism may simply repeat words that they have just heard (echolalia). Their speech may be accompanied by gestures that are not related in any apparent way to the topic at hand (Tager-Flusberg, Paul and Lord, 2005).

Many children with autism display repetitive, ritualistic behaviors, such as head rolling, body rocking or hand and arm waving. In some cases, this repetitive behavior may involve injury to themselves, such as head banging or biting the hands. They may repetitively organize objects into piles or rows. They may become upset if even some minor aspect of their environment is changed, such as the arrangement of furniture. Children with autism may fixate their attention on a single object for extended periods of time (Bodfish and Lewis, 2002; Bodfish et al., 2000). One of the most intriguing mysteries of autism, *savant skills*, may relate to this tendency because of the focused attention to detail (Rutter, 2011). As was noted by pioneers in the field since Kanner (1971), some people with autism are outstanding at an isolated skill, such as memorizing the dates of the calendar of the following 5 years. Rutter (2011) observes that the range of such skills is quite broad, sometimes representing genuine talents, sometimes not. Savant skills are more frequent among people with autism than is often thought, perhaps as frequent as a third of people with the disorder (Rutter, 2011). Rutter objects to the use of the term *idiot savant* to describe this phenomenon because the advanced skill belies the classification of intellectual deficiency. He wonders about the form of neural functioning, yet to be identified, that causes some people to have both intellectual disability and superior talents in some areas.

Superior intellectual skills, albeit in isolated areas, are a theme that has recurred in the movement to delineate *Asperger's syndrome* as a distinct condition (e.g., Lyons and Fitzgerald, 2005; Wolff, 2004), as it was in DSM-IV but not in the current DSM-5. Asperger identified a group of people with the disorder in whom there were often remarkable abilities in math or science in contrast with marked difficulty in the area of social and personal relationships as well as physical clumsiness. These people display very adequate mastery of language but use language in atypical ways. Hans Asperger, the Austrian pediatrician who identified the disorder, as well as eminent contemporary Cambridge psychologist Simon Baron-Cohen, have considered Asperger's syndrome a variation of typical male intelligence (Baron-Cohen, 2003). The syndrome has been seen as both a gift and a curse (Lyons and Fitzgerald, 2005). Indeed, there has been speculation that people with achievements as ground-breaking as those of Einstein, Michelangelo, Thomas Jefferson and Isaac Newton may have had Asperger's syndrome (James, 2006), although conclusive scientific evidence of this cannot of course be culled from historic documents by themselves. Unconfirmed reports in the press contain speculation that Woody Allen, Michael Jackson and Bill Gates should be added to the list (e.g., Lim, 2011).

In parallel to the glimpses of high intelligence in some people with autism, fundamental cognitive deficits are also very common in autism. According to the *theory of the mind*, one very serious deficiency is in acquiring completely the understanding that other people have separate "minds" that direct their own intentions and thinking. Related to this is understanding how similar one is to another person in terms of attributes relevant to a situation being confronted. Such comparisons are crucial in order to "anchor" one's understanding of who one is. Recent research reveals that many children with autism spectrum disorders do acquire a rudimentary sense of other people's minds but much later than their peers without autism. Even so, there are often gaps in their understanding of other people's feelings of

intention, leaving the child with autism with a very egocentric outlook on the world (Lombardo and Baron-Cohen, 2011; Vivanti et al., 2011).

Autism in DSM and ICD

Given the heterogeneity in the symptoms of people commonly described as having autism, it is logical to question whether autism really constitutes a cohesive syndrome (Rutter, 2011). There have been many suggestions for more specific diagnostic categories, for example differentiating fixed gaze and restricted interests from repetitive motor behaviors (Lam, Bodfish and Piven, 2008). Box 17.1 contains a summary of the changes between the DSM-IV and DSM-5 criteria for autism spectrum disorder. The ICD-10 criteria, which are similar to those in the old DSM-IV appear in Box 17.2; these will surely be replaced in ICD-11 by criteria similar to those in DSM-5.

Asperger's syndrome becomes a specifier of the broader category of autism spectrum disorder

In DSM-5, a single descriptor, *autism spectrum disorder*, covers all the specific component conditions mentioned in DSM-IV, that is, autistic disorder (autism), Asperger's disorder, childhood disintegrative disorder and pervasive developmental disorder not otherwise specified. The defining features of autism spectrum disorder are persistent deficits in social communication and social interaction that impair everyday functioning. This decision was taken in order to improve the reliability of diagnosis. Although there has been impressive inter-rater reliability for autism spectrum disorders as a whole but relatively poor inter-rater reliability for the specific component conditions. As well, greater inter-rater reliability should be facilitated by the requirement that the diagnosis will be based on multiple sources of information. The elimination of Asperger's syndrome as a separate condition has provoked controversy and even anger, although there is no doubt that diagnosticians have often been unable to make reliable distinctions between autistic disorder and Asperger's syndrome.

Box 17.1 | **Differences between DSM-IV and DSM-5 criteria for autism spectrum disorder**

- In both DSM-IV and DSM-5, the individual must display communication deficits and engage in restricted, repetitive behaviors, interests or activities.
- In DSM-5, in order to improve specificity, all of the symptoms under the social/communication domain must be present in the individual. These symptoms include deficits in social-emotional reciprocity, non-verbal communication and the development and maintenance of relationships. These symptoms are also present in DSM-IV, but they are organized differently.
- In DSM-IV, only one symptom in the fixated interests and repetitive behaviors domain is required. In DSM-5, however, two symptoms are required. These symptoms include repetitive speech, movements or use of objects; strong adherence to routines and rituals; fixated interests; and unusually high or low sensitivity to sensory input.
- In DSM-IV, it is noted that the symptoms should not be better explained by Rett's disorder (a neurodevelopmental disorder characterized by small head size and small hands) or childhood disintegrative disorder (a neurodevelopmental disorder characterized by late onset). However, in DSM-5, this criterion has been removed because Rett's disorder has been deleted, and childhood disintegrative disorder has been subsumed by autism spectrum disorder.
- In both versions, deficits must be present in early childhood. In DSM-IV, early childhood is considered to be before age 3. In DSM-5, however, no minimum age is included; it is noted that the symptoms usually do not clearly present until the demands put on the child surpass his or her limited ability.
- In DSM-5, it is specified that the symptoms must seriously affect daily functioning.
- In DSM-5, new specifiers have been included: Clinicians may note whether intellectual impairment, language impairment, known genetic or medical conditions, other mental disorders or catatonia are present in the individual.

Source: DSM-5 and DSM-IV-TR consulted June 6, 2013.

Box 17.2 | **ICD-10 Diagnostic criteria for childhood autism**

A. Presence of abnormal or impaired development before the age of 3 years, in at least one out of the following areas:
   1. receptive or expressive language as used in social communication;
   2. the development of selective social attachments or of reciprocal social interaction;
   3. functional or symbolic play.

B. Qualitative abnormalities in reciprocal social interaction, manifested in at least one of the following areas:
   1. failure to adequately use eye-to-eye gaze, facial expression, body posture and gesture to regulate social interaction;
   2. failure to develop (in a manner appropriate to mental age, and despite ample opportunities) peer relationships that involve a mutual sharing of interests, activities and emotions.
   3. a lack of socio-emotional reciprocity as shown by an impaired or deviant response to other people's emotions; or lack of modulation of behavior according to social context or a weak integration of social, emotional and communicative behaviors.
C. Qualitative abnormalities in communication, manifest in at least two of the following areas:
   1. a delay in, or total lack of, development of spoken language that is not accompanied by an attempt to compensate through the use of gesture or mime as alternative modes of communication;
   2. relative failure to initiate or sustain conversational interchange (at whatever level of language skills are present) in which there is reciprocal to and from responsiveness to the communications of the other person.
   3. stereotyped and repetitive use of language or idiosyncratic use of words or phrases;
   4. abnormalities in pitch, stress, rate, rhythm and intonation of speech.
D. Restricted, repetitive and stereotyped patterns of behavior, interests and activities, manifest in at least two of the following areas:
   1. an encompassing preoccupation with one or more stereotyped and restricted patterns of interest that are abnormal in content or focus; or one or more interests that are abnormal in their intensity and circumscribed nature although not abnormal in their content or focus;
   2. apparently compulsive adherence to specific, non-functional routines or rituals;
   3. stereotyped and repetitive motor mannerisms that involve either hand or finger flapping or twisting, or complex whole-body movements;
   4. preoccupations with part-objects or non-functional elements of play materials;
   5. distress over changes in small, non-functional details of the environment.
E. The clinical picture is not attributable to the other varieties of pervasive developmental disorder.

Source: World Health Organization (1993), The ICD-10 Classification of Mental and Behavioral Disorders: Diagnostic criteria for research. Geneva, WHO.

Prevalence and stability

For reasons that are largely a matter of speculation, the prevalence of autistic spectrum disorder seems to be increasing over the past few decades. In documenting this, Wazana, Bresnahan and Kline (2007) cited, first of all, a study from Middlesex, England indicating a rate of 2.5 children per 10,000 people in 1996 (Wing et al., 1976), using the criteria proposed by Leo Kanner. A study conducted in the English Midlands in 2001, using DSM-IV criteria, indicated a rate of 16.8 per 10,000 (Chakrabarti and Fombonne, 2001). Summarizing the results of twelve studies on time trends in the diagnosis of autism over periods of 9–13 years, Wazana et al. (2007) showed that the reported changes range from a very slight decrease to an eleven-fold increase. They suggest that the changes may well be attributable to nothing more than changes in the diagnostic criteria together with greater familiarity with autism by professionals, resulting in a propensity to diagnose it more often. Studying special-education records in the province of British Columbia, Canada, Coo and her colleagues (2008) found that the autism code was used for 12.3 children in 10,000 in 1996. The rate increased to 43.1 per 10,000 in 2004. However, fully half of the increase was attributable to a change in the diagnosis from another condition to autism. Elaborating on the changes in diagnostic practice, Rutter (2005) notes that many of the children now diagnosed with a condition on the autism spectrum would not have been diagnosed formally only a few years ago, but would have been described as displaying some autistic features. As well, as discussed in Chapter 3, comorbidity in general and in this instance is increasingly recognized by diagnosticians, many of whom would have ruled out the diagnosis of autism a generation ago because of the presence of another disorder. Credible as these arguments are, Rutter and others do not dismiss the possibility that there is a true increase in the incidence of autism.

Many environmentalists, however, are not as ready as many mainstream mental health professionals to attribute the increase to changes in diagnostic procedures and familiarity with them. There has been some suggestion that the increase is due to mercury in the water and food supply (Bernard et al., 2002). In a review paper published in the *Journal of Alternative and Complementary Medicine* in 2008, Curtis and Patel noted that, in addition to mercury, high levels of lead, increased smoking by pregnant women and pesticides have been implicated in some but not all studies (2008). Perhaps the most vociferous claim made about the etiology of autism is that the increase in the disorder is attributable to widespread vaccination against measles, mumps and rubella, which is usually conducted when infants are just over a year old. Speculations about this link were raised by then-eminent physician-researcher Andrew J. Wakefield in an article based on twelve case studies (Wakefield et al. 1998). This led to a number of lawsuits against the standard practice of vaccination. Scientists became increasingly skeptical when, after vaccination was discontinued in Japan and in Scandinavia (largely for reasons other than the increase in autism), the rates of autism in those countries failed to drop (e.g., Honda, Shimizu and Rutter, 2005; Rutter, 2011). The debate has largely ended with the discovery that the data in Wakefield's article were totally fabricated, as documented in a 2011 editorial in the *British Medical Journal*. Wakefield's medical license in the UK was then revoked (Godlee, Smith and Marcovitch, 2011). Nevertheless, Wakefield still speaks about the issue to some very attentive audiences in the United States (Dominus, 2011). As dead as the issue is for scientists and research-oriented practitioners, they are not reluctant to recognize that there may be some subtle, unknown, environmental factor that may interact with other causal agents in the etiology of autism spectrum disorder (Rutter, 2011). Some recent data suggest, for example, that the increase in autism may be associated with air pollution (Dawson, 2013).

Gender

As discussed earlier, autism has been associated with a deviant manifestation of male intelligence, although there are many girls with autism. The ratio of boys to girls overall is about 4:1. However, in high functioning cases of autism spectrum disorder without intellectual disability the male:female ratio is higher, in the range of 5:1 to 6:1. Conversely, the gender ratio comes closer to even when autism is comorbid with severe to profound intellectual disability (Fombonne, 2005).

Comorbid conditions

The most common comorbid condition is intellectual disability, to the point that many authorities consider autism a form of intellectual disability. This comorbidity rate is estimated at about 70 percent (Fombonne, 2005; Chakrabarti and Fombonne, 2001). Obviously, this means that about 30 percent of children with autism are of average or even superior intelligence.

Recent studies, conducted since awareness of the comorbidity of different forms of psychopathology has increased, demonstrate very high rates of comorbidity with other mental health disorders. According to a study by Simonoff et al., (2008), the most common comorbid disorders are social anxiety disorder (29.2%), attention deficit/hyperactivity disorder (28.1%) and oppositional defiant disorder (28.1%). As well, 13.4 percent of children with autism also display the symptoms of generalized anxiety disorder, with 10.1 percent diagnosable with comorbid panic disorder. Smaller numbers of children with autism spectrum disorders are also classified as having major depressive disorder (0.9%) or conduct disorder (3.2%).

Culture

There appear to be no reliable data on cross-national differences in the prevalence of autism. Some recent reports indicate higher incidence among some immigrants, such as in the West Indian and African immigrant communities in the UK. There are no known reasons that could explain this trend even vaguely, if this trend is indeed confirmed. When some earlier reports documented similar findings for adult schizophrenia in immigrant groups, hypotheses as esoteric as changes in the production of Vitamin D because of differences in sunlight between the host country and the country of origin were offered. Not surprisingly, such theories were subsequently disproven (Keen, Ried and Arnone, 2010).

However, there has been cross-cultural replication of some research on several features of the disorder. For example, Baron-Cohen's research documenting sex differences relative to theory of mind and lack of empathy, originally supported by research in the UK, has been replicated in Japan (Wakabayashi et al., 2007). The presence of distinct patterns of insistence on sameness and repetitive, ritualistic behaviors has been confirmed in Greece (Papageorgiou, Georgiades and Mavreas, 2008).

In an interesting ethnographic account of autism in Korean society, Hwang and Charnley (2010) reported that traditional Korean beliefs in fatalism and shamanism may be reflected in speculation that a child with autism is born into a family as punishment for past sins, perhaps including the improper placement of houses and graves. The disease may be attributed to the work of evil ghosts. As in other East Asian societies, saving face is an important aspect of Korean culture. Consequently, having a child with autism may bring shame to the family. Strong, pejorative words are used frequently in Korea to describe a child with autism. Fortunately, the scientific progress that has occurred in recent years is lessening the stigma. An important facilitator of progressive attitudes was the 2005 Korean film, *Malaton*, about a Korean marathon runner with autism.

This Korean study underscores some other research indicating that, whether or not there are any cross-cultural differences in the prevalence of autism, there may be important cross-cultural differences in its impact. For example, Blacher and McIntyre (2006) found that US mothers of Latino heritage who had children with autism were more depressed than other US mothers whose children had autism as well.

Early signs

Although many cases of autism remain undiagnosed for years, careful research has shown that the early signs of autism are usually evident among infants and toddlers. At least a dozen analyses of family videotapes of children who would later be diagnosed have been published (Yirmiya and Charman, 2010). For example, in a retrospective analysis of videotapes recorded on children's first birthdays, Osterling and Dawson (1994) found that children later diagnosed with an autism spectrum disorder already displayed four distinctive signs: They looked at others less often than do most infants their age, they displayed no reaction when their name was called, they failed to show objects to birthday guests and did not point to people or things. In fact, infants have been found to show the early signs of autism as early as 6 months, at which time they rarely smile at other people and fail to make eye contact. It is important to note that these retrospective research methods are not without their shortcomings. Parents often record atypical events, such as birthday parties, during which behavior may be atypical. As well, it is impossible for the researchers to "test the limits" of their findings by trying to elicit the behavior they are seeking if the infant fails to display it simultaneously (Barbaro and Dissanayake, 2009).

It is unfortunate that these early signs are not recognized. One of the reasons is that many of the behaviors specified in DSM-5 and ICD-10 do not occur very early, such as repetitive behavior, stereotyped, ritualized behavior and limited range of interest (e.g., Gray and Tonge, 2001). Some researchers distinguish between the *prodrome* of autism – early precursors that often occur together – and the syndrome itself (Yirmiya and Charman, 2010). Another reason is that many medical and mental health professionals are not familiar with ways of detecting autism in infancy or simply do not do so (Barbaro and Dissanyake, 2009).

Given the frequent early appearance of at least some signs of autism and the importance of intervening early, which is discussed later in this chapter, some researchers have developed questionnaires for parents in order to facilitate early diagnosis. These instruments have proven useful in identifying most but not all cases of autism spectrum disorders long before they would probably have been brought to the attention of professionals. Another promising technique for early detection is brain scan, because children who are later diagnosed often (but not always) display enlarged head circumference and enlargements of the brain amygdala. Another frequent early sign of autism that is important to recognize is regression to an earlier stage of development, which often occurs, either suddenly or gradually (Yirmiya and Charman, 2010). Rutter (2011) emphasizes the importance of this feature, which violates every basic principle of child development that has been proposed by researchers since Piaget.

Stability

As autism is usually attributed to biological origin, many professionals believe that no one ever recovers from it. However, as introduced briefly in Chapter 1, isolated case studies have appeared over the years of people who have recovered from it. These are often greeted with skepticism, with many questioning whether the people involved were diagnosed properly in the first place. Probably the first reference to systematic recovery with treatment was made by Lovaas in relation to applied behavior analysis, an intervention based on learning theory that is discussed later in this chapter (Lovaas, 1987). Although that treatment has a clear record of success, claims of recovery after treatment are not readily accepted, a reflex reaction by experts who are weary of the many fads and fakes that have plagued this field (see Helt et al., 2008 for a review of research on the recovery from autism). A recent report by Fein (2013) contains thirty-four case studies of people of all ages who were carefully diagnosed and rediagnosed. The people seem to be free of the diagnostic symptoms and all features of the disorder and are able to interact socially and professionally. Together with earlier case studies, this report is leading a substantial portion of the professional community to believe that autism is not necessarily a lifelong debilitating condition, which many experts still maintain (Ozonoff, 2013).

Interestingly, it has been found that the very first person in history who was diagnosed with autism has recovered! Donald Triplett, identified as Donald T. or Case 1 in Kanner's (1943) treatise, was followed by curious scholars and journalists for years. Donald's case history, including his institutionalization, and his diagnosis were well documented by Kanner. Donald did not, of course, receive the intensive Lovaas treatment, which did not yet exist. However, he did benefit from the devotion of his parents, who, for example, refused to have him join a sensationalist road show in which his *idiot savant* number skills would have been showcased. Subsequently, he was helped by caring members of his Mississippi rural community. He was able to progress within a few years of diagnosis to the point where he was socially adept enough to become a member of a fraternity at his university. When interviewed at age 77, he was living alone after the death of his parents, providing some hope to parents who worry about what will happen to their children with disabilities after the parents die. As a senior, Donald remained idiosyncratic and quirky. However, his daily routine included golf (by himself except when assigned to a team by the golf club) and coffee with friends (Donvan and Zucker, 2010). Donald's case provides many intriguing stories about the lives of individuals with autism who are relatively high-functioning intellectually and socially. Another such story is that of the talented artist Nadia (see Figure 17.1 for an example of her creative work).

Possible causes and correlates

Genetics

Twin and sibling studies have been used to examine the genetic basis of autism. The concordance in autism status for monozygotic twins across the many studies on this issue ranges from 60 to 90 percent, compared to less than 10 percent concordance for dizygotic twins and anywhere from 4 to 8 percent among other siblings (Bonora et al., 2006; Fombonne, 2005; Hurley et al., 2007; Volker and Lopata, 2008; Yirmiya and Charman, 2010). These rates can be compared to the current prevalence of autism in the general population of about 0.4 percent, as reported by Coo et al. (2008; see section on "Prevalence and Stability" earlier in this chapter). Thus, substantial research over several years suggests a heritability rate (see Chapter 4) of about 90 percent (Rutter, 2011). Rutter (2011) notes that at least three or four genes, but possibly many more, are likely to be implicated in the etiology of autism. Evidence available also suggests that spontaneous mutations of genes may be involved in addition to inherited variations. This may possibly involve rare mutations in a large number of genes, although mutations of even a single gene have been linked with the disorder in a relatively small number of cases. These mutations may explain why autism has not died out over time even though people with autism very rarely have children (Rutter, 2011).

Chromosomal abnormalities have been detected in some cases of autism spectrum disorder, including duplications and deletions (Yirmiya and Charman, 2010). Despite the overwhelming support for the genetic route, it is important to remember that even identical twins with identical genes often display very different manifestations of autism spectrum disorders (Rutter, 2011). Given this considerable evidence for the genetic basis of autism spectrum disorders, there is optimism that the methods of molecular genetics will provide further clarification of the genetic mechanisms involved. In the future, enough information may accrue to permit prenatal genetic counseling (Yirmiya and Charman, 2010).

Neurological correlates

As already mentioned, enlarged head and brain size are very common among children with autism spectrum disorders. Rapid brain growth usually begins soon after birth, usually subsiding before the child is 2 years old. After that point, the child's brain grows at about the same rate as in typically

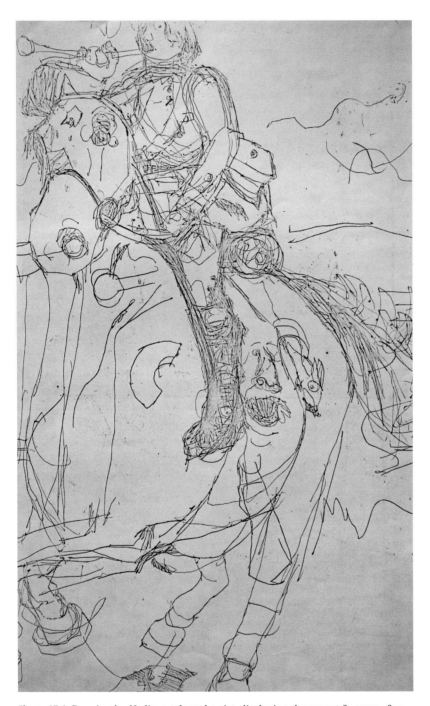

Figure 17.1 Drawing by Nadia, a talented artist, displaying the savant features often associated with higher-functioning autism spectrum disorder.

developing children. Accordingly, about 90 percent of 2- to 4-year-old boys with autism have brain volume greater than the average for boys their age. In 2- to 3-year-olds with autism, overall cortical white matter averages 18 percent greater than average; with cortical gray matter 12 percent greater than average and 39 percent greater than average cerebellar white matter (Aylward et al., 2002; Courchesne, 2004; Volker and Lopata, 2008). By middle childhood or early adolescence, the average brain volume for children diagnosed with autism spectrum disorders tends not to be higher than that of typically developing adolescents. Among the remaining mysteries about autism are the implications of the enlarged head and brain size, which are not currently known.

Atypical patterns of amygdalar development have also been identified in recent studies, with an enlargement in childhood and decreased number of neurons in adulthood. These amygdalar abnormalities have been linked with idiosyncratic patterns of eye contact (Schumann et al., 2004; Schumann and Amaral, 2006; Dalton et al., 2005).

Elevated serotonin levels

Elevated levels of blood platelet serotonin are common. PET scans have revealed diminished serotonin synthesis in the frontal cortex of boys with autism spectrum disorders and increased levels of serotonin synthesis in their cerebella (Mulder et al., 2004: Volker and Lopata, 2008).

Prenatal risk factors

A number of prenatal factors and obstetrical complications are associated with autism. These are summarized in an authoritative meta-analysis by Gardener, Spiegelman and Buka (2009). Their review was based on forty original studies. Subsequent autism has been linked with the following risk factors: gestational diabetes; maternal bleeding during pregnancy; and mother's use of medication, including psychotropic medication, during

pregnancy. Evidence is less conclusive regarding nausea or vomiting during pregnancy, maternal smoking during pregnancy and poor prenatal health in general.

These and other factors co-occur with the age of the parents. The chances of having a child with autism are 27 percent greater if the mother is 30–34 years old in comparison with mothers 25–29 years old. The risk is 106 percent greater if the mother is over 40 years old, compared with mothers under 30. Risk also increased with the age of the father according to some trends in the data analyzed by Gardener, Spiegelman and Buka.

Family factors

In history, the formal identification of autism and the discovery of many of its features co-occurred with the heyday of belief in environmental causation, particularly faulty parenting and, especially, faulty mothering. Looking backwards, it may not seem surprising that parenting was once believed to be the root of the disorder, even though whatever poor parenting there might be would have to have an early and gargantuan effect. Kanner's work emerged in the 1940s, a time when psychoanalysis was highly influential. Reflecting the ideas of his time, Kanner rejected the notion that autism stemmed from any kind of brain dysfunction, although he did believe that genetics was part of the cause. He also observed that many of the parents of children with autism were highly educated, aloof, uninvolved and quite demanding. He believed that this mode of parenting was somehow linked to the children's autism. These ideas entered the vernacular of the time. Looking backwards in 1997, Lorna Wing expressed astonishment at how many of the parents subjected themselves to hundreds of hours of psychoanalysis while no one thought of evaluating the effectiveness of the treatment – or of the lack of treatment for that matter (Wing, 1997).

This concept of the *refrigerator mother* as the cause of her children's autism is now most unmistakably a museum piece. Nevertheless, there is a trend – and no more than a trend – for *some of* the parents of children with autism to have few friends themselves. They also are somewhat more subject to depression and other mental health problems than are the parents of typically developing children, although no higher than the rate of depression among parents of children with other forms of psychopathology (see meta-analysis by Gardener, Spiegleman and Buka, 2009). In any case, their children's autism could be the cause of the depression, not vice versa. The stress and time involved in caring for a child with autism may affect the parents' friendship network. Thus, parental social isolation could also be the result rather than the cause of the disorder.

In recent research, careful observations of the interactions between children with autism and their mothers have not corroborated the image of the refrigerator mother, although the interactions differ somewhat from those between typically developing children and their mothers. In a study by Freeman and Kasari (2013), the parents of children with autism were actually more active than the parents of typically developing children in eliciting play behaviors. However, the parents of the children with autism tended to respond to their children's play with play behaviors that are more mature than those of their children. In contrast, the parents of typically developing children matched and responded at the same level as their children's play. The parents of the children with autism may have responded with the play behaviors they hoped to see but did not. Freeman and Kasari suggest that it may be profitable in therapy to help parents of children with autism respond to their children's play with greater awareness of child cognitive development.

Although poor parenting has been dismissed as a cause of autism, parents still play a vital role in determining how far their children with autism spectrum disorders progress. One important parental role is that of advocate for the child's education and care. In many places, parents have advocated, sometimes in the courts, to obtain for their children the intensive, expensive treatments that have emerged in recent years and that have been found useful, as discussed later in this chapter. Indeed, many authors attribute the increased understanding of autism in recent years and the concomitant improved access to education and care to the incessant efforts of parent advocacy groups (Wolff, 2004).

As well, parents are crucial in the implementation of treatments to deal with problem behaviors, which is also discussed later. This is not because the parents are the causes of the challenging behaviors but because, being faced with behavior problems more severe than those of most children, the parents simply must become more proficient than most parents at managing children's behavior.

Unfortunately, the burden of parenting a child with autism spectrum disorder is highly stressful. Parental stress has been shown to be correlated in a linear fashion with number and severity of the autistic symptoms (Bebko, Konstantareas and Springer, 1987) and with the severity of problem behaviors displayed by the child (Abbeduto et al., 2004) Perry, Harris and Minnes, 2004). However, as documented in a study by Hoffman et al. (2009), parents of children with autism still tend to feel close to their children despite the burden and stress. A number of the personal stories of parents raising children with autism spectrum disorders were recently published in a book by Anderson and Forman (2010). One of the stories, by Kristen Spina, describes the angst experienced by the parents when their child is invited to a birthday party. Accepting the invitation means risking disruptive behavior whereas declining it means isolating the child and perhaps missing out on an opportunity for integration with the peer group. It is important to note that having a child with autism has been linked with higher levels of parental stress than having a child with intellectual disability only or a child with a disruptive behavior disorder (Blacher and McIntyre, 2006).

Child–parent attachment

With the notion of the "refrigerator mother" in the backs of the minds of many, the nature of the attachment bonds between children with autism spectrum disorders and their mothers has become an intriguing area of research. Children with autism usually do not reciprocate affection in ways similar to those of most other children and may not evoke sensitivity on the part of their mothers. Nevertheless, several case studies that appeared early in the literature on autism described secure attachment bonds, inspiring a series of authoritative, methodologically rigorous group-comparison studies. Some of the research involves comparisons between the attachment bonds of children with autism and typically developing children. Other research features comparison of the child–mother attachment of children with autism spectrum disorders and other disorders, often intellectual disability without comorbid autism. These studies were reviewed by Rutgers et al. (2004). Sixteen studies were discussed in the review, of which ten contained data suitable for quantitative meta-analysis. Overall, just over half of the children with autism spectrum disorders who participated in the studies displayed secure attachment bonds with their mothers, with the percentages ranging from 40 to 63 percent in the different studies reviewed. Obviously, this indicates that secure child–mother bonds are not only possible but also very frequent. However, the percentage is lower than for typically developing children. Not surprisingly, very few of the children with autism greeted their mothers actively when the mothers returned to the room in which the Strange Situation procedure was being conducted: 5 percent of children with autism, compared to 35 percent of children with intellectual disability only and 80 percent of typically developing children. Thus, even if the attachment bonds are secure, they may translate into behavior in atypical ways. Unfortunately, only one of the studies reviewed included a measure of the mother's emotional sensitivity, leaving an important aspect of the mother's role unclear.

Peer relations

The behaviors, and probably the thinking, of children with autism spectrum disorders appear to deter potential friends. In a study by Bauminger and Kasari (2000), who worked with twenty-two high-functioning children with autism and nineteen typically developing children, the self-reports of the children with autism indicated that they felt lonelier than the members of the control group and that their friendships brought them less companionship, security and support. Somewhat concerning is the fact that loneliness and friendship ratings were not as highly correlated in the ratings of the children with autism as in the control group. This may mean that the participants with autism may not have understood the concepts of friendship and/or loneliness very well. Some confirmation of this was obtained in a study by Solomon, Bauminger and Rogers (2011), who found that the proficiency in abstract reasoning among high-functioning children with autism was correlated with the quality of their friendships. However, in interviews conducted by Daniel and Billingsley (2010) with seven high-functioning boys with autism 10 to 14 years of age, the boys indicated that they did have friends; their responses did not suggest lack of understanding of the concept. The participants described particular difficulty in establishing new friends, indicating that they did not want to be the one to initiate contact. Some of the respondents were perceptive enough to recognize that there was a social hierarchy in their schools and that they were not rated near its peak. There is probably some basis for this according to a recent study by Chamberlain, Kasari and Rotheram-Fuller (2007), which featured analysis of the group networks in the elementary schools in which seventeen children with high-functioning autism were enrolled. The children with autism were at the periphery of most social groups and experienced little peer companionship. Perhaps because they are aware that they are often rejected by peers, children and adolescents with autism who had friends were actually more likely to experience anxiety than participants with autism who had no friends according to the results of a large-sample study of anxiety and autism by Mazurek and Kanne (2010). One important determinant of the quality of the friendships of high-functioning children with autism seems to be whether or not the friend has autism. In a study by Bauminger and her colleagues (2008), friendships between one child with autism and a typically developing peer were markedly lacking in sharing, positive social action and coordinated play although the friendships appeared to be genuine and rewarding. Importantly, this research featured direct observation of the friends at play as well as questionnaires. School appears to be the place where children with autism make the friends they have (Daniel and Billingsley, 2010). In terms of recreational activities outside of school, children with autism have been found to be even more excluded than children with intellectual disabilities but no autistic features (Solish, Perry and Minnes, 2010).

Treatment

Intensive behavioral interventions

After decades in which treatments for children with autism were the subject of heated controversy but little clarity, interventions based on the principles of *applied behavioral analysis* have emerged as effective in most but not all studies. The fact that there is at last a treatment that probably works if started early enough is in itself a very good reason to rejoice. However, this apparent victory, which many members of the mental health professions are in no hurry to proclaim, comes at a cost: Most of the behavioral interventions proven effective are lengthy, intensive and expensive. Furthermore, they lack the mystique of other treatments and "miracle cures" that have promised to unlock in some creative way the secretive block interfering with the contact between children with autism and the people around them (see below). Instead, the behavioral treatments that are now known to be the most helpful require painstaking effort and patience. It is interesting to note that the research community has resisted recognizing the effectiveness of the intensive behavioral interventions. Part of the reticence may

be a matter of reflex, with many experts conditioned to react negatively to the unwarranted claims of success that have plagued this field. The mechanical, rote nature of the intervention contrasts with the intriguing, rich research on autism as a deficit in basic thinking, language and emotion. However, as evidence accumulates, it is becoming difficult to refute the fact that intensive early applied behavior analysis meets the criteria for a "well-established treatment," as discussed in Chapter 11 (Rogers and Vismara, 2008).

Maurice, Green and Foxx (2001) summarize the core features of the most common forms of applied behavior analysis, known commonly by the acronym ABA. The first element is intensity of treatment, typically 20–40 hours per week that are typically complemented by practicing the skills learned during virtually every waking hour of the child's existence. This may go on for several years. The intervention is individualized to the communication and living skills of the individual child, and sometimes basic academic skills as well. Usually, a wide range of skills are included in the intervention for each child. Skills, such as greeting others or asking for a drink, are broken down into very tiny steps. The goals are sequenced to approximate the normal developmental patterns of typically developing children. The skill is first prompted, then reinforced in some way, perhaps with praise, hug, "rides through the air" or a small bit of food. Several different procedures are used with each child. Treatment starts on a one-to-one basis but is continued in a small-group, family or classroom setting to facilitate generalization of what is learned. Parents become active co-therapists whose role is to help prompt and reinforce the skills that are learned. It is important to note that for the past several decades, positive reinforcement has been used exclusively. The developer of the ABA prototype program, Professor O. Ivar Lovaas of the University of California at Los Angeles, used punishment methods, including mild physical punishment, in his work with children with autism in the 1960s. However, Lovaas later repudiated punishment, stating that his use of it was based on inaccurate scientific information (Lovaas, 1989).

ABA interventions have often been evaluated using the *within-subjects designs* typical of the behavioral movement, with specific, observed behaviors charted at *baseline*, that is, before any reinforcement or intervention is introduced, and then tracked using the same observational procedures as the intervention and reinforcement are introduced. However, there have also been some rigorous controlled group trials conducted, importantly, by researchers outside of the laboratories where the interventions were first developed and tried (see Chapter 11). Virués-Ortega (2010) conducted a meta-analysis of twenty-two studies on the effects of ABA. Eleven of the studies were comparisons of ABA with a control group of some kind, usually a control group receiving another form of intervention. Only a few of these controlled studies featured random assignment of participants to treatments, meaning that it cannot be conclusively established in most of the other studies that the participants in the experimental and control groups were similar in all important ways. Virués-Ortega (2010) reported effect sizes in the range of 1 to 1.5 standard deviation units, which indicates a large effect for most areas of functioning targeted, with the largest effects for language and communication skills. More intensive interventions, that is, those delivered for more hours per week, were more effective than briefer interventions. In a more recent study in which children with autism 18 to 30 months old were randomly assigned to either intensive behavioral treatment or usual community care, the success of applied behavior analysis that was reported in less rigorous studies was confirmed (Dawson et al., 2010). Although the behavioral interventions are of some benefit to older children, there appears to be a critical period between ages 3 and 4 years, after which optimal benefits in language development often fail to appear (Hourmanesh,

2007). Another review of the effects of early behavioral interventions, by Howlin, Magiati and Charman (2009), was based more heavily on changes in IQ. The conclusion was that the early intensive behavioral interventions are indeed effective for most but not all preschoolers with autism. Most of the studies in their review indicated that the experimental groups, who received the intensive treatment, improved more than did the control groups. This was, however, more evident for children who had higher IQs to begin with. Importantly, Howlin, Magiati and Charmin concede candidly that IQ need not be the central outcome measure. They call for more studies of higher methodological quality, especially more studies with random assignment of participants to conditions.

The findings about the general success of ABA and age differences in its effectiveness have led to legal battles between government authorities in some places and the parents of children who have been denied funding for this treatment. The immense costs of the intensive treatment have led to legal disputes even with regard to the younger children who are known to profit from it, as in the legal action that was taken as high as the Supreme Court of Canada by parents who challenged, unsuccessfully, the refusal of the Province of British Columbia to fund applied behavior analysis for their children (Tiedemann, 2008). The Supreme Court refused to rule that ABA was an essential health service, which would have had to be funded according to Canadian law. The decision, though disappointing to many parents of children with autism, did in fact lead to the funding of ABA by some Canadian provinces, sometimes voluntarily, sometimes after legal action. For example, after a series of legal cases in the province of Ontario, the province has agreed to fund ABA for children up to 6 years old. The courts have upheld the province's refusal to fund ABA for older children (Canadian Broadcasting Corporation, 2006).

CASE STUDY: Anne-Marie and Michel, siblings helped by ABA

Perry, Cohen and DeCarlo (1995) present the case study of two siblings, Anne-Marie and Michel. They have one older brother, Daniel, who developed typically without symptoms of autism spectrum disorder. For the first 12–15 months of her life, Anne-Marie's development appeared normal for the most part. She exhibited the normal eye contact and social smile at age-appropriate times and spoke a few single words at age 1 year. She greeted her parents warmly, for example by smiling and saying "Hi, Daddy" when Daddy came home. However, starting at about age 6 months, she began to isolate herself and look serious. She had to be coaxed to play. She would stare at her toys and push them around with a finger rather than play with them. By age 15 months, she displayed the developmental regression, described above, that often occurs in young children with autism. She became irritable and cried frequently. During a 4-day family trip, she maintained her body in an identical position for all waking hours. She became attached to a red toy shovel and tantrumed if it was taken away. At times, she would stare into space or look at her fingers for periods as long as 7 minutes. At age 21 months, Anne-Marie was diagnosed as having autism by a team of mental health professionals.

Anne-Marie's brother Michel, 21 months younger, also showed many signs of developing normally during the first year of life, demonstrating age-appropriate social contact and mastery of single words. By the time he was 18 months old, he was using two-word combinations in an appropriate manner, such as "come here," "sit down" and "bath time." However, at about the same time, he began to withdraw from social contact, became irritable and threw temper tantrums frequently. He began to run back and forth in a corridor at home, looking fixatedly at the wainscoting. When he was 24 months old, Michel screamed uncontrollably at a restaurant for over 30 minutes. His social withdrawal increased and his behavior became increasingly unmanageable. Michel was diagnosed as having autism at that point.

Therapy using applied behavior analysis began when Anne-Marie was 23 months old and when Michel was 25 months old. Trained behavior therapists worked individually with each of the siblings for up to 25 hours a week for 23 and 28 months, respectively. An intensive individualized profile of verbal and non-verbal communication skills, play and cognitive skills was established for each child. Each skill was broken down into numerous small subgoals. The siblings' mother was trained as a parent therapist.

When she was 30 months old, Anne-Marie was able to attend a regular community nursery school. When re-evaluated at age 30 months, the mental health team considered that her symptoms no longer corresponded with the full-blown diagnosis of autism. Anne-Marie continued in regular schools and summer camps throughout the 4-year post-treatment follow-up by Perry and his colleagues. Starting at age 33 months, Michel attended a nursery school that had some special resources to assist children with disabilities. Because of his continued tantrums, Mrs. Maurice remained in the classroom to help manage his behavior. However, by the time he was 4 years old, Michel was able to attend a regular community nursery school; the diagnosis of autism was deemed no longer applicable at that time. By the end of the follow-up period, his reading in school was rated by his teachers as 2 years ahead of the average for pupils his age.

This case study is remarkable, first of all, for its portrayal of parallel developmental regression of two siblings. It of course documents the success of applied behavior analysis. Success to this extent is not at all unusual but not all children participating in the treatment progress to the point that their symptoms are no longer diagnosable, as mentioned earlier in this chapter. Indeed, what some have seen as an implicit claim that autism has been "cured" in some cases has incurred the wrath of many. Probably Lovaas and other proponents of applied behavior analysis should never have reported case studies in which the fact that children who have participated in treatment are no longer diagnosable. This does not necessarily mean that their autism has been "cured" in the sense that no remaining symptoms are present. Nor does it necessarily mean that these behaviorists believe that they can "cure" autism: Many behaviorists do not believe in the concept of disease, so the concept of "cure" has no real meaning to them.

Family interventions

Attachment-based interventions

Interest in the child–parent attachment bonds of children with autism spectrum disorders is beginning to inspire intervention attempts divorced from the concept of the refrigerator mother. In a rigorous study featuring random assignment of participants to either an experimental treatment involving the promotion of parental sensitivity and communication or a usual-treatment control group, Green and his colleagues (2010) found that the parenting skills targeted were significantly improved by the experiment. However, the seventy-seven children in the treatment group, who were preschoolers in major urban areas of the UK, did not improve measurably in language or adaptive skills. Perhaps this kind of training is more suitable for a multicomponent intervention.

Family participation in behavioral and cognitive-behavioral interventions

As described in the previous section on intensive behavioral interventions and in the following section on social skills training, parents play a fundamental role in implementing these techniques and in the maintenance and generalization of the progress made.

Social skills training and cognitive-behavior therapy

Although no other form of intervention for autistic children can rival the success of applied behavior analysis, no other major intervention is as time-intensive or costly. Briefer interventions are, understandably, more successful with children and adolescents who are relatively high-functioning despite being diagnosed as having autism. For example, cognitive-behavioral interventions, which typically consist of direct instruction, role-playing, modeling, performance feedback and rehearsal of new skills, have sometimes been successful in such ways as increasing social interaction, face recognition and solving social problems (LeGoff, 2004; Lopata et al., 2006; Solomon, Goodlin-Jones and Anders, 2004; Thiemann and Goldstein, 2004; Webb et al., 2004). The results of *social skills training* have varied enormously from study to study, providing highly inconsistent support for the effectiveness of social skills training for children and adolescents with autism (see meta-analysis by Wang and Spillane, 2009). Frankel and his colleagues (2010) recently demonstrated that their parent-assisted group treatment for friendship problems was effective for high-functioning children with autism. This intervention, better known for its earlier success with cases of attention deficit/hyperactivity disorder (see Chapter 14), consists of social skills training for the participating children, administered in group format for twelve weekly sessions. During these sessions, the children are taught to approach peers in appropriate ways, initiate conversations and join their play. They also learn how to avoid conflicts. Meeting at the same time, the parent groups learn how to arrange "play

> ## Box 17.3 Social story written to help a child with autism understand and use the concept of helping
>
> ### How I Can Help Children in My Classroom
>
> My name is Juanita. Sometimes, children help me. Being helpful is a friendly thing to do. Many children like to be helped. I can learn to help other children.
>
> Sometimes, children will ask for help. Someone may ask, "Do you know what day it is today?" or "Which page are we on?" or maybe something else.
>
> Answering that question is helpful. If I know the answer, I can answer their question. If I do not know the answer, I may try to help that child find the answer.
>
> Sometimes, a child will move and look all around, either under their desk, in their desk, around their desk. They may be looking for something. I may help. I may say, "Can I help you find something?"
>
> There are other ways I can help. This is my list of ways I can help other children . . .
>
> *Source*: Attwood, T. (2000). Strategies for improving the social integration of children with Asperger's syndrome. *Autism*, 4, 85–100.

dates" for their children and solve any problems that may have arisen during the "play dates." Compared to members of a control group, the program participants improved significantly in teacher-rated social skills, self-control and social participation. Computer-assisted interventions have also been successful, especially with higher-functioning children and adolescents with autism (e.g., Silver and Oakes, 2001).

Attwood (2000) suggests a broader array of methods than has traditionally been included in social skills training programs. One of the methods he proposes is making classmates aware of the nature of the problem so that they can better understand, and hopefully accept, the idiosyncratic behaviors of one of their peers. Another method he emphasizes is direct training of "theory of mind" skills – helping the child with autism spectrum disorder appreciate that other people think about people and situations in ways that are different from theirs. Comic-strip and paragraph-length social stories are useful tools for teachers (see Box 17.3).

Peer-mediated interventions

In many successful attempts to help accommodate children with autism, classroom peers from preschool on have volunteered as mediators. They have been taught to prompt social contact in many ways and to include children with autism in the play activities of typically developing classmates (Kohler, Strain and Goldstein, 2005).

The lure of unproven treatments

Stress-ridden, overburdened and desperate parents are, unfortunately, attracted sometimes passionately to treatments that do not work or that have never been proven to work. These treatments are sometimes expensive. One of the most popular treatments to emerge in the past few years is *facilitated communication*. It is typically used with children with autism who have little or no spoken language. While the child's hand is held by an adult, the child uses a keyboard or points to symbols or images. Thus, the child is essentially communicating through the adult holding the hand. Proponents of the technique purport that it allows communication by children who cannot express themselves verbally. This claim has been clearly refuted by researchers, who have established in many studies that it is actually the adult who initiates the communication in most cases (Kavale and Mostert, 2004). A detailed evaluation by Bebko, Perry and Bryson (1996) indicated that there were a small number of cases, perhaps one in fifteen, where the child initiates the communication. This conclusion is supported by many professional organizations, including the American Psychological Association (1994). However, it is disputed by advocates of the technique, who claim that the procedure is too complicated to be evaluated by empirical research (Emerson, Grayson and Griffiths, 2001; Mostert, 2010). In contrast, there were a substantial number of cases in which some children who are capable of some communication using language or signing communicate more poorly using facilitated communication. This means that they are actually harmed by facilitated communication because their communication abilities are not developed as fully as they could be. Other possible harmful effects include children being transferred to school settings that are not realistic for them on the basis of typed transcripts of what is thought to be their language. As well, there are concerns that unfounded allegations of sexual abuse have emerged through the technique (Howlin and Jones, 1996). Facilitated communication seems to remain in widespread use, despite the lack of research support. Mostert (2010) observes that the continued appeal of the technique demonstrates that many parents and practitioners are not guided by research in their choice of treatments for children with autism.

New unproven treatments continue to appear as the appeal of some of those in vogue a few years ago wanes. One recent technique, condemned by experts in the field, is called *packing*. Packing, which is mostly practiced in France, consists of first wrapping the child, dressed only in underwear, in towels soaked in cold water, then in blankets to help the individual warm up over a period of 45 minutes. This may go one for weeks or months. This is supposed to help rid the child of unhealthy defense mechanisms. This treatment was recently condemned at an international meeting of experts (Amaral et al., 2011).

Pharmacological interventions

Although there is in general no established pharmacological treatment for the core symptoms of autism spectrum disorder, there have been successful psychopharmacological interventions for comorbid attention and aggression problems. There has been some use of antipsychotic and antidepressant medication to reduce stereotyped, repetitive behavior but there is considerable concern about harmful side effects (Rutter, 2011; Volker and Lopata, 2008).

Conclusions and future directions

The alarm raised in some circles about the possibility that autism is an emerging epidemic is not without its benefits. Teachers, psychologists and physicians have become increasingly aware of autism. Many sources credit parent advocacy groups with raising awareness both in the general public and the scientific community (Chakrabarti and Fombonne, 2001; Wolff, 2004). Scientific research on autism has increased dramatically in recent years. Perhaps this momentum will result in a swift, sweeping discovery of the cause of the disorder, leading to a treatment that will address its true cause. The most likely way for this to happen is probably through some new discovery in molecular genetics. However, the comings and goings of ideas in this field and treatments backed up only by creative theories suggest that an earthshaking revelation may not appear. In its place, ongoing, painstaking, step-by-step effort will probably shed light slowly on some of the mysteries about this disorder and its treatment. The popular press does not always reflect this sad reality. Press reports about possible causes and possible new treatments often appear without mention of the very preliminary nature of the research that supports them.

Pending the final outcomes of many of the questions being tackled by researchers, there have been some isolated appeals for a reappraisal of the symptoms of autism spectrum disorder. For example, as illustrated in several case studies described by Cook (2012), a focus on small detail without detraction by the social environment can indeed be an asset in certain work settings, including some that involve sophisticated technological production.

Summary

- Autism spectrum disorders are a heterogeneous group of disorders characterized by neurologically based deficits in social communication and social interaction. Children with autism may also have dysfunctions in the basic understanding and expression of emotion, delayed and deviant language patterns, idiosyncratic intonation and uncoordinated language. Some children with autism repeat words often (echolalia).
- Other typical behaviors for children with autism include repetitive and ritualistic behaviors, repetitive organizing and becoming upset even when a minor aspect of their environment is changed. They may fixate their attention on an object for an extended period of time. This may be why some people with autism are very talented in very specific skills, called savant skills.
- The decision by the DSM-5 Commission to eliminate Asperger's disorder as a separate disorder generated considerable controversy. Many individuals who would have been diagnosed as having Asperger's disorder are now identified by specifiers as having autism without intellectual disability. These individuals master language and engage in social interaction but in atypical, idiosyncratic ways.
- The theory of the mind refers to the developmental ability to distinguish their mind from the minds of other people, with their own intentions and thinking. Those with autism spectrum disorders acquire this basic ability to some extent but much later than their peers. This results in an egocentric view of the world and gaps in the awareness of other people's feelings and intentions.
- The increase over time in the prevalence of autism may be a result of changes in diagnostic criteria and greater familiarity with the disorder by mental health professionals, leading to clinicians diagnosing it more often than before.
- Some scholars, on the other hand, attribute the increase to environmental changes, such as mercury in food and water, high levels of lead, increased smoking by pregnant women, pesticides, vaccination against measles, mumps and rubella; the latter being disproven by research.
- The majority of autism disorders are in boys but there are many girls with autism.
- Common comorbid disorders include intellectual disability, social anxiety disorder, attention deficit/hyperactivity disorder, oppositional defiant disorder, generalized anxiety disorder, panic disorder, major depressive disorder and conduct disorder.
- Cross-culturally, no reliable studies on the differences in prevalence of autism have been conducted. However, some scholars believe that there are important cross-cultural differences in the consequences of having autism.
- Early signs of autism in infants include: looking at others less often, not reacting when their name is called, failure to show objects to people, and not pointing to people or things. Other signs include failing to make eye contact and rarely smiling. As the diagnostic criteria do not include these behaviors, researchers often distinguish the prodrome of autism (i.e., early precursors) from the disorder itself.
- Children with autism often display enlarged head circumferences and enlargements of the amygdala.

- Some young children with autism are known to regress to earlier stages of development, which is very unusual in human development.
- Prevalence rates have increased dramatically in recent years, from 0.1 to 0.2 percent 20 or 30 years ago to at least 0.4 percent now and probably more. The reasons for this increase are the subject of considerable speculation.
- The heritability of autism is high, with at least three or four genes implicated in its etiology.
- Other genetic influences that may cause autism include chromosomal abnormalities, such as duplications and deletions, spontaneous mutations and inherited variations.
- Neurological correlates of autism include: enlarged head and brain size, atypical patterns of amygdala development and elevated levels of blood platelet serotonin.
- Prenatal factors and obstetrical complications, such as gestational diabetes, maternal bleeding during pregnancy and mother's use of medication, can be risk factors for children. The age of the parents is also a major risk factor: The older the mother and father, the more likely the child will have autism.
- The term "refrigerator mother" refers to the idea that the mother is responsible for the child's psychological disorder. This has now been disproved. However, the mother's depression may be caused by the stress inherent in rearing an autistic child.
- Parental stress has been found to be correlated with the number and severity of the autistic symptoms and with the severity of the problem behaviors displayed by the child. This stress is higher among parents of autistic children than parents of children with either intellectual disability or disruptive behavior disorder.
- Secure child–mother attachment even when the child has autism is not only possible, but quite frequent. However, attachment is frequently less secure than with typically developing children. This secure attachment may be shown in distinct ways, though, with very few autistic children actively greeting their mothers.
- With regard to peer relations, children with autism usually feel lonelier than others. Their friendships usually bring them less companionship, security and support. Friendships between two children with autism do not develop as typically as do friendships between two children where only one of them has the disorder.
- The principles of applied behavioral analysis used in intensive behavioral interventions are lengthy, intensive and expensive. This method features intense individualized treatments to teach social skills by breaking down the actions into very tiny steps and reinforcing the positive behavior.
- Research to evaluate ABA often uses within-subjects designs, where observed behaviors are measured at baseline, then after the intervention and reinforcement are introduced. The more intensive the intervention and the higher the IQ of the child before the intervention, the more effective the treatment, provided that treatment started before the critical age of 3–4 years.
- Family interventions, such as attachment-based interventions (involving the promotion of parental sensitivity and communication) and family participation in behavioral and cognitive-behavioral interventions, have been used with some success.
- Cognitive-behavioral interventions, parent-assisted group treatment (i.e., social skills training) and computer-assisted interventions, while less effective than applied behavioral analysis, are briefer, cheaper interventions that have some success among high-functioning children with autism.
- Facilitated communication, involving a facilitator, e.g. a parent, holding the hand of a child and facilitating the communication on a message board, is an example of an unproven technique. It has also been shown to compromise improvement and, in rare cases, invoke accusations of sexual abuse. Packing is another unproven technique involving wrapping the child in cold wet towels to rid the child of unhealthy defense mechanisms.

Study questions

1. Do you agree with the decision to eliminate the category of Asperger's syndrome from the DSM? Why or why not?
2. What are some possible reasons for the apparent recent increase in the prevalence of autism spectrum disorders?
3. What causes autism?
4. How can parents best help their children with autism spectrum disorders?
5. What is the most effective treatment for most children with autism spectrum disorders?

There are two scientific reasons learning problems are considered mental health disorders. One reason is that learning disabilities probably share with many other forms of mental illness an underlying neurobiological basis. Another reason is that learning problems are linked with other forms of psychopathology such as attention deficit, depression and anxiety, and disruptive behavior disorders. When learning problems and other forms of psychopathology co-occur, the learning problems often exacerbate behavioral and emotional difficulties. At the same time, the behavioral and emotional difficulties make it harder for teachers to help with the learning problems.

This chapter begins with a short section on basic terminology. In the section that follows, several case examples from literary sources illustrate the interplay of learning and social/emotional problems. Diagnostic categories are then presented, followed by information about the prevalence. Cultural and gender issues are discussed as moderators of the prevalence rates. Possible causes are considered next, with emphasis on the neuropsychology that is thought to be at the root of learning disabilities. After a discussion of the family bases of learning disorder and peer factors, the final section of the chapter is devoted to treatment issues, with emphasis on the role of the psychologist. The assessment and remediation of academic skills per se are beyond the scope of this book. The reader is referred to textbooks oriented to the school-based professional, such as *Learning Disabilities: Characteristics, Identification and Teaching Strategies* (sixth edition, Bender, 2008).

Terminology: plain English vs. fancy Greek

Confusing terminology has plagued this area at least as much as any other form of psychopathology.

However, the issue is of particular importance here because an operational definition that evokes brain pathology could not be useful in clinical diagnosis because the underlying brain pathology that is hypothesized simply cannot be identified in most individuals affected. The nomenclature has followed trends over the years in beliefs about the way the brain affects children's learning and related processes. At times, experts have been accused of using, if not hiding behind, excessive and inappropriate jargon. The term *specific learning disorder* is used in DSM-5, with specifiers to indicate both the academic area affected (i.e., reading, writing or mathematics) and the degree of severity.

Nevertheless, terms like "reading disorder" have never garnered widespread appeal. One knee-jerk reaction to their simplicity is to question the inclusion of basic school-subject material in a taxonomy of mental disorders. The term *learning disabilities* is currently the most common in schools in most parts of the world; it applies to specific learning problems that are not best explained by intellectual disability. However, in the UK, that expression is often used synonymously with intellectual disabilities. The classic terms *dyslexia* and *dyscalculia* are still used widely around the world in writings in the fields of neuropsychology and special education. Scientific as they may sound, these terms are nothing more than combinations of two Greek words that indicate difficulty in reading and mathematics, respectively.

Crippling effects of learning disabilities depicted in literature and film

Novelists and filmmakers have helped sensitize the public to the scope of the effects of learning disabilities. The best-known example is Ruth Rendell's novel *A Judgment in Stone* (1977), which was the basis of the 1986 film *The Housekeeper,* and the far more successful 1995 film *La Cérémonie* by renowned French director Claude Chabrol. Unable to recognize the learning disabilities of their daughter Eunice, the parents mistreat her and consider her stupid. She never learns to read, which she has to conceal when applying even for jobs as a domestic cleaner and servant. Embroiled with rage, she eventually kills her employers. She is convicted of the crime because she cannot read a note which ended up being used as evidence against her.

A happier fate awaits Ishaan, 8 years old, the protagonist in the award-winning 2007 Bollywood film *Taare Zameen Par* (Like Stars on Earth). Though nominated as the Indian entry for the Academy Award for best foreign film, the film was not a commercial success. However, the film is credited for raising awareness about learning disabilities and other learning disorders in India (Naithani, 2008). Within weeks of its release, the school authorities in Mumbai, where the action takes place, began suddenly to improve educational provision for children with learning disabilities. Ishaan is the youngest son of a well-educated, successful family that has high aspirations for him. His older brother Yohaan is a star athlete and top student. Ishaan is sent to a private boarding school in an effort to improve his academic achievement. He is despondent and lonely there until his stellar artistic talent is noted by a new art teacher. The teacher takes an interest in Ishaan's situation and concludes that the boy probably has learning disabilities. Nikumbh, the teacher, manages to convince Ishaan's father that Ishaan is not just lazy. Nikumbh confides in Ishaan that he too had learning disabilities in his school days. Nikumbh also helps improve Ishaan's reputation among his peers by explaining in class what learning disabilities are and by mentioning the names of celebrities who have gone on to exceptional professional stature despite their learning disabilities (of course, Nikumbh was also explaining learning disabilities to the Indian public). With individual tutoring by Nikumbh, Ishaan begins to do better in school. In a classic Bollywood happy ending replete with joyous, celebratory music, Ishaan wins the prize for artistic achievement in an elaborately staged contest judged by a prominent Indian artist. At the award ceremony, he is congratulated warmly by his parents, who express eternal gratitude to Nikumbh.

Although they are not portrayed as helping Ishaan's transformation, Ishaan does find supportive friends among his peers at boarding school. Unfortunately, that is not always the case for children with learning disabilities and other learning disorders, as will be discussed in the section on peer factors later in this chapter.

CASE STUDY: Jane, struggling with a non-verbal learning disability

Rourke et al. (1990) provide the interesting case study of Jane to illustrate the challenges faced by children with a relatively rare form of learning disabilities, a non-verbal learning disability (see discussion of subtypes later in this chapter). This form of learning disability pertains to children and adults who are quite skilled in using language but have great difficulty on visuo-spatial tasks such as understanding diagrams and performing complex psychomotor tasks. Their attention span is quite good when listening to spoken language or for learning simple, rote material. They remember what they have heard very well but have difficulty remembering what they have seen. They may have difficulty in mathematics and science but often do well in spelling or in reading isolated words. However, they may have problems understanding social situations or the meaning of extended passages they have read. They may have problems relating to others, in part because of difficulties maintaining eye contact and using appropriate facial expressions and body language. Because the school curriculum is so heavily based on language abilities rather than non-verbal abilities, this form of learning disabilities is often undetected by teachers.

Jane, age 9 years, was first referred to the clinic by her family doctor primarily because of problems at school in writing assignments and basic arithmetic skills. Her teachers reported that her fine and gross motor skills were weak but that she did well in reading and spelling. Jane's mother reported that Jane had difficulty concentrating on things and relating to others.

The health history compiled by the clinic professionals noted no substantial irregularities during the pregnancy, birth or early development. However, a specialist was assessing Jane for possible allergies. Jane was seen by a neurologist, who found only some small irregularities, such as nystagmus (involuntary eye movement) when gazing to the left. The neurologist also noted mild ataxia (poor coordination of one's muscle movements) and mild apraxia (the inability to use one's body to perform some movements that the person wants to perform). It was concluded that Jane's learning problems were probably not related to these issues.

Jane participated in a series of neuropsychological tests. These tests were repeated 2, 4 and 6 years later to assess Jane's progress. Jane responded to the test questions in an immature, sing-song voice. Her eye-hand coordination was quite poor. Standard intelligence testing during the initial assessment revealed verbal abilities at about the average for pupils her age but non-verbal abilities at about the first percentile, meaning that in a typical group of 100 pupils her age, ninety-nine would have scores higher than Jane's. Her reading scores were well above average, as was her spelling. However, she was a year and a half below her age level in arithmetic. Importantly, a questionnaire revealed a high degree of social immaturity. Adults who worked with her noted that she related fairly well with adults but responded to other children without much emotional expression in a fairly automatic way. Because of her immaturity and the range of her deficits, Jane's parents and the clinic team decided that Jane should be enrolled in full-day special education. Reassessment at 2-year intervals indicated steady improvements in all areas. However, even 5 years after first being referred, the consensus of professional opinion was that Jane was still not functioning socially at the level of maturity that she would need in order to function successfully in a regular secondary-school situation. Rourke et al. (1990) concluded that this problem persisted because of the strength and pervasiveness of the effects of Jane's non-verbal learning disability.

Diagnostic criteria

As is the case for all definitions of these conditions, the definitions in standard diagnostic schemes represent the compromises designed to define the disorders in the clearest possible manner that would facilitate reliable diagnosis. The definitions have been constructed to avoid notions of causality in general for all disorders and, in the case of learning problems specifically, the invocation of possible causes not

> ## Box 18.1 | Major changes in the diagnostic criteria for learning disorders from DSM-IV to DSM-5
>
> 1. DSM-IV included separate categories for different learning disorders, such as Specific Reading Disorder, Specific Arithmetic Disorder. Recognizing that these learning problems often occur together, the single category of Specific Learning Disorder was introduced in DSM-5.
> 2. DSM-IV specified a statistical discrepancy between IQ and achievement. This has been discarded in DSM-5. The diagnosis of Specific Learning Disorder in DSM-5 requires: (1) that the individual's academic achievement be considerably below average; and (2) that the problem is not better explained by another diagnosable disorder.
> 3. The language used in DSM-5 reflects more of a lifespan perspective than the language of DSM-IV, which contained expressions most relevant to schoolchildren.

well supported by research. When they first appeared, these simple definitions were dismissed by some major authorities in the field as attempts to define learning disability by defining "what it is not" (e.g., Cruickshank, 1975).

The minimalist diagnostic criteria for specific learning disorder in DSM-5, summarized in Box 18.1, are that, first of all, the individual's academic skills must be below the level that would be expected for the person's age, education and level of intelligence. It is further specified that these reading problems must interfere with the person's academic achievement or performance at work. Finally, the difficulty must not be better explained by another mental disorder such as intellectual disability (American Psychiatric Association, 2000).

The ICD-10 category of *specific reading disorder* is similarly minimalist in its defining characteristics. However, there is a semantic difference in the ICD-10 use of the qualifier "specific" rather than specifying a discrepancy between academic achievement and general intellectual disability. The current diagnostic criteria for developmental arithmetic disorder and other learning problems are very similar to those that pertain to reading problems.

Importantly, the DSM-5 criteria stop short of specifying a gap between academic achievement and IQ, which appeared in early editions and in some documents on the categorization of pupils receiving special education. The diminished importance of IQ reflects the weight of increasing evidence that measured IQ, especially full-scale IQ, is not as good a predictor of academic performance in specific areas as was believed in the past (Gresham and Vellutino, 2010; see meta-analysis by Stuebing et al., 2002). As well, it is impossible to measure intelligence in ways that are not influenced to some extent by the individual's previous education and cultural background. Therefore, defining learning disabilities on the basis of this discrepancy can unwittingly lead to inaccuracies in diagnosing the learning problems of members of cultural minority groups (e.g., Siegel, 1999).

Subtypes

It is often found useful to subdivide the heterogeneous population of children with learning disorders for research. Subtyping may also facilitate remedial interventions. Several different classification systems have been developed. Several classification schemes were inspired in the 1970s by the cybernetic or language processing approach espoused by Samuel Kirk and his colleagues, as discussed later in this chapter. The most enduring distinction that has influenced thinking and research over several decades is between children whose learning problems can be attributed mostly to poor verbal skills and those whose learning problems are linked to non-verbal weaknesses (Goldstein and Schwebach, 2009; Rourke, 1989). Non-verbal learning disorders can include such deficits as "visual-spatial-organizational, tactile-perceptual, psychomotor, and nonverbal problem-solving skills" (Forrest, 2004). Aside from the implications of the distinction between verbal and non-verbal disabilities for academic remediation, it is possible that children with non-verbal learning disabilities experience greater difficulties than other children in social interaction with their peers. Galway and Metsala (2011) found that children with non-verbal learning disabilities have difficulty generating appropriate solutions to social problems. They also tended to attribute negative intent to characters in vignettes read to them. Petti et al. (2003) found that children with non-verbal forms of learning disorders tended to have difficulty recognizing the facial cues that convey emotion. It has also been suggested that children with non-verbal learning disabilities are at greater risk for a variety of mental health disorders than children with other types of learning disorder. However, research support for this contention has been somewhat inconsistent (Forrest, 2004: Petti et al., 2003). Children who are affected by the non-verbal subtype are also considered more likely to be socially inept than are children with other forms of learning disabilities (Galway and Metsala, 2011; Rourke, 1995). Logically, an inability to recognize the emotional expressions of others might be behind this, because this skill involves the decoding of non-verbal stimuli. However, the limited research on this issue has failed to identify consistent differences between adolescents with non-verbal and other forms of learning disabilities in the recognition of facial features that convey emotion (Bloom and Heath, 2010).

Prevalence

As with any other disorder, calculating prevalence estimates depends on an accepted standard definition. As already discussed in this chapter, definitional issues here are among the most complex in the field of psychopathology. As well, many of the epidemiological studies of the prevalence in the population of learning disabilities are based in large part on the mathematical discrepancies between IQ and achievement (e.g., Rutter and Yule, 1975), which, as just mentioned, is increasingly criticized. Another probable source of inconsistency is the fact that the DSM and ICD do not specify how the impaired academic subject matter, such as reading, is to be measured. Reading, for instance, might be measured by school marks, tests of reading comprehension or tests of the reading of separate letters and words. Furthermore, the issue of dimensional versus categorical models of psychopathology is very applicable to enumerating the population of persons with learning disorders because these diagnoses could be applied to large segments of the school population whose academic achievement is below average. In a longitudinal study conducted in Connecticut by Shaywitz and her colleagues (Shaywitz, 2003), 17.4 percent of the participants were reading at levels below what would be expected on the basis of their ages and measured intellectual levels. The 2007 report of the Office of Special Education Programs of the US Department of Education (2010) indicates that 14 percent of 6–11 year olds and fully 25.5 percent of pupils 12–17 years old were receiving services after being identified as having specific learning disabilities, a very dramatic increase from figures in the same annual report even 5 years earlier. However, there has been some concern that these educational classifications are being overused, in part to avoid using labels that many people find more stigmatizing (Kavale and Forness, 1998; MacMillan and Siperstein, 2002).

In an authoritative study of children's mental health problems conducted on the Isle of Wight, Rutter and Yule (1975) estimated the incidence of "reading retardation" at just over 3 percent of the population. The incidence statistics in impoverished areas of central London are fully twice as high (Rutter and Maughan, 2005). Similar discrepancies in prevalence data have been reported in different US states for reasons that are not entirely clear. For example, Reschly and Hosp (2004), in a study of prevalence rates in all fifty states, found a threefold difference between Kentucky (2.85%), the state with the lowest identification rate, and Rhode Island (9.85%), the state with the highest identification rate.

Sex differences

It was reported in previous chapters for many of the most common forms of child psychopathology (i.e., disruptive behavior disorders, attention deficit/hyperactivity disorder and autism spectrum disorder) that there is a high disproportion of boys in the diagnostic category. Depending on the nature of the data being considered, many more boys than girls appear to be diagnosed as having learning disabilities or at least enrolled in special programs for pupils with these difficulties. For example, it is estimated that three out of four pupils receiving special education assistance for learning problems in the United States are boys (Coutinho and Oswald, 2005). There is, however, some lingering doubt that males represent three-fourths of the true population incidence of learning disorders even though it is commonly believed that a somewhat higher number of boys are struggling to achieve in school than are girls (Shaywitz, Morris and Shaywitz, 2008). Ample data suggest that many teachers are biased in their referrals of children for assessment and remediation of learning problems. They tend to refer boys for attention and learning problems even when their attention and learning are very similar to those of girls who are not referred (Gillberg, 2003; Rivard et al., 2007; Shaywitz, 1996). Shaywitz, Morris and Shaywitz (2008) speculate that girls' learning problems are manifest in more subtle ways than those of boys, in ways that attract less teacher attention and concern. Not surprisingly, when more objective

measures of academic progress are used, there appears to be less of a teacher-referral bias against girls than with measures that are less precise, asking only for teacher's general impressions of whether or not the child has a learning problem rather than specific data about the child's learning (Flannery et al., 2000). In any case, the social and political implications of the gender imbalance have been debated widely. The contention that schools are not designed to accommodate the bodies and brains of boys (Sommers, 2000) is voiced in counterpoint with concern that real learning problems of girls are being ignored (Jones et al., 2000).

Culture

The incidence of learning disabilities in different countries, as well as the appropriate methods for its diagnosis and remediation, depend in part on the orthographic features of the language used. Spanish, for example, is completely phonetic: The same letters are always pronounced in the same way. For that reason, it is believed that children find it easier to read such languages as Spanish and Italian than English (Smythe et al., 2008; Ziegler and Goswami, 2005). That reason has been offered to explain the apparently lower rate of learning disabilities in Italy compared to the United States (Lindgren, De Renzi and Richman, 1985). This does not apply to English. Chinese, for example, uses symbols to represent complete words, which may mean that the nature of learning disabilities among Chinese speakers is different from learning disabilities among English speakers. However, these language differences do not totally explain the cross-national differences that have been reported. For example, Jimenez and Garcia de la Cadena (2007), using identical diagnostic procedures in two Spanish-speaking countries, Guatemala and Spain, found that the rate of learning disabilities was at least three times as high in Guatemala. They attributed the difference to the discrepancies between the countries in terms of social conditions and environmental stimulation. However, their cross-national comparisons are also valuable in confirming that many of the language and memory deficits associated with learning disabilities occurred in the dyslexic samples of both countries. It is more difficult to interpret cross-national comparisons in which identical diagnostic procedures are not administered because of the differences between countries in definitions of learning disabilities and the professional training of teachers and diagnosticians (Sideridis, 2007a).

Many simultaneous influences affect incidence of learning disabilities among cultural minority groups in complex multicultural societies, including the nature of written language in the child's first language and the trials of mastering the host language. Cultural differences may interact with economic hardship. Whatever the reasons, immigrant children are, for example, disproportionally enrolled in special schools in Germany for pupils with learning problems (Werning, Loser and Urban, 2008). Low socio-economic status by itself is also a risk factor for learning disabilities, as shown in a study of the families of the children attending a special learning clinic near Paris (Melekian, 1990). However, because parents of low socio-economic status tend to have lower educational levels themselves than more affluent parents, it may be the parents' education and not their income that is the important determinant (Melekian, 1990).

Comorbid mental health conditions

Statistical estimates of comorbidity share with other epistemological data the problems entailed by the lack of uniformity in the definitions of learning disabilities. Nevertheless, all data converge to indicate substantial comorbidity rates. Although the components of the now-defunct syndrome of minimal brain damage, discussed elsewhere in this chapter, have now been unpackaged, learning disabilities and ADHD often co-occur. The overlap between learning disorders and ADHD is estimated conservatively at 20–25 percent and, depending on the definitions used, may be considerably higher, to the degree of indicating comorbidity in the

overwhelming majority of cases (Spencer, Biederman and Mick, 2007). Children with this particular comorbidity may be at greater risk for long-term maladjustment than children with only one of these two disorders according to a 5-year longitudinal study by Willcutt and his colleagues (2007), who focused on both academic and social outcomes. Data from a large-scale longitudinal twin study conducted in England suggest that the reason for this comorbidity probably is common genetic influence (Trzesniewski et al., 2006).

The same data, however, do not suggest a genetic link between learning disabilities and disruptive behavior disorders but suggest that learning disabilities and behavior disorders may both be caused by shared environmental factors. The common environmental factors often include an intellectually unstimulating home background, low socio-economic status, maternal depression and child neglect. Trzesniewski and her colleagues (2006) found a reciprocal relationship between reading problems and anti-social behavior: Anti-social behavior led to later reading problems but early reading problems also led to anti-social behavior. Using data from a large-scale longitudinal study in the United States, with a sample size of over 11,000, Morgan et al. (2008) arrived at the same conclusion as did Algozzine, Wang and Violette (2011) with a sample of several hundred US elementary-school pupils. Glassberg, Hooper and Mattison (1999) found that anywhere from one-fourth to one-half of the children and adolescents enrolled in a special educational facility for children with severe behavior problems could be classified as having learning disabilities, depending on the definition used. In elaborating on the mechanisms that might explain the link between learning disorders and disruptive behavior problems, McIntosh et al. (2006) described a *coercive cycle of anti-social behavior*, in which early distaste for the academic demands of the school leads to missing out on instruction, sometimes by being sent out of the class. Having lost access to instruction, the child with learning disabilities falls further behind, finds academics even more aversive and, finally, engages in anti-social behavior as an escape mechanism.

There are several reasons why adolescents with learning disabilities and other learning disorders may choose to engage in such risky behaviors as substance abuse, unprotected sex, shoplifting, gambling and joyriding. One reason could be the poor judgment that may stem from the neurological correlates of learning disorders. Another may be the accumulated frustrations of academic failure. In a study conducted with adolescents with learning disorders in Southern Ontario, McNamara, Vervaeke and Willoughby (2008) found that, in addition to the risk posed by the learning disorder itself, psychosocial factors such as a strained relationship between the adolescents and their mothers and lack of involvement in recreational activity increased the chances of the emergence of risky behaviors. Interestingly, there was little difference in this study between the risky behaviors of participants with comorbid attention deficit/hyperactivity disorder and those diagnosed as having learning disorders only. It is important to remember that risk factors such as those studied by McNamara and his colleagues may interact not only with each other to increase the risk of a child with learning disabilities engaging in substance abuse; these risk factors also interact with risk factors within the child such as genetic vulnerability, prenatal substance exposure and substance abuse in the family (Weinberg, 2001).

The stress of living with a learning problem may trigger a depressive episode, which is one of the possible reasons for the co-occurrence of depression and learning disorders. Another possible cause is the poor coping strategies used by children and adolescents with learning disabilities when faced with problems. Rather than generating effective coping strategies for dealing with difficult situations, they often attempt to avoid the problem altogether (Firth, Greaves and Frydenberg, 2010). Sideridis (2007b) emphasized the enormous tension inherent in constantly seeking to avoid failure as a cause of depressed mood among children and adolescents with learning disorders. Among the Canadian

adolescents with self-reported learning disabilities surveyed by Wilson et al (2009), 14.6 percent also reported that they were depressed.

The cumulative experience of academic failure may also provoke dysfunctional levels of anxiety. On the other hand, dysfunctional levels of anxiety may also lead to academic failure. Finally, a common neurological deficit may lead to both learning disabilities and anxiety (Nelson and Harwood, 2011; Woodward and Fergusson, 2001). In a useful meta-analysis of fifty-eight well-designed studies conducted with over 3,000 participants, Nelson and Harwood (2011) found a significant association between learning problems and anxiety, with an overall moderate effect size of .61 for comparisons between participants with and without learning disorders in the original studies. They were able to estimate statistically that over 70 percent of the participants had to contend with substantial anxiety problems although not necessarily to the extent of the formal diagnosis of anxiety disorder. There was, however, substantial variability among the results of the fifty-eight original studies. This variability had little to do with any characteristics of the participants but was best explained by differences among the sources of information about the anxiety, that is, teacher, parent and self-reports. As in the many other instances in which research in psychopathology is hampered by lack of agreement among informants, more comprehensive, focused research is needed on learning problems among children and adolescents with clinically diagnosed anxiety disorders.

Probable causes and concurrent impairment

One of the many myths about learning disabilities that are slow to die is the belief that they represent some form of *developmental delay* rather than a developmental *deficit*. Perhaps this myth is perpetuated by reports about distinguished individuals who probably had learning disabilities as children but who went on to greatness. The list includes Michelangelo, Beethoven, Hans Christian Anderson, Picasso, Mozart and Tom Cruise (van Kraayenoord, 2002). The cases do not represent the norm.

The brain and children's learning behaviors: a journey in science and science fiction

The neuropsychological basis of learning disabilities has been recognized continuously as fundamental since these problems were first reported in case studies published about 300 years ago (Anderson and Meier-Hedde, 2001). This intriguing history is recounted succinctly in a very readable book by Sylvia Farnham-Diggory (1992). The best-known of the case histories that began to appear in the late 1800s were those reported by Scottish ophthalmologist James Hinshelwood. One of the cases was that of a tailor who, after many years of work at his craft, had forgotten the way common sewing stiches looked and were executed. Hinshelwood noted that the tailor had become an alcoholic and attributed the loss of visual memory to brain damage caused by alcoholism. His belief in the neurological origin of the visual-memory problems was based on his familiarity with other cases where brain damage had undeniably occurred, such as stroke patients. Inferring the cause to the brain was, in the case of the tailor, plausible but by no means proven. Venturing even further, Hinshelwood attributed brain pathology, specifically with regard to visual memory, to the problems of several schoolboys from the same family who were referred by their schoolmasters because they could not remember letters or words despite displaying age-appropriate language and thinking skills (Anderson and Meier-Hedde, 2001; Farnham-Diggory, 1992).

Similar logic continued with the seminal work of pioneers in the early and middle twentieth century. The best-known heroes of the era are Samuel Orton and Alfred Strauss, physicians from very different backgrounds who both worked in state psychiatric hospitals in the United States. Like Hinshelwood, both Orton and Strauss had worked with adults who had clearly experienced brain damage, such as, in Strauss' case, head injuries incurred during wartime. In their work at the state mental hospitals, both physicians were able to identify a group of children whose distractible behavior and learning problems resembled the symptoms demonstrated by people who were known to have suffered brain injuries. This group was distinguishable from the population of people with intellectual disability because the impairment was deemed to be localized and specific, mainly in language functions and focused attention but not abstract reasoning. In fact, the adjective "specific" has often been incorporated in definitions of the disorder. Of course, both eminent neurologists were handicapped by the very limited technology available at the time for studying the workings of the human brain. At the time, the diagnosis of brain damage was usually based on the presence in behavior or in psychological tests of the same symptoms that precipitated the referral for assessment. Although this logic has been widely criticized as tautological (Johnson and Myklebust, 1967; Kavale and Forness, 1985), assessment based on such "soft signs" of brain damage is still practiced, although hopefully with more modest assumptions.

Orton believed that the learning problems were attributable to the lack of complete hemispheric specialization in the brain, expressed frequently in letter reversals after the age at which most children stop making them, and problems with directionality. As many physicians of the era would do when a new condition was being introduced into knowledge, a Latin or Greek title was invoked, in this case dyslexia, derived from the Greek. In contrast, Strauss and his colleague Werner conceptualized the learning problems as part of a wider syndrome that affects the child's basic perceptual processes and that is also reflected in problems of impulsivity and distractibility, which are the core features of attention deficit/hyperactivity syndrome, as discussed in Chapter 14. The condition thus identified was sometimes called *Strauss syndrome* but more often by one of the ubiquitous TLAs (three-letter acronyms) in the mental health field, namely

MBD – *minimal brain dysfunction*. Many similar TLAs such as *minimal brain damage* and *minimal cerebral dysfunction* were also used. Although their hasty invocation of minor brain damage is now considered premature, Orton, Strauss and Werner are remembered because of the many remedial educational techniques that their theories inspired. In order to best accommodate children with minimal brain dysfunction according to the thinking of the time, classrooms were constructed that provided minimal distracting visual stimuli. Efforts were made to have children use simultaneously as many senses as possible – auditory, visual and tactile, such as by tracing the letters of the alphabet in sand (Farnham-Diggory, 1992; Goldstein and Schwebach, 2009; Kavale and Forness, 1985).

Process-oriented or *cybernetic* models and vocabulary, based on psycholinguistics, became prevalent in the 1960s and 1970s. Prominent American psychologist Samuel A. Kirk emphasized the specificity of the problems and introduced the term "learning disabilities" to describe them. Learning disabilities were described according to the language or communication channel or channels that might be impaired, such as auditory memory, verbal expression, perceptual reasoning or visual reception. Techniques such as the Illinois Test of Psycholinguistic Abilities (Kirk, McCarthy and Kirk, 1961; Kirk and Kirk, 2001), in which intelligence is tested via the various channels, were introduced to help pinpoint the learning disabilities that impede individual progress. Remedial exercises were developed to help children practice and improve the modalities in which they were weak. The basic process-oriented vocabulary used and expanded by Kirk and his colleagues has become a standard way of describing language and learning processes in the fields of neuropsychology and special education. However, the educational interventions based on this model turned out to be a dismal failure (Kavale, 1982; Larsen, Parker and Hammill, 1982).

Several other recent approaches in understanding and treating learning disabilities have captured more enthusiasm among researchers than among teachers and parents. These are based on theories of cognitive style and human information processing (Goldstein and Schwebach, 2009). These intriguing ideas have yet to be complemented very extensively by applied interventions based on them.

As awareness of learning disabilities increased, empirical scientists were pitted against enthusiastic proponents of fanciful interventions that, time after time, turned out to be neither effective nor cost-effective. Many scientists and, especially, policy-makers began to describe learning disabilities (the term used in this chapter but not necessarily by them) and related conditions with a minimum of unproven theory and obsolete jargon. A reading disorder began to be called a reading disorder, as in DSM-IV; mathematics disorder and, to a lesser extent, disorder of written expression, followed suit. With perceptual training exercises and dull, stimulus-reduced classrooms long abandoned, reading, arithmetic and writing emerged as the central but by no means exclusive features of the assessment and treatment of these disorders. However, if the neuropsychological basis of learning disabilities and related conditions is totally omitted from the conceptualization of the disorder, it is difficult to define these conditions as distinct disorders because poor achievement in reading, arithmetic and writing can occur for many reasons and can be affected by many different forms of psychopathology.

Therefore, and within the context of a general consensus of experts that learning disabilities and other learning disorders have a neurological basis, research continues. Learning disabilities are still measured to some extent with traditional psychological tests of intelligence and language functioning. There may be significant discrepancies, for example, between a child's processing of information presented verbally and in visual images. Research using traditional psychological tests has yielded many influential findings. For example, there are strong indications that children with learning disabilities are characterized by deficits in both short-term and working memory (see meta-analysis by Swanson, Zheng and Jerman, 2009). Looking more closely at the precise nature of the reading disability, it has been established that a number of core *executive functions*, such as planning ability and working memory (as opposed to short-term memory by itself), may be related to the ability to comprehend a written text even if the individual is capable of reading individual words (Locascio et al., 2010).

Although the results of studies using tests of intelligence, language and academic achievement have been very valuable, the advent of sophisticated imagery techniques for studying the brain more directly has bolstered neuropsychological research in this area as in most forms of psychopathology. Many of the studies conducted to date with structural imaging techniques have been plagued with methodological problems such as small sample sizes, resulting in inconsistent findings pointing to a number of different areas of the brain. The most consistent findings indicate abnormalities in the perisylvian area of the left hemisphere, which contains the circuitry needed for using language (Fletcher et al., 2007). However, there has been some exciting recent research in which *functional imaging* has been used on repeated occasions during the process of remediation of children's reading problems. Functional imaging allows the researcher to observe the functioning of the brain as the child reads. These results suggest abnormalities mostly in the left hemisphere, in several areas. Some studies have shown irregularities in the anterior system in the left inferior frontal region. More consistent evidence has been gathered with regard to dysfunction in two posterior regions of the left hemisphere, in the dorsal parietotemporal system involving the angular gyrus, supramarginal gyrus and posterior portions of the superior temporal gyrus and in the ventral occipitotemporal system involving portions of the middle l gyrus and middle occipital gyrus (Shaywitz et al., 2002). Importantly, the differences between the posterior brain regions of children with and without learning disabilities appear to diminish as the children with learning disabilities improve their reading over several months of remediation (Fletcher, 2009; Meyler et al., 2008).

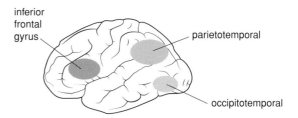

Figure 18.1 Disruption of posterior brain systems for reading in children with developmental dyslexia.

Figure 18.1 depicts the areas of the brain that have been linked with learning disabilities.

In a century of professional work in the area of learning disabilities, the neurological origins of these disorders have not been doubted, although theories about the ways in which biology works to influence reading, writing and arithmetic have been many and diverse. Much more controversial, however, has been the issue of how and, indeed, if these neurological irregularities should be translated into applied interventions. This will be considered later in this chapter.

It is important to remember that the evidence of brain involvement does not at all mean that the family, school and peer environments have no influence on either the academic performance or psychosocial adjustment of children and adolescents with learning disabilities, as will be detailed in subsequent sections.

Genetics

Plomin and Walker (2003) found that over 90 percent of teachers and parents surveyed believe that genetics is at least as important as environmental factors in the causation of learning disabilities. They chide the scientific community, practitioners and policy-makers for not recognizing this scientific fact (Plomin, Kovas and Haworth, 2007; Kovas et al., 2007). In summarizing the evidence indicating strong genetic vulnerability, Plomin and his colleagues (Plomin et al., 2007) emphasize that, in this particular area, it is important to consider the genetic basis of reading, writing and arithmetic ability in general, not only the genetic basis of learning disabilities. Thus, they regard learning disabilities as the extreme points of continua, which is one way of conceptualizing many forms of psychopathology, as discussed in earlier chapters. Furthermore, they emphasize the importance of *multivariate genetic analysis* – the study of how the same genes can affect a variety of traits, such as achievement or disability in several academic subject areas. In the field of genetics, the term *pleitropy* is used to describe the process by which the same gene affects multiple traits. Complicating matters and making research difficult is *polygenicity* – the fact that each trait is affected by several different genes (Plomin et al., 2007).

Twin studies have been the mainstay of the genetic research in this area. Whether diagnosable disorders are considered or the learning abilities across the general population, heritability estimates are very high. In a review of research based on the Twins Early Development Study, in which 13,000 twins from across the UK were studied longitudinally, Oliver and Plomin (2007) reported that the concordance rate for reading disability was 84 percent for monozygotic twins and 48 percent for dizygotic twins. The findings were very similar for mathematics disability: 70 percent for monozygotic twins and 50 percent for dizygotic twins. The conclusions of these behavioral-genetic studies have spurred molecular genetic research in this area (see Chapter 4) focusing on four or five genes that appear to be implicated according to a variety of studies (Plomin et al., 2007; Scerri and Schulte-Körne, 2010).

Family factors

Data about the families of children and adolescents with learning disabilities are highly inconsistent, with some studies revealing very little substantial difference between the families of children with and without learning disorders (Dyson, 1996; Heiman and Berger, 2008; Morrison and Zetlin, 1992). However, other studies have indicated that the parents of children with learning disorders, especially their mothers, tend to be overinvolved with their children, overcontrolling and inflexible (Humphries and Bauman, 1980; Lyytinen et al., 1994; Margalit and Heiman, 1986). Margalit and Heiman (1986) infer a positive nuance to what some researchers see as parental overcontrol, maintaining that this parenting style may be no more than an appropriate response to the needs for structure, stability and organization of their children. Some results also indicate communication problems in the families of children and adolescents with learning disorders (Heiman, Zinck and Heath, 2008) or that adolescents with learning disorders see their relationships with their parents as distant and strained (McNamara et al., 2005). Using a qualitative approach in focus-group interviews with the parents of twelve children with learning disabilities, Dyson (2010) found that the families' reactions varied enormously, ranging from appropriate assertion and coping to stress and exhaustion. Looking at the child–parent attachment bonds of schoolchildren with and without learning disabilities, Bauminger and Kimhi-Kind (2008) found higher rates of insecure attachment among children with learning disabilities (36%) than among their classmates with no diagnosed learning problems (16%). In addition to these studies of the child–parent relationship, it has also been found that children with learning disabilities have a negative effect on their siblings (Lardieri, Blacher and Swanson, 2000).

Some researchers have found it useful to portray the typical if not universal family role in children's learning disabilities in exactly the opposite of the accusatory way that mothers were portrayed in all too many classical socialization studies, as discussed in Chapter 6. Wong (2003) emphasizes the role of supportive parents as an important resiliency resource that helps children learn and adjust despite their learning disorders. In addition to the tangible and emotional support provided to their children, one important parental role is that of advocate for their children in obtaining suitable programming at school.

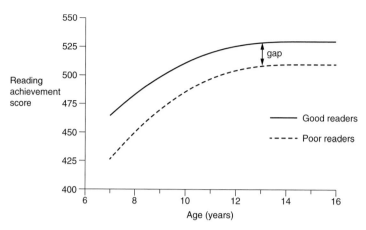

Figure 18.2 The gap between children with learning disorders and their peers increases with age.

Peer factors

Learning disabilities affect much more than schoolwork. Wiener and Schneider (2002) found that children with learning disorders not only had fewer friends than other children but also that their friends were often younger children or other children with learning problems. The friendships were characterized by conflict and little capacity for the resolution of conflict as well as lower levels of support than the friendships of participants without learning problems. The friendships involving children with learning disorders were also less likely than those of other participants in the study to be maintained until the end of the school year. Possibly for the same reasons that explain their inability to grasp the meaning of letters and numbers, many children with learning disorders have difficulty understanding the social cues they receive verbally or non-verbally from their peers, sizing up the situation and responding appropriately to it (e.g., Pearl and Cosden, 1982). In a meta-analysis of research on the acceptance of children with learning disabilities by their school peers, Kavale and Forness (1996) found that 80 percent of them were rejected socially by their classmates. In one of the few studies spanning several successive school years, Estell and his colleagues (2008) found that children with learning disabilities

usually found their way into social groups among their classmates. However, they were rarely at the center of a social group and tended to have negative reputations. None of this changed substantially over the 3 years of their study. Children and adolescents with learning disabilities tend to be lonely (Margalit and Al-Yagon, 2002). Isolated children are often singled out as targets by school bullies. This, together with their often incompetent social behavior, may explain why children with learning disorders are often victimized in school (e.g., Luciano and Savage, 2007; McNamara et al., 2005).

Stability and prognosis

Several longitudinal studies confirm that, without intervention, children who read poorly tend to become adults who read poorly. What usually happens, as in Shaywitz's (2003) longitudinal study of poor readers from age 7 through 16, is that poor readers tend to improve over time as illustrated graphically in Figure 18.2. However, the gap between them and competent readers remains. This is also shown dramatically in the results of a study in which Barbara Maughan and a team of researchers searched for the original participants in the Isle of Wight study, discussed earlier, 45 years after the original data were collected. The majority of the original participants still had difficulty as adults with literacy skills and few of them engaged in regular reading activities (Maughan et al., 2009).

Treatment

Many clinical psychologists are and will remain primarily involved in helping children with learning problems cope with comorbid disorders. In doing so, it is important for the psychologist to bear in mind the ways in which the comorbid depression, anxiety, aggression or attention problems are affected by the processes inherent in learning disabilities, especially with regard to the understanding of the social communication received by the child or adolescent with learning disabilities. Whatever theoretical orientation underlies the intervention being used, the child with learning disabilities may require a more explicit explanation of the social messages received from other people than would other children or adolescents in therapy.

There are many other potential contributions that psychologists can make, whether or not the individual psychologist is involved directly with the academic subject matter that is difficult for the child to master. The psychologist's familiarity with the scientific method constitutes a clear asset to the professional teams whose job it is to help children with learning disabilities. The psychologist may function as a resource person who helps interpret empirical knowledge in this field. Indeed, research is available to guide both assessment and intervention. However, at times, intriguing theories about the workings of the brain, including some that have some basis in research, do not translate into remedial procedures that correct the deficient processes they are supposed to correct. Even if the particular processing deficit targeted in an intervention does improve, improvement in the area targeted may not lead to improvement in the child's academic or social functioning. Besides helping their colleagues appraise the research that pertains to their decision-making, the psychologist may be able to help design and implement research to determine the effectiveness of assessment and intervention techniques.

Until the past 20 or 30 years, practice was guided very extensively by theories that sounded sensible. As special education began to be offered on a more widespread basis in many countries including the United States and Canada, demands for accountability increased. The conclusions reached in a meta-analysis published by Swanson, Carson and Saches-Lee in 1996 represent the thinking of many empirical scientists who reviewed the research basis of interventions in the field at about that time. The Swanson, Carson and Saches-Lee review (1996) is particularly comprehensive, reflecting a wide range of treatment options potentially available to psychologists working in schools. The interventions included techniques as diverse as direct instruction in reading, training of language or perceptual processes, social skills training, reality therapy, relaxation training, conflict resolution, "awareness training" and "responsibility training." The rigorous inclusion criteria resulted in a final sample of seventy-eight well-designed studies. The meta-analysis focused on academic achievement outcomes only. The results indicated clearly that interventions focusing on cognitive processes and direct instruction in school subject areas such as reading, writing and arithmetic are quite effective. Furthermore, interventions designed to improve cognitive processes were most effective if they were supplemented by direct training in reading. Several methodological limitations temper these conclusions. First of all, the effect sizes were lower in the few studies in which participants were randomly assigned to interventions. As well, not all of the researchers took into account variations in the participants' reading achievement prior to the start of the interventions.

In the same year as the Swanson, Carson and Saches-Lee review appeared, Forness and Kavale (1996) published another influential meta-analysis specific to the effects of social skills training for children with learning disabilities. As discussed earlier in this chapter, there is no doubt that children with learning disabilities tend to have poor social skills and poor peer relations. However, social skills training to alleviate these problems requires the child to attend to what is taught during social skills training and apply that learning to other situations and, usually, to other settings. Unfortunately, the meta-analysis, which was based on fifty-three published studies, indicated overall effects that were small, in the area of two-tenths of a standard deviation unit. Neither the authors of the meta-analysis nor other experts who have reflected on the potential benefits of social skills training for children with learning disabilities (e.g., Cartledge, 2005) suggest total abandonment of this effort, although, of course, enthusiasm for it has waned considerably among research-oriented practitioners.

Some practitioners and researchers persist, in spite of these disappointments, in their attempts at improving psychosocial interventions and in attempting to use the results of the latest research in neurosciences in designing training methods for processes found to be deficient, often using the computer (e.g., Lorusso, Facoetti and Bakker, 2011). Others have argued that no single intervention is really applicable to all children with learning disabilities and that the heterogeneity of the population of children with learning disabilities requires tailoring intervention to the specific needs of the individual. This may mean, first of all, that there is little point in studying the overall effectiveness of any form of intervention across this population. Appealing as the idea of custom-tailoring is, it of course poses considerable logistical challenges for teachers. Highly individualized interventions are often difficult to evaluate with traditional research techniques. Fortunately, alternative methods, such as goal-attainment scaling (see Chapter 10) are available for the evaluation of interventions that share common objectives but that differ markedly in their application to individual recipients.

However, rather than trying to improve on the traditional forms of intervention, many policy-makers and practitioners have moved away from interventions that appear to be psychological or neurological. Instead, they emphasize systematic direct work on deficient skills in reading, writing, arithmetic or mathematics. The *responsiveness to intervention (RTI)* approach is now prevalent in many schools in the United States (Unruh and McKellar, 2013). RTI typically consists of three "tiers." In Tier 1, students who are having difficulty in their school subjects are identified using validated measures of academic achievement. These students receive special help, typically in small groups in their own classrooms, in the areas of deficiency. Students who fail to respond to this largely preventive first step are then provided in Tier 2 with more intensive help, often in small seminar rooms at their schools and typically for a substantial portion of the school year. It is only pupils who fail to respond adequately to the Tier 2 interventions who are then formally designated on an individual basis as pupils with special educational needs, including a more elaborate assessment and intervention plan. Depending on local practice, there may or may not be a psychological assessment and/or formal diagnosis of learning disability. Thus, the RTI approach includes, in essence, primary and secondary prevention as well as early treatment, at least of academic problems. Nevertheless, not all authorities in the field have been unequivocal in their support of the responsiveness to intervention approach, which is sometimes seen as bringing about the oversimplification of learning disabilities. Any helpful insight from an individual diagnostic procedure is often lost, especially in the cases of pupils who are simply and globally considered "non-responders." Furthermore, the entire system rests on the scientific validity of the assessment measures and remedial procedures used, which are known to vary enormously from school to school. Another limitation of the RTI approach is that it seems best suited for younger pupils in the first few years of school but may not be very applicable, for example, to adolescents (Berkeley et al., 2009; Fuchs and Deshler, 2007; McKenzie, 2009; Unruh and McKellar, 2013).

Conclusions and future directions

The efficient RTI approach is surely bringing help earlier and to more children in need than previous models would allow. However, as logical as the RTI approach may be, and as commendable as it is for its emphasis on prevention and early intervention, this new approach does not really provide an adequate solution to the many emotional, behavioral and social concomitants of learning disorders. It is, once more, those emotional and behavioral aspects of learning problems that are responsible for their inclusion in the DSM and ICD systems and in this book. Hopefully, the interesting but often frustrating saga of the psychology and biology of learning disabilities will continue with the more complete unraveling of the neurological bases of these disorders. Hopefully as well, those new discoveries will be more amenable to effective applied interventions than the best-informed experts have been able to generate until now.

Summary

- Learning disorder is considered a mental health disorder because it has an underlying neurobiological basis and it is comorbid with other psychopathologies such as depression.
- Dyslexia is Greek for difficulty with reading. This term is widely used in educational circles but not in the DSM or ICD.
- The first cases of dyslexia and other learning disorders were reported about 300 years ago. In early writings, dyslexia was considered a specific visual memory problem. Samuel Orton attributed learning problems to a lack of hemispheric specialization in the brain. The term "minimal brain dysfunction" was originally used to describe together the problems we now call learning disorders and attention deficit/ hyperactivity today.
- Process-oriented or cybernetic models conceptualize learning disorders as a group of individualized communication processing impairments (e.g., auditory memory vs. perceptual reasoning impairments).
- Research with psychological tests shows that children with dyslexia have short-term and working memory problems and difficulties with executive functions such as planning. Working memory is needed to comprehend a text, even if the child recognizes individual words.

- Learning disabilities have been associated with problems in the perisylvian area of the left hemisphere implicated in language, the dorsal parietotemporal system, the supramarginal gyrus, the posterior portions of the superior temporal gyrus and in the ventral occipitotemporal system.
- The DSM system specifies a diagnosis of reading disorder when a child's reading level is below that of other children their age, and when reading difficulties interfere with academic achievement. If there are sensory impairments (e.g., visual), the diagnosis cannot be based on reading difficulties attributed to the sensory impairments. The ICD-10 employs similar diagnostic criteria.
- There are subtypes of learning disabilities such as the non-verbal learning disability. The non-verbal subtype has been associated with difficulties in social interaction.
- Assessing prevalence rates for learning disabilities is complex because reading ability can be measured in different ways (e.g., by school grades, by specific reading comprehension tests).
- Although boys may be more likely than girls to be recommended for help with reading, this may reflect in part teacher biases in recommending more boys than girls for similar reading difficulties.

- Learning disorders are often, but not always, comorbid with other disorders. On their own, learning disabilities are not easily noticed by others, leaving many unaware of their implications.
- Children with learning disabilities often experience social difficulties. These social difficulties may be a result of sensory processing problems that translate into difficulties processing social cues.
- Learning disorders are often associated with attention deficit/hyperactivity disorder (in 20–25% of cases) and anti-social behavior.
- Learning disorders may be associated with anti-social behavior because the learning disorders lead to poor judgment. Learning disorders may lead to frustration which leads to the behavioral misconduct.
- Learning disorders are comorbid with depression in many cases. This comorbidity may be due to a tendency for people with learning disabilities to give up on learning due to fear of failure. Anxiety has been reported in 70 percent of individuals with learning disorders.
- Perhaps because the Spanish language is phonetic (the same letters are always pronounced the same way), there are lower rates of learning disabilities in Spanish-speaking countries than in the USA. However, other social and environmental factors endemic to different regions and socio-economic classes may affect the prevalence of learning disabilities.
- The fact that the same genes may be responsible for the onset of learning disabilities as well as many other traits (pleitropy), and that learning disabilities may be affected by many different genes (polygenicity), complicates the assessment of the biological basis of learning disabilities.
- The concordance rate for learning disabilities for monozygotic (MZ) twins is much higher than the rate for dizygotic twins (DZ), implying heritability in learning disabilities.

- Parents of children with learning disabilities may be overinvolved, overcontrolling and inflexible with their children. However, this may be an appropriate response to, not a cause of, the learning disabilities. Affected adolescents often report a strained relationship with their parents. There are higher rates of insecure attachment between children with learning disabilities and their parents compared to children without learning disabilities and their parents.
- Psychologists involved in the interventions to help children with learning disabilities may often have to deal with the children's comorbid disorders (e.g., depression, anxiety, aggression or social problems).
- One meta-analysis shows that cognitive interventions combined with direct instruction in the academic problem areas are most effective in raising the school performance of children with learning disabilities.
- Another meta-analysis found that social skills training alone did little to alleviate poor academic and social outcomes in children with learning disabilities.
- Some researchers argue that the diversity of the individual cases of learning disabilities should lead to a variety of individual interventions. Such a tailoring of interventions for learning disabilities, however, would pose a strain on the education system.
- The responsiveness to intervention (RTI) approach moves children along a contingency plan of three tiers to address varying levels of reading difficulty in the general population.
- In the first tier of the RTI, children who show difficulties reading are assigned to small groups in their own classrooms for special instruction. In Tier 2, children who did not respond to the Tier 1 intervention are given special instruction in separate classrooms. Those who do not respond to Tier 2 go to Tier 3, which involves highly individualized intervention which may or may not involve formal diagnosis.

Study questions

1. Do you agree with the DSM-5 Commission's decision to use terms like "specific learning disorder" rather than the word "dyslexia"? Why or why not?
2. What are the main reasons learning disorders are considered mental health disorders?
3. How clear and conclusive is the evidence that learning disorders are caused by small abnormalities in the structure or workings of the human brain?
4. What are some explanations of the fact that children with learning disorders are often rejected by their classroom peers and have few friends?
5. Is social skills training the best way for psychologists to help children with learning disorders? Why or why not?

Part IV Less frequent and less clearly defined forms of child psychopathology

19

Eating disorders

Eating disorders are among the most heart-rending of the psychological disorders of young people. As will be explained in this chapter, eating disorders have been attributed to the evils of modern Western society although, as with most other disorders, genetics, family upbringing and peer pressure are important correlates if not causes. What many see as an epidemic affecting adolescent females has been blamed on the pervasive emphasis on thinness, the breakdown of traditional, orderly thinking patterns as well as changes in the traditional roles of women (e.g., Nasser, Katzman and Gordon, 2001). Eating disorders are complex and often misunderstood. They tend to provoke emotional reactions ranging from bewilderment to fear to mistrust because many people cannot understand why a young person would not comply with the fundamental human need to eat or would assign so much importance to personal appearance that it ruins his or her life (Stein, Latzer and Merick, 2009).

In Western countries, mass media portray thinness as an ideal to impressionable young women (see meta-analysis by Groesz, Levine and Murnen, 2002). Young men are bombarded with media images emphasizing a muscular appearance (Agliata and Tantleff-Dunn, 2004). In parallel, "fast food" enterprises are increasingly "supersizing" the food they serve, contributing to a parallel epidemic of obesity among young people male and female. Although the pressures of modern society are often implicated in the probable increase in eating disorders in recent years, case studies indicate that these disorders were of concern even in ancient times. Parry-Jones and Parry-Jones (1991), in a historical account of the emergence of the phenomenon now known as bulimia nervosa, cite the case of Matthew Dakin, which was reported in medical journals in 1745. Matthew was a previously healthy 10-year-old from Black Barnsley, Yorkshire, England who, after an illness of unknown origin, began to display alternations of voracious eating and vomiting. He died, emaciated, shortly after.

This chapter is devoted primarily to the eating disorders that are most common among school-aged children and adolescents. The chapter begins with definitional issues, followed by a section in which developmental issues in the conceptualization of the eating disorders are presented and emphasized. Diagnostic criteria are discussed next. Gender and cultural issues feature prominently in the subsequent section on prevalence. Information is then provided about the stability and prognosis of the different eating disorders. Culture and gender reappear together with intra-individual characteristics in the section on causes and correlates. The chapter closes with a section on the challenges of treating children and adolescents with eating disorders.

Different forms of eating disorder

Anorexia nervosa and *bulimia* are the major eating disorders discussed in the literature, with less attention devoted to *binge eating*. Anorexia nervosa involves, first of all, an overevaluation of the importance of shape and size, including judging one's self-worth almost exclusively on the basis of body weight and living in fear of gaining weight. The fear of gaining weight does not diminish and may even increase after weight loss (Gleaves, Latner and Ambwani, 2009; Walsh and Garner, 1997). Another core feature of anorexia nervosa is the maintenance of low body weight. Bulimia also includes a preoccupation with weight. In bulimia, this preoccupation is expressed through the tendency to alternate between binge eating and draconian efforts to avoid gaining weight, such as very strict dieting and self-induced vomiting (Fairburn and Gowers, 2010). Excessive or compulsive exercise, which is related to the body-image concerns that provoke eating disorders, is beginning to receive attention as well (White and Halliwell, 2010).

There are also less common forms of eating disorder more prevalent among infants and preschoolers; these forms persist only rarely into middle childhood or later. *Pica* is the habitual ingestion of non-nutritive substances, including, very often, sand, insects, animal droppings, paint, plaster, string, cloth or hair. Pica may or may not appear in conjunction with intellectual disabilities, including those in the autism spectrum; it is also associated with cases of severe child neglect. Pica is diagnosed if it persists after the age of 1 year. *Rumination disorder* refers to the enjoyment of voluntary regurgitation and rechewing of food. Finally, there is a condition known as *feeding disorder of infancy or early childhood*, in which a child under 6 years old refuses to eat enough food to gain or maintain weight (Wolf and Collier, 2005).

Eating disorders in developmental perspective

There is no doubt that many eating disorders begin to appear during adolescence, along with normative concerns about one's physical appearance (e.g., Fairburn and Gowers, 2010). However, most experts believe that eating disorders similar to those of adults do occur to some extent in school-aged children. Without denying the existence of eating disorders among children, some authorities in the field have expressed reservations about applicability to young people of the DSM and ICD diagnostic criteria for eating disorders, which were developed, for the most part, with adults in mind. Watkins and Lask (2009) present a comprehensive critique of issues relevant to the definition of eating disorders in

young children. One recurring issue is the extent to which bulimia and anorexia nervosa actually occur in children. Watkins and Lask remark that it would be inappropriate to read pathology into the relatively frequent feeding and weaning problems of infants and preschoolers. During those early years many children are picky about the foods they eat; others develop "food fads." Watkins and Lask argue that such feeding problems are part of the normal developmental process in which children experiment with tastes and textures and discover their role in their relationships with the adults who provide their food. Some theorists believe that anorexia nervosa is a maladaptive reaction to puberty; thus it could not occur in pre-pubertal children (Crisp, 1983). Indeed, many definitions of eating disorders include reference to disruptions of the female menstrual cycle or, less frequently, low levels of serum testosterone for males (Nicholls, Chater and Lask, 2000; Watkins and Lask, 2009). These provisions would render eating disorders impossible before puberty. However, excluding pre-pubertal children from conceptualizations of eating disorders would make it impossible to account for the substantial number of case studies describing anorexia nervosa before the onset of puberty (e.g., Jacobs and Isaacs, 1986). Therefore, it has also been argued that although anxiety nervosa and, very occasionally, bulimia do sometimes exist before puberty, their symptoms are not identical to those of anorexia nervosa and bulimia in adults, limiting the applicability of standard diagnostic schemes such as the DSM. Another major difference is that adults with eating disorders display excessive concern about their body weight and shape whereas children with eating disorders are not necessarily affected by such apprehensions (Watkins and Lask, 2009).

Diagnostic criteria

Boxes 19.1 and 19.2 contain summaries of the recent changes in the DSM criteria for anorexia nervosa and bulimia. The changes from DSM-IV to the

Box 19.1 | **Differences between DSM-IV and DSM-5 criteria for anorexia nervosa**

- In both DSM-IV and DSM-5, the diagnosis is based on the assumption of reduced food intake. This results in a lower than normal body weight, based on what is minimally expected according to normal weight tables.
- In both DSM-IV and DSM-5, the individual must also experience a distorted perception of the body; or an excessive effect of body weight or shape on self-evaluation; or an inability to appreciate the dangers associated with low body weight.
- In DSM-IV, a fear of weight gain or becoming large despite being underweight must be present. This criterion has been retained in DSM-5; however, engaging in behaviors that prevent weight gain despite being underweight is now sufficient to satisfy this criterion.
- In DSM-IV, amenorrhea (i.e., the disappearance of menstruation) is a necessary symptom for postmenarcheal females. However, in DSM-5, this requirement has been removed, in part due to the fact that this criterion in not applicable to children.
- In both versions, the subtype must be specified as either "restricting type," to be used if the individual has not displayed binge eating or purging behavior, or "binge-eating/ purging type," to be used if the aforementioned behaviors have occurred.
- In DSM-IV, the subtype must be applicable to the current episode. However, in DSM-5, the subtype must be applicable to the last 3 months.
- In DSM-5, clinicians may also specify whether the disorder is in partial or full remission. These remission specifiers apply in cases in which the full criteria were previously met but now are partially or no longer satisfied. In DSM-5, severity must be specified based on current body mass index (BMI) for adults or BMI percentile for children and adolescents.

Source: DSM-5 and DSM-IV-TR consulted June 5, 2013.

Box 19.2 | **Differences between DSM-IV and DSM-5 criteria for bulimia nervosa**

- In both DSM-IV and DSM-5, bulimia nervosa involves frequent binge eating. Binge eating is defined as large food intake during a relatively short period of time as well as a lack of control over the eating behavior.
- In both DSM-IV and DSM-5, an individual must engage in inappropriate strategies to compensate for the high food intake in order to avoid weight gain. These include self-induced vomiting, misuse of medications, fasting or excessive exercise.
- In both versions, the individual's self-evaluation must be overly influenced by the state of his or her body.

- In DSM-IV, binge eating and measures taken by the individual to compensate for binge eating must both occur at least twice a week for a period of 3 months. In DSM-5, the criterion has been broadened to include individuals who engage in such behaviors at least once a week for 3 months.
- In DSM-IV, the subtype must be specified (i.e., purging type or non-purging type). This is to differentiate between individuals who use vomiting or medications to avoid weight gain and individuals who solely exercise excessively or fast. However, in DSM-5, the non-purging subtype has been removed; individuals with this subtype might be better described as having binge eating disorder.
- In DSM-5, clinicians may specify whether the disorder is in partial or full remission. These remission specifiers apply in cases in which the full criteria were previously met but now are partially or no longer satisfied. In DSM-5, severity must be specified based on the frequency of inappropriate compensatory behavior.

Source: DSM-5 and DSM-IV-TR consulted June 6, 2013.

DSM-5 criteria for anorexia nervosa and bulimia are relatively few. As detailed in the boxes, many of the changes involve less stringent criteria for diagnosis. However, a new category has been added: *binge eating disorder*. Binge eating disorder is a condition characterized by repeated episodes of binge eating. Binge eaters typically eat much more than most other people would. They may feel that their binge eating is not under their conscious control. Their binge eating causes them distress. The addition of this category means that there could be an increase in the number of children and adolescents whose eating problems are at the level at which they could be diagnosed as having eating disorders.

Prevalence

Establishing the prevalence rates of eating disorders and confirming the widespread impression that they are becoming more prevalent has been difficult because of the lack of well-developed diagnostic instruments (Watkins and Lask, 2009). As well, the secrecy surrounding binge eating and subsequent purging likely results in many cases not being diagnosed (Gleaves et al., 2009). Despite these obstacles, there have been a number of attempts to estimate the prevalence of these difficulties, often using DSM criteria, yielding various estimates. Although improved questionnaires have appeared in recent years, some critics have noted that the vocabulary used in questionnaires may not always be explicit enough or fully understandable to children (Wolf and Collier, 2005). Food diaries (Crowther and Sherwood, 1997) completed daily by children and/or parents provide information of higher quality, including not only the frequencies of eating-related behaviors but also the emotions experienced as they occur. As noted in Chapter 9, semi-structured clinical interviews provide an opportunity for the clinician to probe responses obtained, which cannot usually be done with self-report questionnaires. Such interviews have been developed for the assessment of eating disorders (see, e.g., Bryant-Waugh et al., 1996 and Fairburn and Cooper, 1993). However, most of the studies discussed in this chapter are based on self-report questionnaires.

Estimates based on medical records indicate a prevalence rate of diagnosable eating disorders below 1 percent, perhaps as low as 0.3 percent (Hoek, 2006). In contrast, Zaider, Johnson and Cockell (2000) administered diagnostic interviews to 403 US adolescents in the New York City community. They estimated the prevalence of eating disorders at 3 percent, of whom two-thirds were girls, not including those who might be diagnosed as having an eating disorder not otherwise specified. Similar prevalence rates for adolescent girls (boys did not participate in the studies) were reported in recent epidemiological studies conducted in Italy (Cotrufo, Gnisci and Caputo, 2005), Spain (Ruiz-Lazaro et al., 2005), Iran (Nobakht and Dezhkam, 2000) and Greece and Germany (Fichter et al., 2005). Several of these studies are relevant to the anthropological theories about eating in Mediterranean cultures, which will be discussed later in this chapter.

In all the epidemiological studies, the rates of risky nutrition-related behaviors that do not correspond fully with diagnostic criteria have been much higher than the rates of formal diagnosis, typically as high as one adolescent in seven. Thus, eating problems surely represent a greater source of psychological distress for many more children and adolescents than the rate of formal diagnosis suggests. Given the problems in achieving clear estimates of the prevalence of eating disorders, it is particularly difficult to support with data the widespread contention that this "epidemic" has increased dramatically in recent years. Based on the best data available, Hoek (2006) maintains that the incidence rates of eating disorders among young people in Western countries increased dramatically from the 1930s through the 1980s and have leveled off since then.

Most individuals of all ages who suffer from eating disorders also suffer from other forms of psychopathology. The most common comorbidities are with mood and anxiety disorders, which affect at least half the population whose eating disorders have been formally diagnosed. Other very common comorbid conditions include substance abuse and obsessive-compulsive personality disorder (Zaider et al., 2000).

Gender

The reasons why many more girls are identified as having eating disorders than boys are discussed more fully in the subsequent section of the possible causes of eating disorder. Although eating disorders are much more frequent among girls and women than among boys and men, it has been found in some studies that about a third of male adolescents have demonstrated some symptoms of disordered eating and that about a third of boys desire a thinner but still muscular body shape (Ackard, Fulkerson and Newmark-Sztainer, 2007; Heatherton and Baumeister, 1991; McCabe and Ricciardelli, 2003; Polivy and Herman, 1987). A substantial number of other boys wish to gain weight in order to achieve a muscular appearance. Boys have been found to be as susceptible as girls to messages about ideal male body image from the media, their peers and their parents, especially fathers (Field et al., 2001). Some experts believe that the image of the ideal male has increased in muscularity in recent years, as represented in G.I. Joe action figures and centerfolds of the magazine *Playgirl* (Leit, Pope and Gray, 2001). The psychological consequences of eating disorder appear to be as severe for boys as for girls (Keel et al., 1998; Ray, 2004). Among adults at least, males of minority sexual orientation appear to be at greater risk than others (e.g., Siever, 1994; Wiseman and Moradi, 2010). Eating disorders among men of minority sexual orientation have been attributed to the same preoccupations with appearance and attractiveness that plague other men and women as well as repressed homophobia and to recollections of having been taunted during childhood and adolescence for non-conformity with gender stereotypes (Wiseman and Moradi, 2010).

Culture

There are many studies confirming high rates of eating disorder among children and adolescents outside the United States and other Western cultures. Many of the researchers involved embarked on their cross-cultural journeys to prove the simple fact that eating disorder is a worldwide problem. The results leave no doubt about that fact. The exact prevalence rates reported in different studies may not be readily comparable because of the aforementioned difficulties with the instruments used in identifying study participants. However, according to an authoritative review chapter by Anderson-Fye (2009) prevalence rates at least as high as those found in the United States have been found in both Eastern and Western Europe, Australia, many parts of Asia, the Middle East and the Pacific Islands. Eating disorders appear to be rare in sub-Saharan Africa, probably because there are few places there characterized by food intake that is greater than the level needed for basic subsistence.

Moving beyond the tallying of prevalence rates, some research has been conducted to determine in a more articulate manner the ways in which culture might affect food-related behavior, healthy and pathological. At the most basic level are culturally ingrained values regarding weight and body shape. Not all cultures share the esteem accorded in young people's culture in Western countries to slim, svelte women. African-American girls, for example, have been found to prefer a larger body size than their peers of Western European origin and, conversely, not to endorse a thin-body ideal to the same extent as children of majority culture backgrounds (Ruiz, Pepper and Wilfley, 2004). However, African-American mothers, more than mothers of other ethnic groups in the United States, are known to teach their children to have pride in their bodies. This does not appear to be manifest in high rates of anorexia nervosa or bulimia, although results vary sharply from study to study. However, binge eating has been found to be a substantial problem among African-American boys (George and Franko, 2010; Ruiz et al., 2004; Striegel-Moore et al., 2003). In their careful review of research on the prevalence of eating disorders among US children and youth of minority cultural origin (i.e., African-American, Hispanic, Asian and Native American), George and Franco (2010) emphasize that the most salient feature of this body of data is the inconsistent results across studies

with no obvious explanation for the inconsistencies. They advocate more comprehensive research in which culture is studied as it interacts with other possible causal factors, especially socio-economic status, which will be discussed shortly. It is also important to consider eating disorders as a function not only of cultural minority status but also as a function of the contact – actual and desired – between the member of the minority cultural community and the host culture. Eating disorders have been found to emerge quite often when a child or young person of minority culture is the "token" representative of that culture in a group consisting of members of the cultural majority, which often emphasizes body thinness more than the minority culture (Smolak, Levine and Striegel-Moore, 1996).

Globalization

Westernization and, especially, ubiquitous exposure to Western media such as film and television have been implicated in what many see as an increase in eating disorders in non-Western countries. Anderson-Fye's (2009) review includes several studies in which eating disorders among children and adolescents appear to have increased with exposure to Western culture and Western media, as in Sri Lanka (Perera et al., 2002) and Fiji (Becker, et al., 2003). Social class differences have been reported in many studies, leaving the impression that eating disorders are a plague of the privileged. Similarly, several studies conducted with Mexican and Mexican-American youth have linked exposure to majority US culture to body-image dissatisfaction and eating disorder (Ayala et al., 2007). Although Anderson-Fye (2009) reports that in several countries, increasing Westernization seems to account for an increase in eating disorders in children and youth from negligible to substantial levels, it is important to remember that the ideal of body thinness is not exclusive to Western culture. Chisuwa and O'Dea (2010) found evidence of the thinness ideal in traditional Japanese teachings that are expressed in particular in the conversations between Japanese mothers and their children. These traditional teachings about idealized body image may explain the reports of eating disorders contained in Japanese writings from as early as the seventeenth century.

In an elaborate account of such processes as they occur around the Mediterranean basin, Ruggiero (2003) attributes the emergence of eating disorders to the "partial modernization" of girls and women who are leaving behind a traditional culture of honor and shame, in which females are socialized to be attractive to men and submissive to them. In some parts of the Mediterranean, as in some Arab countries, "plumpness" is thought to convey the impression of fertility (Apter et al., 1994). Ruggiero relates eating disorder to the complex internalized conflicts experienced by girls and women in contemporary Mediterranean societies, who must deal simultaneously with their own wishes and aspirations and the traditional teachings of their families. In their attempts at reconciling these conflicting drives, they may have to deal with overinvolvement by mothers who attempt to hold them back from modernization and/or the social isolation that may ensue from the abandonment of traditional values.

Pinhas and colleagues (2008) studied the rates of eating disorders among Jewish and non-Jewish adolescents in Toronto, Canada. The Jewish adolescent girls, but not boys, displayed higher rates of eating-disordered behaviors than the general population. There was no support for the idea that the risk for eating disorder in this population might have to do with their religious observances because festive meals are an integral part of many aspects of Jewish religious observance. Pinhas and her colleagues speculated that part of the problem may have to do with family messages about nutrition that stem from the Holocaust experiences of the participants' families. Many of their grandparents had been subjected to near-starvation experiences during World War II. After immigration to Canada, many of the parents initially experienced the economic problems that are common among most newcomers who arrive without economic resources. By the time of the study, however, most of the Jewish parents were well established in the country and able to provide food for their children. The contrast in the availability of food across only a few generations may be behind some of the attitudes transmitted about eating.

Social class and urban/rural differences within cultures

As was mentioned in Chapter 8, socio-economic differences within cultures can be as substantial as differences between cultures. Eating disorders, especially anorexia nervosa, are sometimes thought to be particularly prevalent among girls and women of middle to high socio-economic status. This contention, however, has not been confirmed consistently in recent studies (Gard and Freeman, 1996; Fisher et al., 2001). In fact, it is sometimes found that bulimia nervosa is more prevalent in individuals from families of lower socio-economic status (Gard and Freeman, 1996; Gleaves et al., 2009). Anderson-Fye (2009) disputes this contention with data from recent studies showing eating disorders across the spectrum of socio-economic levels. Just as it may be misleading to generalize about individuals of a particular culture, it may be important to explore distinctions among members of a particular social class. Upward mobility, the transition to a higher socio-economic level, seems to be associated with increased eating disorders in several societies, ranging from the United States (Yates, 1989) to Afro-Caribbeans in Britain (Soomro, Crisp and Lynch, 1995) to such non-Western nations as Belize (Anderson-Fye, 2004), Fiji (Becker, 2004) and Zimbabwe (Buchan and Gregory, 1984). Finally, Anderson-Fye (2004) notes that rates of eating disorder are often higher in urban areas than in rural areas of the same countries. This may have to do with Westernization, media influences or upward social mobility.

Stability and prognosis

As with many other aspects of eating disorders among children and adolescents, much more is known about the stability of disorders and their long-term prognosis for girls than for boys. The most authoritative study to date was conducted in Oregon by Measelle, Stice and Hogansen (2006) with a large sample of 493 female adolescents who were followed annually from age 13 to 18. Fortunately, these researchers focused not only on eating disorders but also on a number of other disorders, including several, such as depression, that frequently co-occur with eating disorders. They noted that different causal pathways may conceivably govern the covariance between eating disorders and depression. One possibility is univariate causation, either that eating disorders cause depression or that depression causes eating disorders. Of course, there could be reciprocal causality, with both causal directions operating simultaneously. It is also very conceivable that both eating disorders and depression are the result of the same external risk factor or cause. For example, dysfunctional cognitions such as self-deprecation might be the cause of both (Measelle et al., 2006; Zoccolillo, 1992). Common underlying physiological processes are another possibility (see review by Maxwell and Cole, 2009).

Measelle, Stice and Hogan found that both eating-disordered behavior and depression increased in a linear fashion over the 5-year course of the study, with eating disorders increasing by 0.5 standard deviation, which is substantial; eating disorders increased more than depression did. Importantly, the patterns of change in the data were most consistent with univariate causality, with depression leading to subsequent eating-disordered behavior. Most other studies are not as comprehensive as the research by Measelle, Stice and Hogansen. However, some research has included adolescent males as well as females, confirming not only that boys with eating disorders are likely to be depressed as well, but also that eating disorder often follows earlier depressed feelings (see review by Rawana et al., 2010).

Other research on adolescents who have been diagnosed formally as having eating disorders indicates a highly variable trajectory over time, with many adolescents recovering and maintaining their recovery while many others, unfortunately,

recover and then relapse (e.g., Fairburn et al., 2000). Long-term follow-up of people diagnosed with eating disorders indicates that highly negative outcomes are possible, including death from either suicide or from the physical consequences of eating disorders themselves. Exact statistics regarding the prognosis and outcome of eating disorders in children and adolescents are difficult to establish because of the relative rarity of formal diagnosis and the consequent small sample sizes of many studies. Steinhausen (2002, 2009) contributed a very informative meta-analysis of 119 original studies on the long-term prognosis of adolescent anorexia nervosa; the combined sample size of the studies reviewed was over 5,000. The more refined analysis reported in Steinhausen's 2009 paper includes specific findings regarding 784 adolescents diagnosed with anorexia nervosa in data collection sited in Germany, Switzerland, Bulgaria and Romania. The meta-analytic statistics indicated that, at 10-year follow-up, approximately 73 percent of the adolescent samples demonstrated recovery, with another 8.5 percent having improved substantially. However, 13.7 percent were still suffering from anorexia and about 9.4 percent had died (percentages exceed 100% because these are not statistics about a particular sample but an average of studies with different sample sizes). Review papers in which adult and adolescent data are combined suggest that the prognosis is somewhat better for bulimia nervosa in general than for anorexia nervosa, although the relapse rates remain very troubling. For example, according to a review paper by Agras (2001), most studies indicate a relapse rate of about 10 percent at 10-year follow-up. Unfortunately, exact statistics regarding the specific prognosis for adolescents with bulimia nervosa or binge eating do not appear to be available in the published literature (Steinhausen, 2009). In addition to efforts at tracking the general course of eating disorders, there have been some efforts at identifying factors that are linked to both positive and negative outcomes. A good child–parent relationship is associated with a more favorable prognosis. As well, the outcome tends to be better if the eating-disordered behavior starts early in life and lasts for only a short time (Steinhausen, 2009). On the other hand, among the population of individuals with eating disorders, those who have a history of childhood sexual abuse and those who demonstrate an avoidant personality – which consists of avoidance of social interaction and fear of being evaluated negatively by others – are prone to a more pessimistic outcome (Vrabel et al., 2010).

Although the psychological aspects and outcomes of childhood obesity are beyond the scope of this chapter, it is worth remembering that obesity is a health, and, often, mental health problem that far eclipses anorexia nervosa and bulimia nervosa in terms of the number of children and adolescents affected. The reader is referred to a very comprehensive review of the literature on weight stigma in childhood and adolescence by Puhl and Latner (2007).

Possible causes and correlates

Objectification theory is a recurrent theme in the feminist literature on eating disorders. The theory is based on the view that men treat women as sexual objects and that women are led to do whatever is necessary to increase their attractiveness as such (Fredrickson and Roberts, 1997). According to objectification theory, women are defined by both themselves and by males according to their bodies and appearance. The cumulative effect of socialization by parents and by peers causes girls and women to internalize society's expectations regarding the ideal female body shape. The concept of *objectified body consciousness* includes a number of ideas about the control of one's body, including the fundamental belief that body shape can and should be controlled. This often leads to unhealthy behaviors aimed at body modification (McKinley and Hyde, 1996; Moradi, 2011). *Self-objectification* results in excessive body surveillance and monitoring. The unhealthy by-products of such constant monitoring of one's own body shape often include anxiety,

shame and reduced awareness of body states such as hunger and fullness. At the same time, there may be reduced sensation of psychological states that are associated with well-being, fulfillment and energy (Moradi, 2011). Several other theories, such as the *dual pathway model* (Stice and Agras, 1999) and the *tripartite pathway model* (van den Berg et al., 2002) are similar in many ways to objectification theory but emphasize the individual's *perception* of society's pressures to be thin and the individual's *translation* of many forms of pressure from families, peers and society at large into a driving internal pressure to change their body shape (Moradi, 2011). Empirical support for the basic elements of objectification theory was obtained in a study conducted with Australian boys and girls 12 through 16 years old by Slater and Tiggemann (2010). These researchers found that girls scored higher than boys on measures of body shame, body surveillance, appearance anxiety and disordered eating. However, the basic tenets of objectification theory, namely the roles of body shame, body surveillance and appearance anxiety in the emergence of disordered eating behaviors, appeared to apply to boys as well as girls.

Genetic vulnerability and physiological correlates

The limited research available to date on eating disorders during childhood and adolescence suggests some degree of genetic transmission of eating disorders, with adolescents appearing particularly susceptible (Klump, McGue and Iacono, 2003). Several twin studies have traced the genetic roots of eating disorders. These studies provide greater evidence of a genetic basis for anorexia nervosa than for bulimia. For example, Bulik et al. (2000) found a concordance rate of 55 percent for eating disorders in monozygotic twins. In probably the first study to explore the genetic roots of eating disorder with adoptive children, Klump et al. (2009) confirmed the impression of moderate genetic transmission that is evident in twin studies. It is unlikely that there is a specific genetic route to each form of eating disorder, but rather a common genetic susceptibility that may be manifest in subsequent generations, for example, as anorexia even if a parent has bulimia (Mazzeo et al., 2006; Strober et al., 2000). Part of the genetic route to eating disorders may have to do with a genetic susceptibility to depression (Lilenfeld et al., 1998). Although most experts believe that child and adolescent eating disorders are moderately heritable (Smolak, 2009), they also note the many limitations of the existing research. First of all, most of the studies have been conducted with clinic samples, which may yield conclusions that do not apply to the overall population (Fairburn and Gowers, 2010). Importantly, most researchers have failed to consider possible interactions between genetic and environmental factors (Smolak, 2009). Given the positive findings of several studies using the methodological tools of behavior genetics, there have been some preliminary efforts at applying molecular genetics (see Chapter 4) to research on early-onset eating disorders (Fairburn and Gowers, 2010). Given the persistence of societal interest in eating disorders and the emerging sophistication of methodologies in molecular genetics, clearer answers about the genetic basis of eating disorders is certain to emerge over the next few years.

Central nervous system neuropeptides and the central nervous system neurotransmitters of serotonin, dopamine and norepinephrine are thought to be involved in the regulation of eating behavior. However, their role in the emergence of eating disorders remains unclear because any physiological changes could easily be the result rather than the cause of malnutrition and irregular eating behavior (Kaye, 2008; Stein et al., 2009). A similar problem emerges in the interpretation of neuroimaging studies, which have shown irregularities in several regions of the brain which could, once again, be no more than a consequence of prior eating-disordered behavior. It has, however, been argued that the neurotransmitter alterations that have been found are indeed evident even in people whose eating-disordered behavior has not caused significant nutritional impairment at the time of testing. The elevated dopaminergic and serotonergic activity that has been recorded may exert

its influence not only directly, that is by affecting eating behavior, but also by influencing personality structure, bringing about the personality traits that are commonly associated with eating disorder, as will be discussed in the next paragraph (Kaye, 2008; Klump et al., 2004, Stein et al., 2009).

Temperament/personality and distorted thinking patterns

Another way in which genetics probably influence the emergence of eating disorder is by influencing the child's temperament or personality. Although personality patterns typical of children and young people with eating disorders have been identified, methodological shortcomings limit the confidence that should be placed in most studies linking personality to eating disorders. The primary problem is that the personality profiles studied are often those of children and youth who have already been diagnosed and who are receiving treatment (Stein et al., 2009). As is the case with many other disorders, it may be relatively easy to identify ways in which diagnosed people differ from the "normal" undiagnosed population. However, delineating such differences is not at all the same as identifying a personality profile that typifies the population of people with eating disorders but without other forms of psychopathology. Another issue is the very small numbers of children and adolescents who are diagnosed as having eating disorders, resulting in very small samples in many studies of personality factors.

Notwithstanding this important methodological caveat, identification of a personality or temperament profile that is linked with eating disorders may have important implications for the success of psychotherapy. There is some evidence for links between personality profiles and eating disorders among children and adolescents. *Perfectionism* is often invoked as a maladaptive aspect of personality than can lead to eating disorders. Perfection may involve not only the belief that one must be perfect, including the possession of an attractive body, but also the belief that other people will only grant social acceptance to a perfect person (Hewitt and Flett, 2007). Other personality factors that are thought to be associated with eating disorders include the *lack of interoceptive awareness*, or confusion about the nature of one's internal psychological state and persisting feelings of personal ineffectiveness. Kerremans, Claes and Bijttebier (2010), working with a community sample of Belgian adolescents, confirmed the link between these personality patterns and eating-disordered behavior. In a study conducted with 120 adolescents diagnosed as having eating disorders, Thompson-Brenner and colleagues (2009) found that three distinct personality patterns characterized the participants: they identified a perfectionistic group, an anxious/depressed group and an emotionally dysregulated group. Emotional dysregulation consists of irregularities of mood and the absence of appropriate regulation of the expression of one's emotions, resulting in situationally inappropriate responses ranging from explosive outbursts to the total repression of one's feelings.

In ways that reflect the personality styles that have been linked with the disorder, dysfunctional thinking plays a role in disordered eating behavior. Poor self-concept, feelings of worthlessness and chronic self-criticism are seen as leading to perfectionism, obsessionality (with regard to weight and appearance), rigid thinking, inability to tolerate unhappy experiences or emotions, and thinking of people and events as either totally good or totally bad (Fairburn, Cooper and Shafran, 2003; Stein et al., 2009).The most recurrent themes in the literature on the cognitive bases of eating disorders in young people are a tragically poor self-concept, the inability to achieve an autonomous self-identity and the fear of being rejected by others (e.g., Cozzi and Ostuzzi, 2007; Pilecki and Jozefik, 2008). Although thinking patterns have been studied more extensively in adult women with eating disorders than with children and adolescents, they have been applied with some success to interventions designed for adolescents, as will be discussed later in this chapter.

Poor social skills

Establishing harmonious peer relationships, resisting inappropriate or excessive peer pressure and solving problems in effective and undamaging ways are among the skills needed to establish rewarding and supported relationships with others. It has been suggested that many children and adolescents with eating disorders are deficient in such skills. Some evidence for this comes from a study by Strober, Freeman and Morrell (1997), who conducted an important long-term (10–15 year) follow-up study of people who had been treated for eating disorders during their adolescence. Satisfactory interpersonal relationships were among the factors that most strongly differentiated young people who had maintained their recovery from those who had relapsed. However, social skills training by itself seems unlikely to reverse the complex causal chain that leads to eating disorders. This was established, for example, by an unsuccessful attempt at using interpersonal factors as the core of a prevention program against eating disorders among Canadian adolescents (McVey and Davis, 2002).

Family influence

Parents are the child's first and primary source of food. As such, they create a set of routines about eating and send important and enduring messages about it. As well, most parents communicate their aspirations for their children, which may include aspirations for their children's body sizes and body shapes. They communicate their expectations about eating not only verbally but also by example. Parents also determine the settings in which food is served and the people who are present, including peers, siblings and other relatives who will also transmit directly and by example behaviors and attitudes associated with eating. It is important for parents to provide a healthy degree of structure to their children's eating experiences, encompassing both parental direction and a progressive, age-appropriate level of autonomy. Such parental socialization should, ideally, lead in time to the children learning to self-regulate their eating behavior (Fisher, Sinton and Birch, 2009).

Fisher et al. (2009) enumerate the possible consequences of both excessive parental restriction and parental pressure on their children to eat. Excessive restriction of the child's choice of foods may turn some of them, fruits or otherwise, into "forbidden fruit," whose pursuit may lead in some way to problematic feeding behaviors. For example, one study revealed a high rate of problematic overeating and overweight among the 7-year-old daughters of mothers who restricted their daughters' food intake more extensively than most mothers when their daughters were 5 years old (Birch, Fisher and Davison, 2003; Faith et al., 2004). Relatively little is known about the consequences of excessive pressure *to* eat. However, preliminary data indicate that such pressure is counterproductive, leading to decreased interest in the foods the child is pressured to consume (Galloway et al., 2006). As their daughters, especially, enter adolescence, parental messages about the acceptability of body weight and shape play a primary role in influencing body image and, in some cases, contributing to the onset of an eating disorder (Bencdikt, Wertheim and Love, 1998).

A more systemic perspective has also been utilized in conceptualizing the family dynamics of the child or adolescent with an eating disorder. Their families have been described as more likely than other families to be insensitive, hostile to the individual needs of the child and hypercritical. Parents are prone to be controlling and to intrude excessively on the child's private life. In many cases, the families are enmeshed – excessively close, as discussed in Chapter 6 (Polivy and Herman, 2002).

Peer influence

Messages about the importance of physical appearance come not only from the media and from parents but also from friends and other family members. With the onset of adolescence, close friends and other peers wield considerable influence over attitudes about eating and appearance, as for many other issues. Some longitudinal research has demonstrated that peer pressure is among the sources of influence that lead to increases in disordered eating among adolescents according to data collected during follow-up measurement, typically 6 months to a year after the peer pressure was first recorded (Shomaker and Furman, 2009; Stice, 1998). Because self-report measures are typically used to measure peer influence, it is difficult to determine whether the peer pressure is real or only perceived. However, the potent influence of peer pressure was demonstrated in a recent study conducted with adolescents by Shomaker and Furman (2009), in which parents and close friends participated along with the adolescents providing the self-reports.

Prevention and treatment

Prevention

Increased awareness of the true extent of eating-disordered behavior has spurred investment into prevention programs of many types. Efforts at prevention range from single-session presentations at school assemblies to web-based programs (e.g., Brown et al., 2004) to multi-session group work, the latter being delivered mostly as secondary or target prevention programs aimed at children and adolescents who already show some degree of eating-disordered behavior. Prevention programs have been directed not only at adolescents and adults but also at children of primary-school age, which is earlier than the onset of most eating disorders. Neumark-Sztainer (2005) has argued that it is possible to work toward preventing eating disorders and obesity at the same time.

When primary prevention programs were first introduced with the aim of reducing subsequent onset of eating disorders, some fears were expressed that, perhaps by drawing attention to issues of thinness among children and adolescents, prevention programs might actually do more harm than good (Carter et al., 1997). Indeed, many efforts at prevention do result in small effects or gains that fail to weather the test of time. However, research has shown that well-designed prevention programs can and do work. Stice, Shaw and Marti (2007) presented a very useful meta-analysis of sixty-six published and unpublished evaluations of prevention programs conducted with participants of all ages. The findings indicated that, overall, there was statistical evidence of program-related change. Although the average effect sizes were statistically significant, they were, on the whole, quite small. Encouragingly, 51 percent of the programs were found to be successful in reducing risk factors associated with eating disorders, whereas 29 percent were successful in reducing future eating pathology. However, certain programs tended to be more effective than others. Effects were actually stronger if the intervention was delivered to participants 15 years old or older, perhaps because adolescents are better able to understand and make use of the content presented than are younger children. It was demonstrated that change takes time: Multi-session interventions worked better than brief, single-session efforts. Intervention was also more successful if the participants played a more active role than that of mere listeners by interacting, discussing, questioning, learning new skills or working through problems. Programs offered by trained professionals appear to be more successful than programs delivered by classroom teachers. Targeted interventions provided to young people who already showed some signs of eating-disordered behavior were found to have larger effect sizes than universal, primary prevention programs, which does not at all mean that primary prevention is not worthwhile. Prevention programs have been found to be more effective in enhancing knowledge about the nature of eating disorder than in actually modifying disordered behavior according to a meta-analysis by Fingeret and colleagues (2006). Stice et al. (2007) were able to identify the typical components of the most successful programs: reducing the idealization of thinness, diminishing body dissatisfaction and reducing negative emotions. Some recent programs have also

focused on prevention by media literacy – learning to think critically about the images and messages conveyed by the media (Wilksch, 2010). Another innovation implemented with the hope of improving the success rate of prevention programming is dissonance-based intervention – getting the participants to articulate actively principles that are inconsistent with the dysfunctional cognitions that lead to eating-disordered behavior. Preliminary data indicate that dissonance-based interventions have a greater success rate than other forms of prevention programming (Stice et al., 2008). In contrast, programs aimed at psychoeducation, that is providing participants with basic information about eating disorders, etc., appear to be less effective than other forms of preventive intervention (Stice and Shaw, 2004).

Treatment

This section provides a description of several forms of treatment that have proven successful in helping adolescents with eating disorders. Unfortunately, the data base on the success of these treatments is very limited. Notably few are studies in which different forms of treatment are compared to each other using rigorous methodology, although there are a small number of studies in which treatment groups have been compared with control groups of several kinds. Some attempts at randomly assigning participants to different treatments have failed because the participants wanted to choose the course of their own therapy (Fairburn and Gowers, 2010). In other studies, participants refused to provide the follow-up data needed to establish the long-term effectiveness of the treatments being tried.

Individual and group psychotherapy

Cognitive-behavioral therapy is the best-established modality of individual and group therapy for people with bulimia and binge eating but not necessarily for anorexia nervosa. There have been a few successful randomized control trials of this approach with adolescents suffering from bulimia (e.g., Schmidt

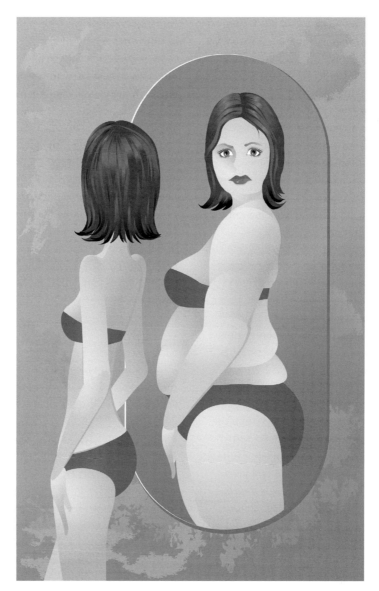

Figure 19.1 Distorted body image is a common cognitive feature of both bulimia and anorexia nervosa.

et al., 2007). Otherwise, it is important to note that the specific evidence of the effectiveness of cognitive-behavioral interventions for adolescents is very limited; most experts base their assumptions about its effectiveness on studies conducted with adults (e.g., Gleaves et al., 2009). The main focus of cognitive-behavioral approaches to eating disorders is, of course, dysfunctional and distorted beliefs about body image and about oneself, which are depicted in Figure 19.1. In its application to eating disorders, focus on strictly cognitive content must be complemented by systematic monitoring of eating and weight (Cooper, Fairburn and Hawker, 2003). In an influential study by Schmidt et al. (2007), eighty-five adolescents with either bulimia or eating disorder not otherwise specified were randomly assigned to receive either family therapy or individual cognitive-behavior therapy. Six months after the start of therapy, results were superior for the group that received the cognitively based therapy. Although the difference disappeared at 12-month follow-up, Schmidt and her colleagues concluded that the individual therapy was preferable because it seems to bring more rapid results. Providing further evidence of the rapidity, there have even been some successful internet-based applications of cognitive-behavioral therapy with adolescents suffering bulimia (Pretorius et al., 2009). The more modest success of cognitive approaches in helping people with anorexia nervosa may be attributable to their fear of change and to the fact that the need to gain weight quickly may be a more pressing issue than the restructuring of the cognitions that are associated with it (Stein et al., 2009).

Interpersonal therapy is, like cognitive-behavioral therapy, a time-limited psychotherapy that is most often delivered on an individual basis, often twelve to twenty sessions (e.g., Rieger et al., 2010). When applied to eating disorders, interpersonal psychotherapy includes a systematic review of the individual's life events, self-esteem and mood, which is also typical of cognitive-behavioral psychotherapy. However, interpersonal psychotherapy is based on the assumption that it is an interpersonal relationship or set of interpersonal relationships, or the loss of them, that play a central role in the individual's eating-disordered pathology. Eating problems may be a substitute that is used to make up for deficiencies in the person's social life (Rieger et al., 2010). Although some studies indicate that interpersonal psychotherapy is as effective in treating adolescent eating disorders as cognitive-behavioral therapy, other results suggest that it takes longer for the interpersonal approach to work (Rieger et al., 2010; Wilfley et al., 2002). This may be very important given the imminent health dangers of eating disorders (Agras et al., 2000; Rieger et al., 2010; Wilfley et al., 2002).

Family treatment

Many authorities believe that family treatment is more applicable to children and adolescents with eating disorders, especially anorexia nervosa, than is individual psychotherapy. There is some empirical support for family treatment, including several randomized trials with follow-up components, although these have often been conducted with small samples (Eisler et al., 2007; Gleaves et al., 2009; Lock and Fitzpatrick, 2009). An important exception is a recent study by Lock and his colleagues (2010) in which 120 adolescents with anorexia nervosa were randomly assigned to receive 24 hours of either family treatment or individual therapy. Therapy-related improvement was tracked at 6-month and 1-year follow-up. Although both treatments were somewhat successful, family therapy led to superior results on most measures, especially at follow-up. It should be noted that, in a similar study conducted with forty-eight participants with bulimia nervosa, family therapy was not found to be clearly superior to individual supportive therapy (Le Grange, Crosby and Lock, 2008). As mentioned in the previous section of this chapter, Schmidt et al. (2007) did not find family therapy superior to cognitive-behavior therapy.

The eminent systemic family therapist Salvador Minuchin described what he considered the typical *psychosomatic family* and demonstrated, with considerable success, ways in which systemic family treatment could be tailored to the characteristics of these families. In a very radical approach, Selvini Palazzoli, pioneer of the Milan school of systemic family therapy, went as far as employing paradoxical directions, such as telling parents to ignore their daughters' self-starvation, in an effort to alter the fundamental role of eating pathology in the interactions of rigid families (Selvini Palazzoli, 1978). Minuchin and Selvini Palazzoli proposed that anorexia nervosa is linked to family rigidity, overprotectiveness, overcontrol and avoidance of conflict (Minuchin, Rosman and Baker, 1978). However, subsequent research has shown that many families of children with eating disorders do not display these characteristics (Stein et al., 2009). Nevertheless, some of Minuchin's techniques were expanded by a team of therapists at London's Maudsley Hospital, who developed a form of family treatment that is supported by considerable research. The detailed procedures manual (Lock et al., 2001) facilitates accurate application and clinical research.

The Maudsley approach does not focus heavily on the family as a system, especially at the start of therapy. In fact, one of the fundamental therapeutic goals expressed to the participants coming for help is getting the family to believe that they are not at fault for the eating disorder of one of its members but that they have the responsibility for bringing about change. The primary objective of early stages of the Maudsley intervention is to restore appropriate nutrition. Once that has been accomplished, any family problems found to interfere with the implementation of appropriate nutrition are addressed. The final phase of the intervention is focused on healthy relationships between parents and children in which eating problems are not the central issue (Le Grange, 1999).

CASE STUDY: Bella and her family in treatment for binge eating

Loeb and colleagues (2009) present an interesting case study of Bella, a 17-year-old who was helped by the Maudsley method. Bella's treatment was instigated by her mother at the suggestion of two professionals who were working with Bella – a pediatrician and a psychotherapist who had been seeing Bella individually. Bella had started individual psychotherapy because of anxiety about her school performance, which was actually excellent, and her excessive standards for herself in several areas. However, the therapist became concerned when she noticed that Bella was losing weight rapidly. In the several months before starting specialized treatment for her eating problem, Bella's weight had dropped by 14 pounds (1 stone, or over 6 kilograms) because of her dieting. She was not only restricting the quantity of food she consumed but also avoiding any carbohydrates except fruit. She occasionally interrupted her dieting with episodes of binge eating followed by excessive exercise. Bella occasionally made remarks about her wide hips and huge thighs. When encouraged to eat healthy meals by her parents, Bella accused them of trying to make her fat. When she came to the hospital for treatment, Bella presented as somewhat introverted. She said that she had excellent relationships with both her parents, her twin sister Kayla and a number of good friends. Bella's parents also indicated that they had good marital relations; they said that they were united in their desire to help Bella overcome her eating problem. The psychotherapist seeing Bella individually had previously advised the parents to pay little attention to Bella's eating, in line with the approach of classic family therapists, as mentioned earlier in this chapter.

The hospital therapist followed the manual for family-based treatment closely. Accordingly, she began the first session by reminding the family of the seriousness of eating disorders. The therapist also informed them that the cause of the eating disorder is not known, alleviating any fears the parents might have that they were to blame. In describing Bella's eating disorder, she offered the metaphor of an octopus, whose tentacles were grasping Bella with increasing tightness. At the end of the first session, the family was instructed to bring a picnic meal to the next session, including foods that Bella used to enjoy but had stopped eating.

Bella continued her dieting and lost more weight before the next session. Bella ate about one-fourth of the chicken salad and bread roll that was her share of the picnic meal. She picked at the fruit salad, eating only the watermelon. Noticeably absent from the menu were brownies, which were previously one of Bella's favorite foods. Bella cried when it was suggested that brownies should be included. The therapist counseled against negotiating with Bella about food. She asked the parents to try to convince Bella to eat one more bit of the picnic meal. Kayla offered to eat it for her twin sister. However, with gentle encouragement from the therapist, who coached them in blending firmness with kindness, Bella finally agreed to eat just a bit more.

In subsequent sessions, Bella's father agreed to reduce his business travel so that he could participate more regularly in regulating Bella's eating. Bella's mother also reduced her work schedule. An unintended change occurred in Kayla, Bella's twin, who began to join Bella in angry outbursts during the therapy sessions, followed by expressions of guilt. Bella tended to use Kayla's weight as a comparison point, accusing her parents of wanting her to become fat like Kayla. Kayla's non-productive attempts at supervising the eating behavior of her twin sister had to be curbed. It became obvious to the therapist that not all of Kayla's problems would be resolved within the framework of the manualized therapy. Therefore, Kayla was referred for adjunct individual therapy. Dad wanted a higher target for Bella's food intake than Mom did; the therapist encouraged them to reconcile this in private. Another temporary setback occurred when Bella discovered that her parents tried to conceal from her some of the ingredients in the foods that were served. The parents stopped doing this, either providing honest information or by reminding Bella that they were temporarily taking over the decisions about food until Bella developed the skills needed to do this for herself. As these changes emerged, Bella began to gain weight.

The second phase of therapy began with the eighth session. Bella contracted with her parents that she could join a soccer (football) team if her weight continued to increase. Bella was able to continue on course with only some of her meals being supervised by her mother. Bella's social life improved, including dates and activities with friends. After another brief period of weight loss, Bella achieved the expected weight for a girl of her age and size by the termination of treatment after the twelfth session. Bella went on to university, where she was able to maintain her weight with some monitoring by her parents during vacation periods. Bella's case illustrates not only the effectiveness of family-based treatment but also some of the many challenges encountered in making it work. The case also indicates the wisdom of the systemic family therapists who have contextualized eating disorders, even if many of their assumptions and techniques have not weathered the test of time.

Other forms of psychotherapy

Although cognitive-behavior therapy and systemic family therapy are the best-established forms of treatment, there has been some success with alternative psychotherapeutic modalities. Juarascio and her colleagues (2013) propose *acceptance and commitment therapy* as an alternative that may be particularly useful for young people who resist the direct "attack" on problematic eating patterns that is usually an integral part of the more established treatment modalities. Young people participating in acceptance and commitment therapy clarify their personal values and set for themselves goals that help lead to more fulfilling lives. Once their personal values are clarified and their personal goals, they become more willing to have negative internal experiences that may interfere with their goals and that may be inconsistent with their values. Jurascio et al. demonstrated empirically that this treatment approach leads to somewhat greater success than the usual treatment the participants would receive in the community, although both treatment groups improved. Importantly, the gains were still evident at follow-up 6 months after the termination of the therapy.

Residential care and partial hospitalization

Not every case of child and adolescent eating disorder can be treated in the community, where not every family can succeed in helping to stabilize eating patterns, which is the most urgent aspect of the treatment that is needed. Nutritional management is, therefore, the primary goal of in-patient care. In-patient care is used more frequently for anorexia nervosa than for bulimia, and often for cases that have reached the final stages of the disorder or for young people with comorbid suicidal ideation. As is the case for most other disorders, the typical length of in-patient stay has decreased dramatically over the past few years, with few patients admitted for longer than a few weeks. Most follow-up studies indicate success for about half the adolescents with anorexia nervosa, a statistic that must be interpreted in light of the fact that the young people admitted are probably those whose disorders are quite severe. Controlled scientific studies of in-patient treatment are unlikely to appear because not many children or families are likely to agree to participate in a study in which they might randomly be assigned to in-patient treatment (Fairburn and Gowers, 2010; Gleaves et al., 2009; Patel, Pratt and Greydanus, 2003; Robin, Gilroy and Dennis, 1998).

Pharmacological interventions

Current medical guidelines do not support the use of psychotropic drugs for children and adolescents with eating disorders (e.g., Fairburn and Gowers, 2010). However, antidepressants are sometimes prescribed for comborbid depression (see Chapter 13). This appears to be more successful for bulimia nervosa than for anorexia nervosa although relapses are reported when the medication is discontinued (Shapiro et al., 2007; Stein et al., 2009). A recent survey of adolescents with eating disorders in the UK revealed that 27 percent were on some form of medication (Gowers et al., 2010).

Conclusions and future directions

Eating disorders among children and adolescents are complex, difficult to treat and more common than was previously believed. As mentioned throughout this chapter, sound research on the etiology and treatment of eating disorders among children and adolescents is only beginning to emerge. Compared to other disorders that, in the end, are probably no more common than eating disorders, there is a dearth of well-designed, authoritative research to serve as a guide for clinicians. The advent of DSM-5 is likely to allow for the formal diagnosis of some cases that were previously either undiagnosed or diagnosed under the vague rubric of Eating Disorder – Not Otherwise Specified. Hence, this may be one condition for which improvements in diagnostic classification may truly live up to their essential purpose of facilitating life-saving research and treatment.

Summary

- Anorexia nervosa involves an overevaluation of the importance of shape and size, as well as the maintenance of low body weight. Bulimia, on the other hand, involves preoccupation with weight by alternating between binge eating and efforts to avoid gaining weight, such as dieting and vomiting. Excessive, compulsive exercise may also be a way to achieve this.
- Some less common forms of eating disorder are more prevalent among infants and preschoolers.

Pica refers to the habitual ingestion of non-nutritive substances (e.g., sand, string, hair). Rumination disorder involves the voluntary regurgitation and rechewing of food. Feeding disorder of infancy or early childhood refers to a child under 6 years old who refuses to eat enough food to gain or maintain weight.

- The normal developmental trajectory of children must be considered when diagnosing eating disorders. Children may be picky about the foods they eat, or they may develop food fads. Some argue that eating disorders cannot appear until after puberty, when disruptions of the female menstrual cycle and low levels of serum testosterone in males would explain the disorders. Others, however, disagree and point to the substantial number of case studies describing eating disorders in pre-pubescent children, although their symptoms sometimes differ slightly from those in adulthood.

- DSM 5 contains a new category, *binge eating disorder*, which refers to repeated episodes of overeating that are often uncontrolled. Many expect this addition to increase the number of children and youth diagnosed as having an eating disorder.

- Prevalence rates are difficult to estimate due to the lack of well-developed diagnostic instruments and lack of reporting. The collection of data with children is difficult, as the language used in the questionnaires may not be explicit enough or fully understandable. Sometimes, food diaries and semi-structured clinical interviews provide insight into eating disorders in children, yet the majority of researchers use questionnaires.

- Although many children and adolescents do not meet full criteria for an eating disorder, approximately one in seven exhibits risky nutrition-related behaviors.

- Comorbid psychopathologies are common among those diagnosed with eating disorders, especially mood and anxiety disorders, substance abuse and obsessive-compulsive personality disorder.

- Studies on eating disorders and depression have revealed two different causal pathways between the two disorders, involving univariate causation (one causing the other) or reciprocal causality (both causing each other). Both disorders may also be the result of the same external risk factor or cause.

- The outcome of having an eating disorder varies and can be extremely negative, including death from suicide or from the physical consequences of the eating disorder itself. The prognosis is somewhat better for bulimia nervosa in general than for anorexia nervosa, although the relapse rates for both are high.

- A good child–parent relationship and the absence of an extensive history of eating problems are both associated with a more favorable prognosis. A history of sexual abuse and an avoidant personality are associated with more negative outcome.

- Objectification theory, the notion that women are men's sexual objects, includes the concept of objectified body consciousness, a term that refers to the idea that people can and should control their own body shape. Self-objectification results in excessive body surveillance and monitoring, leading to anxiety, shame and reduced awareness of hunger and fullness.

- Research indicates greater evidence of a genetic basis for anorexia nervosa than for bulimia. Scholars believe the genetic route to eating disorders is one of common genetic susceptibility, perhaps linked to a genetic susceptibility to depression.

- Central nervous system neurotransmitters, such as serotonin, dopamine and norepinephrine, may be involved in the regulation of eating behaviors. Elevated levels of dopaminergic and serotonergic activity have been found. Some suggest this may be linked to personality structures bringing about certain personality traits commonly associated with eating disorders.

- Research on the role of personality in eating disorders is limited by the failure to consider the co-existence of other forms of psychopathology.
- Perfectionism is thought to be a maladaptive aspect of personality than can lead to eating disorders. Other personality factors associated with eating disorders include lack of interoceptive awareness (confusion about internal psychological state or feelings of ineffectiveness) and emotional dysregulation (irregularities of mood and the absence of appropriate regulation of emotional expression).
- Many children and adolescents with eating disorders are deficient in certain social skills such as establishing harmonious peer relationships, resisting inappropriate or excessive peer pressure, and solving problems in effective and undamaging ways. However, social skills training does not seem to be very effective.
- Many developed countries around the world seem to have similar prevalence rates of eating disorders among children and adolescents. However, not all cultures ingrain values of weight and body shape to the same extent. Within cultures, socio-economic factors are often linked to prevalence rates for eating disorders.
- Westernization of non-Western cultures, media influences and upward social mobility (i.e., the transition to a higher socio-economic level) have been found to be associated with increased prevalence of eating disorders.
- Parental influences are very important for children in fostering good eating habits. At young ages, parents are responsible for the time and place of meals. They determine who is present to show exemplary eating behaviors. Both excessive parental restriction and parental pressure on their children to eat may lead to poor eating behaviors later in life.
- Families in which a child or adolescent presents with an eating disorder are often seen as excessively close. The parents are prone to be controlling and to intrude on the child's private life.

- Especially in adolescence, close friends and peers have a marked influence on attitudes regarding eating and appearance.
- Prevention techniques, ranging from school assemblies to web-based programs to multi-session group work, have been directed at schoolchildren. Primary prevention programs, while effective, have been shown to be less effective than targeted prevention programs. In addition, dissonance-based interventions, in which participants receive information inconsistent with their previous thinking, have shown much greater success rates than psychoeducational programs.
- Due to methodological limits and errors, most studies are not conclusive as to which treatment option is best for children and adolescents with eating disorders. However, the general consensus is that adolescents respond much better to treatment of anorexia nervosa than do adults.
- Cognitive-behavior therapy (i.e., modifying dysfunctional and distorted beliefs about body image while monitoring eating behaviors) seems to be the best treatment for people with bulimia and binge eating, but not necessarily for anorexia nervosa.
- Interpersonal therapy deals with the individual's life events, self-esteem and mood, with a focus on the interpersonal relationships (or loss/lack of them) that play a role in the disordered eating.
- Systemic family treatment is based on the observations of systems theorists about the families of young people with eating disorders. Recent family-based treatment does not focus as heavily on the family as a system, but instead attempts to change the family's belief that they are at fault for the eating disorder. While restoring appropriate nutrition, this method places responsibility on the family to help bring about change.
- Current medical guidelines do not endorse the use of psychotropic drugs for children and adolescents with eating disorders, although antidepressants are sometimes prescribed if there is comorbid depression. This is more successful when dealing with bulimia nervosa than with anorexia nervosa.

Study questions

1. What is objectification theory, and how does it explain eating disorders among girls and young women?
2. Can eating disorders be considered one of the easier forms of child and adolescent psychopathology to treat? Why or why not?

20

Bipolar disorder in childhood and adolescence
A modern-day epidemic?

Bipolar disorder or *manic-depressive disorder* is characterized by unpredictable mood swings, in which the individual shifts from depression to an elated, euphoric mood. Bipolar disorder is also known as *bipolar depression*. Few debates about child psychopathology are as contentious as the current controversy about the extent of this disorder among children. The moods of many children change frequently and their mood changes are not always predictable. Many people find it jarring when the reactions of others in their environments cannot be predicted. Irritable moods and the behaviors they provoke appear to be particularly disturbing to parents and teachers. The question is how bad it needs to be before it needs treating or is to be considered beyond what it developmentally typical.

Manic-depressive illness among adults is a severe disorder that has been recognized since ancient times, when melancholy and mania were described as sometimes constituting two phases of the same disease by the influential first-century Greek physician Aretaeus. Case studies of patients at La Salpêtrière Hospital (Paris) in the nineteenth century were presented in the psychiatry literature to illustrate this dual form of mood disorder. However, for a period at the beginning of the twentieth century, the distinction between unipolar and bipolar depression slipped from the nomenclature, to be resurrected from the 1960s on (Angst and Marneros, 2001). It is now considered a common and serious form of mental illness among adults. Bipolar disorder constitutes a strong risk factor for adult suicide (Bostwick and Pankratz, 2000).

Although there are many doubts about the clarity of the diagnostic category and much wariness about excessive diagnosis, there may be serious risks in *not* diagnosing child and adolescent bipolar disorder.

In the adult literature at least, it is people with untreated bipolar disorder that have been found to be the most likely to commit suicide (Baldessarini, Tondo and Hennen, 2003). Esposito-Smythers and her colleagues (2010) found that, among 432 children and adolescents who had been diagnosed with bipolar disorder, 22 percent of the children and 22 percent of the adolescents reported some form of self-injury that did not lead to death during their last manic episode. Duffy (2009) speculates that delaying treatment may lead to neuroanatomical damage, more serious symptomatology and an increase in comorbid forms of psychopathology. She further speculates, however, that children and adolescents who are treated early may respond better to their treatments than their counterparts who are not diagnosed until the disorder has progressed considerably.

In this brief chapter, emphasis is placed on the reasons for which this disorder is so controversial, namely the diagnostic criteria and prevalence rates. The chapter follows the same sequence as the other chapters on the various disorders: diagnostic criteria, prevalence and stability, possible causes and correlates and, finally, prevention and treatment.

Diagnostic criteria

Many clinicians are firmly convinced that bipolar disorder in children and adolescents is a highly debilitating condition and one that differs from adult bipolar disorder. In the DSM-IV, they had no alternative but to diagnose many children as having bipolar disorder who did not really fit the criteria stated for both children and adults except, of course, to make no diagnosis at all. Therefore, they made most of their diagnoses of bipolar disorder among children either without reference to formal DSM-IV criteria or by using modified criteria, of which several versions have been proposed and adopted for standard use in some clinical settings (e.g., Axelson et al., 2006; Saxena et al., 2009).

One of the most controversial decisions of the DSM-5 Commission was to add a new disorder called *disruptive mood dysregulation disorder.* It shares much of the flavor of bipolar disorder but is listed as a depressive disorder. It can only be diagnosed if the outbursts begin before age 10 years and only for individuals from 6 through 18 years, constituting one of the few situations in which DSM has a totally distinct provision for the problems of children and adolescents. Mood dysregulation disorder is characterized by recurrent fits of temper that are out of proportion to anything that might have provoked them. The outbursts must occur at least three times a week. The diagnostic criteria refer to three settings: home, school and peer interaction. The temper flare-ups must occur in at least two of these settings and must be severe in at least one of them. Only time will tell whether clinicians are able to differentiate reliably between bipolar disorder and disruptive mood dysregulation disorder. As discussed in Chapter 12, there is also a disorder in DSM-5 called *intermittent explosive disorder.* These changes in the DSM were made not only to recognize a clinical condition that has aroused considerable concern but also to increase inter-rater reliability. Research results will hopefully confirm that inter-rater reliability is at the level envisaged by the DSM-5 Commission.

Children and adolescents can be diagnosed as having bipolar illness in DSM-5. There is, however, an additional category, cyclothymic disorder, that is exclusively for adults. The DSM-5 description of a manic episode depicts a heightened state of arousal in general, characterized in many cases by racing thoughts, little need for sleep and constant talkativeness. Unlike DSM-IV, DSM-5 extends the diagnosis of bipolar illness to changes in energy or activity as well as changes in mood. DSM-5 makes a distinction between Bipolar I disorder and Bipolar II disorder. Bipolar I is a disorder characterized by at least one *manic* or mixed episode, although individuals with Bipolar I may also have had one or more major depressive episodes. Bipolar II is defined as a disorder with at least one major depressive episode plus at least one *hypomanic episode.* The criteria for manic disorder are at least three of the following symptoms in general, but four if the person exhibits an irritable mood: inflated self-esteem or grandiosity; lack of sleep; constant talkativeness; frequent shifts of ideas; distractibility; sudden intensive engagement in a goal-directed work or leisure activity; and sudden excessive involvement in a pleasurable activity with high stakes, such as a buying spree, a risky investment or sexual promiscuity. These symptoms are severe enough to cause substantial impairment of the person's daily functioning. The criteria for a hypomanic episode are very similar and involve the same symptoms, but the episode is not as severe and crippling. This criterion, which is almost identical to the parallel DSM-IV criterion, has been seen as arbitrary and not supported by data (Parker, Graham and Synnott, 2014). The clinician using DSM-5 can add many specifiers including "with anxious features" and "with mood-incongruent psychotic features." By adding this degree of detail, DSM-5 became similar to the ICD-10 in terms of the complexity of the bipolar diagnosis. Figures 20.1, 20.2 and 20.3 illustrate the ways in which the diagnostic features of bipolar disorder are distinct from those of ADHD, anxiety disorder and autism, as well as the areas of overlap and potential confusion.

Prevalence and subsequent consequences

Bipolar disorder is now diagnosed in children and adolescents in the United States at least ten times and perhaps as many as forty times as often as it was diagnosed as recently as 10 to 15 years ago (e.g., Blader and Carlson, 2007; Moreno et al., 2007). It is highly unlikely that there has been a ten- to

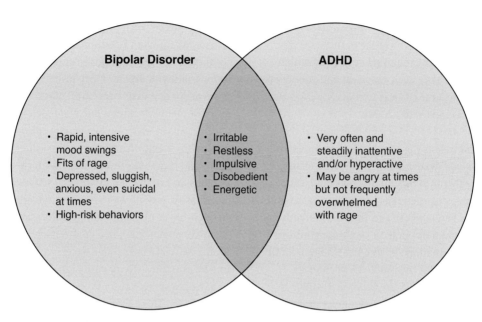

Figure 20.1 Similarities and differences between childhood bipolar disorder and ADHD.

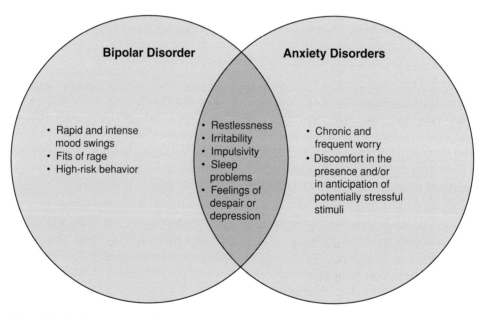

Figure 20.2 Similarities and differences between childhood bipolar disorder and anxiety disorders.

forty-fold increase in the actual incidence of the disorder. Making the current rates of diagnosis even more suspect is the fact that the mood swings involved are often difficult to recognize completely and accurately unless and until the diagnostician spends extended periods of time with the child or adolescent in question (Jenkins et al., 2011; Marchand, Wirth and Simon, 2006).

If the formal DSM-IV criteria for bipolar disorder are applied to community samples of children, no

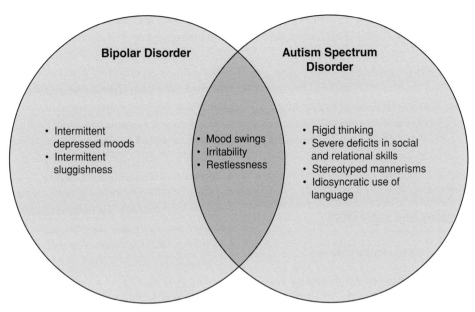

Figure 20.3 Similarities and differences between childhood bipolar disorder and autism spectrum disorder.

more than one child in 100 would be diagnosed and perhaps no more than one in 500 (Costello et al., 1996; Lewinsohn, Klein and Seeley, 1995). However, many diagnosticians now use far less stringent criteria in the case of bipolar disorder, which makes it appear like there is an epidemic with dimensions that are difficult to determine with any degree of precision. As with most other disorders, new research using DSM-5 criteria is needed and may indicate different prevalence rates than appear in previous studies.

Because the diagnosis of bipolar disorder has mushroomed in recent years, longitudinal research of its course and consequences has not been able to keep pace with research on its prevalence. There has been, however, some research on the rates of bipolar illness among the children of parents with bipolar illness. In a 12-year follow-up of the adolescent offspring of Dutch parents diagnosed with bipolar illness, 13 percent of the offspring developed some form of recognizable bipolar illness. However, 72 percent of the offspring developed some form of mental illness, often major depression (Mesmen et al., 2013).

Comorbidity

The rates of comorbidity are extremely high. Comorbidity of childhood bipolar disorder and attention deficit/hyperactivity disorder is consistently reported in epidemiological studies as occurring in at least two-thirds of diagnosed cases of bipolar disorder. There is more fluctuation among the studies in terms of comorbidity with other forms of child psychopathology. Results of different studies indicate that anywhere between one-sixth and two-thirds of children diagnosed with bipolar also have substance abuse, oppositional defiant disorder and/or an anxiety disorder (Axelson et al., 2006; Dickstein et al., 2005; Wozniak et al., 2005). These comorbidity rates and the "drug cocktails" that are used in attempts to treat all the different symptoms involved are part of the current controversy about pediatric bipolar disorder. A poignant account of this was the story of Kyle, published in the *New York Times* on September 1, 2010 (Bickford, 2010). Kyle's medication started with the antipsychotic Risperdal when he was 18 months old. By the time he was

3 years old, he was also taking sleep medication and a psychostimulant to control his attention problems. When he was 6, however, it was apparent that attention deficit was the primary problem and he was weaned off all the other medications. The author of the newspaper article lambasts physicians who prescribe drug "cocktails" for preschool children that have never been shown to work in systematic research, even in the drug trials conducted by pharmaceutical companies.

Possible causes and correlates

Biological factors and family risk

Children with at least one parent diagnosed as having bipolar disorder are at very high risk of developing some form of psychopathology such as major depressive disorder or attention deficit/hyperactivity disorder. This has been demonstrated in a number of studies, although it is important to note that in these longitudinal studies none of the offspring was found to have full-blown diagnosable bipolar disorder before puberty. However, the risk increases greatly from adolescence on. In fact, when onset during adolescence or afterwards is considered, bipolar disorder has been shown to be one of the most heritable forms of psychopathology, with heritability estimates higher than those for schizophrenia (Duffy, 2009). Twin and family studies indicate a heritability estimate of 59–87 percent (Smoller and Finn, 2003), with the very high rate of 57 percent concordance for identical twins (Alda, 1997). It is important to note that although the twin and adoption studies consistently point to substantial heritability, these studies are based on the full formal DSM-IV diagnostic criteria and have often been conducted when many of the twins or adoptees were adults. Therefore, the degree to which genetics account for the current "epidemic" of bipolar disorder that does not correspond with standard diagnostic criteria is not clear. Moving beyond behavioral genetics, there have been a number of molecular genetic studies in recent years. The results so far are highly

variable, pointing to a number of different genes and different genetic-transmission mechanisms (Kelsoe, 2003; Miklowitz and Chang, 2008). Modern MRI technology, including functional MRI, has been employed in recent efforts to pinpoint any brain abnormalities. The results vary from study to study as well. However, the most consistent findings indicate reduced amygdala volume and increased amygdala activation (Blumberg et al., 2005; Delbello, Adler and Strakowski, 2006; Rich et al., 2006).

Strong as the evidence of genetic origin may be, there is also evidence that adverse family background may influence or trigger the emergence of bipolar disorder in children, interacting with genetic predisposition. As with much of the other research on bipolar disorder, most of the data come from studies conducted with adults. Therefore, the results may be affected by errors of memory in the retrospective recollections of the childhood experiences of adults suffering from bipolar disorder. Nevertheless, the consistency of the findings is notable, with early sexual abuse and neglect by parents emerging as predictors of later bipolar disorder (Dienes et al., 2006; Liu, 2010; Miklowitz and Chang, 2008; Mowlds et al., 2010; Post and Leverich, 2006).

Some preliminary research indicates that dietary deficiencies may contribute to the emergence of mood disorders in vulnerable children. The deficiencies implicated include omega-3 fatty acids and Vitamins B, D and E. Some authorities suggest that dietary supplements should be part of secondary prevention programs conducted with children known to be at risk of developing bipolar disorder (McNamara et al., 2010).

A few studies have documented the effects of childhood bipolar disorder on children's daily lives. Goldstein and her colleagues (2009) interviewed 446 children and adolescents who were diagnosed with bipolar disorder, as well as their parents. The participants' ages ranged from 7 to 17 years. The results indicated marked impairment in the work/school domain and in interpersonal relationships, with less impairment of recreational activities. Consistent with the results of several other studies, impairment was greatest during periods of depressed mood. Adolescent participants reported greater impairment of their daily lives than did younger participants. The participants tended to express dissatisfaction with their life functioning. Importantly, other studies have confirmed that the daily functioning of children and adolescents who have been diagnosed with bipolar disorder is more seriously impaired than the functioning of children with other common forms of child psychopathology. Geller and her colleagues (2000) worked with children and early adolescents. Their study showed that interpersonal relationships with both parents and peers were more dysfunctional among the participants with bipolar disorder than among either non-diagnosed control group participants or among participants with attention deficit/hyperactivity. Similarly, Lewinsohn et al. (1995) found that the academic and social functioning of older adolescents diagnosed with bipolar disorder was more impaired than the functioning of a comparison group diagnosed as having unipolar depression. Unfortunately, even after their symptoms have abated, only the minority of adolescents with bipolar disorder appear to reach levels of interpersonal functioning similar to those of typically developing adolescents according to a 1-year follow-up by Delbello and her colleagues (2007).

Prevention and treatment

Prevention

As will be detailed in the following sections, the treatment of pediatric bipolar disorder is difficult and controversial. As argued most articulately by Miklowitz and Chang (2008), future progress in this area may depend not only on the development of better treatments but also on earlier intervention with children who are vulnerable because of family risk. More specifically, they advocate the applications of the major components of family-oriented cognitive-behavior therapy, described

below, to prevention programs. Hopefully, this will avoid the need for intervention with the medications described in the following section, which have strong side effects. Miklowitz and his colleagues (2013) demonstrated success with a 4-month early family-focused intervention for forty youths at risk for bipolar disorder because of family history of bipolar illness. Compared to a control group, which received only an intervention consisting of basic education about the disorder, the child and adolescent participants in the family intervention displayed more rapid recovery from early bipolar symptoms and more weeks with no such symptoms. More research with longer-term follow-up is needed to determine the true impact of early family intervention.

Pharmacotherapy

In most cases, psychotropic medication is prescribed for ever-growing numbers of children and adolescents. The main basis for this until now has been research conducted with adults showing the benefits of the medications. However, physicians are permitted to prescribe these medications "off-label" – to treat conditions for which the drug in question has not been approved officially by any government agency. This is very common and may represent the majority of prescriptions for psychotropic medication with people of all ages. The bodies of children do not necessarily react to medications in the same ways as the bodies of adults do. This practice is far more controversial in attempts at helping children, sometimes as young as 4 years old, than it is with adolescents (Pfeiffer, Kowatch and DelBello, 2010). Nevertheless, this off-label prescription for the treatment of pediatric bipolar disorder is not without scientific basis.

In a 2010 review paper in the journal *CNS Drugs*, Pfeiffer and colleagues (2010) present a useful review of the medications that are usually prescribed for children and adolescents with bipolar disorder. These include, first of all, *lithium*, a mood-stabilizing drug that has been used in adult psychopharmacotherapy for at least 150 years. *Anti-seizure medication* is also used at times. The most recently developed medications mentioned in the review are *atypical antipsychotics*, of which the best known is *risperidone*, often sold as Risperdal. As their name indicates, the atypical antipsychotics were first developed for the treatment of adult schizophrenia. The benefits of these medications have been confirmed in some studies conducted with relatively small samples, as documented in the articles reviewed. The adverse side effects listed include nausea, fatigue, weight gain and even diabetes. Pfeiffer et al. underscore the need for more research featuring random assignment of participants to treatments. However, they conclude that, at present, these medications may be useful. They suggest to practicing physicians that they begin with a single medication, adding additional medications if the response to the first is insufficient.

Although Pfeiffer, et al. present an accurate and helpful summary of the published literature, they do not discuss the raging controversy about that literature. McKinney and Renk (2011) maintain that adverse side effects are probably under-reported by a very substantial degree. The reason often attributed to this is that much of the research is paid for by large pharmaceutical companies, who sometimes pay more money to university researchers to "test" their products than the same researchers receive in salary from their universities. For example, in a highly publicized case, Harvard University disciplined three eminent researchers in 2011 for not meeting the university requirements for reporting potential conflicts of interest pertaining to outside income received from pharmaceutical companies (Yu, 2011). As reported in a *New York Times* article entitled "Side Effects May Include Lawsuits" (published October 2, 2010; Wilson, 2010), these practices are under investigation by the United States Congress. Several leading psychiatrists quoted in the article believe that, at the behest of the pharmaceutical companies, researchers have exaggerated the

benefits of the new antipsychotics. In an editorial entitled "Antipsychotics for Children: Can We Do Better?" published in the May 2010 issue of the *Journal of the Canadian Academy of Child and Adolescent Psychiatry*, Normand Carrey (2010, p. 71) acknowledges the "vertiginous rise" in the prescription of antipsychotics and asks whether this practice has kept pace with the research support for it. Regarding the influence of the pharmaceutical companies, he comments that: "Without demonizing Big Pharma, the bottom line is that they are in the business of making money while we are in the business of providing the best clinical care possible" (p. 71).

In a paper published in the well-regarded *Clinical Psychology Review*, McKinney and Renk (2011) provide useful safety guidelines for the use of atypical antipsychotic medication with children and youth who display a variety of conditions including bipolar disorder. They suggest, first of all, that pharmacotherapy should only be considered if a child's condition has been assessed thoroughly, to the point where a reasonably plausible etiology has been established. The next guideline specifies that, at the current state of knowledge, medication should only be used if psychosocial interventions have been tried and, after ample implementation, proven unsuccessful. Then, if the problem condition is clearly and substantially interfering with the child's well-being, medication can be tried. Its effects must be evaluated regularly. Importantly, medication should not be used any longer than it is clearly needed. An additional safeguard is proposed by Panagiotopoulos (2010) and her colleagues in an article entitled "First Do No Harm [a basic tenet of the medical profession]: Promoting an Evidence-Based Approach to Atypical Antipsychotic Use in Children and Adolescents," published in the *Journal of the Canadian Academy of Child and Adolescent Psychiatry*. In light of the known side effects such as weight gain, waist circumference, dysglycemia (disturbance of the regulation of blood sugar) and hypertension, they propose regular metabolic monitoring of children on these medications.

Psychosocial interventions

Although the guidelines proposed by McKinney and Renk (2011) suggest that medication only be tried if psychosocial interventions have failed, it is a sad reality that not much research has been conducted on psychosocial interventions for pediatric bipolar disorder either. Furthermore, the mood swings encountered in bipolar disorder are sometimes so severe that the children or adolescents simply cannot focus on psychotherapy. Therefore, it has been suggested that psychotherapy be added as a complement to pharmacotherapy as soon as the child's mood has stabilized (e.g., Kowatch et al., 2005).

A specific application of cognitive-behavior therapy has been developed to assist children with bipolar disorder and their parents. Pavuluri and her colleagues at the University of Illinois developed a program called family-focused cognitive-behavior therapy. The components of the program, which is delivered to all family members, include establishing a regular routine; regulating emotions, thinking positively but recognizing and accepting negative emotions when they occur; problem-solving; taking the initiative in making friends; and learning to seek help and support when needed. In an initial trial with thirty-four participants, 8 through 12 years old, the program was well accepted by the children and parents. Symptom rating scales indicated improvement in all areas measured (Pavuluri et al., 2004). A similar intervention administered in group format to twenty-four children and their families has led to significant improvement in many but not all symptoms (West et al., 2009). Despite these initial successes, much work remains to be done. If childhood bipolar disorder is as common and crippling as the recent literature suggests, as much research on its treatment as has been conducted with regard to other major forms of child psychopathology is desperately needed.

Psychoeducational psychotherapy has also been implemented successfully with children and adolescents with bipolar disorder. Psychoeducational psychotherapy focuses heavily on providing children and their parents with a clear understanding of the nature of the disorder and of the properties of the medications that are usually prescribed together with the psychotherapy. The therapist also equips the child and family with strategies for coping with the symptoms of bipolar disorder, including how to work with the child's school (Fristad et al., 2009). Advice about sleep, exercise and diet are provided in recent versions. Therapy typically continues for sixteen to twenty sessions. Parents might remain in the room for only the first and last few minutes of the child sessions. However, the child sessions alternate with sessions for the parents only. There may also be one or more sessions in which siblings participate (Leffler, Fristad and Klaus, 2010). In evaluations of psychoeducational psychotherapy, the interventions have been found to lead to improved family life and better coping skills (Fristad, 2006).

CASE STUDY: Jane, coping with bipolar illness, parental divorce and parental mental illness

Leffler et al. (2010) present the case of Jane, 11 years old, who has been diagnosed with bipolar disorder. At the time of her initial contact with the psychotherapist, Jane's moods were highly unstable, with intermittent displays of sadness, irritability, restlessness and fatigue. At other times, however, she displayed hyperactivity in her physical movements, rapid speech and a degree of pomposity. She washed her hands excessively and picked her skin. Her parents reported that she used to be regarded as popular and fun-loving; now, she has no friends. Aggravating the situation was the conflict between Jane's parents and their subsequent divorce. Another probable complication is the history of mental illness in the lives of both of Jane's parents, including her father's current diagnosis of bipolar disorder.

By the time treatment started, Jane had become verbally and physically aggressive with her parents. In a precipitating incident, Jane was upset because her mother had to leave her for a short time to run an errand. When Jane insisted, her mother allowed her to enter the car. However, Jane tried to jump out of the car window. When other family members tried to calm her, she hit them with a bar. She then went to a window of the upper floor of their home and tried to jump out of it. For over a year prior to coming for psychotherapy, Jane's physicians prescribe several different types of medication for her. Initial results indicated little improvement; the medications were changed at about the time that psychotherapy began. Jane had previously refused to enter psychotherapy. A behavior analyst at Jane's school worked with the school staff to help manage her behavior there.

Jane did not communicate well with the therapist at the beginning of her treatment. She insisted that she would not participate at all. Nevertheless, the therapist was able to communicate the motto of psychoeducational therapy to her: "It's not my fault but it's my challenge." By the second session, Jane became more cooperative. She was able to recognize that she did have a few positive traits. The next several sessions were devoted to her diet and sleep. Jane learned to imagine herself coping well with some stressful experiences. The therapist had to work hard to get her to express her thoughts and feelings. Jane rarely completed the projects that were assigned as "homework" between sessions. However, by the end of treatment, the parents reported seeing some improvement in Jane's behavior. Jane's younger brother and her school behavior analyst participated in a few of the sessions.

The parent sessions were similarly challenging for the therapist. Jane's mother attributed Jane's problems to her shifting moods but her father believed that Jane's behavior was caused by her mother's inconsistent limit-setting. The therapist was able to get the parents to understand Jane's behavior. They were also able to agree on parenting strategies, with reduced attribution of blame and consistent expectations. By the end of treatment, the therapist observed considerable improvement, although all of the problems of Jane and her family had not been resolved. Using standard questionnaires about child mood and family functioning, there was a clear improvement between the beginning and end of therapy (Leffler et al., 2010).

Conclusion and future directions

One important area in which improvement is both needed and very possible is in the training of mental health professionals in the assessment of bipolar disorder in children using scientifically valid methods. Jenkins and colleagues (2011) have developed effective methods for the training of clinicians in the assessment of pediatric bipolar disorder. The professionals participate in the training during professional-development seminars. These researchers found that, when presented with anecdotal case material, clinicians were extremely likely to overdiagnose bipolar disorder in child and adolescent cases. Diagnostic accuracy improves greatly once the clinicians are equipped with *nomograms*, or structured checklists of symptoms that are linked to statistical norms.

If the hype and panic about bipolar disorder in childhood have served any purpose, it has been to sensitize the public and the mental health community about the severity of this disorder. The refinements in the diagnostic criteria promised by the DSM-5 Commission will hopefully provide the foundation for greater scientific rigor in research on all aspects of pediatric bipolar disorder. Hopefully, new research will elucidate safer and more effective treatment methods. Perhaps the greatest hope, however, lies in the development and evaluation of secondary prevention and early-intervention programs.

Summary

- Bipolar illness is characterized by unpredictable and problematic shifts between depressed and elevated moods.
- The diagnosis of bipolar disorder in children and adolescents is controversial in part because the moods of many typically developing children and youth can fluctuate dramatically.
- Many diagnosticians use less stringent criteria than those identified in the DSM when diagnosing bipolar disorder in children.
- Bipolar I is characterized by at least one manic or mixed episode, although individuals may also have had one or more major depressive episodes.
- Bipolar II is defined as a disorder with at least one major depressive episode plus at least one hypomanic episode.
- In child and adolescent bipolar disorder, irritability rather than euphoria is by far the most prevalent form of "mania."
- The most salient prevalent feature of the children currently being diagnosed as having bipolar disorder is the extremely rapid shifts in their moods.
- Two new conditions have been added to DSM-5 that will hopefully allow for greater precision in diagnosis and will not be confused with bipolar disorder: disruptive mood dysregulation disorder and intermittent explosive disorder.
- The daily functioning of children and adolescents who have been diagnosed with bipolar disorder is more seriously impaired than the functioning of children with other common forms of child psychopathology.
- There may be serious risks in *not* diagnosing child and adolescent bipolar disorder, including self-injury, suicide and neuroanatomical damage.
- The rates of comorbidity are extremely high. Comorbidity of childhood bipolar disorder and attention deficit/hyperactivity disorder is reported in at least two-thirds of diagnosed cases of bipolar disorder.
- These comorbidity rates and the "drug cocktails" that are used in attempts to treat all the different symptoms involved are part of the current controversy about pediatric bipolar disorder. However, the off-label prescription of medication for the treatment of pediatric bipolar disorder is not totally without scientific basis.
- Bipolar disorder has been shown to be one of the most heritable forms of psychopathology.

- The most consistent MRI findings indicate reduced amygdala volume and increased amygdala activation among individuals identified as having bipolar disorder.
- Adverse family background may influence or trigger the emergence of bipolar disorder in children, interacting with genetic predisposition.
- Some preliminary research indicates that dietary deficiencies may contribute to the emergence of mood disorders in vulnerable children.
- Not much research has been conducted on psychosocial interventions for pediatric bipolar disorder. It has been suggested that psychotherapy be added as a complement to pharmacotherapy as soon as the child's mood has stabilized.
- A specific application of cognitive-behavior therapy, family-focused cognitive-behavior therapy, has been developed to assist children with bipolar disorder and their parents.
- Psychoeducational psychotherapy focuses heavily on providing children and their parents with a clear understanding of the nature of the disorder and of the properties of the medications prescribed.

Study questions

1. Compare the reasons often invoked for the increases in recent years in the diagnoses of bipolar disorder and autism spectrum disorder.
2. How likely is it that drugs are usually prescribed for children and adolescents with bipolar disorder only when it is clear that psychotherapy cannot help? Explain your answer.

21 Substance use disorders

At what point does substance use become substance abuse and at what point does substance abuse become substance use disorder (the term chosen by the DSM-5 Commission to replace the DSM-IV category of *substance abuse disorder*)? Almost every disorder could be conceptualized as the extreme of a continuum of problematic behavior rather than a discrete entity, as discussed in Chapter 3. This applies very clearly to substance use disorder, which in the DSM and ICD systems represents substance abuse that exceeds a certain degree of experimentation with dangerous substances. This brief chapter begins with information about the diagnostic criteria for substance abuse disorder, followed by data on its prevalence. The section that follows is devoted to the very substantial literature on the factors that make children and youth susceptible to substance abuse problems and the processes involved. Causes and correlates are discussed next, followed by a section on prevention and treatment.

Diagnostic criteria

There have been repeated arguments that the DSM-IV criteria for substance abuse disorder were developed with adults in mind and are not really applicable to children (Martin et al., 1995; Chung and Martin, 2005). Box 21.1 illustrates how this issue has been tackled by the DSM-5 Commission. As shown, the diagnostic criteria in DSM-IV and DSM-5 are based on the same concepts. However, there has been considerable fine tuning of the specific diagnostic criteria. Hopefully, research results will confirm over the next few years the predictive validity of the new DSM-5 criteria.

Prevalence

Substance abuse is quite rare among preadolescent children but unfortunately quite common among adolescents (Chassin et al., 2001). Engaging in risky behavior on some occasion is very typical among adolescents and very often a by-product of their curiosity, their search for identity and their exploration of their ever-expanding social worlds. By the end of secondary school, fully one-half of US adolescents report having tried an illegal drug (Tarter, Vanyukov and Kirisci, 2008). Of course, most of these young people go no further than occasional experimentation. However, a significant minority of adolescents will become dependent on illegal drugs or alcohol, compromising their educational and vocational futures and daily well-being. It has been estimated that 11 percent of adolescents in the United States meet the DSM-IV diagnostic criteria for substance abuse disorder (Winters et al., 2007), although nowhere near that number are ever actually diagnosed.

Adolescent substance abuse by itself (i.e., without any comorbid disorder) is linked with a number of unfavorable outcomes in life, including criminal offenses as an adult (Odgers et al., 2008). However, substance use disorders in adolescence are usually accompanied by other mental health problems. It is estimated that anywhere from 40 to 70 percent of adolescents diagnosed as having substance abuse behavior engage in disruptive behavior diagnosable as a

Box 21.1 | Differences between DSM-IV and DSM-5 criteria for substance use disorders

- In DSM-5, substance abuse and substance dependence have been combined into a single category called "substance use disorders." The reliability of the DSM-IV diagnosis of substance dependence is high, but the reliability of the DSM-IV diagnosis of substance abuse is lower and variable.
- In both DSM-IV substance dependence/abuse and DSM-5 substance use disorders, the use of a substance must lead to impairment or distress.
- In DSM-5, however, substance use disorders are diagnosable if at least two of the listed symptoms are present. The symptoms of DSM-5 substance use disorders include failure to meet one's obligations due to the use of a substance, use of a substance in physically dangerous situations, use of a substance despite its link to interpersonal difficulties, tolerance and withdrawal, use of a substance in larger amounts and for a longer time than was planned, dedication of excessive time to activities related to the substance, continued use of the substance even though the individual is aware of the problems it causes, and the presence of cravings for the substance (this symptom is new in DSM-5).
- In DSM-5, the legal problems criterion (included in the DSM-IV criteria for substance abuse) has been removed because it was found to have very low prevalence compared to other criteria. Removing this criterion will have little effect on the prevalence of substance use disorder.
- In DSM-IV substance dependence, a clinician must specify whether the individual presents "with physiological dependence" or "without physiological dependence." This requirement has not been retained in DSM-5.
- In DSM-IV, the remission-related course specifiers include "early full remission," "early partial remission," "sustained full remission" and "sustained partial remission." These remission-related specifiers are all defined as abstaining from substance use either fully or partially for specific time periods. In DSM-5, only two remission-related specifiers are present: "in early remission," to be used when someone who previously met criteria has met none of the criteria (with the exception of the craving criterion) for 3 months; and "in sustained remission," to be used if someone fails to meet any of the criteria for a year (again, not including the craving criterion).

Source: DSM-5 and DSM-IV-TR consulted June 28, 2013.

disruptive behavior disorder. The comorbidity rate may be as high as 90 percent in samples of adolescents treated at mental health clinics. This particular comorbidity is seen as one of the most common in adolescent psychopathology (e.g., Bukstein, 2000). However, many forms of psychopathology other than conduct disorder also co-occur with substance use disorder, including other externalizing disorders, especially attention deficit/hyperactivity disorder.

Depression and anxiety also accompany substance use disorder in many cases. About 30 percent of adolescents with depression are likely to use illegal substances compared to half that rate among children not diagnosed with major depression. Depression is also linked to early onset of substance abuse within the adolescent years (Cornelius and Clark, 2008). Female adolescents with substance use disorder are more likely than their male counterparts to suffer simultaneously from depression whereas male adolescents are more likely than females to experience comorbid substance abuse and externalizing behavior problems (Chung, 2008).

As a general rule, other comorbid mental health problems precede the onset of substance use disorder. This may or may not mean that the other problems *caused* the adolescent to begin experimentation with an illegal or harmful substance. The exception to this rule may be comorbid depression, which occurs very often after a pattern of substance abuse is already evident according to some studies. In many cases, the depressed mood may be caused by the substance being abused (Chung, 2008; Costello et al., 1999). However, the research findings here are by no means clear: For example, in a retrospective study (i.e., one in which the participants were interviewed after the fact about the sequence of their problems), Rohde, Lewinsohn and Seeley (1996) found that 53 percent of adolescents diagnosed as having alcohol abuse and dysthymia (depressed mood) reported that they felt depressed before they began consuming alcohol in excess.

The presence of comorbid mental health disorders among adolescents who abuse toxic substances is known to intensify the adolescent's involvement with illegal drugs or alcohol and to increase the chances of relapse (McCarthy et al., 2005). Several explanations have been proposed for this. For example, comorbid conditions such as conduct disorder may increase the likelihood of the adolescent coming into contact with deviant peer groups, where substance abuse may be common and rewarded. For several reasons, adolescents suffering from both substance use disorder and other mental health problems are known to be particularly deficient in the coping skills they would need to deal with their problems in life in healthier ways. Adolescents who are depressed may turn to substance abuse as a form of self-medication to relieve their dysphoric moods (Brown and D'Amico, 2003). Chung (2008) emphasizes that it is important to consider underlying dysfunctional personality and temperament as comorbid conditions that aggravate substance abuse problems.

Susceptibility to substance abuse

Although, as already mentioned, substance abuse per se does not typically begin until adolescence, the path toward substance abuse often starts much earlier. It has been noted that children from 6 to 11 years old have fairly clear "risk images" – mental pictures, good or bad, of young people who use dangerous substances (Gibbons et al., 2008). It is thought that television and other mass media influence the development of risk images. There may also be era effects in the perception of risk. As several countries and some US states are legalizing the sale and use of marijuana, perceptions of risk may be changing. Consumption is related to the perception of risk, as illustrated in Figure 21.1. It must be remembered that the excessive consumption of substances such as wine and marijuana, which may not be harmful when consumed in small amounts, may still be addictive or harmful if consumed in excess and before operating motor vehicles.

Preyde and Adams (2008) argue that the simultaneous juxtaposition of opportunities and internal conflicts that occurs during the adolescent years paves the path for vulnerability to substance abuse. On the one hand, the adolescent years provide an opportunity for enjoyment, excitement, new experiences and experimentation. On the other hand, adolescence is often seen as a period of internal conflict, self-doubt and alienation from

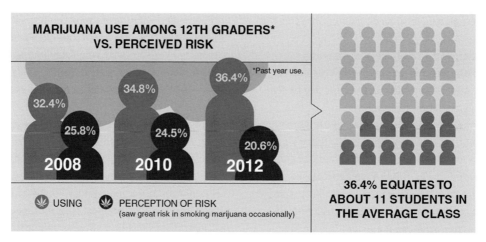

Figure 21.1 Marijuana use among 12th graders vs. perceived risk.

the institutions created by the adult world. The physiological changes that occur in adolescence sometimes create confusion; the emerging adult-like physical body may be the subject of anxiety and doubt. During the adolescent years, adult authority not only wanes in most cultures but also becomes the target of the rebelliousness that is commonly associated with this stage of human development. As all of this takes place, risky substances are often circulating among some of the adolescent's peers. Many of these substances are inexpensive and easy to obtain and try (Preyde and Adams, 2008; Tarter et al., 2008). Researchers have invested considerably in tracing the trajectories over time that often lead to substance use disorder, providing excellent insight into the individual and family factors associated with increased risk for the disorder. It is only occasionally that the stereotyped "innocent" adolescent with no predisposing risk factors succumbs to the temptations offered by deviant peers to the extent of developing substance use disorder. This is not to say that deviant peers do not play a role in the emergence of the disorder, as will be discussed later in this chapter. It is sometimes thought that the properties of the substances themselves propel users to become addicted but this is only true in very exceptional circumstances (Tarter et al., 2008).

Susceptibility: individual differences

The family and peer processes discussed later in this chapter may interact, first of all, with the inherent constitution of the child. In addition, as mentioned in the next section of this chapter, certain types of temperament and personality are associated with susceptibility to adolescent substance abuse. Particularly vulnerable to the negative influences of parents and peers are children who have undergone stressful experiences in early life. Many forms of early environmental stress have been implicated, including physical abuse, sexual abuse, parental divorce, economic hardship, death of a parent and mental illness of a parent (see review by Enoch, 2011). Early physical maturation may enable an adolescent to associate with an older peer group without the psychological maturity needed to feel secure in the group and filter its pressures (Kirillova et al., 2008).

Possible causes and correlates

Several methodological considerations affect the interpretation of research on the genetic and environmental influences on adolescent substance abuse problems. These are discussed in a comprehensive review of genetic influences by Lynskey, Agrawal and

Heath (2010), to which the reader is referred for greater detail about the etiology of adolescent substance use disorder in general. One problem is that most research, by necessity, is based on adolescent self-reports of substance abuse. Many adolescents, understandably, may be reluctant to disclose their own substance abuse problems. However, the researcher has little choice: Parents may not be aware of their children's flirtations with illegal substances and, even if they are aware, may not wish to indicate them to professionals. Urine analysis is beyond the scope of most large-scale studies of risk factors. Of course, this problem affects not only research on the possible causes of substance use disorder but also research on any aspect of the disorder, including research on its treatment.

Another important problem, again not limited to this disorder, is that of determining whether or not a particular correlate or possible cause of substance use disorder is specific to this disorder. Given the high rates of comorbidity between substance use disorders and other diagnosable mental health problems, it is not surprising that the issue of *equifinality* (see Chapter 13 and Enoch, 2011) – the same antecedent condition predicting a number of different end states – arises frequently in this literature.

Biological factors

In this section, research on biological, familial and contextual factors is presented in separate sections. It is important to bear in mind, however, that this distinction is somewhat artificial. For example, precocious physiological maturation, an intra-individual biological factor, may enable an adolescent to circulate freely in peer groups consisting of older children, some of whom may engage in risky behaviors (Kirillova et al., 2008). As well, certain environmental influences, such as early stressful experiences or child abuse, may affect the child physiologically as well as psychologically (Enoch, 2011).

Behavioral genetics
One difficulty in estimating the heritability of substance abuse disorder is the reliance on adoption studies. This problem is of course not limited to research on substance abuse disorder. The problem (i.e., for research) is that social agencies screen adopting parents very carefully, making the best attempts to allow adoption only by parents who are well adjusted themselves. This limits the usefulness of studies in which adopted children are compared with their biological and their adoptive parents because the social agencies have made it almost impossible for substance abuse patterns by adoptive parents to match those of their children (Lynskey, Agrawal and Heath, 2010). Nevertheless, several important adoption studies, especially those conducted in Iowa (Cadoret et al., 1986) and Sweden (Cloninger et al., 1985) do provide very substantial indications of genetic causation.

Strong heritability is also indicated in twin studies of several types. There have even been a few studies involving twins reared apart, which is very rare and very revealing (Grove et al., 1990). As well, there have been several informative studies based on rates of substance abuse among the biological children of twins. The *children-of-twins design* constitutes a particularly informative research strategy because it not only permits the comparison of monozygotic and dizygotic twins but also allows for consideration of environmental risk, by allowing, for example, the study of children whose parents display no substance abuse disorder but whose parents' monozygotic twin is affected by the disorder. Such a child is at no risk because of his or her immediate family environment but is at risk from a genetic point of view (Jacob et al., 2003; Lynskey, Agrawal and Heath, 2010).

In earlier studies, the twins participated in the research when they were already adults. However, recent twin studies have included younger twins. In many of the twin studies, the same genetic route has been shown to lead to both substance use disorder and other forms of externalizing disorder, especially disruptive behavior disorders. This emerged, for example, in a large study conducted by Bornovalova et al. (2010) with over 1,000 twin pairs and their parents.

Behavior-genetic research conducted with adult samples indicates that the abuse of different substances – alcohol, tobacco and illegal drugs – often co-occurs and displays strong evidence of a common genetic risk factor. There are only a few studies on this issue conducted with adolescents, with results that lead to a similar conclusion (Lynskey, Agrawal and Heath, 2010; Rhee et al., 2006; Young, Mufson and Davies, 2006).

Temperament: an indirect genetic link to susceptibility

Some of the temperament or personality styles that are associated with early susceptibility to substance abuse problems are thought to be hereditary. It is recalled that *temperament* can be defined as stable individual differences, thought to be inherent to the individual, in reaction to the outside world, in responding to unfamiliar individuals and in regulating emotions. Temperament can be evident in an individual's emotional expression, motor activity and attention (Rothbart and Posner, 2006). Personality and temperament may also be reflected in differences among individuals in terms of what they find rewarding or motivating (Williams et al., 2010).

Individual differences in sensitivity to reward or reinforcement have been linked with susceptibility to substance abuse problems. Some people find risk-taking by itself a rewarding experience. Being prone to negative affect or negative moods is another risk factor, because such individuals may resort to substance abuse for relief. In a comparison of adolescents referred to mental health clinics for help with substance abuse problems and a control group, Willem et al. (2011) found that low levels of positive affectivity or moods together with low levels of self-control differentiated the clinical and the control groups.

In an important longitudinal study that began when the participants were only 4 months old, Williams and her colleagues studied the long-term links between *behavioral inhibition* in early life and substance abuse problems in adolescence (Williams et al., 2010). Behavioral inhibition, an antecedent of shyness, consists of negative affect and avoidance in novel situations, especially those involving unfamiliar people (Fox et al., 2005; Kagan and Snidman,

1991). The researchers found a complex pattern in the implications of early behavioral inhibition for subsequent substance abuse problems, with important sex differences. Among boys, behavioral inhibition was linked to greater risk of substance abuse; the exact opposite emerged for girls. The differences may have occurred because boys who are behaviorally inhibited do not conform to the pattern of outgoing and dominant behavior that is normally expected of male adolescents. Unable to impress their peers with their social skills, they may attempt to impress their peers by flirting with dangerous substances. Another possibility is that boys who depart from these gender-role expectations may be made so miserable by their social groups that they resort to dangerous substances to escape the negative affect that this social rejection may generate.

Genomics

In future years, greater insight about the genetic roots of substance abuse disorders is likely to emerge from research designed to trace the specific gene variants that may be related to substance use disorders among adolescents. This technology has undergone considerable development but does not appear to have been applied until now to the study of this particular disorder among adolescents (Lynskey, Agrawal and Heath, 2010).

Family factors

There is no doubt that some adolescents who engage in repeated and problematic substance abuse have parents who do the same. In addition, adolescents whose parents have been diagnosed with a wide range of mental disorders are known to be at particularly high risk of substance use disorder. This family risk may represent not only direct modeling by parents who themselves abuse substances but also genetic influences or the transmission of patterns of thinking and behaving that lead to substance abuse (Winters et al., 2008).

Parents also have very important indirect effects on substance abuse through their roles as regulators of adolescents' free-time behavior and the company their adolescent sons and daughters keep. Many studies have indicated that *parental monitoring* – being aware of what their adolescents do when they are in the community – is a powerful negative correlate of substance abuse problems. This finding has been replicated many times in the United States (e.g., Dishion and McMahon, 1998; Wang et al., 2009; Yabiku et al., 2010) and has now been replicated in many countries including Australia (Hayatbakhsh et al., 2008), Norway (Breivik, Olweus and Endresen, 2009), Thailand (Sooraksa, 2009), Mexico (Becerra and Castillo, 2011) and Venezuela (Cox et al., 2010). In the academically oriented cultures of East Asia, parents' monitoring of their children's study habits may indirectly reduce substance abuse by minimizing the free time during which young people might have the freedom to associate with peers who engage in substance abuse (Wu et al., 2007). Adolescents who report that their parents fail to monitor their activities are known to visit websites that promote drug addiction (Belenko et al., 2009). It is important to note that other aspects of parent–child relations are linked with substance abuse to some extent. Harmonious, supportive relationships are correlated with lower rates of problematic substance abuse whereas parent–child conflict is correlated with substance abuse problems (Mrug et al., 2010). However, it has consistently been found that parent monitoring is the strongest correlate among the aspects of parenting examined by researchers (e.g., Breivik, Olweus and Endresen, 2009).

As in most areas of problem behavior, negative influence by parents is often implicated, side by side with negative peer influence, in the emergence of adolescent substance abuse problems. Understudied as sibling influences are, they appear to be very strong. This was demonstrated, for example, in a large-scale longitudinal study conducted by Pomery and her colleagues (2005), which encompassed parent, sibling and peer influences.

Peer influences

As noted by Allen and Antonishak (2008), peer influence among adolescents has acquired a very

negative reputation that is mostly, but not entirely, justified. "One-shot" correlational studies of substance abuse by mutual friends or by members of the same social group do provide an inflated estimate of peer influence. This is because the correlations may indicate not only the extent of influence by friends or peers but may also reflect the very real possibility that young people who already abuse substances are attracted to each other as friends because of their shared activity of seeking and using dangerous substances. However, more sophisticated statistical procedures such as structural equations modeling can be useful in separating the homophily effect – the tendency to befriend people with similar characteristics – from the extent of influence. Indeed, even after the homophily effect has been controlled statistically, peers appear to exert a substantial influence on substance abuse by young people. In particular, having friends who engage in the abuse of substances is likely to increase the risk of an adolescent beginning to abuse multiple dangerous substances and of developing a substance abuse disorder that is comorbid with other mental disorders (e.g., Glaser, Shelton and Van den Bree, 2010). Peer pressure resulting in substance abuse is massive among children living in the company of a deviant peer group, as shown in a recent study of street children in Mumbai, India (Gaidhane et al., 2008).

Importantly, Allen and Antonishak emphasize that peers can also steer each other *away* from substance abuse and toward social groups with norms of prosocial behavior (2008). In fact, it has been found that a great many adolescents say that they would intervene to stop a close friend from engaging in substance abuse or other dangerous behavior (Buckley, Sheehan and Chapman, 2009).

Mechanisms of peer influence

The mechanisms underlying family and peer influence have been compared by theorists and researchers. Gibbons et al. (2008) note that there are four major modalities of influence that form the basis for these comparisons. The first modality is *provision*, which involves making the substances available, whether intentionally or not. Either parents or peers may exert influence in this way. Another direct modality of influence is *modeling*, the imitation of substance abuse that the adolescent has observed. Either parents or peers may exert influence in this way, for example by consuming alcohol or marijuana at a social gathering, sending, perhaps unwittingly, the message that people use substances to be social. In contrast, the third modality, *active encouragement*, usually applies more to peer than to parent influence. The infamous phenomenon of negative peer pressure embodies this modality of influence. Active encouragement of substance abuse is, of course, intentional although it is only effective if practiced on a peer who succumbs. Gibbons and colleagues (2008) maintain that the fourth modality – the shaping of basic beliefs, cognitions and attitudes – is the most potent modality. One important example is the transmission of the belief that the negative consequences of using the substance in question are not likely or that, for whatever reason, the particular individual is immune to them. Thus, these authors emphasize that although both peers and parents may at times make conscious efforts at promoting or preventing substance abuse by the adolescents who relate to them, it is far more common for peers to do so in unwitting and unconscious ways.

There are important differences between individual adolescents in terms of their susceptibility to peer influence. Rejection by peers and social marginalization are *not*, contrary to popular belief, markers of susceptibility. Indeed, peer influence toward substance abuse is very strong among socially popular adolescents, probably stronger than among adolescents who are socially rejected or marginalized. However, other aspects of peer relations are indeed linked with susceptibility. Dominant, articulate members of the peer group tend to be very effective in influencing submissive members of the group. Adolescents who have difficulty forming close friendships have been found to be susceptible to negative peer influence, as are those who are prone to feeling depressed (Allen and Antonishak, 2008). As a

general rule of human behavior, it has been proposed that individuals who feel that their social needs are unfulfilled are likely to do what they think they must in order to fit in (Williams, 2007). Donlan, Lee and Paz (2009), social workers who implement prevention programs with groups of Hispanic adolescents in the southwestern United States, include identification with one's culture as one of these basic social needs. They attribute substance use problems and acting-out behavior to an inability to identify with both their Hispanic roots and the majority culture. They advocate prevention programs in which pride in cultural heritage is fostered, together with skills in being successful in the majority culture.

Contextual factors: neighborhood and school effects

Although peer influence operates wherever young people interact, there are important differences among schools and neighborhoods in the extent to which substance use and abuse constitute a norm that is transmitted widely. These effects may occur because when substances are commonly used in a setting, substance abuse becomes normative, acceptable and even prestigious (Kuntsche and Jordan, 2006). Unlike the data pertaining to many other forms of child and adolescent psychopathology, it is by no means clear that lower socio-economic status is linked with substance abuse problems. This issue has been studied many times, with different results obtained in different studies even though the populations are similar, as documented in a review chapter by Gardner, Barajas and Brooks-Gunn (2010). In fact, it has been reported in a number of US studies that adolescents from well-to-do homes are more likely to engage in problematic alcohol abuse than others (e.g., Botticello, 2009). Even in neighborhoods with schools of similar socio-economic status to one another, school climate has been shown to predict rates of problematic substance abuse. Studies conducted both in the UK and in the United States indicate that pupils are less likely to abuse dangerous substances in schools where there are positive

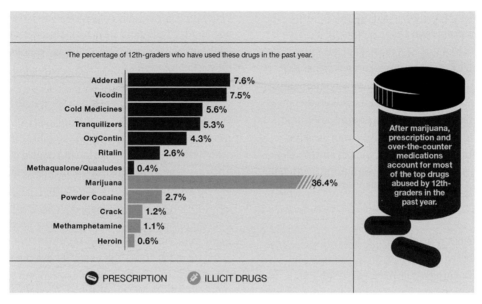

*The percentage of 12th-graders who have used these drugs in the past year.

Adderall	7.6%
Vicodin	7.5%
Cold Medicines	5.6%
Tranquilizers	5.3%
OxyContin	4.3%
Ritalin	2.6%
Methaqualone/Quaaludes	0.4%
Marijuana	36.4%
Powder Cocaine	2.7%
Crack	1.2%
Methamphetamine	1.1%
Heroin	0.6%

After marijuana, prescription and over-the-counter medications account for most of the top drugs abused by 12th-graders in the past year.

● PRESCRIPTION   ◉ ILLICIT DRUGS

Figure 21.2 Prescription/over-the-counter vs. illicit drugs.

teacher–pupil relationships, where attendance rules are enforced and where academic engagement and academic achievement are highly valued (Bisset, Markham and Aveyard, 2007; Fletcher, Bonell and Hargreaves, 2008). In an interesting recent study conducted with middle-school students in the United States, Mrug and colleagues (2010) found that school and parenting effects interacted to increase the risk of early substance abuse problems. Early adolescents who experienced poor parenting (i.e., lack of monitoring and lack of emotional support) were more likely than other schoolmates to be influenced by school-level substance abuse norms.

Societal effects

Mass media may convey images suggesting to young people that alcohol consumption, for example, is linked to enjoyable time spent with peers. In some societies, children and adolescents may experience stress due to pressures for academic achievement and/or social conformity. This may explain the results of Izutsu et al. (2006), who found high rates of self-harm among Japanese middle-school students that were linked to both substance use and to some

of the symptoms of attention deficit/hyperactivity disorder. Another contextual factor is the burgeoning use and misuse of psychotropic drugs that are prescribed to both parents and children, as discussed in several previous chapters. Figure 21.2 reveals the extent of the misuse of prescription drugs.

Prevention and treatment

Prevention

Although substance use disorder does not usually appear before adolescence, many experts on its prevention insist that prevention efforts must begin during the childhood years. Typically, these prevention efforts target the psychological vulnerabilities that may lead to the misuse of alcohol, tobacco or illegal drugs. Given the scope of adolescent substance abuse and the very limited access to treatment, much attention has been given to primary prevention programs. Many of these programs are delivered in schools, where information about the consequences of substance abuse is provided, typically with advice about resisting peer pressure. Unfortunately, these prevention programs have met with only limited success overall (see, e.g., meta-analyses by Ennet et al., 2004 and by Tobler et al., 2000). In a rigorous meta-analysis of over 200 studies, Tobler et al. (2000) calculated an overall effect size of only .15 of a standard deviation unit. Effectiveness was somewhat higher when there was active interaction between the group leaders and the students as opposed to passive transmission of information. The search for the key to effective prevention programming is a continuing challenge.

Treatment

Early treatment research, conducted from the 1970s on, was plagued with inconsistent findings and severe methodological problems (Williams and Chang, 2000). In fact, some intervention researchers were appalled to find that treatment groups for youth with substance abuse and conduct disorders were actually harmful because, despite the best intentions of the therapists, the group participants would acquire new anti-social behaviors from each other (Dishion, McCord and Poulin, 1999). The discouraging effectiveness data contrasted sharply with a growing awareness of the need for effective interventions, leading to a new generation of better-planned treatments that were evaluated in a more rigorous manner than their predecessors (Slesnick, Kaminer and Kelly, 2008). The methodological advances include treatment manuals that describe the interventions clearly, large samples and, in some studies, random assignment to treatment and appropriate control conditions. Despite innovations in practice and growing indications that treatment can be successful, it is apparent that only a minority of adolescents with substance use disorders receive any form of treatment (Dembo and Muck, 2009).

The major established forms of intervention are either family-based or individual treatment techniques fashioned closely on treatments designed for adults with substance abuse problems. The uncritical adaptation of adult treatment methods has been the subject of considerable criticism and debate because they may fail to take into account the realities of adolescent social and family life. For example, therapists working with adults often use sharp confrontational techniques; little is known as to whether this is appropriate for adolescents (Winters et al., 2009).

Treatment can be delivered in several different contexts. Group and individual out-patient therapy has been successful in many but not all cases. Special schools and residential treatment are also common and sometimes indicated. Logically, there should be a continuum starting from prevention, continuing to less-intensive psychotherapy as needed and thence to more intensive treatment such as in a residential institution. However, neither treatment nor research is organized well enough to clarify exactly when more intensive intervention is needed and useful (Plant and Panzarella, 2009).

Family treatment can be either direct or indirect. Direct approaches are inspired by the behavioral tradition and may include, for example, behavioral contracts between the adolescents and their parents, with stipulations of rewards for abstinence and consequences for non-compliance with the provisions of the contract. Pioneering studies by Azrin and his colleagues in the 1990s demonstrated the effectiveness of this approach (e.g., Azrin et al., 1996). More indirect family-treatment modalities address such family issues as poor communication in the family, lack of cohesion and support and the family's inability to tackle problems (Waldron et al., 2001). More recent efforts have included both a combination of family-treatment strategies and multidimensional interventions involving both family therapy and individual cognitive-behavioral therapy for the adolescents. A sizeable number of rigorous controlled studies have documented the success of various family-treatment strategies (Austin, MacGowan and Wagner, 2005; Winters et al., 2009).

The *12-step-based treatment* is founded on the core principles of the well-known Alcoholics Anonymous groups for adults. As such, the participating adolescents attend meetings at which they admit that they need help and are powerless to fight their addiction. They then come to realize that a force bigger than themselves can help reverse their predicaments. Having made a firm decision to change, they benefit from the support of the group in doing so. Relatively little data are available to confirm the value of the downward extension of this well-established adult intervention. There is some evidence that the program is helpful to adolescents who commit fully to it (Winters et al., 2009).

The *therapeutic-community model* can be applied to out-patient groups, day treatment or residential treatment. This concept is interpreted somewhat differently by different groups of professionals. One version, quite prevalent in the UK but also espoused by some developmental psychologists in the United States who study moral development, emphasizes the therapeutic value of participation in the governance of a democratic community that is overseen by professionals who provide supervision and guidance but who do not completely set and enforce the rules (e.g., Adlam and Scanlon, 2011). The version most prevalent in US treatment for adolescent substance abuse also focuses on identification of a community as the main vehicle for change. Within the US communities, there may be self-help groups, behavioral contracting and values education. At least one well-designed evaluation, by Morral, McCaffrey and Ridgeway (2004) confirmed the superiority of the therapeutic-community approach in comparison to a control condition in which the substance abusers received whatever treatment was usually prescribed in their communities.

Brief interventions – sometimes as short as a single 10-minute session but usually a few sessions long – are sometimes based on the charismatic personalities of the adult therapists involved. These practitioners may be able to convince the adolescents they work with of their own potential in a drug-free life. Once convinced, the adolescents proceed to self-help interventions of various kinds. This uplifting *motivational enhancement therapy* has been found effective in some cases but not for "career" drug abusers (Winters et al., 2009). The final major model of treatment is *cognitive-behavioral therapy*. Some data do indicate that CBT is effective

on its own. However, it is usually combined with the group, family or community treatments described earlier (Winters et al., 2009).

Thus, a variety of treatment options exist. This in no way means that all treatment modalities are equally useful. As a guide to the choice of treatment options, Dembo and Muck (2009) point out that no single treatment is appropriate to all individuals. They also emphasize that treatment must address the whole person and not just substance abuse. More specifically, they distinguish in a very useful manner between treatments that do and do not have an established track record of effectiveness. The proven treatments are those that have been mentioned previously in this section. However, several forms of treatment are still in common use despite the fact that they clearly do not work. The best-known examples of ineffective treatment modalities that remain popular are supportive counseling and unfocused "talk" groups.

Pharmacotherapy: substances that treat substance abuse

Management of substance abuse with medication is more common among adults than among adolescents. However, preliminary results of several medications are largely positive although the sample sizes are small and the number of studies is few. Medications like disulfiram can evoke an aversive sensation when the targeted problem substance is present in the body. Other medications can reduce cravings or alleviate withdrawal symptoms (Winters et al., 2009). Even if pharmacotherapy is further developed, it is likely to be most useful as a short-term initial component of a more comprehensive "package" intervention (Dembo and Muck, 2009).

Treatment with emphasis on comorbid conditions

As mentioned earlier, substance use disorders in adolescents are usually accompanied by other comorbid conditions. Treating all of the adolescent's psychological problems provides a formidable challenge for clinicians.

CASE STUDY: Sammy, in treatment for substance abuse, PTSD and dissociative experiences

Jaffee, Chu and Woody (2009) discuss treatment challenges in the case study of a 15-year-old adolescent male referred for professional help because of chronic substance dependence as well as post-traumatic stress syndrome and dissociative experiences. Dissociative disorders, which sometimes are found among children and adolescents as well as adults, are defined by sudden or gradual disturbances in the integration of a person's consciousness, identity or perception. Individuals affected by these disorders may lose parts of their understanding of who they are (American Psychiatric Association, 2000; Dell and O'Neill, 2009). Sammy was 15 years old when he was admitted for brief residential treatment after an accidental overdose of oxycodone, a semi-synthetic opioid that is usually prescribed for the treatment of chronic pain. He also had experimented with alcohol, marijuana and sedative drugs often prescribed for people who have sleep problems. Both at school and at home, Sammy was described as angry and irritable much of the time. At school, he often withdrew from social contacts.

There was no known history of substance abuse or mental illness in his family. Sammy lived with his biological parents and younger sister. He had a close relationship with his mother but was more distant emotionally from his father and younger sister. The major risk factor noted at the time of referral was a rape at knifepoint when he was 13. Sammy was raped in a university men's room.

As the first step in Sammy's treatment, the psychologist established a behavioral contract with Sammy and his parents. Sammy's compliance with the contract was verified by means of periodic urine checks. Although the medication clonazepam was prescribed to deal with Sammy's anxiety, it failed to turn up in a subsequent urine specimen. At about the same time, his parents reported that a quantity of the opioid painkiller that had precipitated Sammy's hospitalization was missing.

The implementation of the behavioral contract continued for several weeks, resulting in Sammy losing privileges from time to time as a consequence of his failure to live up to the commitments he had made. After several weeks, however, Sammy became engaged in psychotherapy sessions. Sammy professed a strong desire to improve. Nevertheless, he resisted any of the brief cognitive-behavioral interventions the psychologist attempted, including deep breathing, identification of the events that triggered his anger and anxiety, and reinterpretations of some of the inferences he made about people or events. Sammy said that such things simply do not work for him.

At the same time, Sammy was involved in Alcoholics Anonymous, the well-known self-help group. At one of the group's meetings, he self-disclosed more than he intended to, revealing the details of his rape at knifepoint. This led to further setbacks, with his urine checks revealing a variety of harmful substances. Dissociative experiences began, including some in which he was disoriented at home for an extended period during which he would just stare into space. His mother reported that, during one such incident, Sammy taped bamboo skewers to his fingers and, in a conversation with "Freddy" (perhaps the serial killer in the *Nightmare on Elm Street* series), maintained that Freddy could not harm him.

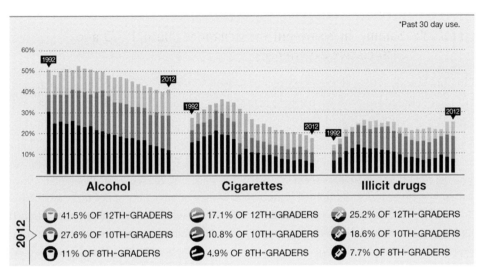

Figure 21.3 Last two decades of alcohol, cigarette and illicit drug use.

The psychologist eventually discovered several ways of helping Sammy end these dissociative episodes. These included deep breathing, changing the sounds in the room he was in, and teaching Sammy how to change the topic and focus of his thinking when he felt that an episode was imminent. Subsequently, Sammy was able to discuss the rape incident frankly with his therapist and to begin to discuss and deal with the sources of his anger and anxiety. Although Sammy eventually remained substance-free for a considerable time, psychotherapy continued for an extended period, as necessitated by the gravity of the trauma and the multiple symptoms and disorders. This intriguing case study illustrates the complexity and difficulty of treating persistent substance use disorder that is comorbid with other serious forms of mental illness.

Conclusions and future directions

Just as nations are finding it difficult to cope with the problem of pervasive importation and sale of dangerous substances, families and schools are finding the challenge of steering young people away from these substances a formidable one. Children and adolescents seem to be using and abusing substances at an increasing rate, as illustrated in Figure 21.3. Given the scope of the problem, better prevention programs are clearly needed, as is better access to treatment. Even if the outcomes of some prevention programs are discouraging, efforts must be redoubled to find ways of increasing the success rate, perhaps by a systematic series of baby steps. An analogy exists in the treatment of cancer, which has gradually improved, resulting in a progressive increase in survival rates even in the absence of revolutionary new discoveries that could eradicate the disease.

Summary

- Substance abuse is much more common in adolescents than in preadolescent children. Of those adolescents that experiment with different drugs, a significant minority will become dependent on them.

- Adolescent substance use disorder and disruptive behavior disorder are considered one of the most common comorbidities in adolescent psychopathology. Other psychopathologies are known to co-occur with substance use disorder, including other externalizing disorders such as attention deficit/hyperactivity disorder.

- Depression and anxiety accompany substance use disorder in many cases. Those with depression are more likely to use illegal substances and display early-onset substance abuse within the adolescent years.

- The DSM and ICD systems portray substance abuse as exceeding a certain degree of experimentation with dangerous substances. Some scholars believe that the diagnostic criteria were not adequately developed for children or adolescents.

- Certain mental health problems usually precede substance use disorder in adolescents, such as conduct disorder, dysfunctional personality and sometimes depression. However, some studies suggest that depression does not usually occur until after the pattern of substance abuse has set in.

- Some researchers believe that children influenced by television and mass media may develop risk images of people who use dangerous substances.

- Vulnerability to substance abuse is acute among adolescents due to the developmental processes they undergo at this time, including the physiological changes to their body, pressures to become or want to become more autonomous, and new opportunities for enjoyment and excitement.

- Individual differences among adolescents, such as their exposure to stressful experiences in early life or early physical maturation, may be associated with susceptibility to adolescent substance abuse.

- Methodological problems exist in studying the causes and treatment of adolescent substance abuse, specifically the fact that most research must rely on self-report methods. The adolescent may be reluctant to disclose use. Parent reports are also limited by the fact that parents may be unaware of their children's activities. A second issue is the fact that many comorbid disorders may co-occur with adolescent substance abuse, which makes it difficult to specify the causal direction. *Equifinality* refers to the idea that the same antecedent condition may predict a number of different end states.

- Biological, familial and contextual factors, while sometimes studied separately, often have a complex inter-relationship with one another.

- With adoption studies, it is difficult to accurately study the heritability of substance use disorders, as adopted parents are usually screened and only chosen if they are relatively well-adjusted. The children-of-twins design, on the other hand, allows researchers to study the genetic factors in the emergence of this disorder.

- Research has shown a common genetic risk factor in adults and adolescents with regard to the co-occurring abuse of different substances.

- Some personality types or temperaments may lead to increased susceptibility to substance abuse in adolescents, specifically sensitivity to reward or reinforcement. People prone to negative affect or negative moods are also at risk.

- *Behavioral inhibition* refers to negative affect and avoidance in new situations, especially those with unfamiliar people. Early behavioral inhibition for boys may lead to subsequent substance abuse problems.

- Children whose parents have mental health issues may be at risk for substance abuse in a variety of ways. They may imitate their parents' behavior. Genetic influences may interact with certain patterns of thinking and behaving to make them more susceptible.

- Parental monitoring, being aware of what their adolescents do when they are in the community, has been negatively correlated to substance abuse problems. Along the same lines, harmonious, supportive relationships are correlated with lower rates of substance abuse.

- The *homophily* effect, which refers to the tendency to befriend people with similar characteristics, is a methodological concern that must be taken into consideration when studying peer influences on substance use disorder in adolescents. Controlled for this effect, peer influence appears still to be a substantial influence on substance abuse.

- Four modalities of influence form the basis for the mechanisms of peer and family influence: provision (substance availability), modeling, active encouragement (intentional peer pressure) and shaping of basic beliefs, cognitions and attitudes to encourage substance use.

- Social rejection is not a marker of susceptibility; however, the inability to form close friendships may be.

- Adolescents in individualistic societies, such as the United States, have been found to be more susceptible than their counterparts in other cultures to peer pressure to use dangerous substances. This may be due to individuals needing to establish their identities by validating their self-worth through comparisons with others. In some cultures, such as those of Eastern Asia, parents monitor their children's neighborhood activities very closely. This may minimize negative peer influences leading to substance use problems.

- The normalization, acceptance or prestige of illegal substances in certain schools or neighborhoods may lead to higher adolescent substance use. However, lower socio-economic status is not linked clearly with substance abuse problems.

- Although not very effective, primary prevention programs target children and adolescents, demonstrating the consequences of substance abuse and giving advice about resisting peer pressure.

- Only a small number of adolescents with substance use disorder receive any form of treatment. Early research suggested that adolescents acquire new anti-social behaviors from others in the participant groups. More recent research suggests that this risk is not substantial.

- The two major forms of intervention are family-based and individual treatment techniques. Direct family treatment includes behavioral contracts, whereas indirect family treatment addresses such family issues as poor communication and lack of support and cohesion.

- The 12-step-based treatment, based on the core principles of Alcoholics Anonymous, appears to be helpful for adolescents who fully commit to them, although research is very limited.

- The therapeutic-community model, emphasizing the therapeutic value of participation in the governance of a democratic community and identifying the community as the main vehicle for change, is an effective approach for the treatment of substance use disorders.

- Motivational enhancement therapy helps adolescents realize their own potential in a drug-free life so that self-help interventions prove effective. Cognitive-behavioral therapy is not usually effective on its own; it is usually combined with group, family or community treatments.

- Although more common among adults, pharmacotherapy is somewhat effective among adolescents. Some medications evoke an aversive sensation to the substances; others reduce cravings or alleviate withdrawal symptoms.

Study questions

1. Which types of temperament and/or personality have been linked to substance abuse in young people?
2. What is the major conceptual limitation of one-shot correlational studies showing that affiliating with "bad" peers is associated with substance abuse?

22 School refusal

Undoubtedly, many cases of school refusal have been treated as simple truancy since the advent of compulsory public education in Western countries in the past two centuries. Even today, authorities in some parts of the United States and the UK sometimes launch campaigns to raise school attendance, often with the intent of enhancing the school achievement of members of underprivileged minority groups, without considering the many reasons for absence from school that are discussed in the small but growing professional literature on school refusal (Sheppard, 2011).

This brief chapter begins with a section on the nebulous status of school refusal in the literature on child and adolescent psychopathology. The subsequent sections are devoted to issues of prevalence, stability, possible causes and correlates, prevention and treatment.

Diagnostic criteria

School refusal and *school phobia* are not recognized diagnostic entities in DSM-5 or ICD-10, largely because of the heterogeneity of the problem and the reasons that lead to it. Persistent refusal to attend school because of anxiety about separation from parents is, however, listed in DSM-5 and ICD-10 as a possible symptom of separation anxiety disorder. The term "school phobia" is used less frequently than "school refusal" in current nomenclature because it implies that anxiety about the school is necessarily the core feature, which it can be but often is not. Last and Strauss (1990) suggest a distinction between school refusal caused by anxiety and school refusal that can be considered truancy. Truancy may be seen as a form of oppositional defiant

behavior. In an influential review of the literature, Kearney (2008) notes that the major problem with this simplistic dichotomy is that there is too much overlap between its two components. Even if the dichotomy makes sense theoretically, children's motives in not attending school may not be so easily distinguishable. Even delinquents whose initial absenteeism is unrelated to anxiety may become anxious about returning to school after a period of truancy. Another problem is that some physical ailments often provoke absence from school although there are of course somatic complaints related to anxiety, making a clear delineation quite difficult.

Kearney proposes instead classification of the functions that might be served by being absent from school, with elements that may not be mutually exclusive. One possible function is in fact the avoidance of school, common especially among younger children. The discomfort in this case may have to do with a major feature of the school but might pertain, for example, to incidents that occur on a school bus or in the corridors as students make the transition from one school activity to another. The second function of school refusal identified by Kearney is the specific avoidance of being evaluated at school. The third function has nothing to do with school itself; the child simply prefers to remain in the company of parents. Finally, Kearney notes that school refusal sometimes makes available to the child activities or objects that seem more appealing or reinforcing than what is available at school. In contrast with the wide range of possible causes elaborated by Kearney, Pellegrini (2007) observes that the heterogeneity of the problem of school refusal may have been overstated in the epidemiological literature, resulting in inattention to school features that may be linked to most instances

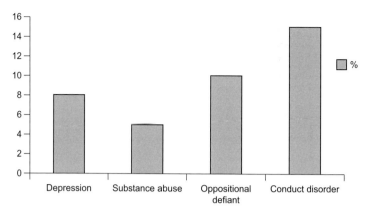

Figure 22.1 Disorders among youth in treatment for anxiety-based school refusal.

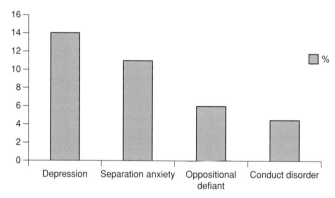

Figure 22.2 Mental health conditions associated with youth truancy from school.

of school refusal in some way, even in cases where individual anxiety is present. He speculates that the alienation of male pupils, especially those of lower socio-economic background, from the school systems of contemporary Western societies may be a contributing factor. Without attributing school refusal to any shortcomings of this nature in the school system, Thambirajah, Grandison and De-Hayes (2008) summarize the various operational definitions of school refusal that researchers have adopted as consisting of two components: a behavioral component involving non-attendance at school and some degree of emotional distress evoked by the prospect of being at school.

Prevalence

Given the nebulousness of the terminology involved and the lack of distinct status as a diagnostic category, it is understandable that relatively little is known about the prevalence and course of anxiety-based school refusal. However, school attendance records confirm that many pupils do not attend school regularly. The best estimate of the prevalence rate of school refusal ranges from 1 to 5 percent of the school population (King et al., 2001). If these estimates are accurate, school refusal merits much more attention by researchers than it has received to date. As mentioned above, some theorists have

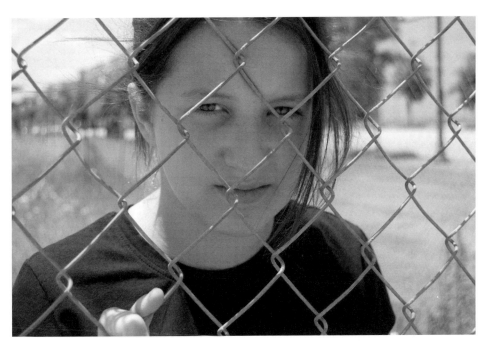

Figure 22.3 Many psychological problems may underlie non-attendance at school.

linked resistance to school with the Western school system's failure to provide adequately for the needs of male pupils. However, this appears not to translate into any sex difference in the frequency of school refusal, which is typically found to be equal among boys and girls (Beidel and Alfano, 2011). Problems of school refusal are discussed frequently in the writings of psychologists in countries where great value is placed on education and where individual expression of emotion is commonly discouraged, as in East Asia. However, there is no evidence that school refusal is more common in those societies than elsewhere. In fact, in some North American research, resistance to school has been found to be strongest in ethnic groups known for educational underachievement, such as Aboriginal peoples in Western Canada (Nakhaie, Silverman and LaGrange, 2000).

Complicating the issue is the fact that, although anxiety disorders are the most frequent mental health condition associated with school refusal, there is a substantial number, about one-third of children referred to mental health professionals for school-refusal issues,

who are identified as not having any diagnosable form of psychopathology at all (Kearney and Albano, 2004). King and his colleagues (2001) report that most cases first emerge either after the start of elementary school at about age 6 years or after the transition to middle school in early adolescence. Although systematic cross-cultural data are lacking, concern about school refusal is expressed very frequently in professional writings in Japan, perhaps because of the emphasis on school achievement there and because of the school climate, which is often described as competitive and stressful (Inoue et al., 2008; Pellegrini, 2007).

Possible causes and correlates

Kearney (2008) invokes contextual risk factors that may interact with individual risk factors. These include homelessness, poverty, school violence, lack of engagement and challenge at school and lack of parental involvement in children's schooling. Research on all aspects of school refusal is very limited, including research on the possible causes of this problem. The scarcity of research is probably attributable at least in part to the conceptual ambiguity of many of its manifestations. In order to facilitate progress and clarity, some researchers simply identify the population in their studies as having *anxiety-based school refusal*, eliminating any other known causes and correlates.

Thambirajah and colleagues (2008) summarize the very heterogeneous causal factors that have been evoked in the limited research literature on school refusal. They note that multiple causes are often responsible for individual cases of school refusal. School refusal occurs when the "pull" to stay away from school becomes stronger than the "push" to attend, when stress becomes stronger than support. Possible causes include child factors, family factors and school factors. Child factors may include difficulty separating from parents, which is probably the most frequent cause mentioned in the literature. The child may also experience anxiety about relations with peers or may be generally immature. The parents may encourage the child, subtly or overtly, to cling to them. They may be overinvolved with the child and/or overprotective. There may have been an experience of loss in the family or a transition to a new community. At school, the child may be a victim of bullies. The child may be experiencing difficulty in a transition from a more supportive elementary school to a more academically oriented upper-level school. The child may also be experiencing some type of learning disability or emotional problem. The child might also be anxious about some part of the school routine, such as public speaking or physical activity. With regard to how these causes interact and contribute to both emotional stress and school failure, Thambirajah et al. (2008) describe a vicious circle. Absence from school, even if caused by some child or family factor, soon exacerbates the problem as the child misses out on the continuity of the academic lessons missed. The peer group also becomes puzzled by the child's absence, exacerbating negative peer relations. This vicious circle makes a return to regular school attendance all the more difficult. Furthermore, chronic absence from school deprives a child of opportunities to learn from peers the social skills that, ironically, are most needed to anchor him or her into the social network of school peers (Beidel and Alfano, 2011).

Although there is little doubt that chronic school absenteeism is linked with psychopathology, it is not entirely clear whether absenteeism leads to psychopathology or psychopathology leads to absenteeism. In a large, longitudinal study in the United States, Wood (2012) found evidence for both causal pathways. However, in adolescence, there was more evidence that psychopathology causes absenteeism than vice versa.

Stability and prognosis

There have been a few longitudinal studies of the long-term implications of school refusal, with smaller samples than those who participated in longitudinal studies of other forms of psychopathology that affect large numbers of children and adolescents. In a follow-up study of 117 referred adolescents who received professional assistance for problems of school refusal, McShane, Walter and Rey (2004) found that one-fourth to one-third of the participants demonstrated substantial maladjustment 3 years after treatment. Buitelaar et al. (1994) followed twenty-five Dutch adolescents who had been referred to a clinic for school refusal. At follow-up an average of 5 years later, thirteen of the cases still had some form of psychiatric disorder. Ten-year outcome data are available in an Irish study based on only thirteen cases, of whom about one-third were in need of mental health treatment at 10-year follow-up (McCune and Hynes, 2005). Thus, the combined results of the small-sample follow-up studies indicate that even with mental health treatment, school refusal has long-term consequences for children and adolescents.

Prevention and treatment

Given the many possible causes and correlates of school refusal, psychological assessment must be particularly comprehensive (King et al., 2000). Although some specific questionnaires pertaining to school-refusal problems have been developed, these instruments should constitute only part of the assessment. Treatment for anxiety-based school refusal is not very different from the general approaches used in the treatment of anxiety disorders.

The cognitive-behavioral interventions discussed earlier are the most common and the best supported by research. Pharmacotherapy with SSRIs is also used in some cases (Kearney, 2008; King et al., 2000). However, there has been some criticism of the exclusive focus on the individual child in the treatment of school refusal. Inasmuch as contextual factors often play a role in the emergence of school refusal, teachers, families and the community at large could be more extensively involved in prevention and treatment than they usually are at present (Kearney, 2008; Lyon and Cotler, 2009).

Preventing school refusal: primary prevention strategies

Given the wide range of possible causes and manifestations of school refusal, a myriad of prevention strategies are conceivable. Many of these strategies involve improving schools in a number of general ways that improve pupil–teacher attachment, cooperative (as opposed to competitive) learning experiences and better peer relations among pupils. Thus, prevention might also entail restructuring the school so that one specific teacher or school staff member has increased responsibility for monitoring the progress of each pupil and providing counseling to that pupil and his or her parents. More and better contact between teachers and parents in general may also constitute a viable prevention strategy (Kearney and Hugelshofer, 2000). School attendance may either be the specific focus of a preventive intervention or one of the many desired outcomes of a prevention program. For example, improved school attendance could be one of the desired outcomes of a primary prevention program that includes in-class instruction in social skills and problem-solving. More specific

preventive programming to combat school refusal has also been attempted. Even small, secondary (see Chapter 10) preventive measures such as displaying in the school the photographs or good schoolwork of a pupil who has missed school for some time can be helpful (Kearney and Hugelshofer, 2000).

Tailoring treatment to the heterogeneous nature of school refusal

In an effort to make treatment more applicable to children whose school-refusal problems are not caused completely or even partially by anxiety, Kearney (2008) has developed treatment modules based on the four functions of school refusal described earlier. In a preliminary evaluation of a modular intervention for adolescents referred for problems of school refusal, Heyne and his colleagues (2011) developed the "@school" program. This program is typically delivered during ten to fourteen sessions with the young person and ten to fourteen sessions with the parents. Because of the individualization, the program is delivered on a one-on-one basis. Some of the component modules are compulsory. For both parents and adolescents, modules on keeping things in perspective and setting goals were compulsory. The compulsory modules for the adolescents also include solving problems and managing stress. The compulsory modules for the parents include giving effective instructions and responding to their children's behavior. Optional modules are selected by the therapists based on their knowledge of each case. These include a module on dealing with social situations for the adolescents and a module on bolstering parents' confidence in their parenting.

Twenty school-refusing adolescents participated in the evaluation. After the program, school attendance improved significantly; this was maintained through follow-up 2 months after the end of treatment. There were similar improvements in anxiety and depression and in both the adolescents' and the parents' confidence in their ability to improve school attendance. These impressive results merit replication in a larger-scale study with a control group.

CASE STUDY: Becky, school refusal as a message to an absent father

Laszloffy (2002) describes her successful intervention with a family that included Becky, age 13, the younger daughter. Laszloffy is a systemic family therapist whose policy it is to see the whole family together. The two older daughters were at university out of town and were, therefore, unavailable. Becky's Mom, Janet, came willingly for therapy but her Dad was often too busy; he attended only two of the ten therapy sessions. During the initial interview, Mom expressed her frustration at the daily ordeal of reminding Becky to get ready in time to catch the school bus, which she often missed. Mom would then drive her to school, with Becky crying all the way. During discussions that took place in the evenings, Becky promised repeatedly to attend school willingly but almost always broke the promise.

Given the chronicity of the situation and Mom's desperation, Laszloffy reluctantly began therapy without Bill, the father, who would be too busy at work for another month. Becky stated that she hated school, had no friends there and was teased constantly. Many of the taunts of Becky's peers had to do with Becky being overweight. However, Laszloffy expected that there were other causal factors at work because Becky's school refusal seems to have started at a time when her Mom had an accident, falling from a ladder at the shop where she worked, and subsequently resigned from that job, becoming unemployed. When questioned about her early school experiences, Becky said that she had been teased since as early as she could remember but that the teasing did not bother her that much.

A critical incident of the kind often mentioned in the family-therapy literature occurred when Lazloffy asked Becky whether she was any more or less absent from school than Dad was from the family. Becky demonstrated a reaction different from any previous response: She got a bit angry at Lazloffy. Becky subsequently clarified that she was not angry at Lazloffy but at Janet, who always made excuses for her Dad. Janet recognized that she was constantly making excuses both for Becky's school refusal and her husband's absence from the family. Bill, the father, appeared for the next session. Janet reported that she and Bill had discussed the situation. Bill had agreed to take over the task of driving Becky to school, changing his work schedule to suit. Although the therapeutic breakthrough occurred at the time of the critical incident, therapy continued for three more sessions. However, the focus was more on Janet's loneliness than Becky's school refusal. From the time of the critical incident through follow-up a year later, Becky attended school regularly and willingly.

Clinicians commenting on this case study have congratulated Lazloffy on both her success and her application of systemic family therapy. However, Stith, Rosen and McCollum (2002), writing from a feminist perspective, observed that the therapeutic progress might have been achieved without following the classic pattern of blaming the mother.

Conclusions and future directions

The nebulous diagnostic status of school refusal has surely hindered progress in understanding and coping with this problem. The heterogeneity of the phenomenon of school refusal and its heterogeneous causes have also served as an impediment to progress in understanding and treating this condition. It is encouraging that contemporary experts are accepting rather than resisting this heterogeneity. The need to develop treatments that are flexible enough to address different manifestations of school refusal has been recognized. These treatments are still in their infancy and require evaluative research conducted, as far as possible, with the same methodological rigor as the studies designed to evaluate and refine interventions for the more common forms of child psychopathology that have been discussed in earlier chapters.

Summary

- School refusal refers to the persistent refusal to attend school, usually because of anxiety about separation from parents. The term "school phobia" is used less frequently in current writings because it implies that anxiety about the school is necessarily the cause.
- School refusal is not a disorder in either the DSM or ICD schemes.
- The vast majority of children demonstrating school-refusal problems extensive enough to require the attention of professionals also suffer from anxiety disorders, depression and/or oppositional defiant disorder.
- For greater clarity, some researchers suggest using the term "anxiety-based school refusal" when anxiety appears as a very prominent element of the school refusal, as opposed to school refusal characterized by opposition/defiance or no known psychopathology.
- School refusal can be associated with avoidance of particular incidents that occur at transition times, fear of evaluation, or a preference for remaining close to parents. Some parents may make available objects or activities that are more appealing than school.
- School refusal has been linked to maladjustment and mental health treatment later in life.
- Cognitive-behavioral therapies are the most common and the best supported by research, although pharmacotherapy has also been used in some cases.

Study questions

1. In what important way is the term "school refusal" a misleading name for the disorder?
2. Given the heterogeneous causes of school refusal and the different forms of psychology that may accompany it, is it still useful to consider this phenomenon as a psychological disorder? Why or why not?
3. Is there anything schools can do to reduce the rates of school refusal?

Post-traumatic stress disorder (PTSD) is a severe and long-lasting reaction to a traumatic event that involves intense fear, horror and feelings of hopelessness (American Psychiatric Association, 2000). Common traumata vary considerably, including war, sexual abuse, physical abuse and natural disasters such as earthquakes, floods and tidal waves. Such traumatic experiences are, unfortunately, very common: It is estimated that one child in four experiences a significant traumatic event before reaching the adult years (Costello et al., 2002). Many children who live through a traumatic event will show some symptoms of PTSD immediately after the event (Aaron, Zaglul and Emery, 1999). Indeed, it would probably be abnormal for them *not* to react. Moderate psychological distress shortly after the trauma can thus be considered normal (Cohen, D. et al., 2010). However, on the average, about 30 percent of sufferers continue to have symptoms of PTSD one month after the traumatic event (Kessler et al., 1995; Cohen, D. et al., 2010).

Mental health professionals were as slow to recognize the clinical significance of PTSD in childhood and adolescence as they were to acknowledge the extent and severity of anxiety disorders. Awareness increased largely as the result of widespread knowledge of several important historical events that affected children that were brought to public attention by authors, journalists and photojournalists. This chapter begins with a section on the slow process leading to the recognition of PTSD as a real and serious problem for children and adolescents. Information on diagnostic criteria follows. The section on prevalence includes information about the factors that have been found to differentiate children and youth who are most and least likely to develop PTSD after a potentially

traumatic incident. The section on causes and correlates is devoted primarily to biological processes that are thought to influence individual reactions to traumatic events. The chapter closes with a section on treatment.

Emerging recognition of PTSD in childhood and adolescence

Psychoanalyst Lenore Terr has devoted much of her career to describing the reactions of children to various traumatic events. Her most influential writings are based on her interviews with the twenty-three kidnapping victims involved in a famous incident in Chowchilla, California on July 15, 1976. Ranging from 5 to 14 years of age, they were being transported by school bus after a recreational swim that was a break from their summer-school classes. Three masked men stopped the school bus at gunpoint and transferred the children to two vans, with windows covered over, to be driven for 11 hours to an underground hiding place. Two of the oldest and strongest boys dug them out to find that the kidnappers had fled; they were arrested while attempting to escape to Canada, never having had the chance to deliver their ransom letter. The children suffered no physical harm during their 27 hours of captivity (Miller and Tompkins, 1977; Terr, 1979, 1981).

Reflecting the prevailing ideas of the times, which maintained that children usually recover from traumatic incidents without long-term effects, the mental health physician at the local clinic predicted that probably only one of the kidnapped would be emotionally affected in the long term. His prediction was based on the vague ideas about the prevalence of such traumata, not on any knowledge of the children. However, 5 months later, several of the parents sought psychiatric help for their children. The psychiatrist they consulted knew of Terr's interest in trauma and arranged for her to meet the parents and children as well. The children had begun to react in different maladaptive ways. Sheila, 11 years old, changed from being a sweet if slightly bossy preadolescent to an angry, obstinate and difficult person. Fourteen-year-old Bob, one of the two heroes who helped dig his schoolmates out, developed a pervasive fear of strange vehicles, which he expressed by shooting a BB gun at the car rented by Japanese tourists who were stopped at the side of the road when the car broke down. Several of the siblings began to fight and argue with each other. Some developed anxious reactions to moving vchicles, including 10-year-old Alison, who would not venture into the front seat of her family's new car. Alison and several others developed a fear of fear – anxiety about becoming perturbed in some new way in the future. The children's dreams were replete with other kidnapping incidents, some similar to the one that had happened but with more dire outcomes such as being lined up, shot and killed. In their dramatic play, the children re-enacted the incident. Many expressed the fear that they could be kidnapped again. In her remarks to the professional community, Terr urged greater attention to traumata of this sort. She noted that even psychoanalysts had moved away from the study of trauma, even though early traumata were emphasized by Freud (Terr, 1981). Perhaps they developed a fear of studying trauma in reaction to the ridicule they received for what some critics saw as the attribution of subtle trauma in a very facile manner to a wide variety of problems far less serious than those of the Chowchilla victims (e. g., Meehl, 1973).

Terr also pioneered in raising awareness about the psychological effects of child-battering. Her efforts in this area included an influential publication in *The American Journal of Psychiatry* based on her interviews with ten battered children (Terr and Watson, 1968). In that publication, she sensitized

her peers to the traumatic effects of not only the battering but also the adversarial legal process. In her paper, that was aptly entitled "The Battered Child Rebrutalized," she lambasted professionals who failed to report the injuries. Since her times, sensitivity to both physical and sexual abuse has resulted, for example, in legislation requiring professionals to report cases in which abuse of children is suspected. At the time of Terr's writings, no one suspected the extent of child abuse. The Children's Bureau of the United States government reported that in 2009, 1,770 children died as the result of physical and psychological abuse and neglect, with 81 percent of the incidents committed by parents and 6 percent by other relatives. Over three million incidents were reported in that year, involving over six million children. Only about a third of the cases were substantiated by the authorities (US Department of Health and Human Services, 2010). Unfortunately, the statistics also indicate a substantial problem of false accusations. However, that leaves approximately two million confirmed child victims each year. Record-keeping in the UK is less comprehensive but the child abuse registers indicate that almost 47,000 children are listed as of March 31, 2010 (Department for Education, 2010). In interpreting this figure, it is important to remember that experts believe that no more than 5 percent of cases of child abuse, and perhaps no more than 1–2 percent, are reported to regulatory authorities (Edwards et al., 2003). Detailed retrospective interviews with adolescents and young adults across the UK indicate that about one in four reports having been abused in some way as a child (NSPCC, 2011). It is important to note that many children, about a third of those who have suffered any form of abuse, experience more than one form of abuse (Kearney et al., 2010). In any case, these statistics are highly alarming, especially since an unknown but very large number of abuse cases certainly remain unreported.

Natural disasters such as tsunamis and earthquakes have dominated headlines in recent years, including a tsunami in Sri Lanka, Hurricane Katrina in New

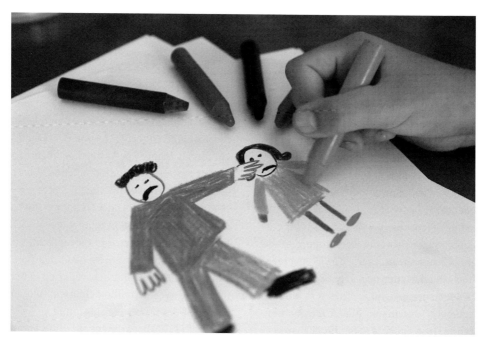

Figure 23.1 Traumatic experiences are sometimes depicted in children's artwork.

Orleans and an earthquake in Haiti. War and the experience of becoming a refugee also exact a toll on millions of children, some of whom are already vulnerable because of other psychological problems. Indeed, the recognition of PTSD in DSM-III is often attributed to public awareness in the United States of the psychological needs of returning veterans of the Vietnam War (Brett, 1996; Salmon and Bryant, 2002). At that time, revealing photographic details of the suffering of the children in that war sensitized the American public to their plight. Since those years, the public has been shocked by such incidents as the mass shooting of schoolchildren in Colombine, Colorado and the attacks on the World Trade Center towers in New York City.

When these disasters occur in countries with well-developed mental health services, professionals participate in the rescue team and researchers are deployed to learn about the effects on children. In other places, physical survival needs take precedence (Berger and Gelkopf, 2009; Cohen, 2008; Nemeroff

and Goldschmidt-Clermont, 2011; Salloum et al., 2011). In a long-term follow-up of children who had experienced war-related trauma during World War II, Strauss and her colleagues (2011) found that many of them still experienced psychological effects, especially depression, even as they entered old age.

Although the suffering of children who have been abused arouses profound and widespread concern, diagnosing the victims is not without its critics. In a perceptive review of the societal ramifications of the growing awareness of victimization, Best (1997) chronicles attacks by commentators of all political persuasions. Critics condemn a wide range of abuses that they see occurring as a way of combating abuse, ranging from what they see as alarmist inflation of the numbers of people actually affected, to the unjustified use of the "abuse excuse" (Dershowitz, 1994) to avoid being blamed for delinquency, to the emergence of a "victim industry" that derives benefit in terms of credibility and/or income from exaggerating the numbers of victims and using unproven techniques to treat them. As a sociologist, Best highlights the problem of ignoring the broader social forces that cause PTSD as a by-product of identifying and "medicalizing" individual cases.

Diagnostic criteria

In the 1987 revision of the DSM-III (i.e., the DSM-III-R), it was recognized for the first time that children's reactions to traumatic experiences might be different from those of adults. Children may indeed react with fear and horror, as may adults, but they may also display agitated, disorganized or defiant behavior. Their traumatic experiences may be re-enacted in nightmares and may be expressed repeatedly in their dramatic play. They may develop stomach aches or headaches without known physical cause (American Psychiatric Association, 1987; Salmon and Bryant, 2002). The diagnostic category of post-traumatic stress disorder pertains to a wide range of trauma, some of which are unpredictable, some of which involve familiar people and some of which are linked to political events in the countries in which children and adolescents live and grow. All data on the prevalence, course and consequences of PTSD must be interpreted with the understanding that they may not apply to all causes and manifestations of the disorder.

PTSD is one of the few diagnoses in DSM that is based on an identifiable cause, the precipitating trauma. This exception is entirely logical. However, some concern has been expressed that the diagnostic procedures often used entail the elicitation of the details of the traumatic event even though one of the prominent features of PTSD (Cohen, D. et al., 2010) is often the avoidance of recounting the event, if not the total repression of its memory.

There is some recognition that children may display PTSD in distinct ways unlike the reactions of adults. Importantly, the criteria reflect the understanding that children may relive their traumatic experiences through repetitive play and/or somatic symptoms. However, far greater attention

to developmental differences has been advocated by many. In a paper on developmental factors in PTSD, Salmon and Bryant (2002) point out, first of all, that there are differences between the ways children and adults encode the traumatic event. Young children, especially, encode less completely and more slowly than do older children and adolescents. Therefore, they simply retain less information for recall later on. Furthermore, unlike many adults, children usually appraise the traumatic event with little background knowledge. The unfamiliarity by itself may evoke a strong emotional response and may lead to incredible misinterpretations of it. Children's language development may impede verbal reports of trauma that affect them profoundly. Subsequent language development may not necessarily enable them to verbalize traumatic experiences that occurred before they mastered the language needed to encode them. However, traumatic events have been identified in the non-verbal language of children with immature language development up to a year after the event (De Bellis et al., 2009; Kataoka et al., 2009; Salmon and Bryant, 2002).

PTSD often has wide-ranging effects on the lives of children and adolescents. Their sleep patterns, school functioning and family lives are often affected. It is not surprising, therefore, that comorbid major depressive disorder is often diagnosed. For example, in their study of the diagnoses of adolescents after a catastrophic cyclone in India, Kar and Bastia (2006) reported that almost half of the victims who had been diagnosed with PTSD also suffered from other diagnosable disorders, with depression evident in a third of the cases. Other frequent comorbid conditions include attention deficit/hyperactivity disorder, oppositional defiant disorder and other anxiety disorders (Kearney et al., 2010). It is often found that victims with comorbid diagnoses are more difficult to treat than those with only a single diagnosis (e.g., Dixon, Howie and Starling, 2005).

In DSM-5, PTSD constitutes the major portion of a distinct chapter "Trauma and Stress-Related Disorders." That chapter also includes *reactive attachment disorder*, in which the child reacts with depression or social withdrawal to such trauma as parental neglect or frequent changes of caregivers and *disinhibited social engagement disorder*, in which the child reacts to the same traumatic experiences with caregivers with a lack of inhibition that might be displayed by becoming overly familiar with unknown adults, venturing off away from adult care, or unhesitatingly going off with an unknown adult. Thus, PTSD is no longer considered a form of anxiety disorder as it was in DSM-IV. This emphasizes the traumatic origin of the syndrome and reflects new research documenting the patterns of reaction to traumatic experiences by children and adults. The diagnosis of PTSD in children older than 6 years or in adults requires, first of all, exposure to a potentially traumatic experience in some way, be it experiencing the trauma directly, witnessing it or learning about it. The event must also intrude into the current experience of the victim in one of several ways, such as memories of the event, distressing dreams, flashbacks, distress at the location of the event or at similar locations, or untoward reactions in the presence of cues that bring back the memory. The victim avoids stimuli associated with the trauma. His or her moods and thoughts assume a negative tone. After the event, the victim's arousal and/or reaction patterns change. For example, he or she might become angry, irritable, aggressive, distracted or reckless. These changes must be evident for at least 1 month and must significantly affect the individual's social daily functioning. New to DSM-5, there is a separate list of criteria for children under the age of 6 years. The criteria are quite similar to those for adults but with increased emphasis on such manifestations as flashbacks and intrusions of the traumatic event into the child's dramatic play (American Psychiatric Association, 2013). Comments from practicing mental health professionals include some laudatory remarks. For example, Canadian pediatrician and child psychiatrist Harriet L. MacMillan observes that removal of PTSD from the anxiety disorders section constitutes an overdue recognition of the fact that PTSD symptoms go far beyond fear-based anxiety. She wonders, however, whether the expansion of the criteria has gone so far that it is no longer a single disorder that is being diagnosed. This expansion may also result in treatment being delivered to children who would recover anyway without any extended special intervention (www.biomedcentral.com/1741-7015/11/202/, retrieved February 28, 2014).

The ICD-10 diagnosis is conceptually similar, although the specifics of the diagnostic criteria do vary considerably. The differences between the two diagnostic symptoms may be reduced for this and most other disorders with the next revision of the ICD. Some proposals for ICD-11 advocate, however, more specific criteria than those of DSM-5, directing professionals to the truly central features of PTSD, as noted in comments by Australian psychology professor Richard A. Bryant and Simon Wessely, a psychiatrist who works at the Maudsley Hospital and King's College, London (www.biomedcentral.com/1741-7015/11/202/, retrieved February 28, 2014).

Prevalence

Fortunately, many children who experience traumatic events react for only relatively short periods of time. This is especially true of reactions to natural disasters, which typically reach the level of diagnosable PTSD in fewer than 5 percent of cases according to the best information available. The rates of PTSD among children who lived through the devastation of Hurricane Ike in the Southeastern US states were studied by Lai and colleagues (2013). Although fully 13 percent suffered from post-traumatic symptoms 8 months later, only 7 percent suffered post-traumatic symptoms 15 months after the hurricane. Many of the children suffered from both PTSD and depression. Children in the comorbid group were less likely to recover over time than children with PTSD only. The results of Lai and her colleagues, like those of most other research on post-disaster PTSD, are limited because no data were available on the participating children's mental health before the hurricane.

However, PTSD is far more likely to occur if a child has experienced war, where as many as a third of children affected are likely to develop PTSD. Similarly, about a third of the children who have experienced violent crime are typically diagnosed with PTSD afterwards. Understandably and tragically, PTSD is believed to affect all children who have been exposed to the sexual assault or murder of their mothers. Estimates of the rate of PTSD following sexual abuse vary enormously, with most credible studies indicating that anywhere from 50 to 90 percent of child victims of sexual abuse will develop PTSD (Kiser et al., 1988; Salmon and Bryant, 2002; Timmons-Mitchell, Chandler-Holtz and Semple, 1997; Wolfe, Gentile and Wolfe, 1989). The risk of developing PTSD increases dramatically with exposure to multiple traumatic events (Suliman et al., 2009).

Data on the prevalence of PTSD in the general population are somewhat suspect because children and their parents are likely to under-report some forms of trauma, especially sexual abuse. Reported incidence rates range from 1.6 percent in a study conducted in Germany (Essau, Conradt and Petermann, 2000) to anywhere from 5 to 9.2 percent in influential studies from the United States (Breslau et al., 1991; Cohen, D. et al., 2010; Kilpatrick et al., 2003). The differences may reflect differences in diagnostic practice and self-report bias rather than any true cultural difference. Surprisingly few data on the long-term prognosis are available. However, many reports indicate that the effects of a trauma often last for many years (e.g., Arias, 2004), whether or not the formal diagnosis remains stable over time.

Research on the risk factors associated with developing PTSD after a traumatic experience has been wide-ranging, including characteristics of the individual child, the family network and the surrounding culture. There has been some interesting research aimed at pinpointing the differences between children who develop PTSD after a traumatic event and those who manage to recover without reactions of diagnosable proportion. Although more girls than boys are diagnosed with PTSD, boys are more likely

to react behaviorally than are girls (Yule, Perrin and Smith, 1999). A parental history of mental illness and, especially, parental history of PTSD, can double the risk of exposure to traumatic events that may lead to PTSD (Costello et al., 2002). This may occur because of reaction patterns that are transmitted genetically or by the learning that occurs when children observed their parents reacting to difficult events (Dyregrov and Yule, 2006). A troubled family background prior to the precipitating event is a potent risk factor (Dyregrov and Yule, 2006; Meiser-Stedman, 2002; Pine and Cohen, 2002). A host of family problems are thought to leave children vulnerable to PTSD after a traumatic event: insecure child–parent attachment, conflict, lack of family cohesion, coercive child-rearing, divorce and family economic hardship (Afifi et al., 2009; Dyregrov and Yule, 2006; Kearney et al., 2010). Another way in which parents may unwittingly increase the risk of PTSD for their children is by allowing extensive television viewing of disaster-related events (Hoven et al., 2005; Thienkrua et al., 2006). As well, PTSD is more likely to emerge later on if the child has a history of mental disorder prior to the trauma (Cohen, D. et al., 2010; Sinclair, Salmon and Bryant, 2007; Pine and Cohen, 2002; Pfefferbaum et al., 2006).

Identification of the protective factors associated with resilience in the face of trauma could be very helpful in illuminating the processes of human resilience in general. Researchers have examined a wide range of possible protective factors, with results that vary sharply across the types of traumatic events that may lead to PTSD and, even then, from study to study. Social support networks including supportive siblings and friends have been linked with reduced PTSD after a traumatic event in some studies (Cohen, 2010; Laor et al., 1997; Milan et al., 2013; Peltonen et al., 2010; Stevens et al., 2013). Older children who have the ability to understand the situation they are facing tend to fare better than less mature children (Punamaki and Puhakka, 1997).

General intellectual capacity is thought to work as a protective factor against the suffering that occurs when the child or adolescent engages in repetitive rethinking about the traumatic event (Saltzman, Weems and Carrion, 2006). Certain specific thinking skills, such as abstract reasoning and memory, may operate in a similar protective manner (Eisen et al., 2007; Kearney et al., 2010). Creative thinking may also be an asset to coping, as shown in a study of Middle Eastern children who have experienced political violence by Punamaki, Qouta and El-Sarraj (2001).

Culture

Culture may work as a risk factor, protective factor or moderating factor. Obviously, living in a country at war is associated with increased risk. It has also been suggested that positive cultural identification, which may be linked to unified families, participation in religious activities and social gatherings, may function protectively (Kearney et al., 2010), perhaps by means of social support. Religious beliefs themselves may be thought of as either a risk or a protective factor. If the religious beliefs lead to fatalism and pessimism, they may aggravate the situation (Kearney et al., 2010; Shen, 2009). However, religion can also bring hope and faith in a better future.

As is often the case in writings about cultural differences in psychopathology (see Chapter 8), cultural differences are often interwoven with differences in socio-economic status (e.g., De Bellis et al., 2010). Poverty exerts an effect on family life. Economic hardship and neighborhood risk have been linked to PTSD in children and adolescents (Kearney et al., 2010).

Gender

Based on a meta-analysis of fifty-two separate male–female comparisons, Tolin and Foa (2008) report that girls and women are about twice as likely as are boys and men to be diagnosed with PTSD. However, the cumulative data suggest that the difference in diagnosable PTSD probably does not occur because of sex differences in the actual

frequency of traumatic events. In fact, boys and men are significantly more likely than girls or women to report a potentially traumatic event. Looking more closely at the data, it appears that there is no sex difference in potentially traumatic events occurring during childhood. There are, however, sex differences in the types of trauma reported by boys and girls. Girls report more incidents of sexual assault than do boys, well over twice as many. Boys tend to experience more accidents, non-sexual physical assaults, fires and other disasters. Even when the difference in the experience of traumatic events is taken into account, girls appear to suffer more frequent or more intense PTSD than do boys. More importantly, girls and boys tend to display their PTSD in different ways: Boys often act out aggressively whereas girls tend to experience internalizing symptoms such as anxiety and depression. This is demonstrated most clearly by studies in which the reactions of boys and girls to the same traumatic event are compared, as was found in a study of the long-term consequences of the Buffalo Creek Dam collapse in 1972 (Green et al., 1994; Tolin and Foa, 2008).

Possible causes and correlates

PTSD is the one disorder in the DSM system in which a cause, that is a traumatic event, is identified as a requirement for diagnosis. Some research illuminates the ways in which the trauma comes to affect individuals. According to the *developmental traumatology model* (De Bellis et al., 2010), maltreatment leads to PTSD by affecting children's biological stress systems, the developing brain and cognitive functioning. The precipitating maltreatment activates several neurotransmitter and neuroendocrine systems, which, under normal circumstances, would result in adaptive behavior that would maximize the organism's ability to survive and adjust. However, excessive and prolonged arousal may cause a number of untoward effects in a number of specific, vulnerable

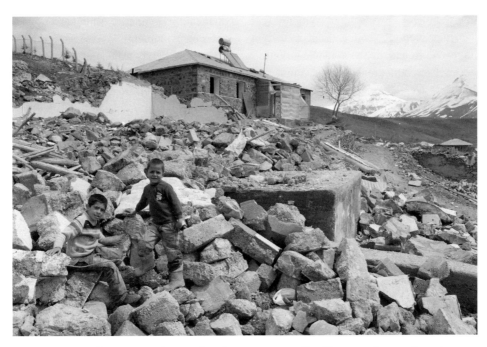

Figure 23.2 Natural disasters such as earthquakes are an unpredictable traumatic experience to which some children are particularly vulnerable.

areas of the brain. These changes may occur at crucial periods in brain development, affecting growth and development in ways that may not be reversible (Charmandari, Tsigos and Chrousus, 2005; Pervanidou, 2008). The secretion of cortisol becomes dysregulated, as illustrated in a number of studies showing either higher or lower levels of cortisol in children with PTSD as compared to other children. The hippocampus, which is associated with attention and memory, may be affected according to several recent studies. In other studies, although there was no evidence of abnormal hippocampal volumes, the memory capacities of children with PTSD were shown to be impaired. Other areas of the brain may also be affected, including the corpus callosum, prefrontal cortex and cerebral lobes. Some studies suggest that biological alterations immediately after the traumatic event, including immediate reduction in cortisol level, are linked to the severity of subsequent PTSD symptoms (De Bellis et al., 2010; Jackowski et al., 2009; Pervanidou, 2008). The trauma itself may interact with pre-existing

genetic factors linked to these biological processes (Pervanidou, 2008; Villarreal et al., 2004). Much more research is needed to clarify these issues and to resolve the many inconsistencies among studies on the biology of PTSD.

Treatment

It is probable that only a small proportion of the children and adolescents with PTSD are ever seen by mental health professionals. This is highly unfortunate, because treatment can be quite helpful. The strategies that have been attempted by psychotherapists are very diverse, including CBT, art therapy (see Figure 23.1), hypnotherapy, social skills training, graduated exposure, narrative retelling of the trauma, relaxation training, training in the expression of emotion, training in the interruption of dysfunctional thoughts, non-directive child-centered therapy, eye movement desensitization and psychoeducation about the nature of PTSD.

Exposure treatment typically involves a hierarchy of stress-invoking situations, leading gradually to the ability to remember and discuss the most serious traumatic experiences. Both group and individual treatment formats have been implemented. There is some limited evidence that individual psychotherapy is superior to the group format (Trowell et al., 2002). In some successful therapies, children maintain a journal of their thoughts and experiences (Cohen, D. et al., 2010; Kearney et al., 2010).

Not all forms of psychotherapy are equally effective with children and adolescents with PTSD. Interventions that focus specifically on the traumatic event or events have been found more effective than indirect approaches, such as relationship-based child-centered psychotherapy (Cohen, D. et al., 2010; Cohen, J. A. et al., 2004; Feather and Ronan, 2006; Liberman, Van Horn and Ippen, 2005; Trowell et al., 2002). As with other forms of anxiety disorder, cognitive behavior therapy, as adapted specifically to PTSD, has been found more effective than other approaches (Cohen, Mannarino and Deblinger, 2006; Saunders, Berliner and Hanson, 2004). However, in a comprehensive meta-analysis of twenty-eight studies focusing specifically on sexual abuse, Hetzel-Riggin, Brausch and Montgomery (2007) found that the effectiveness of psychotherapy depended on the specific outcome and manifestation of PTSD being considered. For example, group cognitive behavior therapy was most effective for relieving psychological distress but not necessarily for

enhancing self-concept. Although more research is needed to pinpoint the therapeutic approaches that are optimal for achieving specific objectives, it is comforting to note that enough research has been conducted to allow several careful reviewers to conclude with confidence that cognitive behavior therapy is an established, effective intervention (e.g., Saunders et al., 2004). Typical of the results of meta-analyses on the general effects of psychotherapy are those of Harvey and Taylor (2010), whose meta-analysis of thirty-nine separate studies on psychotherapy for victims of sexual abuse revealed typical global treatment effects in excess of one standard deviation, with smaller but still significant effect sizes for some specific outcomes. Some but not all effects were still evident at follow-up measurement months and years after the end of treatment.

There is evidence that parent involvement in treatment tends to enhance effectiveness. As with child psychotherapy, a wide range of interventions have been used successfully with parents of children and adolescents with PTSD. Many therapists help parents with parenting skills, dealing with their children's emotions and solving conflicts. Sometimes therapists working with parents also focus on personal problems of the parents such as depression. Some therapists emphasize the value of conjoint sessions in which the therapist works with the parent and child during the same session (Cohen, D. et al., 2010; Kearney et al., 2010).

CASE STUDY: Marc, struggling with abuse at home and from his peers

A case study by Grasso and colleagues (2011) illustrates the techniques of trauma-focused CBT and the ways in which it differs from other applications of CBT. "Marc," 11 years old, came to the attention of a community mental health outreach program after an incident in which he was assaulted by other children. Screening for child abuse is a routine part of the procedures of the outreach program. Marc's responses indicated a history of physical abuse by his biological father, both to him and to his mother. Marc described vividly being grabbed by his father and shoved against an outdoor dog cage during a family barbecue. When Marc tried to run away, his father hit and kicked him. Following the incident, Marc and his biological mother, Sandra, moved to Marc's grandmother's house. Afraid of having nightmares, Marc insisted on sleeping in the room where his mother slept. He would tremble whenever he saw a truck that resembled his father's. He expressed his anxiety by chewing his clothing. Subsequent professional assessment confirmed the diagnosis of PTSD, with no diagnosable comorbid condition.

During the initial sessions, the therapist provided Marc with a foundation of knowledge about PTSD, basic relaxation skills and basic coping skills such as using a computerized mood chart to identify and manage his emotions. Marc learned to understand PTSD as a condition in which a person's body goes into alarm mode but the alarm does not get turned off. Marc's therapist assisted Marc in preparing a baseline narrative in which he described the most salient incident of abuse and his feelings about it. Marc learned about "mindfulness" – being aware of what is going on around him at the present time. The therapist engaged in parallel work with Sandra, who was emotionally burdened by a series of abusive relationships with men as well as a history of experiencing and witnessing domestic violence during her childhood. Sandra's adult life was characterized by maladaptive dependence on others and alcoholism. One of the men beat her during the eighth month of pregnancy, causing her to lose the child. The therapist helped Sandra relax, to recognize her feelings of guilt and to use positive methods of child-rearing. By the tenth session, Marc was ready for a conjoint session with Sandra at which they discussed his narrative together. In the final phase of therapy, the therapist help Marc articulate the end of his personal story by describing on the computer his goals for the future. Marc described a future in which he suffers no more abuse, gets good marks in school and awards for his achievement, and has more friends. Mark's future projection includes no contact with his father or people like his father. Marc goes on to become a successful veterinarian. Follow-up at 3, 6 and 12 months indicated the maintenance of the gains made in therapy. Sandra's plans for her own future included a divorce and more intensive personal psychotherapy. A year after treatment, Marc phoned the therapist to inform him that his Mom had started drinking again. Marc and his mother decided to resolve this problem without further therapy.

Although most experts consider psychotherapy the treatment of first choice for PTSD, sometimes pharmacotherapy is used as an adjunct. SSRIs, which have been used successfully with adults with PTSD, have been tried with children as well, as have a wide range of other medications. A few studies indicate that psychotropic medication is effective with children and adolescents with PTSD. One drawback is that there are also strong effects for placebo tablets in some of these studies (Cohen, D. et al., 2010; Cohen, J. A. et al., 2007; Robb et al., 2008). Furthermore, as noted earlier in this chapter and in Chapter 13, there are many concerns about the side effects.

In addition to the interventions supported by science, there are a number of dramatic and controversial therapies that have been used with children and adolescents with PTSD, arousing the dismay and concern of many experts. Some therapists have attempted to generate a "rebirth" experience by holding or binding children, or restricting their access to food or water (American Academy of Child and Adolescent Psychiatry, 2005). Another controversy in the mental health and legal professions pertains to the emergence and possible therapist elicitation of "repressed memories" by children in therapy for PTSD. These memories may or may not be accurate, which is consistent with research on the effects of PTSD on memory processes (Zoellner et al., 2000).

Conclusions and future directions

Although media reports of alarming incidents of child abuse have surely raised public awareness of PTSD, the prevailing cloud of secrecy still impedes an accurate estimate of extent of this disorder. Better research is now being conducted about the treatment of childhood PTSD but evidence remains very limited, in large part because of limited access to information about some traumatic events and the unpredictable nature of others. The new, expanded DSM-5 criteria may facilitate research but may turn out to be so expansive that they will not be regarded as criteria for a single disorder.

Western media are now documenting the traumata related to war and terrorism. Improved communication and transportation have facilitated the work of dedicated professionals and non-professionals who do their best to help child victims. Progress still depends heavily, however, on the dedication of professionals like Lenore Terr, who act quickly after the unpredictable trauma that often, but not always, leads to PTSD.

Summary

- Post-traumatic stress disorder (PTSD), a severe and long-lasting reaction to a traumatic event involving fear, horror and feelings of hopelessness, can occur among children and adolescents, although it is often deliberately concealed by adults.
- Children who have suffered one form of abuse are also likely to experience other forms.
- PTSD may also occur in children following natural disasters, such as tsunamis and earthquakes, during times of war (e.g., experience of becoming a refugee), or during mass shooting incidents at school.
- Some critics concerned with the politics behind psychopathology downplay the effect of PTSD on children, indicating that the numbers of people actually affected are inflated, that delinquency is being overly excused and that a "victim industry" is emerging.
- It was not until the DSM-III-R that the diagnosis of children with PTSD differed from that of adults. Particularly, children may not only react with fear and horror, but they may also demonstrate agitated, disorganized or defiant behavior. They may also develop stomach aches or headaches without known physical cause.
- PTSD is one of the few disorders in the DSM where the etiology is necessary for the diagnosis.
- In DSM-5, PTSD is including in a separate section on disorders related to stress or trauma. In DSM-IV, PTSD was considered a form of anxiety disorder.
- Some critics believe that the DSM-5 criteria are so broad that they may apply to more than a single disorder. The new criteria may also result in the diagnosis of children with symptoms not severe enough to need extended professional help.
- Not only may traumatic experiences in children be relived differently than adults (e.g., through repetitive play), but the way in which children encode the traumatic event differs from that of adults. Since children encode less completely and more slowly; the unfamiliarity of the situation may be misinterpreted later on, affecting them even more. Children may not have the language proficiency to describe their experiences, although skilled therapists become attuned to non-verbal language and work with the child's artwork.
- Importantly, most children who have lived through traumatic experiences do not develop PTSD.

- DSM-5 includes, for the first time, separate diagnostic criteria for children younger than 6 years. The criteria, however, are not very different than those developed for use with older children and adults.
- Comorbid disorders are often diagnosed along with PTSD, including major depressive disorder in the majority of cases, attention deficit/hyperactivity disorder, oppositional defiant disorder and other anxiety disorders. Patients with comorbid disorders are often more difficult to treat.
- The risk of a child developing PTSD is higher when the child has been exposed to the sexual assault or murder of their mothers, suffered sexual abuse, experienced violent crime or war. Risk is lower when a child has experienced a natural disaster.
- Due to differences in diagnostic practices and self-report bias (especially in sexual assault cases), true incidence rates are not fully known.
- Risk factors for children include: parental history of mental illness (especially PTSD), a troubled family background prior to the event, insecure child–parent attachment, conflict, lack of family cohesion, coercive child-rearing, divorce, family economic hardship, extensive viewing of disaster-related events on television and a history of mental disorder in the child before the event.
- Protective factors include: social support networks (supportive siblings and friends), age (older children are better able to understand the situation), general intellectual capacity, abstract reasoning and memory and creative thinking.
- Culture may be a risk factor (regions of war), protective factor (positive religious beliefs, social gatherings, positive cultural identification or social support) or moderating factor. Socio-economic status and economic hardship may be associated with PTSD in children and adolescents as well.
- Girls and women are more likely to be diagnosed with PTSD (and more intensely) than boys and men. However, this is probably not due to sex differences in diagnostic practice but to the frequency of traumatic events. Males are more likely to report a potentially traumatic event. Girls report more incidents of sexual assault, whereas boys report more accidents, non-sexual physical assaults, fires and other disasters. Boys act out aggressively in reaction to PTSD, whereas girls experience internalizing symptoms such as anxiety and depression.
- The developmental traumatology model refers to the idea that maltreatment leads to PTSD by affecting children's biological stress systems and the development of the brain and cognitive functions. This is due to excessive or prolonged arousal in the sympathetic nervous system, dysregulating natural cortisol levels. Major impairments in certain regions of the brain, such as the hippocampus, corpus callosum, prefrontal cortex and cerebral lobes, are also associated with PTSD.
- Treatment options vary for children with PTSD and include: cognitive-behavioral therapy (CBT), art therapy, hypnotherapy, social skills training and graduated exposure, among others. Interventions that focus specifically on the traumatic event have been found to be more effective than indirect approaches. CBT has been found to be more effective than other forms of treatment.
- Treatment may also benefit the parents, as some therapists will work with parents to teach parenting skills, also focusing on mental health issues such as depression.
- Psychotropic medication is sometimes used for children with PTSD. However, strong effects for placebo tablets appear in some of the research. In addition, clinicians need to be concerned about the side effects of the medication.
- Some interventions exist without any scientific support, such as restricting access to food and water for children with PTSD. Controversies surround the accuracy of information elicited during therapy in the form of repressed memories.

Study questions

1. Some children are more likely than others to develop PTSD after a potentially traumatic event. Aside from any feature of the event itself, what factors tend to differentiate children who develop PTSD from those who do not?

2. What are the typical features of successful psychotherapy for children and adolescents with PTSD?

Gender dysphoria in children
Or, what is psychopathology?

Deciding whether *gender dysphoria* is or should be a mental disorder invokes many of the fundamental issues about the nature of psychopathology that were considered in the first chapters of this book. As discussed in Chapter 1, a disorder may be delineated in several ways, each of which poses major conceptual problems along with distinct advantages. One way is to consider patterns of behavior that are atypical in the population as disorders. Another option is to define pathology on the basis of the assumption that the body and mind of the person involved are affected by some kind of illness that may or may not be curable. A final approach usually considered is to delineate disorder or pathology when a pattern of behavior interferes with the person's adaptation to the environment or successful daily life functioning. In addition, the diagnostician is responsible ethically to ensure that the person is better off at the end of the process. There is the growing recognition that in contemporary Western society, being diagnosed as having a mental disorder can itself contribute to the public stigma of people being diagnosed. Thus, diagnosis could actually compromise their well-being and daily life functioning, the very opposite of what helping professionals are supposed to do. These issues have been in the forefront of the debate that has raged over the past 40 years about the diagnostic status of homosexuality and, more recently, of gender dysphoria. The term "gender dysphoria" is new in DSM-5; it replaces the DSM-IV term "gender identity disorder." The current debate about whether to delete gender identity issues from the lexicon of mental illness is considered by many a continuation of the polemics that led to the progressive deletion of homosexuality in the 1970s and 1980s.

In this chapter, as much attention is devoted to the debate about the place of gender variance in the list of psychological disorders as to information about the disorder, if it indeed should be considered a disorder. By finishing with consideration of these issues, the book concludes with a review and test of the limits of the concepts of disorder and pathology. The current controversy cannot be understood without the context of the earlier debate about the status of homosexuality as a mental disorder, which is discussed first. The second part of the chapter is more similar to the previous chapters on other disorders. Information about diagnostic criteria is followed by sections devoted to prevalence, possible causes and correlates, stability and prognosis. The chapter closes with a brief section on the very little that is known about the treatment of the distress associated with gender variance.

Historical perspective

Drescher (2010) presents a comprehensive discussion of the parallels between the current debate about the diagnostic status of gender variance and the events leading to the elimination of homosexuality per se from the DSM scheme, which he lumps together under the rubric of "queer diagnoses" (p. 427). Inherent in the inclusion and eventual elimination of homosexuality as a mental health diagnosis are theories about the origins and causes of homosexuality. Drescher groups these theories into three types: *normal variation theories*, *pathology theories* and *immaturity theories*, as summarized in Table 24.1.

Theories of normal variation contain the assumption that homosexuality is a phenomenon that

Table 24.1 Theories about the origin of homosexuality, compared

Theory	Origin of Sexual Orientation	Implications for Psychopathology	Implications for Psychotherapy
Normal variation theories	Probably innate	Not a disorder	Psychotherapy needed by some, the same as some members of the population of majority sexual orientation
Pathology theories	Organic defect, inappropriate parenting hormone imbalance or trauma	Pathological	Needs to be "cured" if possible
Immaturity theories	A developmental phase that typically ends with maturity	Depends on individual's developmental level	Probably difficult to change

occurs naturally. Homosexuality is probably innate, just like left-handedness. Indeed, several authors intentionally offer the analogy of left-handedness because it was regarded as sinister in past eras, when children were often punished in school for writing with their left hands (Drescher, 2010). However, such superstitions about left-handedness have largely disappeared, as should, in the opinions of many, pathologization of homosexuality. In any case, if homosexuality falls within the range of the normal biological variation of the human species, there is no basis for considering it a mental disorder even if it is infrequent. The best-known historical figure associated with normal variation theories is Havelock Ellis (1859–1939), a well-known English physician and psychologist who authored the first English textbook on homosexuality, published in 1897 (Ellis and Symonds, 2008).

In contrast, pathology theories contain the idea that homosexuality is caused by some internal defect of the organism or by some pathogenic agent that causes the organism to malfunction. Such pathogenic agents could include inappropriate parenting, sexual abuse or intrauterine exposure to certain

hormones. Drescher observes that many people who harbor biases against homosexuals believe these pathological theories, either as the cause or the result of their prejudice. Writing at about the same time as Havelock Ellis' textbook appeared, German psychiatrist Richard von Krafft-Ebing described homosexuality as a degenerative disease. Homosexuality is grouped together in Krafft-Ebing's 1886 *Psychopathologia Sexualis* with sadomasochism and several forms of fetishism. Krafft-Ebing considered these conditions as both pathological and immoral, and this reflected his Catholic background and his attraction to Darwin's theory, which he interpreted as indicating that the purpose of sexual activity is procreation and, thence, the survival of the species (Rosario, 2002).

Finally, immaturity theories feature the assumption that homosexuality is a phase of human development that is not necessarily pathological when it first appears but that normally is outgrown. This was Freud's position, which he held emphatically, rebuking colleagues who argued that homosexuality was anything other than a very common aspect of normal human sexual development and rebuking anyone who would treat homosexuals with anything but compassion (Drescher, 2010). Freud expressed his views succinctly in a public letter to the mother of a young gay man in 1935. In that letter, Freud assured the mother that while homosexuality surely provides no advantage in life, it is nothing to be ashamed of. He responded to the mother that sexual orientation can be altered only rarely in psychoanalysis (Freud, 1951).

The influential American psychiatrist Harry Stack Sullivan incorporated similar ideas into his interpersonal theory of psychiatry (Sullivan, 1953). In that theory, same-sex relationships during adolescence, whether non-sexual or sexual to the extent of mutual masturbation, were seen as paving the way for males to enjoy healthy heterosexual relationships as adults (Sullivan, 1972). Sullivan even encouraged same-sex relationships among male employees of hospitals, which he felt would help them mature and express their desires more freely. Few readers of Sullivan's work when it was published in the mid-twentieth century were aware that Sullivan's views reflected not only his scientific observations but also his personal experience. It is now known that Sullivan, although he helped the US army develop methods for detecting homosexuality among its new recruits, enjoyed same-sex relationships in his private life (Wake, 2008).

In tracing the patterns of adherence to these three competing sets of theories, Drescher (2010) observes that Freud's views probably represented the opinions of most psychiatrists from the 1920s to the 1950s. With the decline of classic Freudianism and the emphasis on medical model thinking and taxonomies of mental illness, most psychiatrists then shifted to the belief that homosexuality is a disease.

The saga of "queer diagnoses" in DSM

Reflecting the belief common among psychiatrists of their time, homosexuality was listed as a disorder, indeed a "sociopathic personality disturbance," in the first edition of DSM-I, which appeared in 1952. In DSM-II, published in 1968, homosexuality was retained as a form of mental illness but reclassified as a "sexual deviation." As detailed in Drescher's (2010) review of the history of homosexuality, the social climate of the times began to change soon after that. Indeed, as early as the 1950s, psychological studies appeared that indicated that gay men and women are on the whole no more maladjusted than their heterosexual counterparts. The best-known of these studies was by Evelyn Hooker, a psychology professor at the University of California at Los Angeles. In an influential paper presented to the American Psychological Association in 1956 and published in 1957 (Hooker, 1957), Hooker reported on the Rorschach inkblot responses of gay and straight study participants, obtained with funding from the National Institute of Mental Health. The anti-psychiatry movement and the emerging gay rights movement targeted the stigmatization of gay people by the profession of psychiatry starting in the late 1960s. Street demonstrations in favor of gay rights were held in New York and other places, including the well-known Stonewall riot of 1969. In 1973, the Board of Trustees of the American Psychiatric Association voted for the declassification of homosexuality per se as a mental illness. That decision was ratified by the membership of the association, with 58 percent of the votes in favor. In deference to the substantial minority, the diagnosis "ego-syntonic homosexuality" – homosexuality that a person does not like – was adopted for the DSM-III, which appeared in 1980. However, by the time the text revision of DSM-III appeared in 1987, that diagnosis was eliminated. Since that time, the professional community has implicitly endorsed the natural, even though some right-wing political and religious groups in the United States and elsewhere still see homosexuality as a sickness.

It is important to define some of the terms that are used frequently in this literature and often confused; these definitions are articulated very clearly by Dragowski, Scharron-del Rio and Sandigorsky (2011). *Biological sex* refers to the anatomical and reproductive structures, usually based on the external genitalia present at birth. Although usage varies widely, the distinction between the terms "sex" and "gender" made in the American Psychological Association is widely used. *Sex* refers to biology and is used when biologically based differences are being discussed. *Gender*, in contrast, refers to culture and distinctions that relate primarily to societal factors or to socialization by parents or other caregivers (American Psychological Association, 2009). *Gender identity* refers to the individual's subjective sense of congruence with his or her biological sex. *Gender role* refers to the basic expectations in a society for how members of each biological sex should behave. *Transgender* is a broad term that refers to the adoption of behaviors and/or physical features of the biological sex that was not assigned to them at birth. *Transsexuals* are adults who sometimes transform their physical bodies to conform to the gender role that corresponds to their gender identities. Various terms have been proposed to describe children whose behavior does not correspond to the cultural norms for their biological sex, including *gender variant* and *gender non-conforming* (Diamond, 2002; Dragowski et al., 2011; Drescher, 2010). "Gender dysphoria" refers to dissatisfaction and distress about one's biological sex or biological identity; this is the title of the DSM-5 disorder that replaces the term "gender identity disorder" in the previous edition, the DSM-IV. *Sexuality* and *sexual orientation* refer to the gender identity of the persons toward whom an individual's sexual desires are directed. Sexual orientation can be *heterosexual* when a person is attracted to a member of the opposite sex/gender, *homosexual* if the attraction is toward members of the same sex/gender, or *bisexual*, if a person is attracted to members of any sex/gender.

Traditional cultural expectations are that children, adolescents and adults conform to the gender roles prescribed for their biological sex, develop gender identities consistent with their biological sex and be sexually attracted to members of the opposite sex. This happens in the overwhelming majority of the world's cultures. However, there are some North American Aboriginal tribes and some Pacific Island cultures that recognize and respect a special group of people of a given biological sex who assume gender identities and gender roles of the opposite sex, as will be discussed in greater detail later in this chapter (Newman, 2002; Vasey and Bartlett, 2007).

Sometimes a child may assume the gender identity and gender role of the biological sex opposite to the one assigned at birth. Should this continue into adulthood, the person may decide to live as a person of the opposite biological sex. It is important to note that this does not always happen and, as will be detailed later in this chapter, does not happen in the majority of cases in which a child adopts or wishes to adopt the gender identity opposite to his or her biological sex. As pointed out by Diamond (2002) and by Dragowski et al. (2011), it is a common stereotype among anti-gay groups that gay people engage in some form of transgendered behavior and want to be of the opposite sex. In fact, there are many gay men and boys who are very content with their male bodies and male gender identities and whose behavior and beliefs do not reflect gender non-conformity. This also occurs among many lesbian girls and women.

The political debate about gender variance in mental health nomenclature

Some scholars think that both gender variance and homosexuality were stigmatized in the same ways and for the same reasons. Once homosexuality was removed from the DSM, the argument goes, the stigma surrounding homosexuality dissipated. Hence, if gender dysphoria were to be removed from the DSM, stigma associated with gender variance – which may cause much of the dysphoria – would likely dissipate as well (e.g. Ault and Brzuzy, 2009; Drescher, 2010). Drescher (2010) argues that both homosexuality and gender variance were once condemned at least in part on the basis of biblical injunctions. Over time, religious law began to be less universally applied and was increasingly replaced by secular law, and biblical explanations of human and physical phenomena were gradually replaced by scientific and medical explanations. Rather than resulting in an acceptance of homosexuality and gender variance, this resulted in their criminalization and medicalization. Importantly, early proponents of pathology theories, including Krafft-Ebing, failed to differentiate between homosexuality and gender variance although it is by now abundantly clear that many if not most gay and lesbian people do not display gender variant behavior nor any degree of dysphoria about their gender identities.

Some critics and advocates believe that the inclusion of the various versions of "queer diagnoses" (i.e., ego-dystonic homosexuality, gender identity disorder and now gender dysphoria) in successive editions of the DSM has been merely a devious means of repathologizing homosexuality. In other words, the writers of various versions of the DSM have really wanted homosexuality to remain a disorder but have had no means of achieving this (Ault and Brzuzy, 2009).

It has been argued that whether or not gender variance or gender dysphoria are placed in the DSM as a means of pathologizing homosexuality, their presence in the official nosology necessarily reaffirms modern notions of normative gender and sexuality, which, in turn, engenders stigma and maltreatment (Ault and Brzuzy, 2009; Bockting and Ehrbar, 2006; Meyer-Bahlburg, 2010). To be fair, it must be noted that the DSM-5 Commission was in many ways sensitive to critics of previous versions. For example, the diagnosis of gender dysphoria in DSM-5 does not appear in the chapter on sexual disorders but in a chapter of its own. Many experts in the field applaud the addition of the distress criterion, meaning that gender variance without distress is not considered a disorder. Some critics wish that there was also a proviso that the distress constitutes a diagnostic criteria if the distress is not caused

by prejudice (De Cuypere, Knudson and Bockting, 2011). On a broader level, this entire issue raises doubt about the extent to which what is supposed to be an objective, science-based classification system is really a political instrument. Perhaps it is inevitable, however, that the delineation of normal and abnormal reflects, to a considerable extent, the values and norms of a society. If so, this could be acknowledged more candidly.

The pragmatic debate

Of considerable concern in the debate is the question of whether the diagnostic category of gender dysphoria helps or hinders recipients and possible recipients of the diagnosis. Critics note that retaining the diagnostic category increases the likelihood of inappropriate treatment for gender non-conforming individuals (Hill et al., 2007), although many of their arguments are more pertinent to adults than to children.

These criticisms have not gone unchallenged. Regarding concerns of stigma, it has been suggested that the stigma stems not from the fact that gender dysphoria is an official psychological disorder, but from gender non-conformity (Meyer-Bahlburg, 2010). To elaborate, it is not the abstract concept of psychological dysfunction that elicits ostracism, but, rather, the overt behaviors of individuals receiving the label that elicits this stigma (Zucker, 2006). If this is the case, one would expect to see stigma surrounding gender variance remain even if "queer diagnoses" were removed from the official nosology. Going even further, Zucker (2006) notes that receiving a diagnostic label can reduce stigma because it provides an explanation for otherwise incomprehensible behaviors. Even if stigma were to remain after any removal of the "queer diagnoses" from the DSM, argue Bockting and Ehrbar (2006), children displaying gender variant behaviors would still experience significant psychological and social difficulties. Professionals who advocate retention of the diagnosis insist that therapy can be very helpful in protecting children from ridicule and discrimination while fostering resilience (Bockting and Ehrbar, 2006). Relatedly, it has been noted that retaining these diagnostic categories increases access to treatment (Bockting and Ehrbar, 2006), including, in many places, permitting insurance coverage for the services some professionals see as needed (Bockting and Ehrbar, 2006; Meyer-Bahlburg, 2010).

There is no doubt that part of the reason for including gender dysphoria in DSM-5 is that many insurance companies in the United States will only pay for the treatment of recognized forms of illness. Clinical psychologists and other mental health professionals cannot always provide service to anyone experiencing distress, diagnosable or not. This evokes the question of whether the scientific community should be complicit in this. Hein and Berger (2013) argue that, if the purpose is to assist the child with gender dysphoria to function better as a transgendered person, this can or should be accomplished without a stigmatizing diagnosis. If, however, the purpose is to help the child with gender dysphoria move to gender conformity, insurance companies may well refuse to pay for the medical and psychological care involved, whether or not the care is addressed as a disorder.

The ontological debate

Ontology is the study of the nature of being and existence in reality. Applied to classification of mental illness, it can broadly be interpreted as the degree to which a disease entity actually exists and is more than a social construction, which is not to say that it is without social influence. This is perhaps the most pertinent debate within the current controversy.

Opponents to the retention of the diagnosis of gender dysphoria argue that the distress is not inherent to the disorder itself, which they see as part of the natural variation in human sexual functioning. They see the disorder as a consequence of society's reactions and beliefs (Ault and Brzuzy, 2009; Bockting and Ehrbar, 2006). There are a

small number of societies where this does not occur. For example, Vasey and Bartlett (2007) conducted a study of *fa'afafine* people of the Pacific island nation of Samoa. The *fa'afafine* are a group of individuals who are anatomically male but adopt stereotypically feminine gender roles and mannerisms. Some of these individuals self-identify as female but most self-identify simply as *fa'afafine*. The *fa'afafine* are well accepted and integrated within Samoan culture. Given this, Vasey and Bartlett (2007) studied the gender dysphoria within this group to obtain insight into the question of whether gender dysphoria within the West is inherent to the disorder. The authors studied whether *fa'afafine* people recalled strong and persistent cross-gender identification in childhood, a sense of inappropriateness with their male gender roles, gender dysphoria or distress regarding their gender identities. According to the results, many of the *fa'afafine* would not be diagnosed as having gender dysphoria using DSM-5 criteria, although they could have been diagnosed within the previous DSM-IV as having gender identity disorder (Vasey and Bartlett, 2007). Some *fa'afafine* participants reported that, on occasion, a parent or relative would display disapproval of their cross-gender behavior and this did cause distress. Many of the boys also reported dissatisfaction with their genitalia. Nevertheless, no participants reported severe or chronic distress as a result of their cross-gender behaviors or identities. Indeed, many participants indicated that they experienced a sense of extreme joy over their status as *fa'afafine* (Vasey and Bartlett, 2007). The Samoan case may be considered either as an aberrant exception to cultural trends around the world or as a convincing argument that gender dysphoria is more related to social sanctions than to anything else.

Although it constitutes an isolated case, perhaps the proverbial exception that proves the rule, the Samoan example suggests that a certain degree of gender variance may not be inherently distressing or dysfunctional. The problems that may lead children showing gender variance in large Western countries to other comorbid problems such as depression and school refusal may thus be symptoms not of any disorder internal to the child but symptoms of harassment and rejection on the part of the peer groups at school and in the community (Gray, Carter and Levitt, 2012; Meyer-Bahlburg 2010). Some critics suggest that this principle should be revisited to extricate "disorders" that are essentially the result of social stigma. This issue is not relevant to the inclusion of this disorder in the DSM as established by its developers because, as noted in Chapter 3, the DSM has become a taxonomy built on symptoms, not causes.

Perhaps the most important issue from an ontological standpoint is whether gender variance during childhood leads to maladaptive outcomes later on, even though any such maladaptive outcomes could be largely imposed by societal sanctions. There could indeed be some validity in delineating a cluster of symptoms as a disorder if it can be shown that the symptoms lead to maladaptation later in life. The long-term outcome of gender variance during the childhood years will be considered in greater detail later on in this chapter. The general picture emerging from longitudinal studies is that gender variation in children is not associated in the majority of cases with gender variation or gender dysphoria in adulthood. Childhood gender variance is, however, linked with adult homosexuality, which is not a pathological condition.

Proponents of retaining the diagnostic entity retort that gender dysphoria in itself is distressing (Bockting and Ehrbar, 2006) for reasons over and beyond whatever social stigma accompanies it. Therefore, the disorder gains legitimacy because it is not merely a response to social pressures. Behind this position is the argument that there is an inherent element of distress or dysfunction in living as a transgendered person. Doing so often involves a certain degree of stress regarding surgery and hormone treatment, neither of which is without side effects. Another inevitable source of stress is relating as a man to people with whom one has related as a woman, and vice versa. Proponents and opponents of this position duel about the quality of the empirical data illustrating the distress (Meyer-Bahlburg, 2002; Zucker, 2006). In any case, new instruments will have to be developed and new research conducted on stress among people with gender dysphoria using the new DSM-5 criteria.

Diagnostic criteria

The terminology used in the diagnostic criteria convey the degree to which the disorder was considered severe and serious at the time the diagnostic manual was written. In the mid-twentieth century, gender variance was often considered a very severe, pervasive mental illness, even a form of psychosis. This abated somewhat as professionals became aware of individuals who displayed gender variant behavior but who were very successful in life and, from all appearances, free of disturbance and distress (Meyer-Bahlburg, 2010). In essence, the criteria include a pronounced cross-gender identity associated with prolonged and marked distress. The DSM-5 Commission engaged in a long and tortuous debate about the fate of this category, chronicled by Kamens (2010). The initial recommendation was that the disorder be renamed "gender incongruence."

The DSM-5 Commission decided to relabel the disorder "gender dysphoria." It is not called a disorder although, indeed, it appears in a manual of disorders. The criterion of marked distress and impairment was added to those that were originally considered. The obvious parallel between this diagnostic label and the defunct condition of *ego-dystonic homosexuality* that entered and exited the nomenclature a generation ago is uncanny. The changes between the DSM-IV criteria for "gender identity disorder" and the DSM-5 criteria for "gender dysphoria" are summarized in Box 24.1.

Box 24.1 | **Differences between DSM-IV and DSM-5 criteria for gender dysphoria in children**

- In DSM-5, the name of the disorder has been changed from "gender identity disorder" to "gender dysphoria." In both DSM-IV and DSM-5, there must be a discrepancy between an individual's assigned gender and experienced gender.
- In both DSM-IV and DSM-5, the individual must experience significant distress based on the gender discrepancy.
- In both versions, the individual's desire to be of the opposite gender or insisting that he or she is of the opposite gender is mentioned. Optional in DSM-IV, this symptom is required in DSM-5.
- In addition, the individual must display at least five other symptoms. Symptoms include dressing in clothing usually associated with the other gender; taking on roles of the other gender in fantasy play; playing with toys usually associated with the other gender; preferring friends of the other gender; rejecting activities generally associated with the individual's gender; disliking one's sexual anatomy; and desiring that the sex characteristics would match the individual's experienced gender.
- In DSM-5, the term "sex" has been replaced by "gender." This change makes the criteria of gender dysphoria applicable to children with disorders of sex development, which are congenital conditions that involve sex characteristics developing in an atypical manner.
- In DSM-5, the specifier "with a disorder of sex development" (e.g., androgen insensitivity syndrome) has been added.

Source: DSM-5 and DSM-IV-TR consulted June 6, 2013.

CASE STUDY: A boy struggling with both gender identity and attachment issues

Michaud and Boivin (2009) present an interesting case of gender dysphoria in a 7-year-old adopted boy who also demonstrated problems in his attachment to his adoptive parents as well as marked opposition to their authority and that of his school. At the time the parents first sought professional help for their son, they mentioned that they had not specified at the time a preference for the sex of the child they wished to adopt. The boy was adopted at 16 months of age from the Asian region of Russia. When he first arrived at his adoptive home in Canada, he was reticent to form relationships, especially with male adults. Nevertheless, his adoptive father remained committed to including his new son in the family. As he learned to speak, the boy began to speak of himself as a girl. By the time he was 4 years old, he played mostly with girls. He wore make-up and borrowed items of his mother's clothing. He requested that his penis be replaced with a vulva. He kept asking his parents if he was a boy or a girl. At the same time, the boy began to display tantrums, argued constantly and became frustrated very easily. The boy was ostracized by his peers at school. When interviewed by the mental health worker who saw him at age 7, he recognized that he was a boy at that time but was unsure that he would remain a boy. Nevertheless, he had typical male fantasies of a future as a firefighter or police officer. The parents were quite tolerant of the boy's gender-variant behavior, neither encouraging it nor discouraging it. The mother used an affectionate nickname for her son, one that would have been appropriate for a very young girl. The interviewer's impression was that the mother was overly involved with her son. Michaud and Boivin concluded that a combination of gender identity, attachment and oppositionality issues were evident. The clinical team provided counseling to the parents regarding these issues, believing that some intervention with the boy around his attachment issues would be needed as well.

Prevalence

Prevalence data are not yet available for the DSM-5 diagnosis of gender dysphoria. There are some relevant studies based on the DSM-IV criteria for gender identity disorder. As noted by Zucker and Seto (2010), gender identity disorder has not been explored in large-scale epidemiological studies similar to those discussed in the earlier chapters on disorders that occur more frequently. As with all other conditions discussed in this book, there are problems in constructing an arbitrary dividing line between disordered and non-disordered, although the DSM and ICD systems require the professional to do so. The number of children referred for professional diagnosis of gender-variant behavior is very small. However, about 1 percent of children are rated in parent checklists as "behaving like a member of the opposite sex" whereas almost none are reported by their parents as wanting to be a member of the opposite sex. Boys referred to specialized clinics because of gender-variant behavior outnumber girls by at least 3:1 (van Beijsterveldt, Hudziak and Boomsma, 2006; Zucker, Bradley and Sanikhani, 1997; Zucker and Seto, 2010).

About one-half of children formally diagnosed as having gender identity disorder are also diagnosed as having some other mental disorder, about the same proportion as children with other clinical diagnoses such as ADHD (Wallien, Swaab and Cohen-Kettenis, 2007). Comorbid internalizing disorders, such as anxiety and depression, are more common than comorbid externalizing problems. However, although anxiety is intrinsically linked with gender identity disorder in some theoretical writings, the results of a recent study by Wallien et al. (2007) revealed that only about 30 percent of children diagnosed as having gender identity disorder also have anxiety problems at the level required for a DSM-IV diagnosis of anxiety disorder.

Possible causes and correlates

Genetics

The biological processes linked with sex/gender development are thought to begin at the time of conception and to be determined by sex chromosomes. In most cases, XX chromosomes lead to female biological sex and female gender identity whereas XY chromosomes are linked to male biological sex and male gender identity. Biological theories have been proposed to explain the minority of situations where the typical phenotypical pattern does not emerge; several biological processes have been implicated. It is important to note that this body of research is very small and flawed in many ways. One biological process that may be involved is atypical prenatal hormonal influences (Dragowski et al., 2011; Zucker and Seto, 2010). There may also be differences between people who do and do not display gender variance in terms of brain structure. Many post-mortem examinations of the brains of male-to-female transsexual adults reveal atypical volume in a portion of the stria terminalis, a brain area associated with sexual functioning (Dragowski et al., 2011; Zhou et al., 1995).

Several twin studies indicate fairly high rates of heritability (e.g., Coolidge, Thede and Young, 2004). The technology of molecular genetics appears not to have been applied to date to this condition (Zucker and Seto, 2010).

Temperament

In addition to the biological and environmental factors that may be associated with gender-variant behavior, there may be biological and environmental influences on the temperament type that some theorists believe to be associated with gender-variant behavior. Zucker and Bradley (2004) proposed that children who display gender-variant behavior tend to be anxious and overly sensitive to conflict in their environments, especially their home environments.

It is important to reiterate that the fact that there are genetic and environmental correlates of gender variance does not necessarily mean that it should be considered a disorder. There are of course genetic and environmental correlates of many human traits that are not pathological at all.

Family factors

Several patterns of family interaction and socialization by parents have been associated with gender variance among their children. Research on these family processes remains very limited. Possible pathways of family influence include the mother being bisexual; the father being absent or having limited interactions with his son, whom the father may be avoiding because of his effeminate behaviors; close bonds between a son and female members of his family; and a symbiotic relationship in which the mother needs the child as much as the child needs the mother. Parents who really wanted a daughter may reinforce feminine behaviors in their sons. In homes where there is extensive family conflict, parents who are preoccupied with their own problems may not attend to their child's psychosexual development (Coates, 1992; Dragowski et al., 2011; Meyer-Bahlburg, 2002; Zucker and Bradley, 2004).

Peer influence

Clinicians frequently report that children who display gender-variant behaviors are scorned, bullied and rejected by their peers. Peer rejection is known to occur for a variety of reasons that may vary according to the norms of the peer group doing the rejecting (Schneider, 2000). Rejection of effeminate boys is a prominent theme in the interviews of gender-variant children by Green (1976), whose longitudinal studies were influential in shaping professional thinking about gender variance. Such rejection may relate to children's expectations for gender constancy, which are known to be very strong among preschoolers as young as 3 years of age. As part of the process by which young children develop their own understanding of gender, they usually develop the expectation that people will always be of the same sex and gender and behave in ways that are socially sanctioned for their biological sex (Ruble et al., 2007). Although most research does confirm that children who display gender-variant behaviors tend to be rejected by their peers, an important nuance was added by a recent study conducted in the Netherlands. Wallien and colleagues (2010) were able to obtain sociometric measures from the classmates of twenty-eight boys and girls who were referred to a clinic that specializes in work with people with gender identity issues. Although the sociometric data did indicate overall peer rejection of the children who displayed gender-variant behavior, the rejection was mainly by same-sex classmates. In sharp contrast, classmates of the opposite sex tended to accept the children with gender-atypical behavior quite well.

Stability and prognosis

One important element in the decision as to whether
or not gender-variant behavior should be included
in the list of mental disorders is its long-term
prognosis. The landmark longitudinal study by
Green (1987), reported in a book tellingly entitled
*The Sissy Boy Syndrome and the Development of
Homosexuality* was conducted with forty-four boys
who displayed effeminate behaviors and a control
group of thirty other boys. The results indicated
that the boys identified as having gender identity
disorder tended not to display distress about their
gender identity in later life. However, 80 percent
turned out to be adults with either a homosexual
or bisexual sexual orientation. Although the exact
percentages vary, these results have essentially been
replicated in a number of other studies. For example,
in a recent longitudinal study conducted by Wallien
and Cohen-Kettenis (2008) with seventy-seven
boys and girls referred to a specialized clinic in the
Netherlands, almost all of the participants grew up
with a homosexual or bisexual sexual identity. Only
a minority (27%) still experienced dysphoric feelings
about their gender identities.

Treatment

As discussed earlier in this chapter, one of the
arguments advanced for retaining a diagnostic
category for gender-variant behavior is that it would
legitimize the provision of treatment, especially
in jurisdictions where a diagnosis is necessary for
treatment at public institutions or for payment by
insurance companies. For adults, the issue is quite
clear because gender-reassignment surgery is a
very complicated and expensive procedure that
many adults have found to be helpful. Children
and adolescents, however, do not receive gender-
reassignment surgery. Thus, if the diagnosis is to be
retained because it facilitates treatment, the question
arises as to what treatment might consist of if not
some effort at reducing gender-variant behavior.

Indeed, there have been such efforts, especially in the
1970s and 1980s, using the technology of behavior
therapy to reduce cross-gender behavior. In some
cases, the therapist would reinforce gender-typical
behavior during therapy sessions. Once it was found
that any change would not generalize to the child's
environment outside of therapy, such cognitive-
behavioral therapy techniques as self-monitoring
were introduced (Rekers and Varni, 1977; Zucker,
1985; Zucker and Seto, 2010). More recent attempts
at reducing cross-gender behavior have involved the
parents, with the therapist advising the parents on
how to "set limits" (Zucker, 2007; Zucker and Seto,
2010, p. 871) on the child's gender-variant behavior.
Some critics view this use of psychological science
in an attempt to alter what some see as part of the
natural range of sexual expression as paralleling the
"reparative therapy" used in previous years to change
homosexuality per se (Schope and Eliason, 2004), but
that is now condemned by professional associations
including the American Psychological Association.
It is only recently that some clinicians have begun to
advocate for a more supportive form of therapy that
would promote the child's adjustment while affirming
the child's gender-variant behavior (Menvielle and
Tuerk, 2002). Because the question as to whether
diagnosis leads to better treatment is so important in
resolving the status of gender variance as a mental
health disorder, it is highly unfortunate that there
are almost no treatment data to inform the decision.
Although there are some case reports documenting
what the therapists see as progress, there appear to be
no controlled studies and, certainly, no comparisons
of different treatment options and orientations
(Zucker and Seto, 2010).

Conclusion and future directions

This book closes with a chapter about a "disorder"
that is very different in many ways from the other
disorders in this book. Unfortunately, it is a condition
about which there has been very little research
but very heated polemics. The current debate

about the status of gender variance as a mental disorder evokes many of the age-old deliberations about what constitutes psychopathology. Many of these issues are debated not only in professional journals but also in the mass media. The history of the "queer diagnoses" illustrates that mental health professionals, powerful as they are in many ways, can and often do respond to the positions of advocacy groups and to the changing social climate. In the past half-century, many members of the educated public have become very aware of the advantages of diagnoses in terms of access to treatment and its cost in terms of stigma. This has led to the elimination of homosexuality from the diagnostic nomenclature. Time will tell if gender dysphoria will follow the same path. In any event, both accurate information and misinformation about child psychopathology have grown far beyond the confines of the professions that specialize in it. Furthermore, the professions that specialize in it are not, and probably never will be, insulated from the societies of which they are a part if not a pillar.

Summary

- The theories about the origins and causes of homosexuality can be grouped into three types: normal variation theories, pathology theories and immaturity theories.
- Theories of normal variation assume that homosexuality is a naturally occurring, innate phenomenon, falling within the range of normal biological variation of the human species.
- Pathology theories refer to the idea that homosexuality is an internal defect or a malfunction caused by a pathogenic agent, such as inappropriate parenting, sexual abuse or intrauterine hormone exposure.
- Immaturity theories describe homosexuality as a phase of human development that is not necessarily pathological, and may be outgrown.
- Throughout the earlier editions of the DSM, homosexuality was referred to as a sociopathic personality disturbance, form of psychosis or sexual deviation. Ego-dystonic homosexuality, or homosexuality that causes profound distress for the individual, was eliminated from the DSM-III-R in 1987. The professional community now implicitly endorses the natural variation theories.
- Biological sex refers to the anatomical and reproductive structures usually present at birth; sex refers to biologically based differences; and gender refers to sexual identity in the context of culture.
- Gender identity refers to the individual's subjective sense of congruence with his or her biological sex, whereas gender role refers to the basic expectations in a society for how members of each biological sex should act.
- Transgender refers to the adoption by an individual of behaviors and/or physical features of the biological sex that were not assigned to him/her at birth, while transsexuals are adults who transform their bodies to conform to their gender identities. Children whose behavior does not correspond to the cultural norms for their biological sex have been described as being gender-variant and gender non-conforming.
- Gender dysphoria occurs when one is dissatisfied or distressed about one's biological sex or gender identity. This is the term adopted in 2013 for DSM-5.
- Sexuality and sexual orientation refer to the gender identity of the persons toward whom an individual's sexual desires are directed. Orientations include heterosexual (opposite sex), homosexual (same sex) and bisexual (both sexes).
- Traditional cultural expectations in the majority of the world's cultures are that individuals conform to the gender roles prescribed for

their biological sex, develop consistent gender identities and be sexually attracted to people of the opposite sex.

- Similar to the removal of homosexuality, some scholars believe that removing gender dysphoria from diagnostic systems will ultimately reduce the stigma associated with these natural gender variations.

- The pragmatic debate argues that gender dysphoria should remain in the DSM for a number of reasons, most notably the fact that getting professional help may depend on a diagnosis.

- The ontological debate centers on the discussion of whether the disease actually exists or whether it is a social construction. On one side, those who wish to remove gender dysphoria from the DSM argue that the distress of the individuals is not inherent to the disorder itself, but instead a consequence of society's beliefs (see the case of the *fa'afafine* people of Samoa). These critics remark that the diagnosis of gender-identity disorder in DSM-IV was not predictive of late disorder.

- Gender variation in children is not associated in the majority of cases with gender variation or gender dysphoria later in life. However, it is linked to later homosexual behavior.

- Proponents of the diagnostic label of gender dysphoria point to the distress that often accompanies gender-variant behavior. They see this distress as inevitable and not exclusively caused by social stigma.

- The majority of children referred to specialized clinics because of gender-variant behavior are boys.

- Comorbid diagnoses are common, especially internalizing disorders, such as anxiety and depression.

- Atypical prenatal hormonal influences may be involved. Post-mortem examinations of male-to-female transsexual adults show atypical volume in a portion of the stria terminalis, a brain area associated with sexual functioning.

- Gender variance is very hereditable. However, more molecular genetics research needs to be conducted. Temperament may also be linked to gender variance: children who display gender-variant behavior tend to be anxious and overly sensitive to conflict.

- Possible pathways of family influence on gender-variant behavior include: a bisexual mother, an absent father, close son–female bonds in the family, an overly symbiotic relationship between mother and son and extensive family conflict.

- Children who display gender-variant behavior are often rejected by their peers. Some studies show that it is specifically same-sex peers that reject these children. Such rejection reinforces children's beliefs relative to gender constancy i.e., the expectation that people will always be of the same sex and behave in socially accepted ways.

- Proponents of the maintenance of gender dysphoria as a diagnosis insist that it facilitates treatment. However, little is known about how treatment might be delivered in ways that respect the child's wishes and decisions.

- Gender-reassignment surgery is often a fundamental component of the treatment for adults. Very little is known about how to help children struggling with gender identity issues.

Study questions

1. Remembering the basic definitions of psychopathology covered in Chapter 1, do you agree that gender dysphoria should be included among the classifications of mental disorder? Why or why not?

2. In your opinion, what is the most helpful and ethical intervention a psychologist can offer an adolescent referred for problems of gender variance?

GLOSSARY

12-step-based treatment: a treatment based on a set of guiding spiritual principles outlining a course of action for recovery from addiction, compulsion or other behavioral problems. Originally proposed by Alcoholics Anonymous (AA) as a method of recovery from alcoholism (The Free Dictionary, Farlex, n.d.).

Acceptance and commitment therapy: a form of psychotherapy based on the enhancement of awareness and acceptance by the individual of his/her internal events, feelings and experiences, be they positive or negative (Barcaccia, 2008).

Acculturation: the process of, by virtue of direct contact, assimilating the beliefs, ideas, customs, values and knowledges of another culture, typically after immigration.

Acetylcholine: a neurotransmitter secreted from the ends of neurons that functions as the main chemical messenger for motor neurons in the peripheral nervous system, including the autonomic nervous system, and as a significant neurotransmitter in the central nervous system, functioning to excite skeletal muscles and to inhibit cardiac muscle (Colman, 2009).

Adaptive functioning: a person's ability to manage the routines of daily living and to interact socially with others.

Additive model: model explaining how having aggressive friends leads to the development and maintenance of aggression with the negative influence of an aggressive friend occurring independently of any other risk factor.

Adventure therapy: therapy designed to help adolescents overcome their emotional and behavior problems by overcoming the challenges inherent in living in the wilderness.

Affectionate control: parental style in which some overcontrolling parents dominate in ways that convey affection and even overindulgence.

Affectionless control: parental style in which some overcontrolling parents dominate in ways that are devoid of warmth and affection.

Agoraphobia: a phobia or cluster of phobias associated with anxiety or fear of leaving home, being in a crowd, visiting public places such as shopping areas, traveling alone in buses, trains or aircraft, or being in other situations from which escape might be awkward or where a panic attack would be difficult to handle (Colman, 2009).

Alleles: slightly different versions of the same gene.

Allodynamic control: a perspective on the regulation of physiological responses to relevant stimuli (e.g., challenges, threats, rewards) that emphasizes the functional utility of flexibility and variability. A notable difference from earlier models of homeostatic regulation is that allodynamic control does not assume there is one constant set point of arousal that is optimal or to which physiological systems are always trying to return. Following reactivity to a stimulus, adaptive and appropriate recovery might entail reaching a new balance of parasympathetic and sympathetic enervation of the body.

Ambulatory biosensors: unobtrusive devices carried by people undergoing assessment in their natural environments. They are used to measure cardiovascular, physical and/or chemical activity.

Amygdala: an almond-shaped mass of gray matter in the front part of the temporal lobe of the cerebrum that is part of the limbic system involved in the processing and expression of emotions, especially anger and fear (The American Heritage Science Dictionary, from The Free Dictionary, Farlex, n.d.).

Analytic intelligence: involved when the components of intelligence are applied to analyze, evaluate, judge or compare and contrast. It typically is involved in dealing with relatively familiar kinds of problems where the judgments to be made are of a fairly abstract nature (Sternberg and Kaufman, 2011).

Androgen: a male sex hormone.

Anorexia nervosa: a disorder marked by a severe and prolonged refusal to eat with severe weight loss, amenorrhea or impotence, disturbances of body image, and an intense fear of becoming obese. Most frequently encountered in girls and young women (Bhatia, 2009).

Anterior cingulate cortex (ACC): the upper frontal part of the cingulate gyrus, implicated in decisions between competing responses, language processing and monitoring of performance. It shows activity when a person experiences social exclusion or distress (Colman, 2009).

Anti-social personality disorder: a disorder characterized by the inability to get along with other members of society and by repeated conflicts with individual persons and groups. Common attributes include impulsiveness, egocentricity, hedonism, low frustration tolerance, irresponsibility, inadequate conscience development, exploitation of others and rejection of authority and discipline (Bhatia, 2009).

Applied behavioral analysis (ABA): an intervention based on functionally assessing the relationship between a targeted behavior and the environment, then using the methods of ABA to change that behavior (The Free Dictionary, Farlex, n.d.).

Appraisal support: social support that involves the transmission of information in the form of affirmation, feedback and social comparison (European Union Public Health Information System, www.euphix.org).

Arbitrary discipline: discipline that is *not* predictable *or* appropriate to the child's age or personality, and which may be inconsistent (Hoffman, 1983).

Arrested socialization hypothesis: first developed by Patterson (1982), states that children and adolescents who are arrested in development lack a variety of self-regulatory skills needed for successful interpersonal relationships.

Artifactual hypothesis: common explanation of the manner in which DSM and ICD systems are flawed – due to the introduction of many categories which do not truly represent the distinct disease entities.

Asperger's syndrome: a condition listed in the previous DSM-IV as a separate disorder consisting of atypical, idiosyncratic patterns of language usage and social interaction.

Attachment theory: a theory according to which an infant has an inborn biological need for close contact with the mother (or other main caregiver), in a normal bond developing within the first 6 months of life through the mother's responsiveness (Colman, 2009). This bond determines the internal working model that underlies the child's subsequent close relationships with others.

Atypical antipsychotics: a group of antipsychotic tranquilizing drugs used to treat psychiatric conditions. Some atypical antipsychotics are FDA-approved for use in the treatment of schizophrenia. Some are approved for acute mania, bipolar depression, psychotic agitation, bipolar maintenance and other indications, mostly in adults. However, many physicians also prescribe atypical antipsychotics for children with bipolar disorder, sometimes in combination with other drugs.

Atypical behavior: unusual or irregular behavior.

Atypical development: unusual or irregular development.

Auditory cortex: the cortical area that receives auditory information from the medial geniculate body (The Free Dictionary, Farlex, n.d.).

Authoritarian parents: parents who are highly demanding but not responsive to their children, expecting obedience without explanation (Baumrind, 1991; Socolar, 1997).

Authoritative parents: parents who are demanding of their children but also very responsive to them (Socolar, 1997). They are assertive, but not intrusive and restrictive, and use disciplinary methods that are supportive rather than punitive (Baumrind, 1991).

Authority-conflict pathway: pathway along which children begin exhibiting stubbornness and disobedience before age 12 and continue along those lines to more brazen acts of defiance to authority later on.

Autism spectrum disorder: a pervasive neurodevelopmental disorder characterized by gross and sustained impairment of social interaction and communication; restricted and stereotyped patterns of behavior, interests and activities; and abnormalities manifested before age 3 in social development, language acquisition or play. Also called autism, childhood autism, infantile autism, Kanner's syndrome (Colman, 2009).

Autonomic space: a model of autonomic control that incorporates the possibilities for independent, reciprocal or concurrent activation of target organs by the sympathetic and parasympathetic branches of the autonomic nervous system. The extent of activity change in a target organ (e.g., increased or decreased heart rate) depends on combined influences of sympathetic and parasympathetic activation.

Avoidant attachment: type of insecure attachment that occurs when an intimate bond between child and caregiver fails to emerge in the first place.

Axon: elongated extension of a neuron that conducts impulses away from the cell body and toward the synaptic terminals (Grand, 2008).

Baseline: period in which a stable and reliable level of performance is assessed that can be used as a basis for evaluating changes in behavior caused by the introduction of an independent variable (Bhatia, 2009).

Behavioral activation system (BAS): system which motivates the drive to attain rewards, and thus is responsible for activating approach behavior in response to cues that desirable things are available, and also for activating avoidant behaviors when there are cues that punishment might occur but could be escaped. Particularly important in behavior disorders, ADHD and anxiety.

Behavioral assessment: type of psychological assessment, in which, applying the principles of the learning theory, the conditions in the child's environment are assessed in order to find those that sustain the problem behavior (Belloch, Sandín and Ramos, 2008).

Behavioral inhibition system (BIS): system that triggers the drive to avoid loss and harm and thus is responsible for inhibiting ongoing behaviors in the presence of cues that suggest punishment is imminent, or that rewards are not available to be obtained. Particularly important in behavior disorders, ADHD and anxiety.

Behavioral inhibition: the consistent display of fearfulness and withdrawal, especially in unfamiliar situations.

Bidirectional manner: reciprocal influence of child's and parent's behavior.

Bidirectionality of influence: moving or operating in two opposite directions (The Free Dictionary, Farlex, n.d.). In psychopathology, this expression often refers to the influences of both the child's problem on parents' practices and the influence of the parents' practices on the child's problem.

Binge-eating disorder: a condition characterized by recurrent episodes of binge eating, with similar signs and symptoms to bulimia nervosa but without the compensatory behavior intended to prevent weight gain, such as self-induced vomiting, misuse of laxatives or diuretics, enemas, fasting or excessive exercise (Colman, 2009).

Biological sex: the anatomical and reproductive structures, usually based on the external genitalia present at birth.

Biopsychosocial: general model that posits that biological, psychological and social factors all play a significant role in human functioning in the context of disease or illness. Health is best understood in terms of a combination of biological, psychological and social factors rather than purely in biological terms (Santrock, 2007).

Bipolar depression or manic depression: other terms for bipolar disorder, which is characterized by recurrent episodes of depression, often alternating with periods of mania.

Bipolar disorder: a disorder characterized by fluctuations in mood, with manic episodes or mixed episodes and usually major depressive episodes.

Bisexual: sexually attracted to both men and women (Butterfield, 2003).

Bottom-up procedure: a method of building classifying schemes by clustering data about individual diagnoses into categories, often using such statistical procedures as factor analysis (the opposite of a top-down procedure, in which the categories are specified first, with the diagnostic data then fitted to the categories).

Broad-band attachment theory: an interpretation of attachment theory in which it is maintained that early attachment predicts a wide range of cognitive, affective and behavioral processes.

Bulimia: an eating disorder, common especially among young women of normal or nearly normal weight, that is characterized by episodic binge eating and followed by feelings of guilt, depression and self-condemnation. It is often associated with measures taken to prevent weight gain, such as self-induced vomiting, the use of laxatives, dieting or fasting (Morris, 2000).

Categorical models: type of model for classifying disorders of childhood, made up of categories, in which the diagnostician can only indicate the total absence or presence of a problem condition, not the degree to which an individual's problems correspond to the condition.

Categorical-dimensional or mixed models: hybrid models, combining both categorical and dimensional aspects, in which a subject is usually first assessed in a qualitative or categorical way, recognizing the subject's most representative traits, and secondly in a dimensional or quantitative way, representing different grades of clinical relevance (Belloch et al., 2008).

Catharsis theory: a theory according to which it is therapeutic for a person to release strong, pent-up emotions or tensions and/or to bring long-repressed material to consciousness.

Causal model: model according to which the peer-relations deficits themselves are at the root of subsequent processes that terminate in a diagnosable mental health problem.

Central nervous system (CNS): the part of the nervous system that in humans and other vertebrates comprises the brain and spinal cord (Colman, 2009).

Challenge study: study in which researchers intentionally give subjects/patients pharmacological agents in order to induce and study psychiatric symptomatology (Hope and McMillan, 2004).

Children-of-twins design: design that permits the researcher to separate the developmental effects of co-occurring genetic and environmental factors, using control groups that vary in genetic and environmental risk.

Chromosome: thin DNA molecule that consists of two parallel, intertwined chains of molecular building blocks.

Chronosystems: system that represents changes over time in micro-, meso- and macrosystems.

Chumship: in early adolescent years, a close friendship that will prepare for satisfying intimate romantic relationships later on.

Cingulate gyrus: a gyrus within the longitudinal fissure above and almost surrounding the corpus callosum. It is part of the limbic system and is involved in pain sensations, control of visceral responses associated with emotions and the planning of motor actions. Also called the cingulate cortex (Colman, 2009).

Circadian cortisol levels: variations in cortisol levels caused by the everyday cycle of biological activity occurring over a 24-hour period and influenced by variation in the environment, including change between night and day, is called the circadian rhythm. These variations themselves vary from individual to individual.

Client-centered framework: a form of non-directive psychotherapy, created by Carl Rogers, focusing on the patient's thoughts and feelings, which the therapist helps to clarify, using empathy and understanding. Considered more humanistic, this process was created in response to the authoritativeness and interpretation common in more traditional psychotherapies.

Clique: small, exclusive, informal group of people (www.merriam-webster.com/dictionary/clique).

Closed–field or **analogue**: structured observations in which interactions can be more easily observed and recorded. These situations may feature dyadic interaction or group interaction and, like observations in the natural environment, are valuable measures of social performance. Sometimes they require the participation of experimental confederates, and coding systems are used to classify the targeted behaviors (Nangle et al., 2010).

Coactivation: refers to increased sympathetic and parasympathetic action (El-Sheikh et al., 2009).

Coalitions: alliances between members of the family in which some members habitually side with each other in opposition to other family members.

Coercion: the action or practice of persuading someone to do something by using force or threats (Stevenson, 2010).

Coercive discipline: discipline in which parents take advantage of their strength and positions of authority.

Coercive sequences: repeated and correlated coercion actions in child–parent interaction. The child may annoy the parent who "natters" (nags), starting an escalating vicious circle leading often to DBD.

Cognitive-behavior therapy (Cognitive-behavioral therapy): a type of psychological therapy derived from behavior therapy, modified to take the patient's cognition into consideration. It is designed to change both maladaptive beliefs and maladaptive behaviors.

Cognitive-hyphen-behavioral treatments: Meichenbaum's expression that describes Lewinsohn's approach to cognitive-behavioral therapy, in which many complementary behavioral components such as relaxation training, direct instruction in social skills, or working on the client's schedule of pleasant activities are added.

Cohesive families: families in which relationships between members are warm and supportive; there are clear but flexible boundaries that permit access to resources and support by children.

Coinhibition: refers to decreased action of both sympathetic and parasympathetic systems (El-Sheikh et al., 2009).

Collateral model: model to explain how having aggressive friends leads to the maintenance of, or increase in, aggression. The friend does not influence aggression; it is the pre-existing proclivity toward aggression in the child or adolescent that results in *both* the aggression and the selection of an aggressive friend.

Comorbidity: medical term, introduced by Feinstein (1970), referring to the co-existence of more than one illness, be they physical, mental or both; the simultaneous presence of two chronic diseases or conditions in a patient (Stevenson and Lindberg, 2010).

Complete genome scan: systematic scan of a fixed number of genes on each chromosome across the complete sets of DNA of many people to find genetic variations associated with a particular trait.

Computerized tomography (CT): also called computerized axial tomography. A system of examining the body in which a narrow x-ray beam, guided by a computer, photographs a thin section of the body or of an organ from several angles, using the computer to build up an image of the section (Collin, 2007).

Conduct disorder: a childhood disorder characterized by anti-social behavior. The conduct disorders include undersocialized, aggressive and non-aggressive, and socialized aggressive and non-aggressive (Bhatia, 2009).

Confrontive discipline: discipline that involves reasoning with the child, and that can be implemented with different degrees of directness and firmness.

Cortisol: a corticosteroid hormone belonging to the glucocorticoid group secreted into the bloodstream by the adrenal cortex in response to adrenocorticotrophic hormone (ACTH) secreted by the anterior pituitary, especially in response to stress or injury, switching the body from carbohydrate to fat metabolism, regulating blood pressure and having powerful anti-inflammatory effects. The amount of cortisol (and also adrenalin or epinephrine and noradrenaline or norepinephrine) in the blood or urine is sometimes used as a measure of stress (Colman, 2009).

Cortisol awakening response (CAR): an increase of about 50 percent in cortisol levels that may occur shortly after awakening in the morning. Thought to be linked to the hippocampus' preparation of the hypothalamic-pituitary-adrenal axis (HPA) in the presence of anticipated stress.

Cost–benefit analysis: a method of measuring the usefulness of a proposal in terms of the ratio of current benefits to current costs, in order to choose the option with the highest net benefit.

Covert pathway: pathway of escalation toward disruptive behavior, marked by sneaky anti-social behaviors before age 15, leading to property damage and then to moderate to serious juvenile delinquency.

Creative intelligence: manifested while discovering, inventing, dealing with novelty and creating (Gardner, 1993).

Cross-sectional study: The study of a relatively large and diverse group of people at a single point in time (Statt, 2003).

Cue detection: how observers use predictive contextual information to facilitate the detection and identification of visual objects in complex scenes (Bayne, Axel Cleeremans and Wilkin, 2009).

Culture: basic features of different societies and the values and beliefs of their members.

Cybertherapy (syn. computer-based therapy; computer-assisted therapy): a modality in which electronic communication is used to provide all or part of the therapeutic counselling.

Cyclical attractor: phenomenon in which two friends get stuck in talking about deviance, which becomes a predominant feature of their conversations.

Demandingness: a dimension in Baumrind's model describing the levels of competence or effort parents require from children.

Dendrite: slender filaments projecting from the cell body of a nerve cell or neuron. They receive incoming messages from many other nerve cells and send them to the cell body. If the combined effect of these messages is strong enough, the cell body will send an electrical impulse along the axon. The tip of the axon passes its message to the dendrites of the nerve cells (ebrary Inc., 2005).

Developmental cognitive neuroscience: discipline which emphasizes the ontogenesis, or progressive construction, of neural structures that support cognitive capacities (Johnson et al., 2005).

Developmental delay: a noticeable lag in the development, physical or mental, of children relative to their peers.

Developmental epidemiological framework: an integration of the life course developmental orientation with community epidemiology. Joined with experimental preventive trials directed at specific risk antecedents, it provides a scientific framework for testing the etiological role of the targeted antecedent as well as the efficacy of the experimental intervention (Kellam and Van Horn, 1997).

Developmental traumatology model: systemic investigation of the psychiatric and psychobiological impact of overwhelming and chronic interpersonal violence (child maltreatment) on the developing child (Bellis et al., 2001).

Deviance regulation theory: a behavioral decision theory relevant to the maintenance of desirable identities. The theory predicts that actions translate into meaningful identities to the extent that they cause the individual to deviate from reference group norms (Blanton and Christie, 2003).

Deviant talk: conversation in which deviant behavior is legitimized and encouraged by laughing or otherwise reinforcing the remarks of their friends.

Dexamethasone suppression test (DST): a diagnostic procedure in which dexamethasone is injected, and then the degree to which cortisol secretion into the bloodstream has been suppressed is measured. Cortisol secretion will not be suppressed in patients with Cushing's syndrome (overactivity of the adrenal glands) or in some patients with severe depression, melancholia, anorexia nervosa and bulimia nervosa.

Diathesis-stress models: a psychological theory that explains behavior as both a result of biological and genetic factors ("nature"), and life experiences ("nurture"). This theory is often used to describe the pronunciation of mental disorders that are produced by the interaction of a vulnerable hereditary predisposition, with precipitating events in the environment (Zubin and Spring, 1977).

Difficult temperament: describes children who are slow to adapt to change, likely to react negatively and intensely.

Dimensional model: conception of psychopathology and/or classification scheme consisting of dimensions of maladjustment. An individual can be considered closer to the adaptive or maladaptive pole of each dimension. There are not discrete single cutting points that differentiate between diagnosable and non-diagnosable conditions. Dimensional models are the major alternative to categorical models.

Disease: a disorder with a specific cause (which may or may not be known) and recognizable signs and symptoms; any bodily abnormality or failure to function properly, except that resulting directly from physical injury (the latter, however, may open the way for disease) (Martin, 2010).

Disengaged families: families characterized by rigid boundaries and cold, unsupportive relationships among family members.

Disinhibited social engagement disorder: a disorder in which a child reacts to changes in caregiver, child neglect or abuse with an inappropriate loss of the fear of strangers. The child may become excessively familiar with strangers or may become excessively willing to go off with them.

Disorder: in the context of psychological problems, signifies "an illness that disrupts normal physical or mental functions" (Simpson and Weiner, 1989).

Disorder of written expression: a learning disability characterized by substantially below-average writing skills for the given age, intelligence and education, interfering substantially with scholastic or academic achievement or everyday life and not being due merely to a sensory deficit (Colman, 2009).

Disorganized or **controlling attachment:** occurs when a child displays an inconsistent pattern of behavior when separated from the parent, wavering between ambivalent and avoidant styles.

Disruptive mood dysregulation disorder: a disorder introduced in DSM-5 characterized by severe recurrent temper outbursts in response to common stressors. The temper outbursts are manifest verbally and/or behaviorally, such as in the form of verbal rages, or physical aggression toward people or property. The reaction is grossly out of proportion to any provocation and is usually inconsistent with the individual's developmental level.

Dizygotic twins: twins that develop from two separate eggs that are fertilized by two separate sperm.

DNA: Deoxyribonucleic acid.

DNA methylation: a chemical process that leads to changes in the epigenetic code.

Dopamine: neurotransmitter, an intermediate in the formation of adrenalin. There are special nerve cells (neurons) in the brain that use dopamine for the transmission of nervous impulses. One such area of dopamine neurons lies in the basal ganglia, a region that controls movement. Another dopamine area is the limbic system, a region closely involved with emotional responses (ebrary Inc., 2005).

Dorsolateral prefrontal cortex (DLPFC): according to a more restricted definition, is roughly equivalent to a region of the brain labeled Brodmann areas 9 and 46. According to a broader definition DLPFC consists of the lateral portions of Brodmann areas 9–12, of areas 45, 46 and the superior part of area

47. Dopamine plays a particularly important role in DLPFC. DLPFC is connected to the orbitofrontal cortex, and to a variety of brain areas, which include the thalamus, parts of the basal ganglia, the hippocampus and primary and secondary association areas of neocortex. DLPFC serves as the highest cortical area responsible for motor planning, organization and regulation. It plays an important role in the integration of sensory and mnemonic information and the regulation of intellectual function and action. It is also involved in working memory (The Free Dictionary, Farlex, n.d.).

Double-bind theory: the view that contradictory messages or conflicting demands can induce severe stress and even schizophrenia in an individual. Used especially in cases of a dependent relationship, such as that between child and parent, where the child can neither resolve nor escape the psychological dilemmas of the situation (Statt, 2003).

Double-blind study: research design such that both the experimenter and the research participant will be unaware of which experimental treatment has been applied to which individuals, until after the data have been collected. This design allows studies to control for experimenter effects and the influence of demand characteristics. Double-blind studies are used in drug trials, for example, often with a placebo, in order to prevent contamination resulting from biases or preconceptions of the experimenter or subjects.

Down's syndrome: a condition resulting from a chromosomal abnormality most commonly due to the presence of three copies of chromosome 21 (trisomy 21), which is most likely to occur with advanced maternal age. Down's syndrome can also occur as a result of chromosomal rearrangement (translocation) and as part of a mosaicism, which are not related to maternal age (Martin, 2010).

Dual diagnosis: Presence of more than one disorder in a person's symptoms. Used most often to describe the comorbidity of intellectual disability and an emotional or behavioral problem. See comorbidity.

Dual pathway model: model of bulimia which proposes that dietary restraint and negative affect combine as pathways in the development of bulimia (Duemm, Adams and Keating, 2003).

Dynamic cascade model: model to describe how parenting and peer relations affect each other reciprocally over time, according to which, while their children are very young, some parents may be harsh in their discipline and relate to their children without emotional warmth. For that reason, the children fail to develop the social and cognitive skills needed to relate to others.

Dyscalculia: reduced ability to solve mathematical problems, typically as a result of presumed brain dysfunction.

Dyslexia: impairment in reading ability. Dyslexia is usually diagnosed when difficulty in learning to read is clearly not due to inadequate intelligence, brain damage or emotional problems (Sterns, 2008).

Easy temperament: describes children who adjust well to new situations, adapt well to new routines and are cheerful and easy to calm.

Ego-dystonic homosexuality: a controversial term in the old DSM-III for a sexual preference that is experienced as ego-dystonic, i.e., distressing and unacceptable to the individual.

Electrodermal activity: changes in the electrical resistance or conductance of the skin's surface due to changes in perspiration by the eccrine sweat glands, usually measured on the palm or fingers.

Electrodermal response (EDR): technique by which sensors monitor the skin's electrical resistance to treat anxiety disorders, chronic pain, hyperhidrosis and stress. Also called electrodermal activity therapy (Jonas, 2005).

Electroencephalogram: a chart on which the electrical impulses in the brain are recorded (Collin, 2007).

Emotion: at the most basic level, subjective feelings which have positive or negative value for the individual. Theories vary in defining emotion beyond this. Current theories typically consider emotion a psychological response paired with a cognitive evaluation of the situation.

Empowerment movement: a mental health promotion strategy of the 1980s and 1990s that accepted, as a first principle, that individuals in society are able and responsible for taking control of their lives, which means taking control of their mental health (Stark, 1992).

Endogenous disorders: disorders located or originating within the individual.

Endophenotype: a component part of a broad or complex phenotype. The concept was introduced in 1966 by population geneticists B. John and K. R. Lewis to refer to microscopic and internal phenotypes that are not apparent to the casual observer; since then it has been applied in medicine and psychiatry in efforts to unravel the genetic and physiological basis of multifactorial diseases, such as schizophrenia and heart disease. An endophenotype is thus a measurable and genetically determined aspect of a "bigger picture." For example, cortisol secretion is an endophenotype of anxiety. Similarly, in evolutionary biology, complex traits, such as behaviors, can be regarded as the net result of the assembly of various modular endophenotypes (Martin and Hine, 2008).

Enmeshed families: families in which relationships between some of the members become entangled and stifling. Children may receive some affection and support, but in order to do so, they have to give up much of their autonomy and ally themselves with one subsystem in its hostility to another subsystem (Minuchin, 1974).

Environment-centered studies: studies which aim indirectly at changing individuals by changing the environments in which they live and work.

Epigenetic code or **epigenome:** the complete pattern of tissue-specific gene-activation in an individual.

Equifinality: a principle indicating that different early experiences (e.g., parental divorce, physical abuse, parental substance abuse) can lead to similar outcomes (e.g., childhood depression) (The Free Dictionary, Farlex, n.d.).

Era effects: effects in research caused by the particular circumstances of the historical period when the study took place.

Errorless: behavioral methods featuring analysis of the reinforcement patterns at work in the setting in which the behavior occurs, which are modified using positive reinforcement for appropriate behavior exclusively (Ducharme, 2008).

Ethnotypic consistency: describes the assumption that what is referred to as the same disorder (e.g., depression or attention deficit) is actually very much the same in different cultures.

Eugenics movement: movement beginning in the nineteenth century as an attempt at primary intervention, consisting of the study of hereditary improvement of the human race by controlled selective breeding (Morris, 2000).

Event-related potential (ERP): electrical activity produced by the brain in response to a sensory stimulus or associated with the execution of a motor, cognitive or psychophysiological task (Bhatia, 2009).

Executive functions: a collection of brain processes that are responsible for planning, cognitive flexibility, abstract thinking, rule acquisition, initiating appropriate actions and inhibiting inappropriate actions, and selecting relevant sensory information (The Free Dictionary, Farlex, n.d.).

Experience-sampling techniques: recording in "real time" such events as: (a) the frequency and patterning of daily activity, social interaction and changes in location; (b) the frequency, intensity and patterning of psychological states, that is, emotional, cognitive and conative dimensions of experience; and c) the frequency and patterning of thoughts, including quality and intensity of thought disturbance.

Exposure hierarchy: used in the behavior therapy of phobias. A hierarchy of fears (increasingly fearful stimuli) is assembled. Patients expose themselves to a single level of the hierarchy, until habituation occurs, after which the patient proceeds to the next highest level of the hierarchy. Ultimately the patient will be able to cope with the feared object or situation.

Face validity: the degree to which a procedure or psychological test seems to be relevant to the variable it is dealing with. Not necessarily the true validity of a test, only the appearance of validity.

Facilitated communication: a method in which a facilitator supports the hand or arm of a communicatively impaired individual while using a keyboard or other devices with the aim of helping the individual to develop pointing skills and to communicate (The Free Dictionary, Farlex, n.d.).

False negatives: diagnostic errors in which cases that should have been diagnosed with a particular disorder are in fact missed.

False positives: diagnostic errors in which individuals that are diagnosed with a particular disorder do not really have it.

Family sculpture: family intervention technique to gain and deliver insight about the structure of relationships within the family system (Duhl et al., 1973). Each family member is asked to create a physical "sculpture" of what the family might look like by directing the family members to position themselves in the ways that represent their roles.

Family therapists: therapists practicing family therapy, a form of psychotherapy based on the assumption that psychological problems are often rooted in and sustained by family relationships, in which two or more members of a family participate simultaneously (Colman, 2009).

Faulty attributions of intent: maladaptive thinking of children with disruptive behavior disorder. In a social situation where the intentions of an individual are not really clear, children with DBD are more likely than others to believe that another person intends to harm them (Dodge and Frame, 1982; Milich and Dodge, 1984).

Fear: a primitive, intense emotion in the face of threat, real or imagined, which is accompanied by physiological reactions resulting from arousal of the sympathetic nervous system and by a defensive pattern of behavior associated with avoidance, fight or concealment (Bhatia, 2009).

Fearlessness theory: attributes disruptive behavior disorders to deficits in the regulation of emotions. According to this theory, activity of both neuroendocrinological and autonomic systems is attenuated in these children; therefore, they do not perceive the somatic cues that would otherwise lead them to alter their course of action in risky situations.

Feeble-minded: an obsolescent term for mild intellectual disability (Colman, 2009).

Feeding disorder of infancy or early childhood: an eating disorder with onset before 6 years of age characterized by a persistent failure to eat adequately, leading to significant weight loss over an extended period, the behavior not being attributable to a gastrointestinal or other medical condition or lack of available food (Colman, 2009).

Fight–or–flight response: first described by Walter Bradford Cannon, this is the biological and behavioral reaction of animals to threats or challenges. Biologically, it entails increased activity in the two main stress response and regulation systems, the hypothalamic-pituitary-adrenal (HPA) axis and the sympathetic-adrenomedullary (SAM) system, decreased parasympathetic activity and numerous changes in central nervous system activity. These prime the animal for the behavioral response of fighting or fleeing. In the evolution of the human species, fight was manifested in aggressive, combative behavior against challengers, and flight was manifested by fleeing potentially dangerous situations, such as being confronted by a predator. In current times, these biological responses persist, but fight and flight responses have assumed a wider range of behaviors (The Free Dictionary, Farlex, n.d.).

Forebrain: the front part of the brain, divided into the telencephalon and diencephalon. It includes the cerebral hemispheres, thalamus, hypothalamus and associated structures. Also called the prosencephalon, especially in a developing embryo (Colman, 2009).

Formative evaluation: evaluation based on the examination of the delivery of the program or technology, the quality of its implementation, and the organizational processes and communication among the people involved (Putnam, 2008).

Fragile X syndrome: the most frequent inherited cause of intellectual disability, in which an easily damaged X chromosome has a tip hanging by a narrow thread; it is often accompanied by attention deficit/hyperactivity disorder, and other characteristics including enlarged head, long face, prominent ears and (in males) enlarged testicles (Colman, 2009).

Frontal lobes: area in the brain located at the front of each cerebral hemisphere and positioned anterior to the parietal lobes and superior and anterior to the temporal lobes. The frontal lobe contains most of the dopamine-sensitive neurons in the cerebral cortex. The executive functions of the frontal lobes involve the ability to recognize future consequences resulting from current actions, to choose between good and bad actions, override and suppress unacceptable social responses, and determine similarities and differences between things or events (The Free Dictionary, Farlex, n.d.).

Functional magnetic resonance imaging (fMRI): a type of magnetic resonance imaging that measures the increased hemodynamic response seen with neural activity in the brain or spinal cord. fMRI has allowed major advances in brainmapping (i.e., matching sections of the brain with particular behaviors, thoughts or emotions) (Martin, 2010).

Fusiform face area (FFA): a part of the human visual system which might be specialized for facial recognition, although there is some evidence that it also processes categorical information about other objects, particularly familiar ones (The Free Dictionary, Farlex, n.d.).

Gender: sexual identity, especially in relation to society or culture (Morris, 2000).

Gender dysphoria: distress regarding the biological sex one is assigned at birth or about one's gender identity (Colman, 2009).

Gender identity: the role in one's subjective sense of self as male or female of one's own personal negotiation with masculinity and femininity as framed within one's culture.

Gender non-conforming: a phenomenon in which pre-pubescent children do not conform to expected gender-related sociological or psychological patterns, and/or identify with the opposite gender (The Free Dictionary, Farlex, n.d.).

Gender role: a set of behavior patterns, attitudes and personality characteristics stereotypically perceived as masculine or feminine within a culture (Colman, 2009).

Gender variant: an individual who deviates from the expected characteristics of his or her sex.

Gender-intensification hypothesis: hypothesis according to which cultural expectations for conformity to traditional gender roles increase with the onset of adolescence, with girls expected to be dependent and self-effacing.

Gene–environment correlation (rGE): phenomenon whereby environmental experiences are influenced by genes.

Gene–environment interaction (GxE): phenomenon whereby genetic effects vary depending on environmental circumstances, or whereby environmental effects vary depending on genetic factors.

Generalized anxiety disorder: a type of anxiety disorder in which the individual experiences excessive and largely uncontrollable anxiety as a result of everyday activities, such as work or school, rather than focused on any specific circumstances. Symptoms of restlessness, tiredness, difficulty concentrating, irritability, muscle tension or sleep disturbance (insomnia or restless sleep) cause significant impairment in everyday functioning.

Genetic code or **genome:** the complete pattern of DNA sequences (= genetic information) of an individual.

Genetic dominance effect: interaction effect between alleles that are at the same gene location, where the effect of a "dominant" allele completely masks the effect of another "recessive" allele.

Genetic epistasis effect: interaction effect between alleles that are at different gene locations, where the effects of one allele are modified by one or several other alleles.

Genotype: the complete set of DNA sequences (= genetic information) of an individual.

Gentle discipline: discipline in which the lowest possible level of power is asserted.

Glial cells: cells of the nervous system that support the neurons. They can form insulating sheaths of myelin round neurons in the central nervous system, preventing impulses from traveling between adjacent neurons. Other functions of glial cells include providing nutrients for neurons and controlling the biochemical composition of the fluid surrounding the neurons (Martin and Hine, 2008).

Glutamate: a salt of glutamic acid, the main excitatory neurotransmitter for all nerve impulses in the diencephalon and telencephalon and for sensory impulses in the peripheral nervous system (Colman, 2009).

Goal attainment scaling: a method for evaluating programs by assessing the degree to which they achieve their stated objectives.

Halo effects: positive or negative effects in which a positive or negative feature of an individual is generalized to a positive or negative perception of everything that person does.

Heart rate variability (HRV): the time interval between sequential heart beats is not a constant. Heart rate variability is the degree of variation in the time between heart beats (called inter-beat intervals). It can be analyzed to create a measure of parasympathetic influence over cardiac activity (The Free Dictionary, Farlex, n.d.).

Heterosexual: sexually attracted to persons of the opposite biological sex.

Heterotypic continuity: term used to describe the assumption that what is referred to as the same disorder (e.g., depression of attention deficit) is actually very much the same in different stages of development. The prediction of a disorder by another disorder (Ferdinand et al., 2007).

Hierarchical classification system: classification system with fewer, larger categories that are divided into subtypes.

Hikikomori: specific pattern of anxiety reported in Japan, which involves social withdrawal to the extent of becoming a recluse, spending months in parents' homes and refusing to attend school or see other people. Only in some cases is *hikikomori* associated with anxiety.

Hindbrain: the lower part of the brainstem, comprising the cerebellum, pons and medulla oblongata. Also called rhombencephalon (Stevenson, 2010).

Hippocampus: a phylogenetically primitive structure in the limbic system of the brain, folded into the inner surface of each temporal lobe between the thalamus and the main part of the cerebral cortex, having a cross-section shaped like a sea horse, involved in emotion, motivation, navigation by cognitive maps, learning and the consolidation of long-term memory (only declarative memory and not procedural memory). The entire hippocampal formation consists of Ammon's horn (the hippocampus proper) together with the subiculum and the dentate gyrus (Colman, 2009).

Histone modification: a chemical process that leads to changes in the epigenetic code.

Homeostasis: process by which an organism regulates its internal conditions to stabilize health and functioning, regardless of the outside changing conditions (www.biology-online.org/dictionary/Homeostasis).

Homophily: the tendency of individuals to associate and bond with similar others. The presence of homophily has been discovered in a vast array of network studies (The Free Dictionary, Farlex, n.d.).

Homophily principle: is the tendency of individuals to associate and bond with similar others.

Homosexual: a person who is sexually attracted to members of the same biological sex.

Homotypic continuity: the prediction of a disorder by the same disorder (Ferdinand et al., 2007).

Hopelessness theory: theory which emphasizes the importance of cognitive processes in the etiology, maintenance and treatment of depression. This theory posits that some people are vulnerable to depression because they tend to generate interpretations of stressful life events with negative implications for their future and self-worth, a cognitive vulnerability that interacts with stress to produce depression.

Humanistic/existential approach: an approach to psychotherapy in which creativity, humor, play and psychological growth in general are emphasized. It is sometimes considered the "third force," relative to behaviorism and psychoanalysis.

Humor: in ancient Greek writings, a temperament caused by the body fluids that affect human personality, and which, in excess, lead to mental distress (Stevenson and Lindberg, 2010).

Hypercortisolism: condition characterized by elevated cortisol levels which persist for extended periods of time. It can lead to a variety of harmful immunological, physical and psychological side effects.

Hypomanic episode: a state in which an individual displays an abnormality of mood falling somewhere between normal euphoria and mania. It is characterized by unrealistic optimism, pressure of speech and activity, and a decreased need for sleep (Bhatia, 2009).

Hypothalamic–pituitary–adrenal (HPA) axis: one of the body's primary stress response and regulation systems. Through a cascade of hormones, the hypothalamus stimulates the pituitary gland, which in turn stimulates the adrenal glands to release glucocorticoid hormones (cortisol in humans) and an androgen hormone (dehydroepiandrosterone – DHEA). The HPA axis plays important roles in the regulation of stress or fight-and-flight responses, hunger, thirst, sleep, mood, sexual activity, learning and memory (Colman, 2009).

Hypothalamic–pituitary–adrenal (HPA) axis system: a self-regulating system, based on negative feedback, in which hormones are released from the hypothalamus, stimulating the release of a different class of hormones from the pituitary gland, which in turn stimulate secretions of a third class of hormones from the adrenal glands and the testes, or ovaries. The whole cycle plays an important role in the regulation of hunger, thirst, sleep, mood, sexual activity, learning and memory.

Hypothalamic–pituitary–adrenal (HPA) hyperreactivity: hypersensitivity of the HPA axis due to anxiety problems, making people feel afraid more easily, more strongly and in more situations.

Hypothalamic–pituitary–gonadal (HPG) axis: in addition to stimulating the adrenal glands to secrete cortisol, the hormones released by the pituitary gland stimulate the testes and ovaries (gonads) to release androgen and estrogen sex hormones.

Identified patient: the family member initially designated by the family as requiring the psychological care.

Idiot savant: a person with intellectual disability with a high level of ability in some specific domain of intellectual functioning, such as memorizing vast bodies of information, musical or artistic performance, or calendar calculations (Colman, 2009).

Imitation: acting in the same way as another person, either temporarily or permanently. It can be used in therapy (see modeling) (Martin, 2010).

Immaturity theories: theories assuming that homosexuality is a phase of human development that is not necessarily pathological when it first appears but that normally is outgrown.

Impairment (of functioning): loss of physical or mental functioning related to a disorder.

Impairment criterion: criterion applied to filter out cases in which the symptoms are present but general life functioning is not markedly affected.

Impedance cardiography: measuring the flow of blood through the chambers and vessels of the heart by examining changes in their resistance to an electrical current.

Incidental model: model in which an outcome, such as aggression or depression, is caused by an underlying pathology that may not be fully evident in childhood or adolescence (Parker and Asher, 1987).

Inclusive sports: inclusions of persons with intellectual and/or physical handicaps in the normal sports activities of a school or community.

Incremental validity: the additional benefit an instrument provides over those already in use by a psychologist or clinic.

Indicated prevention interventions: preventive interventions for identified individuals who are showing early signs of mental illness.

Individualistic cultures: cultures in which individual competitiveness and autonomy are valued more than cultural norms, social cohesion, cooperation and harmony (which is seen by many as a fundamental distinction between cultures). The USA, Australia, Great Britain, Canada and the Netherlands are considered by Hofstede to be the most individualistic (Hofstede, 1984, 2003). Individualistic cultures are typically low power distance cultures.

Inherent good: Rousseau's view of childhood and human nature, in which children were seen as "noble savages" who would learn and adjust without much need for intervention, if they were given the proper nurturing environment (Curren, 2007).

Insecure and ambivalent relationship: relationship in which the child is very distressed when separated even briefly from the attachment figure, with the distress persisting even after the caregiver returns, and generally wary of strangers.

Instrumental aggression: instrumental aggression involves purposeful behaviors that are implemented with a goal in mind and that are not necessarily linked to emotions such as anger (e.g., a child steals a peer's notebook so the peer cannot do her homework that night). A form of aggression against another person in which the aggression is used as a means of securing some reward or to achieve an external goal such as a victory. Harm to others is incidental and is not the perceived goal.

Instrumental support: the most concrete direct form of social support, encompassing help in the form of money, time, in-kind assistance and other explicit interventions on the person's behalf (European Union Public Health Information System, www.euphix.org).

Intellectual disability: a condition characterized by limitations in mental functioning and in skills such as communicating, taking care of oneself and social skills. These limitations will cause a child to learn and develop more slowly than a typically developing child (www.cdc.gov/ncbddd/actearly/pdf/parents_pdfs/IntellectualDisability.pdf).

Interactive model: model to explain how having aggressive friends leads to the maintenance of aggression. The aggressive friend exacerbates pre-existing proclivities toward aggression within the individual. The influences of the aggressive friend and the predisposition to aggressiveness act in a multiplicative way rather than an additive way.

Intermittent explosive disorder: a disorder introduced in DSM-5 characterized by severe recurrent temper outbursts in response to common stressors.

Internal working model: in attachment theory, an understanding of interpersonal relationships based on early child–caregiver bonds that is later applied to other close relationships.

Interpersonal therapy: a time-limited psychotherapy that focuses on the interpersonal context and on building interpersonal skills. Interpersonal therapy is based on the belief that interpersonal factors may contribute heavily to psychological problems. It is commonly distinguished from other forms of therapy in its emphasis on interpersonal processes rather than intrapsychic processes. Interpersonal therapy aims to change the person's interpersonal behavior by fostering adaptation to current interpersonal roles and situations (The Free Dictionary, Farlex, n.d.).

Inter–rater reliability: agreement among different raters or coders about the category to which an event (e.g., the diagnosis of a mental disorder, an observed behavior or a verbal utterance) belongs.

Intrasubjectivity hypothesis: postulates that the key mechanism underlying peer influence is the intrinsic reinforcement of shared deviant values (thoughts, perceptions, experiences) within an interpersonal context of endorsement and agreement (Prinstein and Dodge, 2008).

Invulnerable: characteristic of some children who, being exposed to *risk factors* that often lead to mental illness, failed to develop adult schizophrenia despite clear signs that they are at risk because of genetic endowment or parental history of psychosis.

Kappa coefficient: statistical measure of inter-rater agreement, based on the number of agreements between observers, considered as a proportion of the total decisions made (i.e., agreements + disagreements), corrected for the number of agreements between raters that might occur purely by chance. An agreement rate of about 80 percent, resulting in kappa of .70 or more (after correction for random agreement), is usually considered acceptable from a scientific point of view.

Kleptomania: the inability to restrain an impulse to steal.

Kumu: a condition common in Northern Uganda found in children who have suffered through war and the experience of becoming refugees and have immigrated to Western countries, where they face the dual challenge of adapting to very unfamiliar cultures and attempting to overcome the trauma of what they have lived through. The central feature is persistent grief or sadness, often manifested by self-isolation, crying, loss of energy and many worries.

Lack of interoceptive awareness: poor interoceptive awareness, often cited as a key feature of eating disorders, in which the precise nature of the deficits and their relationship to eating pathology remain unclear. Interoceptive awareness includes both acceptance of affective experience and clarity regarding emotional responses (Merwin et al., 2010).

Latin American machismo: the cultural expectation that men will be strong, if not chauvinistic, and hold their families together.

Learning disabilities: any of a number of specific difficulties in learning, such as difficulties in learning to read (dyslexia), write (dysgraphia) and calculate (dyscalculia), affecting school-age children of average or above-average intelligence.

Least restrictive setting: one of the six principles that govern the education of students with disabilities and other special needs. It means that a student who has a disability should have the opportunity to be educated with non-disabled peers, to the greatest extent appropriate.

Lithium: an orally administered drug in the form of lithium carbonate or lithium citrate used in prevention and treatment of episodes of mania or recurrent depression in patients with bipolar affective disorder.

Locus: the physical location of a gene on a chromosome.

Lower cortisol levels: insufficient amount of cortisol, which can disrupt metabolism. The overall effect of low cortisol is weakness, dehydration and diminished ability to fight infection, trauma and stress. These issues are often first noticed during periods of extreme stress or trauma.

Macrosystem: system in Bronfenbrenner's model that represents the influence of the surrounding society.

Magnetic resonance imaging (MRI): a non-invasive method of brain imaging or examination of other body organs by recording the responses to radio waves, or other forms of energy, of different kinds of molecules in a magnetic field (Colman, 2009).

Magnetic resonance spectroscopy (MRS): a diagnostic technique that utilizes the phenomenon of nuclear magnetic resonance to obtain a biochemical profile of tissues by exciting elements other than hydrogen in water and other body components. It is particularly useful for biochemical analysis of tissues in the living body. The technique is still largely at the research level (Martin, 2010).

Mainstreaming: the practice of placing students who are below average in educational achievement in at least some classes together with students of average or above-average achievement (paraphrase from Matsumoto, 2009).

Manic episode: a mood episode lasting at least 1 week, characterized by continuously elevated, expansive or irritable mood, sufficiently severe to cause marked impairment in social or occupational functioning or to require hospitalization, during which there may be inflated self-esteem or grandiose ideas or actions, decreased need for sleep (almost invariably), increased talkativeness, flight of ideas, distractibility, increased goal-oriented activity, psychomotor agitation and risky pleasure-seeking activities such as spree shopping, sexual indiscretions or imprudent financial investments (Colman, 2009).

Manic–depressive disorder: another term for bipolar disorder.

Marianismo: an aspect of the female gender role in the machismo of Latin American folk culture. It is the veneration for feminine virtues like purity and moral strength (The Free Dictionary, Farlex, n.d.).

Marker: indicator of the presence of a factor, influence, phenomenon, etc. (Bukowski and Adams, 2005). For example, peer relations are conceptualized as markers of maladjustment, early signs of broader dysfunction.

Masculinity/femininity: the allowance for expressions of emotion and compassion in a culture.

Masked depression: depression that is thought to underlie another form of abnormal behavior, such as disruptive behavior.

Matching law: law discovered by McDowell (1988) according to which aggressive boys tend to match the level and frequency of deviant talk to the level of their friends. The content of the conversations of aggressive boys and their friends may be quite immature.

Mathematics disorder: a learning disability in which the individual exhibits below-average mathematical ability for his or her age, intelligence and education, which interferes substantially with scholastic or academic

achievement or everyday life and is not due merely to a sensory deficit.

Mediated model of the influence of friends: model to explain how having aggressive friends leads to the maintenance of aggression. Based on the belief that pre-existing proclivities toward aggression result in the selection of an aggressive friend and that the negative influence of the aggressive friend makes matters worse from that point on.

Mediating variable: a variable that explains a correlation between two other variables.

Medical model: a conception of psychopathology according to which mental disorders and distress function in the same way as physical diseases. Therefore, they need to be treated in a more or less standard way that is prescribed by qualified professional experts.

Melancholia: originally a term in the Hippocratic tradition, until the end of the nineteenth century it denoted the depressive syndrome. Now archaic in the professional literature.

Mental hygiene movement: a public health perspective within psychiatry, which was influential from 1910 until about 1960. Instead of focusing on the treatment of mental illness, mental hygienists emphasized early intervention, prevention and the promotion of mental health. They focused on parent education and on improving the school system.

Mental retardation: term replaced by "intellectual disability" in DSM-5 and most contemporary writings.

Mental schema: a plan, diagram or outline, especially a mental representation of some aspect of experience, based on prior experience and memory, structured in such a way as to facilitate (and sometimes to distort) perception, cognition, the drawing of inferences or the interpretation of new information in terms of existing knowledge (Colman, 2009).

Mesosystem: system in Bronfenbrenner's model that represents such relatively nearby interactions as those between mothers and fathers or between parents and teachers.

Metacognition: one's knowledge concerning one's own cognitive processes or anything related to them (Flavell, 1976, p. 232).

Methylphenidate: methylphenidate hydrochloride, an analogue of amphetamine, being a mild central nervous system stimulant drug that blocks the reuptake of noradrenaline and dopamine and is often prescribed in the treatment of attention deficit/hyperactivity disorder in children and narcolepsy in adults. Commonly called Ritalin (trademark) (Colman, 2009).

Micro-social analysis: analysis of the social interactions of people and how they react to each other.

Microsystem: system of Bronfenbrenner's model that represents the environmental forces with which the child is in direct contact, including not only the child's relationships with his or her parents but also relationships with peers and teachers.

Midbrain: the middle part of the brain, connecting the diencephalon to the hindbrain, including the tectum, tegmentum, cerebral peduncles and the aqueduct of Sylvius, also called the mesencephalon, especially in a developing embryo (Colman, 2009).

Minimal brain damage, Minimal brain dysfunction (MBD), Minimal cerebral damage, Minimal cerebral dysfunction: Archaic terms for a broader syndrome that included symptoms now considered symptoms of attention deficit/hyperactivity disorder.

Miscue: the parents' failure to recognize the child's emotional needs.

Mixed models: mixing qualitative and quantitative research strategies.

Modeling: providing an example of adaptive or maladaptive behavior that a person can imitate.

Monomania: exaggerated or obsessive enthusiasm for or preoccupation with one thing (Stevenson, 2010).

Monozygotic twins: twins that develop from a single fertilized egg (zygote) that splits and forms two embryos.

Motivational enhancement therapy: a systematic intervention, based on principles of motivational psychology for evoking change. Designed to produce rapid, internally motivated change. Rather than attempting to guide the client through each part of recovery, motivational strategies are employed to encourage the client to mobilize his or her own change resources.

Multifinality: refers to how individuals who start out at essentially the same point, and seem to be developing in the same ways, turn out differently at the end.

Multivariate genetic analysis: the study of how the same genes can affect a variety of traits, such as achievement or disability, in several academic subject areas.

Myelin: white tissue forming an insulating sheath (myelin sheath) around certain nerve fibers. Damage to the myelin sheath causes neurological disease, as in multiple sclerosis (Butterfield, 2003).

Narrow-band attachment theory: an interpretation of attachment theory in which it is maintained that attachment is more strongly linked to intimate relationships than to other possible outcomes.

Naturalism: the doctrine that the world can be understood in scientific terms without recourse to spiritual or supernatural explanations (The Free Dictionary, Farlex, n.d.).

Negative affect: a general dimension of subjective distress and unpleasurable engagement that subsumes a variety of aversive mood states, including anger, contempt, disgust, guilt, fear and nervousness. Low negative affect is characterized by a state of calmness and serenity.

Negative correlation: correlation in which large values of one variable are associated with small values of the other.

Nerve attack (ataque de nervios): a common phenomenon in Latin America (*ataques de nervios*) that involves uncontrolled screaming, crying and trembling, sometimes accompanied by verbal and/or physical aggression, fainting and seizure-like behavior.

Neuron: the cell that constitutes the basic unit of the nervous system (Statt, 2003). Any of the impulse-conducting cells that constitute the brain, spinal column and nerves, consisting of a nucleated cell body with one or more dendrites and a single axon. Also called nerve cell (Morris, 2000).

Neuroticism: enduring tendency to experience negative emotional states. Individuals who score high on neuroticism are more likely than the average to experience such feelings as anxiety, anger, guilt and depressed mood (The Free Dictionary, Farlex, n.d.).

Nomogram: line graphs using a linear scale to relate a given set of variables to others. Relationships are indicated with lines connecting two known variables to a third, unknown variable.

Non-shared environment: environmental influence that affects each family member in a different way and that makes family members dissimilar from each other.

Non-specific electrodermal responses: electrodermal activity which does not seem to be produced in response to an identifiable stimulus.

Norepinephrine: a key neurotransmitter active in many parts of the brain and central nervous system, and also in the nerve endings of the sympathetic nervous system, to cause vasoconstriction and increases in heart rate, blood pressure and the sugar level of the blood. Also called noradrenaline (Morris, 2000).

Normal variation theories: theories that contain the assumption that homosexuality is a phenomenon that occurs naturally and is probably innate.

Normalization: efforts to render the living conditions of people with learning disabilities as similar as possible to those without disabilities, including living outside institutions and encouragement to cope with work, pay, social life, sexuality and civil rights (Martin, 2010).

Nucleotides: molecular building blocks.

Objectification theory: theory which proposes that girls and women are typically acculturated to internalize an observer's perspective as a primary view of their physical selves (Fredrickson and Roberts, 1997).

Objectified body consciousness: a process by which a person develops an image of his/her body on the basis of the body's external appearance to others rather than on what the body can do or how it feels from the inside (paraphrased from McKinley, 1999).

Obsessive-compulsive disorder (OCD): an anxiety disorder characterized by either obsessions or compulsions, recognized by the afflicted person (if an adolescent or adult) as excessive or unreasonable, causing significant distress, wasting significant amounts of time or markedly interfering with everyday life, occupational or academic performance, or social interaction. Also called anankastic neurosis, obsessive-compulsive neurosis (Colman, 2009).

Ontogenesis: the development or progressive construction of an individual from conception forward; can be used to describe physical development, neural development or psychological development (Johnson et al., 2005).

Ontological status: the nature of being and reality (*New Oxford American Dictionary*, 2010). In psychopathology, the nature of a disorder.

Oppositional defiant disorder: a disorder characterized by recurrent negativistic, defiant, disobedient or hostile behavior toward authority figures.

Overt pathway: pathway along which minor incidents escalate into more serious physical aggression and onward to serious violence.

Panic: a sudden unreasoning and overwhelming fear or terror, often affecting a group. It may occur in a state of high anxiety (Kent, 2000).

Panic disorder: an anxiety disorder characterized by recurrent, unexpected panic attacks, followed by persistent apprehension about further attacks, concern about the possible effects of the attacks (such as having a heart attack or going insane) or a significant alteration in behavior brought about by the attacks (such as resigning from a job). Panic disorder may occur with or without agoraphobia (Colman, 2009).

Paradoxical instruction: a technique in systemic family therapy, which consists of telling the family to do the exact opposite of what would be therapeutic for them.

Parasympathetic nervous system (PNS): one of the two major subdivisions of the autonomic nervous system whose general function is to conserve metabolic energy, acting in opposition to and with more specificity than the sympathetic nervous system by slowing pulse rate, stimulating the smooth muscles of the alimentary canal (peristalsis), promoting secretion of salivary and intestinal juices and voiding of urine, constricting the pupils and preparing the eyes for near vision (Colman, 2009).

Parataxic distortion: in Sullivan's theory, a perceptual or judgmental distortion of interpersonal relations resulting from the observer's need to pattern responses on previous experiences and thus defend against anxiety (*McGraw-Hill Dictionary of Scientific and Technical Terms*, 2003).

Parental monitoring: "a set of correlated parenting behaviors involving attention to and tracking of the child's whereabouts, activities, and adaptations" (Dishion and McMahon, 1998, p. 61).

Parenting style: a construct that represents the strategies that parents use in raising their children.

Pathognomonic: term applied to a sign or symptom specifically associated with a particular disease entity. When the symptom is present, the disease is always diagnosed (Bhatia, 2009). There are very few pathognomonic symptoms in DSM or ICD.

Pathology theories: theories containing the idea that homosexuality is caused by some internal defect of the organism or by some pathogenic agent that causes the organism to malfunction.

Pathoplastic effect: compounds the severity of some other conditions. For example, an intellectual disability may act to increase the severity of a comorbid oppositional defiant disorder.

Perfectionism: a belief that perfection can and should be attained. In its pathological form,

perfectionism is a belief that work or output that is anything less than perfect is unacceptable (The Free Dictionary, Farlex, n.d.). Often considered a personality trait.

Permissive parents: parents in Baumrind's (1991) classification who are not very demanding but who are responsive to their children.

Person–centered studies: studies which aim directly at changing individuals.

Personality: a grouping of behavior–response patterns typical of an individual in responding to people and situations.

Personality vulnerability theory: a theory in which certain personality styles are seen as increasing individual risk of becoming depressed; these styles include dependency, self-criticism and excessive need for approval (Zuroff, Mongrain and Santor, 2004).

Phenotype: the outward manifestation of the genetic information.

Physiological hyperarousal: a state of increased psychological and physiological tension marked by such effects as reduced pain tolerance, anxiety, exaggeration of startle responses, insomnia, fatigue and accentuation of personality traits (Dorland, 2007).

Pica: an eating disorder of infancy or early childhood characterized by persistent eating of inappropriate substances such as paint, plaster, string, hair, cloth, animal droppings, sand, insects, leaves, pebbles, clay, soil or other non-nutritive matter, but without any aversion to conventional foods, the behavior not occurring as part of a culturally sanctioned practice (Colman, 2009).

Placebo: a therapy without known specific effect for the condition being treated, used for comparison with another therapy presumed to have specific effect (Shapiro, 1960).

Play therapy: a type of therapy used with children in which the child reveals his or her problems on a fantasy level with dolls, clay and other toys. The therapist intervenes opportunely with helpful explanations about the patient's response and behavior in language geared to the child's comprehension (Bhatia, 2009).

Pleiotropy: multiple phenotypic effects caused by the same gene.

Pleitropy: a situation in which a single gene is responsible for more than one effect in the phenotype. The mutation of such a gene will therefore have multiple effects (Martin, 2010).

Polygenicity: the fact that each trait is affected by several different genes.

Polymorphism: a specific gene variation that occurs very frequently in a population.

Polyvagal theory: a theory developed by Stephen Porges to explain the role of the vagus nerve (also called the tenth cranial nerve, and a key part of the parasympathetic nervous system) in the regulation of emotions and social behaviors. In safe and comfortable situations, greater parasympathetic influence through the vagus nerve helps individuals to calmly engage in positive social interactions. In response to salient cues in the environment, parasympathetic influence through the vagus decreases, which supports the adaptive response of orientation and increased attention toward the cues.

Positive affect: feelings like happiness, excitement, joy, contentment and enthusiasm, reflecting a level of pleasurable engagement with the environment.

Positive connotation: a technique from the Milan school which consists of praising, paradoxically, elements of the family system that maintain homeostasis, even though the elements are not praiseworthy and the therapists intend to challenge and try to change them.

Positive reinforcement: a type of reinforcement in which a reward is provided – something the organism wants, needs or likes. The reward is typically paired to a behavior that the person dispensing the reinforcement wishes to see more often.

Positron emission tomography (PET): a technique for assessing brain activity and function by recording the emission of positrons from radioactively labeled substances, such as glucose or dopamine (Butterfield, 2003).

Post-traumatic stress disorder (PTSD): a severe and long-lasting reaction to a traumatic event that involves intense fear, horror and feelings of hopelessness (American Psychiatric Association, 2000).

Power assertion: parenting, often punitive, based on the parents' position of strength over their children.

Power distance: the degree of authority exercised by authority figures in a culture. In cultures of high power distance, subordinates acknowledge the power of others based on formal, hierarchical positions (The Free Dictionary, Farlex, n.d.).

Practical intelligence: involves individuals applying their abilities to the kinds of problems that confront them in daily life, such as on the job or in the home (Wagner and Sternberg, 1986).

Prader-Willi syndrome: a rare disorder (occurring in about one in 12,000–15,000 people of both sexes) usually caused by deletion, at or soon after conception, of several genes on the copy of chromosome 15 inherited from the father, resulting in hyperphagia, with a risk of morbid obesity. Other signs and symptoms include hypotonia, cognitive impairment, short stature and incomplete sexual development, obsessive or compulsive symptoms and tantrums (Colman, 2009).

Predictive validity: the extent to which a score on a scale or instrument predicts scores on some criterion measures (The Free Dictionary, Farlex, n.d.).

Pre-ejection period: a measure of the influence of the sympathetic nervous system (SNS) over cardiac activity, pre-ejection period is the amount of time (measured in milliseconds) from the beginning of the contraction of the left ventricle of the heart until the aortic valve opens (allowing the blood to be pumped out of the ventricle). A shorter pre-ejection period reflects greater SNS influence over cardiac activity.

Prefrontal cortex (PFC): the frontmost portion of the frontal lobe, in front of the primary and secondary motor cortex, uniquely large in the human brain, involved in anxiety and also in brain functions such as working memory, abstract thinking, social behavior and executive functions such as decision-making and strategic planning, any or all of which are affected by lesions in this area. The right prefrontal cortex is involved in monitoring behavior, resisting distractions and providing an awareness of self and of time (Colman, 2009).

Prevention science: the term "prevention science" has emerged to reflect an empirical perspective on prevention strategies.

Primary prevention: measures taken to prevent the occurrence of a disorder (Colman, 2009).

Primary universal prevention programs: programs which are provided to, and are planned to confer benefit on, all persons in the target population. The interventions are intended to target people before any symptoms become manifest.

Primary–indicated prevention programs: programs which target individuals who show some symptoms of pathology but do not meet full diagnostic criteria for any pathology (Mrazek and Haggerty, 1994).

Primary–selective prevention programs: programs which seek to intervene in the key mediators in the processes known to lead to psychopathology.

Process–oriented or cybernetic models: model which focuses on teaching students perceptual strategies, such as auditory memory, visual perception or visual-motor coordination.

Prodrome: a symptom indicating the onset of a disease (Martin, 2010).

Projective techniques: procedures used to uncover a person's unconscious motivations, conflicts and anxieties. Projective techniques consist of unstructured stimuli, designed to allow individuals to project material that would be inadmissible to consciousness in a direct, undisguised form.

Protective factor: a positive processes or event that helps the individual to become resilient to negative influences. These protective factors include positive interpersonal relationships and the intellectual ability and flexibility needed to succeed in school and to solve problems (Kohlberg et al., 1972).

Provision: mechanism of influence which involves making the substances available, whether intentionally or not. Either parents or peers may exert influence in this way.

Psychoeducation: an intervention that consists of providing information about mental health and about the individual's specific difficulties, with general guidance on how to cope with the problems in question.

Psychodynamic school: an approach to the study of human behavior in which internalized motivation and drives are emphasized; includes but is not limited to Freudian psychoanalysis.

Psychological treatment: interventions directed at a mental health disorder. Some but not all applications of psychotherapy can be considered forms of psychological treatment (i.e., when they are directed at a mental health disorder).

Psychoneuroendocrinology: the study of the roles played by hormones in the production and regulation of behavior.

Psychopathic trait: a personality trait characterized by self-centeredness and a lack of guilt and remorse (APA Dictionary of Psychology, 2007).

Psychosomatic family model: theory proposed by Salvador Minuchin according to which certain unhealthy patterns of family interaction (rigidity, lack of conflict resolution and overprotection) influence the emergence of psychosomatic symptoms in one of the family members (paraphrased from Kog, Vertommen and Vandereycken, 1987).

Psychotherapy: a highly heterogeneous range of verbal techniques that often have as their goal the alleviation of the symptoms of a mental health disorder; other goals may include self-discovery or personal development.

Pyromania: a disorder characterized by experiencing pleasure connected to repeatedly setting fires.

Qualitative methods: an approach to research in which the detail and richness of the data being collected are given higher priority than the control of the research situation and standardization of a research protocol. Often consists of participant observation and open-ended interviews but not questionnaires with known psychometric properties.

Quantitative trait loci: the locations of genes known to contribute to inter-individual differences in a continuous – or quantitative – trait (e.g., weight or height).

Randomized clinical trials (RCT): type of scientific experiment most commonly used in testing the efficacy or effectiveness of healthcare services (such as medicine or nursing) or health technologies (such as pharmaceuticals, medical devices or surgery). The key distinguishing feature of the usual RCT is that study participants, after assessment of their eligibility but before the intervention to be studied begins, are randomly allocated to receive one or other of the alternative treatments under study (The Free Dictionary, Farlex, n.d.).

Rational power assertion: type of power assertion which provides a predictable environment for the child, with clear information provided about the parents' expectations and age-appropriate consequences for misbehavior (Hoffman, 1983).

Reactive aggression: aggression in response to a perceived or real provocation.

Reactive attachment disorder: a disorder in which a child reacts to changes in caregiver, child neglect or abuse with symptoms of depression and/or social withdrawal.

Reading disorder: a disorder marked by faulty oral reading, slow reading and reduced comprehension in which one's reading ability is significantly below what is expected based on age and developmental level. The problem is not due to global intellectual disability, chronologic age or inadequate schooling (Anderson, 2009).

Reciprocal determinism: the idea that a person's behavior and the social learning environment continually influence each other in reciprocal ways; one learns behavior from interactions with other persons, and one's behavior influences how other persons interact with one (Roeckelein, 1998).

Reflecting-team approach: a technique in systemic family therapy in which there is one therapist in the therapy room, while other professionals are observing the therapy and, often, providing insight to the main therapist.

Reframing: a change of "the conceptual and/or emotional setting or viewpoint in relation to which a situation is experienced, placing it in another frame which fits the 'facts' of the same concrete situation equally well or even better, and thereby changes its entire meaning" (Watzlawick et al., 1974).

Refrigerator mother: term coined around 1950 as a label for mothers of children diagnosed with autism or schizophrenia. These mothers were often blamed for their children's atypical behavior, which included rigid rituals, speech difficulty and self-isolation (The Free Dictionary, Farlex, n.d.).

Relational aggression: also known as covert aggression, a subtle non-physical form of aggression, such as spreading nasty rumors and getting other children to exclude the targets of their displeasure from playgroups (Crick et al., 1997).

Relativist position: an approach according to which the basic understanding and definition of pathology must be established in reference to each culture and, hence, must be replicated in each culture.

Resilience or resiliency: a phenomenon or process reflecting positive adaptation despite experiences of significant adversity or trauma (Masten, 2011).

Respiratory sinus arrhythmia (RSA): a normal variation of heart rate, in which breathing heart rate increases during inspiration and decreases during expiration. RSA is sometimes used as a measure of vagal tone and general well-being (Ben-Tal, Shamailov and Paton, 2011).

Response bias: a type of cognitive bias which can affect the results of a statistical survey if respondents answer questions in the way they think the questioner wants them to answer rather than according to their true beliefs (The Free Dictionary, Farlex, n.d.).

Response–styles theory: theory proposed by Susan Nolen-Hoeksema proposing that the way a person habitually responds to depressive symptoms determines the intensity and duration of the depressive episode. The theory proposes two distinct styles of responding to depression: people who tend to focus inward on their symptoms and on the possible causes and consequences of these symptoms – the ruminative style – and people who try to distract themselves from their symptoms through activity or other means – the distracting style (Strauss et al., 1997).

Responsiveness to intervention (RTI): a method of academic intervention designed to maximize the progress of pupils with learning disabilities by pinpointing academic weaknesses, using empirically based methods for remediating them, frequent assessment of progress and, as far as possible, educational decisions based on research data.

Responsiveness: parental warmth, supportiveness and sensitivity to their children's needs (Baumrind, 1971).

Restructuring: in family therapy, the process of addressing the family structure during the therapy, loosening coalitions that are unhelpful.

Risk factors: an attribute, such as a habit (e.g., cigarette smoking) or exposure to some environmental hazard, that leads the individual concerned to have a greater likelihood of developing an illness. The relationship is one of probability and, as such, can be distinguished from a causal agent (Martin, 2010).

Risperidone: a drug belonging to the group of atypical antipsychotics that acts as a serotonin and a dopamine antagonist. Also called Risperdal (trademark) (Colman, 2009).

Rumination disorder: a childhood eating disorder in which the sufferer brings up partially digested food and rechews it before swallowing it or spitting it

out. Rumination disorder typically occurs within 3–12 months of age and can lead to the child becoming malnourished (The Free Dictionary, Farlex, n.d.).

Savant skills: savants' phenomenal or genius abilities, such as limitless mnemonic skills, with many having eidetic or photographic memories.

Scapegoat: a person who is blamed for the wrongdoings, mistakes or faults of others (Stevenson, 2010).

School refusal or **school phobia**: refusal to attend school, often due to emotional distress. School refusal differs from truancy in that children with school refusal feel anxiety or fear toward school, whereas truant children generally have no feelings of fear toward school, often feeling angry or bored with it instead. The term was coined as a more general alternative to school phobia, which is often used to describe school refusal caused by separation anxiety (The Free Dictionary, Farlex, n.d.).

Secondary prevention: steps taken to contain the spread of an existing disorder.

Secure attachment: in attachment theory, a close supportive relationship between child and caregiver in which separation distress is relatively mild and quickly resolved when the child and caregiver are reunited.

Secure base: the trusting, secure, bond formed with the attachment figure, from which the child feels comfortable exploring the surrounding world, and especially other people with whom close, trusting relationships might eventually be formed.

Selective breeding: the artificial mating of organisms with particular genotypes in order to enhance or suppress certain hereditary characteristics (Colman, 2009).

Selective mutism: a mental disorder of childhood or adolescence whose essential feature is a persistent failure to speak in certain social situations in which speaking is expected, such as at school or among peers, despite a proven ability to speak in other situations. Also called elective mutism (Colman, 2009).

Selective prevention interventions: interventions which target subgroups of the general population that are determined to be at risk for mental illness.

Self-construals: the ways in which individuals interpret their identities.

Self-determination theory: a theory of motivation concerned with the development and functioning of personality within social contexts, including sport. The theory focuses on the degree to which human behaviors are made by personal choice. It assumes that people are active organisms with innate tendencies toward psychological growth and development, and that they strive to master challenges and to integrate experiences into a coherent sense of self (Kent, 2000).

Self-instruction training: training derived from Luria and Vygotsky's work, in which the therapist guides the child in using internal language to regulate his or her behavior, typically to remain calm rather than act aggressively out of anger (Foster, 1988; Kendall and Braswell, 1982).

Self-objectification: process by which individuals internalize the cultural norms and beliefs about attractiveness as their own (paraphrased from Moradi, 2011).

Self-selection: indicates any situation in which individuals select themselves into a group. It is commonly used to describe situations where the characteristics of the people which cause them to select themselves in the group create abnormal or undesirable conditions in the group (The Free Dictionary, Farlex, n.d.).

Sense of community: a concept which focuses on the experience of community rather than its structure, formation, setting or other features (McMillan and Chavis, 1986).

Sensitivity: (e.g., of a test or diagnosis) the proportion of people with a disease who are correctly diagnosed.

Separation anxiety disorder: a mental disorder with onset before age 18 years, characterized by developmentally inappropriate and excessive separation anxiety relating to separation from home or from major attachment figures (Colman, 2009).

Serotonin: a chemical produced by the brain that functions as a neurotransmitter. Low serotonin levels are associated with mood disorders, particularly depression. Medications known as selective serotonin reuptake inhibitors (SSRIs) are used to treat disorders characterized by depressed mood (Younger, 2013).

Severe intellectual disability: a level of intellectual disability associated with IQ approximately between 20 and 35 (in adults, mental age from 3 to under 6 years) and very limited capacity for autonomous living.

Sex: the characteristics associated with an individual's reproductive status and sexual organs as male or female (paraphrased from Matsumoto, 2009).

Sexual orientation: a person's sexual identity in relation to the gender to which he or she is attracted; the fact of being heterosexual, homosexual or bisexual (Stevenson, 2010).

Sexuality: concern with or interest in sexual activity (Morris, 2000).

Shared environment: environmental influence that affects all family members in the same way and that makes family members similar to each other.

Shared method bias: methodological problem in which the same conclusion emerges from a number of different measures obtained from the same informant.

Single photon emission computerized tomography (SPECT): a cross-sectional imaging technique for observing an organ or part of the body using a gamma camera; images are produced after injecting a radioactive tracer. The camera is rotated around the patient being scanned. Using a computer reconstruction algorithm similar to that of a computerized tomography scanner, multiple "slices" are made through the area of interest. SPECT scanning is used particularly in cardiac nuclear medicine imaging. It differs from PET scanning in that radioactive decay gives off only a single gamma ray (Stevenson, 2010).

Single-subject design: research done by doing detailed investigating of a single individual or a single organized group. Changes occurring over time in the individual's behavior are usually the focus of the researcher's interest.

Skin conductance level (SCL): level of the electrical conductance of the skin. It is also a method of measuring the electrical conductance of the skin, which varies with its moisture level, also known as galvanic skin response (GSR), electrodermal response (EDR), psychogalvanic reflex (PGR) or skin conductance response (SCR).

Slow-to-warm-up temperament: describes children who have difficulty in social situations at first but adjust better with time.

Social anxiety or **social phobia**: an anxiety disorder characterized by a fear of scrutiny by others or of being the focus of attention in social situations involving strangers (Colman, 2009).

Social argumentation hypothesis: hypothesis according to which the gravitation to an anti-social peer group may become inevitable once a child has been marginalized from the mainstream peer group, perhaps because of aggressive behavior. The marginalized child simply has no other potential friends.

Social diagnosis: a process introduced by Richmond, in which the therapist takes into account the behavior of all members of the family, focusing on the family process rather than the psychopathology of any individual family member.

Social embeddedness: the degree to which individuals or firms are enmeshed in a social network.

Social integration: the inclusion of a social group that was previously separate into a larger entity such as a community.

Social skills: any skill necessary for competent social interaction, including both language and non-verbal communication (Colman, 2009).

Social support: communication, often at times of stress, that results in the belief that one is cared for and loved, esteemed and valued, and belongs to a network of communication and mutual obligations (Cobb, 1976).

Social-learning theory: theory developed by Albert Bandura in an attempt to explain human behavior in terms of reciprocal interaction between the individual and the social context. Modeling and observational learning are key features of social-learning theory.

Sociogenesis: the origin of social behavior that derives from past interpersonal experiences (The Free Dictionary, Farlex, n.d.). Social origin of all higher psychological processes, including thinking, volition and memory.

Specific learning disorder: the DSM-5 category pertaining to problems in reading, writing and/or arithmetic that affect an individual's school progress or occupational functioning.

Specific phobia: an anxiety disorder in which the fear-producing stimulus is a specific type of object (such as spiders), event (such as thunder), activity (such as flying) or situation (such as being in enclosed spaces).

Specific reading disorder: category of the ICD-10, similar to the specific learning disorder diagnosis in DSM-5 with the specifier that the deficit is in the area of reading.

Specificity: a measure of the reliability of a test or diagnosis based on the ability of the measure to indicate the specific diagnosis for which it is intended, not other diagnoses.

Specifier (in DSM): feature that can be used by the clinician to add detail to a broad clinical diagnosis, such as severity or comorbid symptoms.

Stimulation-seeking theory: attributes risky and disruptive behaviors to a physiologically based drive to seek out experiences that are new, thrilling and complex.

Strange Situation procedure: a laboratory test for infants developed by Ainsworth in which the child's attachment behavior system is activated by the unfamiliarity of the situation and in which the mother temporarily leaves the room where she interacted with her child. The return of the mother allows one to see how the child organizes his or her attachment behavior toward her.

Strauss syndrome: another term for the syndrome called *minimal brain damage* or *minimal brain dysfunction*.

Stress–reactive cortisol levels: cortisol levels increase due to stressful events. Stress response involves activation of both the hypothalamic-pituitary-adrenal (HPA) axis and the autonomic nervous system, and, thus, the cortisol secretion (Evers et al., 2010).

Striatum: a large mass of striped white and gray matter of the forebrain or prosencephalon in front of and around the thalamus in each cerebral hemisphere, the afferent part of the basal ganglia, mainly involved in movement planning and control and habit formation. It includes the putamen (connected mainly to the primary somatosensory cortex, the primary motor cortex and the supplementary motor area) and the caudate nucleus (connected to widespread cortical association areas) (Colman, 2009).

Structural equations model (SEM): a statistical technique for testing and estimating causal relations using a combination of statistical data and predictions about cause based on a theory (The Free Dictionary, Farlex, n.d.).

Structural MRI (sMRI): provides detailed pictures of the brain's anatomy which can be used to describe the shape, size and integrity of white and gray matter in the brain.

Summative evaluation: evaluation which examines the effects or outcomes of an intervention (as opposed to examining the process of its implementation).

Sympathetic nervous system (SNS): one of the two major subdivisions of the autonomic nervous system, consisting of nerves originating from the cervical, thoracic and lumbar regions of the spinal cord, supplying muscles and glands, concerned with general activation and mobilizing the body's fight-or-flight reaction to stress or perceived danger. It acts in opposition to and more diffusely than the parasympathetic nervous system, accelerating pulse rate, dilating the pupils of the eyes and preparing them for far vision, causing the sweat glands to secrete and urine to be retained, inhibiting the smooth muscles of the alimentary canal, diverting blood from the skin and intestines to the voluntary striped muscles, and activating the adrenal gland to secrete adrenalin (epinephrine) and noradrenalin (norepinephrine) (Colman, 2009).

Sympathetic–adrenomedullary (SAM) system: one of the body's primary stress response and regulation systems, incorporating the sympathetic branch of the autonomic nervous system and the adrenal medulla, the SAM serves to increase general activation and mobilize the body's fight-or-flight response.

Syndrome: set of signs and symptoms that appear as a clinical picture or disease. Recurrent pattern or grouping of signs and symptoms (Belloch et al., 2008).

Systemic approach: a way of looking at family life that is inspired by systemic thinking in biology and cybernetics.

Tabula rasa or **empty slate**: also known as the blank-slate or white-paper thesis, a name for the radically empiricist view of the mind and knowledge. According to John Locke, the contents of the mind are written on it by experience, as if it were white paper at birth, a view comparable with modern behaviorist theories, which try to account for mental processes as products of external stimuli and behavioral responses.

Taijin kyofusho: commonly found in Japan and Korea, an anxiety condition consisting of excessive fear that one's appearance, gaze or body odor will be offensive to others.

Telepsychology: psychotherapy and psychological assessment and using various electronic means such as videoconferencing, teleconferencing and telephone therapy, psychotherapy and counseling over the internet through various software packages with or without a video camera or webcam, counseling via email or internet chat, using social networking sites like Facebook, etc. (see www.telepsychology.net).

Temperament: an inherent, constitutional predisposition to react in a certain way to stimuli (Bhatia, 2009); "the behavioral response style of a person" (Chess and Thomas, 1996).

Tertiary prevention: used to diminish or eliminate the effects of a disorder that is already present, frequently using rehabilitation.

Theory of the mind: one's ability to understand others' and one's own states of mind, such as beliefs and thoughts.

Therapeutic–community model: participative, group-based approach to long-term mental illness, personality disorders and drug addiction. The approach is usually residential, with the clients and therapists living together. It is based on milieu therapy principles and includes group psychotherapy as well as practical activities (The Free Dictionary, Farlex, n.d.).

Thresholds: the magnitude or intensity that must be exceeded for a certain reaction, phenomenon, result or condition to occur or be manifested (Stevenson, 2010).

Time-out corner: negative intervention which normally consists in sending the child for a few minutes to a corner, where there is little in the way of enjoyable activity and where the child is not likely to receive attention.

Top-down procedure: diagnostic system process in which categories are first sketched on the basis of general theory or experts' opinions, and then validated in empirical field trials.

Trait: any enduring characteristic of a person (Statt, 2003).

Trajectories: the paths followed in an individual's development.

Transgender: appearing as, wishing to be considered as or having undergone surgery to become a member of the opposite biological sex (Morris, 2000).

Transsexual: a person with a powerful desire to adopt the physical attributes, and to play the role, of a member of the opposite sex. A person who has undergone medical and surgical treatment to alter the body's external sexual characteristics to those of the opposite sex (Colman, 2009).

Treatment integrity: the degree to which intervention is implemented as designed and intended.

Triarchical model: theory formulated by Robert J. Sternberg, according to which intelligence is defined as "(a) mental activity directed toward purposive adaptation to, selection, and shaping of, real-world environments relevant to one's life." Sternberg's theory comprises three parts: componential, experiential and practical (Sternberg, 1985, p. 45).

Tripartite model of anxiety and depression: a model positing that the majority of between-person variability in emotional symptoms consists of three underlying affective dimensions: negative affect, anhedonia and low positive affect. Developed by Clark and Wilson.

Tripartite pathway model of eating disorder: model of body image and eating disturbance which proposes that three formative influences (peer, parents and media) affect body image and eating problems through two mediational mechanisms: internalization of the thin ideal and appearance comparison processes (Keery, Van den Berg and Thompson, 2004).

Two-tam: a problem experienced by children from Northern Uganda, meaning having "a lot of thoughts," poor self-esteem, feelings of hopelessness and poor concentration.

Uncertainty avoidance: degree to which members of a society are anxious about the unknown, and, as a consequence, attempt to cope with anxiety by minimizing uncertainty and making expectations explicit (The Free Dictionary, Farlex, n.d.).

Unengaged or **rejecting-neglecting parents:** type of parents in Baumrind's classification (1991), who are neither demanding nor responsive to their children (Socolar, 1997).

Universal prevention interventions: strategies designed to reach the entire population, without regard to individual risk factors, and which are intended to reach a very large audience.

Universalist position: an approach according to which the basic structure of psychopathology, including the classification of the disorders, their definitions, their core symptoms, consequences for the people affected and the degree of overlap between different disorders, is essentially the same for people of all cultures.

Vagal augmentation, or **increased RSA**: young children with disruptive behavior problems who had been exposed to domestic violence actually showed vagal augmentation, or increased RSA, when they were deceived into thinking that a peer had provoked them.

Ventromedial prefrontal cortex (PFC): a part of the prefrontal cortex in the mammalian brain. The ventral medial prefrontal is located in the frontal lobe and is implicated in the processing of risk and fear, and in decision-making (The Free Dictionary, Farlex, n.d.).

Virtual–reality therapy: a method of psychotherapy that uses virtual-reality technology to treat patients with anxiety disorder and phobias. Virtual reality involves the simulation of the setting that evokes the patient's difficulties.

Vulnerable population hypothesis: hypothesis according to which certain people may be particularly vulnerable to psychological problems, perhaps because of environmental and social conditions, personality or temperament problems, physiological factors or any combination of these risk factors (Zachar, 2009).

Within–subjects designs: any research design in which the same research participants or subjects are tested under different treatment conditions (Colman, 2009).

BIBLIOGRAPHY

AACAP. (2007). Practice parameter for the assessment and treatment of children and adolescents with attention-deficit/hyperactivity disorder. *Journal of the American Academy of Child and Adolescent Psychiatry, 46,* 894–921.

Aaron, J., Zaglul, H. and Emery, R. E. (1999). Posttraumatic stress in children following acute physical injury. *Journal of Pediatric Psychology, 24,* 335–43.

Abbeduto, L., Seltzer, M. M., Shattuck, P., Krauss, M. W., Orsmond, G. and Murphy, M. M. (2004). Psychological well-being and coping in mothers of youths with autism, Down Syndrome, or Fragile X Syndrome. *American Journal on Mental Retardation, 109,* 237–54.

Abela, J. R. Z. and Sarin, S. (2002). Cognitive vulnerability to hopelessness depression: A chain is only as strong as its weakest link. *Cognitive Therapy and Research, 26,* 811–29.

Abela, J. R. Z., Skitch, S. A., Adams, P. and Hankin, B. L. (2006). The timing of parent and child depression: A hopelessness theory perspective. *Journal of Clinical Child and Adolescent Psychology, 35,* 253–63.

Abela, J. R. Z. and Hankin, B. L. (2008). Cognitive vulnerability to depression. In J. R. Z. Abela and B. L. Hankin (Eds.), *Handbook of depression in children and adolescents* (pp. 35–78). New York: Guilford.

Abela, J. R. Z., Zinck, S., Kryger, S., Zilber, I. and Hankin, B. L. (2009). Contagious depression: Negative attachment cognitions as a moderator of the temporal association between parental depression and child depression. *Journal of Clinical Child and Adolescent Psychology, 38,* 16–26.

Aberson, B., Shure, M. B. and Goldstein, S. (2007). Social problem-solving intervention can help children with ADHD. *Journal of Attention Disorders, 11,* 4–7.

Abhay, M., Gaidhane, A. M., Zahiruddin, Q. S. and Zodpey, S. (2008). Substance abuse among street children in Mumbai. *Vulnerable Children and Youth Studies, 3,* 42–51.

Abikoff, H. (2009). ADHD psychosocial treatments: Generalization reconsidered. *Journal of Attention Disorders, 13,* 207–10.

Abikoff, H., Courtney, M., Pelham, W. E. and Koplewicz, H. S. (1993). Teachers' ratings of disruptive behaviours: The influence of halo effects. *Journal of Abnormal Child Psychology, 21,* 519–34.

Abikoff, H., Hechtman, L., Klein, R. G., Gallagher, R., Fleiss, K., Etcovitch, J.,…Pollack, S. (2004). Social functioning in children with ADHD treated with long-term methylphenidate and multimodal psychosocial treatment. *Journal of the American Academy of Child and Adolescent Psychiatry, 43,* 820–9.

Abou-ezzeddine, T., Schwartz, D., Chang, L., Lee-Shin, Y., Farver, J. and Xu, Y. (2007). Positive peer relationships and risk of victimization in Chinese and South Korean children's peer groups. *Social Development, 16,* 106–27.

Aboud, F. and Mendelson, M. J. (1996). Determinants of friendship selection and quality: Developmental perspectives. In W. M. Bukowski, A. F. Newcomb and W. W. Hartup (Eds.), *The company they keep: Friendship in childhood and adolescence* (pp. 87–112). New York: Cambridge University Press.

Abramson, L. Y., Alloy, L. B. and Metalsky, G. I. (1988). The cognitive diathesis-stress theories of depression: Toward an adequate evaluation of the theories' validities. In L. B. Alloy (Ed.), *Cognitive processes in depression* (pp. 3–30). New York: Guilford.

Abramson, L. Y., Metalsky, G. I. and Alloy, L. B. (1989). Hopelessness depression: A theory-based subtype of depression. *Psychological Review, 96,* 358–72.

Achenbach, T. M. (1966). The classification of children's psychiatric symptoms: A factor-analytic study. *Psychological Monographs: General and Applied, 80,* 37.

Achenbach, T. M. (2009). Some needed changes in DSM-V: But what about children? *Clinical Psychology: Science and Practice, 16,* 50–3.

Achenbach, T. M. and Rescorla, L. A. (2000). *Manual for the ASEBA Preschool Forms and Profiles.* Burlington, VT: University of Vermont, Research Center for Children, Youth and Families.

Achenbach, T. M. and Rescorla, L. A. (2001). *Manual for the ASEBA School-Age Forms and Profiles.* Burlington, VT: University of Vermont, Research Center for Children, Youth and Families.

Achenbach, T. M. and Rescorla, L. A. (2007). *Multicultural understanding of child and adolescent psychopathology: Implications for mental health assessment.* New York: Guilford Press.

Ackard, D. M., Fulkerson, J. A. and Neumark-Sztainer, D. (2007). Prevalence and utility of DSM-IV eating disorder diagnostic criteria among youth. *International Journal of Eating Disorders, 40*, 409–17.

Acoca, L. (1998) Outside/inside: The violation of American girls at home, on the streets, and in the juvenile justice system. *Crime and Delinquency, 44*, 561–89.

Adam, E. K. (2012). Emotion-cortisol transactions occur over multiple time-scales in development: Implications for research on emotion and the development of emotional disorders. *Monographs of the Society for Research in Child Development, 77*, 17–27.

Adam, E. K., Doane, L. D., Zinbarg, R. E., Mineka, S., Craske, M. G. and Griffith, J. W. (2010). Prospective prediction of major depressive disorder from cortisol awakening responses in adolescence. *Psychoneuroendocrinology, 35*, 921–31.

Adams, R. E., Bukowski, W. M. and Bagwell, C. (2005). Stability of aggression during early adolescence as moderated by reciprocated friendship status and friend's aggression. *International Journal of Behavioral Development, 29*, 139–45.

Adlam, J. and Scanlon, C. (2011). Working with hard-to-reach patients in difficult places: A democratic therapeutic community approach to consultation. In A. Rubitel and D. Reiss (Eds.), *Containment in the community: Supportive frameworks for thinking about antisocial behavior and mental health* (pp. 1–22). London: Karnac Books.

Addis, M. E. (2008). Gender and depression in men. *Clinical Psychology: Science and Practice, 15*, 153–68.

Adleman, N. E., Menon, V., Blasey, C. M., White, C. D., Warsofsky, I. S., Glover, G. H., et al. (2002). A developmental fMRI study of the Stroop color-word task. *Neuroimage, 16*, 61–75.

Adler, P. A. and Adler, P. (1998). *Peer power: Preadolescent culture and identity.* Piscataway, NJ: Rutgers University Press.

Adolphs, R. (2001). The neurobiology of social cognition. *Current Opinion in Neurobiology, 11*, 231–9.

Adolphs, R. (2003). Cognitive neuroscience of human social behaviour. *Nature Reviews Neuroscience, 4*, 165–78.

Adolphs, R. (2010). What does the amygdala contribute to social cognition? *Annals of the New York Academy of Sciences, 1191*, 42–61.

Adolphs, R., Tranel, D., Damasio, H. and Damasio, A. R. (1995). Fear and the human amygdala. *Journal of Neuroscience, 15*, 5879–91.

Adolphs, R., Tranel, D., Hamann, S., Young, A. W., Calder, A. J., Phelps, E. A., …Damasio, A. R. (1999). Recognition of facial emotion in nine individuals with bilateral amygdala damage. *Neuropsychologia, 37*, 1111–17.

Adolphs, R., Gosselin, F., Buchanan, T. W., Tranel, D., Schyns, P. and Damasio, A. R. (2005). A mechanism for impaired fear recognition after amygdala damage. *Nature, 433*, 68–72.

Afifi, T. O., Boman, J., Fleisher, W. and Sareen, J. (2009). The relationship between child abuse, parental divorce, and lifetime mental disorders and suicidality in a nationally representative adult sample. *Child Abuse and Neglect, 33*, 139–47.

Agliata, D. and Tantleff-Dunn, S. (2004). The impact of media exposure on males' body image. *Journal of Social and Clinical Psychology, 23*, 7–22.

Agras, W. S. (2001). The consequences and costs of the eating disorders. *Psychiatric Clinics of North America, 24*, 371–9.

Agras, W. S., Walsh, T., Fairburn, C. G., Wilson, G. T. and Kraemer, H. C. (2000). A multicenter comparison of cognitive-behavioral therapy and interpersonal psychotherapy for bulimia nervosa. *Archives of General Psychiatry, 57*, 459–66.

Aharon, I., Etcoff, N., Ariely, D., Chabris, C. F., O'Connor, E., and Breiter, H. C. (2001). Beautiful faces have variable reward value: fMRI and behavioral evidence. *Neuron, 32*, 537–51.

Ainsworth, M. D. S. (1967). *Infancy in Uganda: Infant care and the growth of love.* Oxford: Johns Hopkins University Press.

Ainsworth, M. S., Blehar, M. C., Waters, E. and Wall, S. (1978). *Patterns of attachment: A psychological study of the strange situation.* Oxford: Lawrence Erlbaum.

Albee, G. W. (1998). The politics of primary prevention. *The Journal of Primary Prevention, 19*, 117–27.

Albee, G. W. (2005). Prevention of mental disorders. In W. E. Pickren and S. F. Schneider (Eds.), *Psychology and the National Institute of Mental Health: A historical analysis of science, practice, and policy* (pp. 295–315). Washington, DC: American Psychological Association.

Albee, G. W., Bond, L. A. and Monsey, T. V. C. (1992). *Improving children's lives: Global perspectives on prevention.* Newbury Park, CA: Sage Publications.

Alda, M. (1997). Bipolar disorder: From families to genes. *Canadian Journal of Psychiatry, 42*, 378–87.

Alexander, D. (1998). Prevention of mental retardation: Four decades of research. *Mental Retardation and Developmental Disabilities Research Reviews, 4*, 50–8.

Alexander, F. G. and Selesnick, S. T. (1966). *The history of psychiatry.* New York: New American Library.

Algozzine, B., Wang, C. and Violette, A. S. (2011). Reexamining the relationship between academic achievement and social behavior. *Journal of Positive Behavior Interventions, 13*, 3–16.

Ali, O. S., Milstein, G. and Marzuk, P. M. (2005). The Imam's role in meeting the counselling needs of Muslim communities in the United States. *Psychiatric Services, 56,* 202–5.

Allen, J. P., Hauser, S. T. and Borman-Spurrell, E. (1996) Attachment theory as a framework for understanding sequelae of severe adolescent psychopathology: An 11-year follow-up study. *Journal of Consulting and Clinical Psychology, 64,* 254–63.

Allen, J. P., Porter, M. R. and McFarland, F. C. (2006). Leaders and followers in adolescent close friendships: Susceptibility to peer influence as a predictor of risky behavior, friendship instability, and depression. *Development and Psychopathology, 18,* 155–72.

Allen, J. P. and Antonishak, J. (2008). Adolescent peer influences: Beyond the dark side. In M. J. Prinstein and K. A. Dodge (Eds.), *Understanding peer influence in children and adolescents* (pp. 141–60). New York: Guilford Press.

Allen, N. B., Gilbert, P. and Semedar, A. (2004). Depressed mood as an interpersonal strategy: The importance of relational models. In N. Haslam (Ed.), *Relational models theory: A contemporary overview* (pp. 309–34). Mahwah, NJ: Lawrence Erlbaum Associates Publishers.

Allès-Jardel, M., Fourdrinier, C., Roux, A. and Schneider, B. H. (2002). Parents' structuring of children's daily lives in relation to the quality and stability of children's friendships. *International Journal of Psychology, 37,* 65–73.

Alpert, R. and Haber, R. N. (1960). Anxiety in academic achievement situations. *The Journal of Abnormal and Social Psychology, 61,* 207–15.

Alvarez Valdivia, I., Schneider, B. H., Lorenzo Chavez, K. and Chen, X. (2005). Social withdrawal and maladjustment in a very group-oriented society. *International Journal of Behavioral Development, 29,* 315–22.

Amaral, D. (2002). The primate amgydala and the neurobiology of social behavior: Implications for understanding social anxiety. *Society of Biological Psychiatry, 51,* 11–17.

Amaral, D., Rogers, S. J., Baron-Cohen, S., Bourgeron, T., Caffo, E., Fombonne, E.,…van der Gaag, R. J. (2011). Against Le Packing: A consensus statement. *Journal of the American Academy of Child and Adolescent Psychiatry, 50,* 191–2.

Ambrosini, P. J. (2000). Historical development and present status of the Schedule for Affective Disorders and Schizophrenia for School-Age Children (K-SADS). *Journal of the American Academy of Child and Adolescent Psychiatry, 39,* 49–58.

American Academy of Child and Adolescent Psychiatry. (2005). Practice parameter for the assessment and treatment of children and adolescents with reactive attachment disorder of infancy and early childhood. *Journal of the American Academy of Child and Adolescent Psychiatry, 44,* 1206–19.

American Educational Research Association, American Psychological Association, National Council on Measurement in Education. (1999). *Standards for educational and psychological testing.* Washington, DC: American Educational Research Association.

American heritage dictionary of the English language (2006). Boston: Houghton-Mifflin.

American Psychological Association. Resolution on facilitated communication. August 14, 1994.

American Psychiatric Association. (1980). *Diagnostic and statistical manual of mental disorders* (3rd edn.). Washington, DC: Author.

American Psychiatric Association. (1987). *Diagnostic and statistical manual of mental disorders* (3rd edn., rev.). Washington, DC: Author.

American Psychiatric Association. (2000). *Diagnostic and statistical manual of mental disorders* (4th edn., text rev.). Washington, DC: Author.

American Psychiatric Association. *DSM-5 development.* Retrieved June 17, 2010 from www.dsm5.org

American Psychiatric Association. (2013). *Diagnostic and statistical manual of mental disorders* (5th edn.). Washington, DC: Author.

American Psychological Association. (2003). Guidelines on multicultural education, training, research, practice and organisational change for psychologists. *American Psychologist, 58,* 377–402.

American Psychological Association. (2005). *Policy statement on evidence-based practice in psychology.* Retrieved from www.apa.org/practice/resources/evidence/evidence-based-statement.pdf

American Psychological Association. (2009). *Report of the APA task force on gender identity and gender variance.* Washington, DC: Author.

Ameringen, M. V., Mancini, C. and Farvolden, P. (2003). The impact of anxiety disorders on educational achievement. *Journal of Anxiety Disorders, 17,* 561–71.

Anderson, C. A., Shibuya, A., Ihori, N., Swing, E. L., Bushman, B. J., Sakamoto, A.,…Saleem, M. (2010). Violent video game effects on aggression, empathy, and prosocial behavior in Eastern and Western countries: A meta-analytic review. *Psychological Bulletin, 136,* 151–73.

Anderson, D. M. (2009). *Mosby's medical dictionary* (8th edn.). St Louis, MO: Mosby/Elsevier.

Anderson, E., and Hope, D. A. (2008). A review of the tripartite model for understanding the link between anxiety and depression in youth. *Clinical Psychology Review, 28,* 275–87.

Anderson, H. and Gerhart, D. (2007). *Collaborative therapy: Relationships and conversations that make a difference.* New York: Routledge.

Anderson, J. C. (1996). Is hyperactivity the product of Western culture? *The Lancet, 348,* 73–4.

Anderson, K. and Forman, V. (2010). *Gravity pulls you in: Perspectives on parenting children on the autism spectrum.* Bethesda, MD: Woodbine House.

Anderson, P., Jacobs, C. and Rothbaum, B. O. (2004). Computer-supported cognitive behavioral treatment of anxiety disorders. *Journal of Clinical Psychology, 60,* 253–67.

Anderson, P. L. and Meier-Hedde, R. (2001). Early case reports of dyslexia in the United States and Europe. *Journal of Learning Disabilities, 34,* 9–21.

Anderson, S. W., Bechara, A., Damasio, H., Tranel, D. and Damasio, A. R. (1999). Impairment of social and moral behavior related to early damage in human prefrontal cortex. *Nature Neuroscience, 2*(11), 1032–7.

Anderson-Fye, E. (2004). A "coca-cola" shape: Cultural change, body image, and eating disorders in San Andres, Belize. *Culture, Medicine and Psychiatry, 28,* 561–95.

Anderson-Fye, E. (2009). Cross-cultural issues in body image among children and adolescents. In L. Smolak and J. K. Thompson (Eds.), *Body image, eating disorders, and obesity in youth: Assessment, prevention, and treatment* (2nd edn., pp. 113–33). Washington, DC: American Psychological Association.

Andersson, G. and Cuijpers, P. (2009). "Psychological treatment" as an umbrella term for evidence-based psychotherapies? *Nordic Psychology, 61,* 4–15.

Andersson, G. and Ghaderi, A. (2006). Overview and analysis of the behaviourist criticism of the Diagnostic and Statistical Manual of Mental Disorders (DSM). *Clinical Psychologist, 10,* 67–77.

Andrews, G., Slade, T. and Peters, L. (1999). Classification in psychiatry: ICD-10 versus DSM-IV. *British Journal of Psychiatry, 174,* 3–5.

Andrews, G., Slade, T., Sunderland, M. and Anderson, T. (2007). Issues for DSM-V: Simplifying DSM-IV to enhance utility: The case of major depressive disorder. *American Journal of Psychiatry, 164,* 1784–5.

Andrews, J. (1998). Begging the question of idiocy: The definition and socio-cultural meaning of idiocy in early modern Britain, Part 1. *History of Psychiatry, 9,* 65–95.

Ang, R. P. and Hughes, J. N. (2002). Differential benefits of skills training with antisocial youth based on group composition: A meta-analytic investigation. *School Psychology Review, 31,* 164–85.

Angier, N. (1994, July, 24). The debilitating malady called boyhood. The *New York Times.* Retrieved from www.nytimes.com

Angold, A., Costello, E. J. and Erkanli, A. (1999). Comorbidity. *Journal of Child Psychology and Psychiatry, 40,* 57–87.

Angst, J. (2001). Bipolarity from ancient to modern times. *Journal of Affective Disorders, 67,* 3–19.

Angst, J. and Marneros, A. (2001). Bipolarity from ancient to modern times: Conception, birth and rebirth. *Affective Disorders, 67,* 3–19.

Ansbacher, H. L. and Huber, R. J. (2004). Adler – Psychotherapy and Freud. *Journal of Individual Psychology, 60,* 333–7.

Anthony, E. J. (1986). A brief history of child psychoanalysis. *Journal of the American Academy of Child and Adolescent Psychiatry, 25,* 8–11.

Anthony, J. and Scott, P. (1960). Manic-depressive psychosis in childhood. *Child Psychology and Psychiatry, 1,* 53–72.

Antshel, K. M. and Remer, R. (2003). Social skills training in children with attention deficit hyperactivity disorder: A randomized-controlled clinical trial. *Journal of Clinical Child and Adolescent Psychology, 32,* 153–65.

APA dictionary of psychology. (2007). VandenBos, G. R. (Ed.), Washington, DC: American Psychological Association.

Appel, A. E. and Holden, G. W. (1998). The co-occurrence of spouse and physical child abuse: A review and appraisal. *Journal of Family Psychology, 12,* 578–99.

Aptel, A., Abu Shah, M., Iancu, I., Abramovitch, H., Weizman, A. and Tyano, S. (1994). Cultural effects on eating attitudes in Israeli subpopulations and hospitalized anorectics. *Genetic, Social, and General Psychology Monographs, 120,* 83–99.

Apter, A., Abu-Shah, M., Iancu, I., Abromovitch, H., Weizman, A. and Tyano, S. (1994). *Cultural effects on eating attitudes in Israeli subpopulations and hospitalized anorectics,* Genetic, Social and General Psychology Monographs, *120,* 85–99.

Aragona, M. (2009). The role of comorbidity in the crisis of the current psychiatric classification system. *Philosophy, Psychiatry, and Psychology, 16,* 1–11.

Araya, R., Montero-Marin, J., Barroilhet, S., Fritsch, R. and Montgomery, A. (2013). Detecting depression among adolescents in Santiago, Chile: sex differences. *BMC Psychiatry, 13,* 1–12.

Arbona, C. and Power, T. G. (2003). Parental attachment, self-esteem, and antisocial behaviors among African American, European American, and Mexican American adolescents. *Journal of Counseling Psychology, 50,* 40–51.

Archer, J. (2004). Sex differences in aggression in real-world settings: A meta-analytic review. *Review of General Psychology, 8,* 291–322.

Arias, I. (2004). The legacy of child maltreatment: Long-term health consequences for women. *Journal of Women's Health*, *13*, 468–73.

Ariès, P. (1962). *Centuries of childhood*. New York : Vintage Books.

Arnarson, E. O. and Craighead, W. E. (2009). Prevention of depression among Icelandic adolescents. *Behaviour Research and Therapy*, *47*, 577–85.

Arnett, J. J. (2006). G. Stanley Hall's Adolescence: Brilliance and nonsense. *History of Psychology*, *9*, 186–97.

Asch, S. E. (1951). Effects of group pressure upon the modification and distortion of judgment. In H. Guetzkow (Ed.), *Groups, leadership and men*. Pittsburgh, PA: Carnegie.

Asher, S. R., Rose, A. J. and Gabriel, S. W. (2001). Peer rejection in everyday life. In M. R. Leary (Ed.), *Interpersonal rejection* (pp. 105–44). New York: Oxford University Press.

Atkinson, L., Niccols, A., Paglia, A., Coolbear, J., Parker, K. C. H., Poulton, L., Guger, S. and Sitarenios, G. (2000). A meta-analysis of time between maternal sensitivity and attachment assessments: Implications for internal working models in infancy/toddlerhood. *Journal of Social and Personal Relationships*, *17*, 791–810.

Atkinson, L., Paglia, A., Coolbear, J., Niccols, A., Parker, K. C. H. and Guger, S. (2000). Attachment security: A meta-analysis of maternal mental health correlates. *Clinical Psychology Review*, *20*, 1019–40.

Attwood, T. (2000). Strategies for improving the social integration of children with Asperger's syndrome. *Autism*, *4*, 85–100.

August, G. J., Braswell, L. and Thura, P. (1998). Diagnostic stability of ADHD in a community sample of school-age children screened for disruptive behavior. *Journal of Abnormal Child Psychology*, *26*, 345–56.

Ault, A. and Brzuzy, S. (2009). Removing gender identity disorder from the Diagnostic and Statistical Manual of Mental Disorders: A call for action. *Social Work*, *54*, 187–9.

Aune, T. and Stiles, T. C. (2009). Universal-based prevention of syndromal and subsyndromal social anxiety: A randomized controlled study. *Journal of Consulting and Clinical Psychology*, *77*, 867–79.

Austin, A. M., Macgowan, M. J. and Wagner, E. F. (2005). Effective family-based interventions for adolescents with substance use problems: A systematic review. *Research on Social Work Practice*, *15*, 67–83.

Australian Psychological Society. (2004). *Guidelines for the provision of psychological services for, and the conduct of psychological research with, Aboriginal and Torres Strait Islander people of Australia*. Melbourne: Author.

Avenevoli, S., Knight, E., Kessler, R. C. and Merikangas, K. R. (2008). Epidemiology of depression in children and adolescents. In J. R. Z. Abela and B. L. Hankin (Eds.) *Handbook of depression in children and adolescents* (pp. 6–32). New York: Guilford.

Axelson, D., Birmaher, B., Strober, M., Gill, M. K., Valeri, S., Chiappetta, L.,...Keller, M. (2006). Phenomcnology of children and adolescents with bipolar spectrum disorders. *Archives of General Psychiatry*, *63*, 1139–48.

Axline, V. (1964). *Dibs: In search of self*. London: Heinemann.

Ayala, G. X., Mickens, L., Galindo, P. and Elder, J. P. (2007). Acculturation and body image perception among Latino youth. *Ethnicity and Health*, *12*, 21–41.

Aylward, E. H., Minshew, N. J., Field, K., Sparks, B. F. and Singh, N. (2002). Effects of age on brain volume and head circumference in autism. *Neurology*, *59*, 175–83.

Azrin, N. H., Acierno, R., Kogan, E. S., Besalel, V. A. and McMahon, P. T. (1996). Follow-up results of supportive versus behavioral therapy for illicit drug use. *Behaviour Research and Therapy*, *34*, 41–6.

Baer, R. A. and Nietzel, M. T. (1991). Cognitive and behavioral treatment of impulsivity in children: A meta-analytic review of the outcome literature. *Journal of Clinical Child Psychology*, *20*, 400–12.

Bagot, R. C., and Meaney, M. J. (2010). Epigenetics and the biological basis of gene × environment interactions. *Journal of the American Academy of Child and Adolescent Psychiatry*, *49*, 752–71.

Bagwell, C. L., Newcomb, A. F. and Bukowski, W. M. (1998). Preadolescent friendship and peer rejection as predictors of adult adjustment. *Child Development*, *69*, 140–53.

Bagwell, C. L., Molina, B. S., Pelham, W. E. and Hoza, B. (2001). Attention-deficit hyperactivity disorder and problems in peer relations: Predictions from childhood to adolescence. *Journal of the American Academy of Child and Adolescent Psychiatry*, *40*, 1285–92.

Bagwell, C. L., Schmidt, M. E., Newcomb, A. F. and Bukowski, W. M. (2001). Friendship and peer rejection as predictors of adult adjustment. In D. W. Nangle and C. A. Erdley (Eds.), *The role of friendship in psychological adjustment: New directions for child and adolescent development* (pp. 25–49). San Francisco, CA: Jossey-Bass.

Bailey, W. (1994). A longitudinal study of fathers' involvement with young children: Infancy through 5 years. *Journal of Genetic Psychology*, *155*, 331–9.

Baker, J., Parks-Savage, A. and Rehfuss, M. (2009). Teaching social skills in a virtual environment: An exploratory study. *Journal for Specialists in Group Work*, *34*, 209–26.

Baker, J. R. and Hudson, J. L. (2013). Friendship quality predicts treatment outcome in children with anxiety disorder. *Behaviour Research and Therapy, 51*, 31–6.

Baker, L. A., Tuvblad, C., Reynolds, C., Zheng, M., Lozano, D. I. and Raine, A. (2009). Resting heart rate and the development of antisocial behavior from age 9 to 14: Genetic and environmental influences. *Development and Psychopathology, 21*, 939–60.

Baker, M., Milich, R. and Manolis, M. B. (1996). Peer interactions of dysphoric adolescents. *Journal of Abnormal Child Psychology, 24*, 241–55.

Baker-Henningham, H., Walker, S., Powell, C. and Gardner, J. M. (2009). A pilot study of the Incredible Years Teacher Training programme and a curriculum unit on social and emotional skills in community pre-schools in Jamaica. *Child Care, Health and Development, 35*, 624–31.

Bakermans-Kranenburg, M. J. and van IJzendoorn, M. H. (2006). Gene–environment interaction of the dopamine D4 receptor (DRD4) and observed maternal insensitivity predicting externalizing behavior in preschoolers. *Developmental Psychobiology, 48*(5), 406–9.

Bakermans-Kranenburg, M. J., van IJzendoorn, M. H., Pijlman, F. T. A., Mesman, J. and Juffer, F. (2008). Experimental evidence for differential susceptibility: Dopamine D4 receptor polymorphism (DRD4 VNTR) moderates intervention effects on toddlers' externalizing behavior in a randomized controlled trial. *Developmental Psychology, 44*, 293–300.

Bakken, J. P. and Brown, B. B. (2009). Principles of peer influence. *Paradigm, 14*, 14–18.

Baldessarini, R. J., Tondo, L. and Hennen, J. (2003). Lithium treatment and suicide risk in major affective disorders: Update and new findings. *Journal of Clinical Psychiatry, 64*, 44–52.

Baldry, A. C., and Winkel, F. W. (2004). Mental and physical health of Italian youngsters directly and indirectly victimized at school and at home. *International Journal of Forensic Mental Health, 3*, 77–91.

Baldwin, J. S. and Dadds, M. R. (2008). Examining alternative explanations of the covariation of ADHD and anxiety symptoms in children: A community study. *Journal of Abnormal Child Psychology, 36*, 67–79.

Banathy, B. H. (1996). *Designing social systems in a changing world.* New York: Plenum Press.

Bandura, A. (1969). *Principles of behavior modification.* New York: Holt, Rinehart and Winston.

Banerjee, T., Middleton, F. and Faraone, S. V. (2007). Environmental risk factors for attention-deficit hyperactivity disorder. *Acta Paediatrica, 96*, 1269–74.

Bank, L., Marlowe, J. H., Reid, J. B., Patterson, G. R. and Weinrott, M. R. (1991). A comparative evaluation of parent-training interventions for families of chronic delinquents. *Journal of Abnormal Child Psychology, 19*, 15–33.

Banks, J. A., and McGee Banks, C. A. (1989). *Multicultural education.* Needham Heights, MA: Allyn & Bacon.

Barbaro, J. and Dissanayake, C. (2009). Autism spectrum disorders in infancy and toddlerhood: A review of the evidence on early signs, early identification tools, and early diagnosis. *Journal of Developmental and Behavioral Pediatrics, 30*, 447–59.

Barcia, D. (2005). The history of Spanish psychiatry. In J. J. Lopez-Ibor, C. L. Cercos and C. C. Masia (Eds.), *Images of Spanish psychiatry* (pp. 37–61) Madrid: Glosa.

Barcaccia, B. (2008, June). Accepting limitations of life: Leading our patients through a painful but healing path. Lecture at Ludwig-Maximilians-Universität, Munich, Germany.

Bardone, A. M., Moffitt, T. E., Caspi, A., Dickson, N. and Silva, P. A. (1996). Adult mental health and social outcomes of adolescent girls with depression and conduct disorder. *Development and Psychopathology, 8*, 811–29.

Bar-Haim, Y., Dan, O., Eshel, Y. and Sagi-Schwartz, A. (2007). Predicting children's anxiety from early attachment relationships. *Journal of Anxiety Disorders, 21*, 1061–8.

Bar-Haim, Y., Lamy, D., Pergamin, L., Bakermans-Kranenburg, M. J. and van Ijzendoorn, M. H. (2007). Threat-related attentional bias in anxious and nonanxious individuals: A meta-analytic study. *Psychological Bulletin, 133*, 1–24.

Barkley, R. A. (1988). The effects of methylphenidate on the interactions of preschool ADHD children with their mothers. *Journal of the American Academy of Child and Adolescent Psychiatry, 27*, 336–41.

Barkley, R. A. (1989). Hyperactive girls and boys: Stimulant drug effects on mother–child interactions. *Journal of Child Psychology and Psychiatry, 30*, 379–90.

Barkley, R. A. (2004). Critique or misrepresentation? A reply to Timimi et al. *Clinical Child and Family Psychology Review, 7*, 65–9.

Barkley, R. A. (2007). School interventions for attention deficit hyperactivity disorder: Where to from here? *School Psychology Review, 36*, 279–86.

Barkley, R. A. (2010). Against the status quo: Revising the diagnostic criteria for ADHD. *Journal of the American Academy of Child and Adolescent Psychiatry, 49*, 205–7.

Barkley, R. A., Karlsson, J. and Pollard, S. (1985). Effects of age on the mother–child interactions of ADD-H and normal boys. *Journal of Abnormal Child Psychology, 13*, 631–7.

Barkley, R. A., Fischer, M., Edelbrock, C. S. and Smallish, L. (1990). The adolescent outcome of hyperactive children diagnosed by research criteria: I. An 8-year prospective follow-up study. *Journal of the American Academy of Child and Adolescent Psychiatry, 29,* 546–57.

Barkley, R. A., Fischer, M., Smallish, L. and Fletcher, K. (2002). The persistence of attention-deficit/hyperactivity disorder into young adulthood as a function of reporting source and definition of disorder. *Journal of Abnormal Psychology, 111,* 279–89.

Barkley, R. A., Fischer, M., Smallish, L. and Fletcher, K. (2006). Young adult outcome of hyperactive children: Adaptive functioning in major life activities. *Journal of the American Academy of Child and Adolescent Psychiatry, 45,* 192–202.

Barlow, D. H. (2004). Psychological treatments. *American Psychologist, 59,* 869–78.

Barlow, J. and Stewart-Brown, S. (2000). Behavior problems and group-based parent education programs. *Journal of Developmental and Behavioral Pediatrics, 21,* 356–70.

Baron-Cohen, S. (2003). *The essential difference: The truth about the male and female brain.* New York: Basic Books.

Baron-Cohen, S., Luctchmaya, S. and Knickmeyer, R. (2004). *Prenatal testosterone in mind.* London: MIT Press.

Baron-Cohen, S., Knickmeyer, R. and Belmonte, M. (2005). Sex differences in the brain: Implications for autism. *Science, 310,* 819–23.

Barrett, P. and Turner, C. (2001). Prevention of anxiety symptoms in primary school children: Preliminary results from a universal school-based trial. *British Journal of Clinical Psychology, 40,* 399–410.

Barrett, P., Farrell, L. J., Ollendick, T. H. and Dadds, M. (2006). Long-term outcomes of an Australian universal prevention trial of anxiety and depression symptoms in children and youth: An evaluation of the Friends Program. *Journal of Clinical Child and Adolescent Psychology, 35,* 403–11.

Barry, R. J., Johnstone, S. J. and Clarke, A. R. (2003). A review of electrophysiology in attention-deficit/hyperactivity disorder: II. Event-related potentials. *Clinical Neurophysiology, 114,* 184–98.

Barry, R. J., Clarke, A. R., McCarthy, R. and Selikowitz, M. (2006). Age and gender effects in EEG coherence: III. Girls with attention-deficit/hyperactivity disorder. *Clinical Neurophysiology, 117,* 243–51.

Bartels, A. and Zeki, S. (2000). The neural basis of romantic love. *Neuroreport, 11,* 3829–34.

Bateson, G., Jackson, D. D., Haley, J. and Weakland, J. (1963). Toward a theory of schizophrenia. In N. J. Smelser and W. T. Smelser (Eds.), *Personality and social systems* (pp. 172–87). Hoboken, NJ: Wiley.

Bauer, A. M., Quas, J. A. and Boyce, W. T. (2002). Associations between physiological reactivity and children's behavior: Advantages of a multisystem approach. *Journal of Developmental and Behavioral Pediatrics, 23,* 102–13.

Bauermeister, J. J., Shrout, P. E., Chavez, L., Rubio-Stipec, M., Ramirez, R., Padilla, L.,...Canino, G. (2007). ADHD and gender: Are risks and sequel of ADHD the same for boys and girls?*Journal of Child Psychology and Psychiatry, 48,* 831–9.

Baughman, F. A. (2006). *The ADHD fraud: How psychiatry makes "patients" out of normal children.* Bloomington, IN: Trafford Publishing.

Baumeister, R. F., DeWall, C. N., Ciarocco, N. J. and Twenge, J. M. (2005). Social exclusion impairs self-regulation. *Journal of Personality and Social Psychology, 88,* 589–604.

Bauminger, N. and Kasari, C. (2000). Loneliness and friendship in high-functioning children with autism. *Child Development, 71,* 447–56.

Bauminger, N. and Kimhi-Kind, I. (2008). Social information processing, security of attachment, and emotion regulation in children with learning disabilities. *Journal of Learning Disabilities, 41,* 315–32.

Bauminger, N., Solomon, M., Aviezer, A., Heung, K., Brown, J. and Rogers, S. J. (2008). Friendship in high functioning children with autism spectrum disorder: Mixed and non-mixed dyads. *Journal of Autism and Developmental Disorders, 38,* 1211–29.

Baumrind, D. (1971). Current patterns of parental authority. *Developmental Psychology, 4,* 1–103.

Baumrind, D. (1991). The influence of parenting style on adolescent competence and substance use. *The Journal of Early Adolescence, 11,* 56–95.

Baumrind, D., Larzelere, R. E. and Owens, E. B. (2010). Effects of preschool parents' power assertive patterns and practices on adolescent development. *Parenting: Science and Practice, 10,* 157–201.

Bayne, T., Cleeremans, A. and Wilken, P. (Eds.) (2009). *The Oxford companion to consciousness.* New York: Oxford University Press.

Beauchaine, T. P., Katkin, E. S., Strassberg, Z. and Snarr, J. (2001). Disinhibitory psychopathology in male adolescents: Discriminating conduct disorder from attention-deficit/hyperactivity disorder through concurrent assessment of multiple autonomic states. *Journal of Abnormal Psychology, 110,* 610–24.

Beauchaine, T. P., Hong, J. and Marsh, P. (2008). Sex differences in autonomic correlates of conduct problems and aggression. *Journal of the American Academy of Child and Adolescent Psychiatry, 47,* 788–96.

Beauchaine, T. P., Neuhaus, E., Brenner, S. L. and Gatzke-Kopp, L. (2008). Ten good reasons to consider biological processes in prevention and intervention research. *Developmental Psychopathology, 20,* 745–74.

Beauchaine, T. P. (2012). Physiological markers of emotion and behavior dysregulation in externalizing psychopathology. In T. A. Dennis, K. A. Buss and P. D. Hastings (Eds.), Physiological measures of emotion from a developmental perspective: State of the science (pp. 79–86). Monographs of the SRCD, 77(2), Serial No. 303.

Bebko, J. M., Konstantareas, M. M. and Springer, J. (1987). Parent and professional evaluations of family stress associated with characteristics of autism. *Journal of Autism and Developmental Disorders, 17,* 565–76.

Bebko, J. M., Perry, A. and Bryson, S. (1996). Multiple method validation study of facilitated communication: II. Individual differences and subgroup results. *Journal of Autism and Developmental Disorders, 26,* 19–42.

Bebko, J. M., Wainwright, J. A., Brian, J. A., Coolbear, J., Landry, R. and Vallance, D. D. (1998). Social competence and peer relations in children with mental retardation: Models of the development of peer relations. *Journal on Developmental Disabilities, 6,* 1–31.

Bebko, J. M., and Weiss, J. (2005). Mental retardation. In R. T. Ammerman (Ed.), Vol. III: *Child Psychopathology* (pp. 233–53). Part of: M. Hersen and J. C. Thomas (Eds.), *Comprehensive handbook of personality and psychopathology.* New York: Wiley.

Becerra, D. and Castillo, J. (2011). Culturally protective parenting practices against substance use among adolescents in Mexico. *Journal of Substance Use, 16,* 136–49.

Beck, A. and Alford, B. A. (2008). *Depression: Causes and treatment, 2nd Edition.* Philadelphia: University of Pennsylvania Press.

Beck, S. J. et al. (2010). A controlled trial of working memory training for children and adolescents with ADHD. *Journal of Clinical Child and Adolescent Psychology 39*(6).

Becker, A. E. (2004). Television, disordered eating, and young women in Fiji: Negotiating body image and identity during rapid social change. *Culture, Medicine, and Psychiatry, 28,* 533–59.

Becker, A. E., Burwell, R. A., Navara, K. and Gillman, S. E. (2003). Binge eating and binge eating disorder in a small-scale, indigenous society: The view from Fiji. *International Journal of Eating Disorders, 34,* 423–31.

Becker, K. and Domitrovich, C. E. (2011). The conceptualization, integration, and support of evidence based interventions in schools. *School Psychology Review, 40,* 582–9.

Beelmann, A., Pfingsten, U. and Losel, F. (1994). Effects of training social competence in children: A meta-analysis of recent evaluation studies. *Journal of Clinical Child Psychology, 23,* 260–71.

Beelman, A. and Schneider, N. (2003). The effects of psychotherapy with children and adolescents. A review and meta-analysis of German-language research. *Zeitschrift fur Klinische Psychologie und Psychotherapie: Forschung und Praxis, 32,* 129–43.

Beels, C. C. (2002). Notes for a cultural history of family therapy. *Family Process, 41,* 67–82.

Beers, C. (1981). *A mind that found itself.* Pittsburgh, PA: University of Pittsburgh Press.

Beesdo, K., Knappe, S. and Pine, D. S. (2009). Anxiety and anxiety disorders in children and adolescents: Developmental issues and implications for DSM-V. *Psychiatric Clinics of North America, 32,* 483–524.

Beevers, C. G. and McGeary, J. E. (2012). Therapygenetics: Moving towards personalized psychotherapy treatment. *Trends in Cognitive Sciences, 16*(1), 11–12.

Befera, M. S., and Barkley, R. A. (1985). Hyperactive and normal girls and boys: Mother–child interaction, parent psychiatric status and child psychopathology. *Journal of Child Psychology and Psychiatry, 26,* 439–52.

Begg, D. J., Langley, J. D., Moffitt, T. and Marshall, S. W. (1996). Sport and delinquency: An examination of the deterrence hypothesis in a longitudinal study. *British Journal of Sports Medicine, 30,* 335–41.

Behrens, K. Y., Parker, A. C. and Haltigan, J. D. (2011). Maternal sensitivity assessed during the Strange Situation Procedure predicts child's attachment quality and reunion behaviors. *Infant Behavior and Development, 34,* 378–81.

Beidel, D. C. (1991). Determining the reliability of psychophysiological assessment in childhood anxiety. *Journal of Anxiety Disorders, 5,* 139–50.

Beidel, D. C., Turner, S. M. and Fink, C. M. (1996). Assessment of childhood social phobia: Construct, convergent, and discriminative validity of the Social Phobia and Anxiety Inventory for Children (SPAI-C). *Psychological Assessment, 8,* 235–40.

Beidel, D. C. and Turner, S. M. (2005). *Childhood anxiety disorders: A guide to research and treatment.* New York: Routledge.

Beidel, D. C. and Alfano, C. A. (2011). *Child anxiety disorders: A guide to research and treatment.* New York: Routledge.

Belenko, S., Dugosh, K. L., Lynch, K., Mericle, A. A., Pich, M. and Forman, R. F. (2009). Online illegal drug use information: An exploratory analysis of drug-related website viewing by adolescents. *Journal of Health Communication, 14,* 612–30.

Bell, R. Q. and Harper, L. V. (1977). *Child effects on adults.* Hillsdale, NJ: Erlbaum.

Bellak, L. and Abrams, D. M. (1996). *The T.A.T., the C.A.T., and the S.A.T. in clinical use* (6th edn.). Needham Heights, MA: Allyn & Bacon.

Belloch, A, Sandín, B. and Ramos, F. (2008). *Manual de psicopatología*. Leon, Spain: Mnemosine.

Belsky, J. and Kelly, J. (1994). *The transition to parenthood*. New York: Delacorte Press.

Belsky, J. and Fearon, R. M. P. (2004). Exploring marriage-parenting typologies and their contextual antecedents and developmental sequelae. *Development and Psychopathology, 16*, 501–23.

Bender, W. N. (2008). *Learning disabilities: Characteristics, identification, and teaching strategies* (6th edn.). Boston, MA: Pearson/Allyn & Bacon.

Benedikt, R., Wertheim, E. H. and Love, A. (1998). Eating attitudes and weight-loss attempts in female adolescents and their mothers. *Journal of Youth and Adolescence, 27*, 43–57.

Benenson, J. F., Apostoleris, N. H. and Parnass, J. (1997). Age and sex differences in dyadic and group interaction. *Developmental Psychology, 33*, 538–43.

Bennahum, D. (1998). Navajo beliefs and end-of-life issues. In New Mexico Geriatric Education Center (Ed.), *Indian elders* (pp. 3–5). Albuquerque: New Mexico Geriatric Education Center.

Benson, M. J., Buehler, C. and Gerard, J. M. (2008). Interparental hostility and early adolescent problem behavior: Spillover via maternal acceptance, harshness, inconsistency, and intrusiveness. *The Journal of Early Adolescence, 28*, 428–54.

Ben-Tal, A., Shamailov, S. S. and Paton, J. F. R. (2011). Evaluating the physiological significance of respiratory sinus arrhythmia: Looking beyond ventilation–perfusion efficiency. *The Journal of Physiology, 590*, 1989–2008.

Benzaquén, A. S. (2006). *Encounters with wild children: Temptation and disappointment in the study of human nature*. Montreal: McGill-Queens Press.

Berganza, C. E., Mezzich, J. E. and Jorge, M. R. (2002). Latin American Guide for Psychiatric Diagnosis (GLDP). *Psychopathology, 35*, 185–90.

Berger, R. and Gelkopf, M. (2009). School-based intervention for the treatment of tsunami-related distress in children: A quasi-randomized controlled trial. *Psychotherapy and Psychosomatics, 78*, 364–71.

Berger, S. L., Kouzarides, T., Shiekhattar, R. and Shilatifard, A. (2009). An operational definition of epigenetics. *Genes and Development, 23*, 781–3.

Bergeron, N. and Schneider, B. H. (2005). Explaining cross-national differences in peer-directed aggression: A quantitative synthesis. *Aggressive Behavior, 31*, 116–37.

Bergmann, M. S. (2004). *Understanding dissidence and controversy in the history of psychoanalysis*. New York: Other Press.

Berkeley, S., Bender, W. N., Peaster, L. G. and Saunders, L. (2009). Implementation of response to intervention: A snapshot of progress. *Journal of Learning Disabilities, 42*, 85–95.

Berkman, L. F. and Glass, T. (2000). Social integration, social networks, social support, and health. In L. F. Berkman and I. Kawachi (Eds.), *Social epidemiology* (pp. 137–73). New York: Oxford University Press.

Bernard, S., Enayati, A., Roger, H., Binstock, T. and Redwood, L. (2002). The role of mercury in the pathogenesis of autism. *Molecular Psychiatry, 7*, 42–43.

Berndt, T. J. (2004). Children's friendships: Shifts over a half-century in perspectives on their development and their effects. *Merrill-Palmer Quarterly: Journal of Developmental Psychology, 50*, 206–23.

Berntson, G. G. and Cacioppo, J. T. (2000). Psychobiology and social psychology: Past, present, and future. *Personality and Social Psychology Review, 4*, 3–15.

Berntson, G. G. and Cacioppo, J. T. (2007). Integrative physiology: Homeostasis, allostasis, and the orchestration of systemic physiology. In J. T. Cacioppo, L. G. Tassinary and G. G. Berntson (Eds.), *Handbook of psychophysiology* (pp. 433–452). New York: Cambridge University Press.

Berntson, G. G., Cacioppo, J. T. and Quigley, K. S. (1991). Autonomic determinism: The modes of autonomic control, the doctrine of autonomic space, and the laws of autonomic constraint, *Psychological Review, 98*, 459–87.

Berntson, G. G., Quigley, K. S. and Lozano, D. (2007). Cardiovascular psychophysiology. In J. T. Cacioppo, L. G. Tassinary and G. G. Berntson (Eds.), *Handbook of psychophysiology* (3rd edn., pp. 182–210). Cambridge: Cambridge University Press.

Berrios, G. E. (1999). Classification in psychiatry: A conceptual history. *Australian and New Zealand Journal of Psychiatry, 33*, 145–60.

Berton, O., McClung, C. A., DiLeone, R. J., Krishnan, V., Renthal, W., Russo, S. J.,…Nestler, E. J. (2006). Essential role of BDNF in the mesolimbic dopamine pathway in social defeat stress. *Science, 311*, 864–8.

Best, J. (1997). Victimization and the victim industry. *Society, 34*, 9–17.

Betancourt, T. S., Speelman, L., Onyango, G. and Bolton, P. (2009). A qualitative study of mental health problems among children displaced by war in northern Uganda. *Transcultural Psychiatry, 46*, 238–56.

Bettencourt, B. and Miller, N. (1996). Gender differences in aggression as a function of provocation: A meta-analysis. *Psychological Bulletin, 119*, 422–7.

Beyer T. and Furniss, T. (2007). Child psychiatric symptoms in primary school: The second wave 4 years after preschool assessment. *Social Psychiatry and Psychiatric Epidemiology, 42*(9), 753–8.

Bhatia, M. S. (2009). *Dictionary of psychology and allied sciences.* New Delhi: New Age.

Bhugra, D. (2007). Hindu and Ayurvedic understandings of the person. In J. Cox, A. V. Campbell and B. Fulford (Eds.), *Medicine of the person: Faith, science and values in health care provision* (pp. 125–38). London: Jessica Kingsley Publishers.

Bickford, C. (2010). Child's ordeal shows risks of psychosis drugs for young. *New York Times*, September 1, 2010.

Biederman, J. (1991). Sudden death in children treated with a tricyclic antidepressant. *Journal of the American Academy of Child and Adolescent Psychiatry, 30*, 495–8.

Biederman, J. (2005). Attention-Deficit/Hyperactivity Disorder: A selective overview. *Biological Psychiatry, 57*, 1215–20.

Biederman, J., Kwon, A., Aleardi, M., Chouinard, V. A., Marino, T., Cole, H.,...Faraone, S. (1996). Response and habituation of the human amygdala during visual processing of facial expression. *Neuron, 17*, 875–87.

Biederman, J. and Spencer, T. (1999). Attention-deficit/hyperactivity disorder (ADHD) as a noradrenergic disorder. *Biological Psychiatry, 46*, 1234–42.

Biederman, J., Kwon, A., AleardiM., Chouinard, V. A., MarinoT., Cole, H.,...Faraone, S. V. (2005). Absence of gender effects on attention deficit hyperactivity disorder: Findings in nonreferred subjects. *The American Journal of Psychiatry, 162*, 1083–9.

Biederman, J., Monuteaux, M. C., Mick, E., Spencer, T., Wilens, T. E., Silva, J. M.,...Faraone, S. V. (2006). Young adult outcome of attention deficit hyperactivity disorder: A controlled 10-year follow-up study. *Psychological Medicine, 36*, 167–79.

Biederman, J., Petty, C., Fried, R., Fontanella, J., Doyle, A. E. and Seidman, L. (2006). Impact of psychometrically-defined executive function deficits in adults with ADHD. *American Journal of Psychiatry, 163*, 1730–8.

Biederman, J., Petty, C. R., Doyle, A. E., Spencer, T., Henderson, C. S., Marion, B., Fried, R. and Faraone, S. V. (2008). Stability of executive function deficits in girls with ADHD: A prospective longitudinal follow-up study into adolescence. *Developmental Neuropsychology, 33*, 44–61.

Biederman, J., Petty, C. R., Monuteaux, M. C., Fried, R., Byrne, D., Mirto, T.,...Faraone, S. V. (2010). Adult psychiatric outcomes of girls with attention deficit hyperactivity disorder: 11-year follow-up in a longitudinal case-control study. *American Journal of Psychiatry, 167*, 409–17.

Bienert, H. and Schneider, B. H. (1995). Deficit-specific social skills training with peer-nominated aggressive-disruptive and sensitive-isolated preadolescents. *Journal of Clinical Child Psychology, 24*, 287–99.

Bierman, K. L., Miller, C. L. and Stabb, S. D. (1987). Improving the social behaviour and peer acceptance of rejected boys: Effects of social skill training with instructions and prohibitions. *Journal of Consulting and Clinical Psychology, 55*, 194–200.

Bierman, K. L., Greenberg, M. T. and the Conduct Problems Prevention Research Group (1996). Social skill training in the FAST Track program. In R. DeV. Peters and R. J. McMahon (Eds.), *Preventing childhood disorders, substance abuse, and delinquency* (pp. 65–89). Newbury Park, CA: Sage.

Bifulco, A., Moran, P. M., Ball, C., Jacobs, C., Baines, R., Bunn, A. et al. (2002). Childhood adversity, parental vulnerability and disorder: Examining inter-generational transmission of risk. *Journal of Child Psychology and Psychiatry and Allied Disciplines, 43*, 1075–86.

Biglan, A., Lewin, L. and Hops, H. (1990). A contextual approach to the problem of aversive practices in families. In G. R. Peterson (Ed.), *Depression and aggression in family interaction* (pp. 103–29). Hillsdale, NJ: Erlbaum.

Bilsky, S. A., Cole, D. A., Dukewich, T. L., Martin, N. C., Sinclair, K. R., Tran, C. V.,...Maxwell, M. A. (2013). Does supportive parenting mitigate the longitudinal effects of peer victimization on depressive thoughts and symptoms in children? *Journal of Abnormal Psychology, 122*, 406–19.

Bimmel, N., van I., Jzendoorn, M. H., Bakermans-Kranenburg, M. J., Juffer, F. and de Geus, E. J. C. (2008). Problem behavior and heart rate reactivity in adopted adolescents: Longitudinal and concurrent relations. *Journal of Research on Adolescence, 18*, 201–13.

Binet, A. (1907) *Les enfants anormaux* [Abnormal children]. Paris: Colin.

Binet, A. and Simon, T. (1907). *Les enfants anormaux.* Paris: Colin.

Birch, H. G. (1964). *Brain damage in children: The biological and social aspects.* Baltimore, MD: Williams and Wilkins.

Birch, L. L., Fisher, J. O. and Davison, K. K. (2003). Learning to overeat: Maternal use of restrictive feeding practices promotes girls' eating in the absence of hunger. *American Journal of Clinical Nutrition, 78*, 215–20.

Bird, H. R. (2002). The diagnostic classification, epidemiology, and cross-cultural validity of ADHD. In P. S. Jensen and J. R. Cooper (Eds.), *Attention deficit hyperactivity disorder: State of the science-*

best practices (Vol. II, pp. 1–16). Kingston, NJ: Civic Research Institute.

Bird, H. R., Davies, M., Duarte, C. S., Shen, S., Loeber, R. and Canino, G. J. (2006). A study of disruptive behavior disorders in Puerto Rican youth: II. Baseline prevalence, comorbidity, and correlates in two sites. *Journal of the American Academy of Child and Adolescent Psychiatry, 45*, 1042–53.

Birkett, M., Espelage, D. L. and Koenig, B. (2009). LGB and questioning students in schools: The moderating effects of homophobic bullying and school climate on negative outcomes. *Journal of Youth and Adolescence, 38*, 989–1000.

Birmaher, B., Arbelaez, C. and Brent, D. (2002). Course and outcome of child and adolescent major depressive disorder. *Child and Adolescent Psychiatric Clinics of North America, 11*, 619–38.

Bisset, S., Markham, W. A. and Aveyard, P. (2007). School culture as an influencing factor on youth substance use. *Journal of Epidemiology and Community Health, 61*, 485–90.

Bittner, A., Egger, H. L., Erkanli, A., Costello, E. J., Foley, D. L. and Angold, A. (2007). What do childhood anxiety disorders predict? *Journal of Child Psychology and Psychiatry, 48*, 1174–83.

Bjork, J. M., Knutson, B., Fong, G. W., Caggiano, D. M., Bennett, S. M. and Hommer, D. W. (2004). Incentive-elicited brain activation in adolescents: Similarities and differences from young adults. *Journal of Neuroscience, 24*, 1793–802.

Blacher, J. and McIntyre, L. L. (2006). Syndrome specificity and behavioural disorders in young adults with intellectual disability: Cultural differences in family impact. *Journal of Intellectual Disability Research, 50*, 184–98.

Blacher, J., and Baker, B. L. (2007). Positive impact of intellectual disability on families. *American Journal on Mental Retardation, 112*, 330–48.

Blachman, D. R. and Hinshaw, S. P. (2002). Patterns of friendship among girls with and without attention-deficit/hyperactivity disorder. *Journal of Abnormal Child Psychology, 30*, 625–40.

Black, D. and Newman, M. (1996). Children and domestic violence: A review. *Clinical Child Psychology and Psychiatry, 1*, 79–88.

Blader, J. C. and Carlson, G. A. (2007). Increased rates of bipolar disorder diagnoses among U.S. child, adolescent, and adult inpatients, 1996–2004. *Biological Psychiatry, 62*, 107–14.

Blair, R. J. (2007). Dysfunctions of medial and lateral orbitofrontal cortex in psychopathy. *Annals of the New York Academy of Science, 1121*, 461–79.

Blair, R. J. (2010). Neuroimaging of psychopathy and antisocial behavior: A targeted review. *Current Psychiatry Reports, 12*, 76–82.

Blair, R. J. and Cipolotti, L. (2000). Impaired social response reversal: A case of "acquired sociopathy." *Brain, 123*, 1122–41.

Blanton, H. and Burkley, M. (2008). Deviance regulation theory: Applications to adolescent social influence. In M. J. Prinstein and K. A. Dodge (Eds.), *Understanding peer influence in children and adolescents* (pp. 94–121). New York: Guilford Press.

Blanton, H. and Christie, C. (2003). Deviance regulation. *Review of General Psychology, 7*, 115–49.

Blashfield, R. K., Keeley, J. W. and Burgess, D. R. (2009). Classification. In P. H. Blaney and T. Millon (Eds.), *Oxford textbook of psychopathology* (pp. 35–57). New York: Oxford University Press.

Blocker, J. S. (2006). Did prohibition really work? Alcohol prohibition as a public health innovation. *American Journal of Public Health, 96*, 233–43.

Bloom, E. and Heath, N. (2010). Recognition, expression, and understanding facial expressions of emotion in adolescents with nonverbal and general learning disabilities. *Journal of Learning Disabilities, 43*, 180–92.

Bloom, M. and Gullotta, T. P. (2003). Evolving definitions of primary prevention. In T. P. Gullotta and M. Bloom (Eds.), *Encyclopedia of primary prevention and health promotion* (pp. 9–15). New York: Kluwer.

Blumberg, H. P., Donegan, N. H., Sanislow, C. A., Collins, S., Lacadie, C., Skudlarski, P., … Krystal, J. H. (2005). Preliminary evidence for medication effects on functional abnormalities in the amygdala and anterior cingulate in bipolar disorder. *Psychopharmacology, 183*, 308–13.

Blum, H. P. (2007). Little Hans: A centennial review and reconsideration. *Journal of the American Psychoanalytical Association, 55*, 750–65.

Bockting, W. O. and Ehrbar, R. D. (2006). Commentary: Gender variance, dissonance, or identity disorder. *Journal of Psychology and Human Sexuality, 17*, 125–34.

Bodenmann, G., Cina, A., Ledermann, T. and Sanders, M. R. (2008). The efficacy of the Triple P-Positive Parenting Program in improving parenting and child behaviour: A comparison with two other treatment conditions. *Behaviour Research and Therapy, 46*, 411–27.

Bodfish, J. W., Symons, F. J., Parker, D. E. and Lewis, M. H. (2000). Varieties of repetitive behavior in autism: Comparisons to mental retardation. *Journal of Autism and Developmental Disorders, 30*, 237–43.

Bodfish, J. W. and Lewis, M. H. (2002). Self-injury and comorbid behavior in developmental, neurological, psychiatric, and genetic disorders. In S. Schroeder, M. Oster-Granite and T. Thompson (Eds.), *Self-injurious behaviour: Gene–brain–behavior relationships*. Washington, DC: American Psychological Association Press.

Bögels, S. M. and Phares, V. (2008). Fathers' role in the etiology, prevention and treatment of child anxiety: A review and new model. *Clinical Psychology Review, 28*, 539–58.

Bögels, S. M., Alden, L., Beidel, D. C., Clark, L. A., Pine, D. S., Stein, M. B. and Voncken, M. (2010). Social anxiety disorder: questions and answers for the DSM-V. *Depression and Anxiety, 27*, 168–89.

Bohlin, G., Hagekull, B. and Rydell, A.-M. (2000). Attachment and social functioning: A longitudinal study from infancy to middle childhood. *Social Development, 9*, 24–39.

Bohnert, A. M. and Garber, J. (2007). Prospective relations between organized activity participation and psychopathology during adolescence. *Journal of Abnormal Child Psychology, 35*, 1021–33.

Boivin, M., Brendgen, M., Vitaro, F., Dionne, G., Girard, A., Pérusse, D., B. Tremblay, R. E. (2013). Strong genetic contribution to peer relationship difficulties at school entry. Findings from a Longitudinal Twin Study. *Child Development, 84*, 1098–1114.

Bond, L. A. and Carmola Hauf, A. M. (2004). Taking stock and putting stock in primary prevention: Characteristics of effective programs. *The Journal of Primary Prevention, 24*, 199–221.

Bond, L. A. and Carmola Hauf, A. M. (2007). Community-based collaboration: An overarching best practice in prevention. *The Counseling Psychologist, 35*, 567–75.

Bonora, E., Lamb, J. A., Barnby, G., Bailey, A. J. and Monaco, A. P. (2006). Genetic basis of autism. In S. O. Moldin and J. L. R. Rubenstein (Eds.), *Understanding autism: From basic neuroscience to treatment* (pp. 49–74). Boca Raton, FL: CRC Press.

Boomsma, D. I., van den Bree, M. B., Orlebeke, J. F. and Molenaar, P. C. (1989). Resemblances of parents and twins in sports participation and heart rate. *Behavior Genetics, 19*, 123–41.

Boonstra, A. M., Oosterlaan, J., Sergeant, J. and Buitelaar, J. (2005) Executive functioning in adult ADHD: A meta-analytic review. *Psychological Medicine, 35*, 1097–108.

Booth, J. R., Burman, D. D., Meyer, J. R., Lei, Z., Trommer, B. L., Davenport, N. D. et al. (2005). Larger deficits in brain networks for response inhibition than for visual selective attention in attention deficit hyperactivity disorder (ADHD). *Journal of Child Psychology and Psychiatry, 46*(1), 94–111.

Borelli, J. L., David, D. H., Crowley, M. J. and Mayes, L. C. (2010). Links between disorganized attachment classification and clinical symptoms in school-aged children. *Journal of Child and Family Studies, 19*, 243–56.

Borenstein, M., Hedges, L. V., Higgins, J. P. T. and Rothstein, H. R. (2009). *Introduction to meta-analysis*. Chichester: Wiley.

Borkenau, P., Riemann, R., Angleitner, A. and Spinath, F. M. (2002). Similarity of childhood experiences and personality resemblance in monozygotic and dizygotic twins: A test of the equal environments assumption. *Personality and Individual Differences, 33*, 261–9.

Bornovalova, M. A., Hicks, B., Iacono, W. and McGue, M. (2012). Longitudinal twin study of borderline personality disorder traits and substance use in adolescence: Developmental change, reciprocal effects, and genetic and environmental influences. *Personality Disorders: Theory, Research, and Treatment, 4*, 23–32.

Bosch, N. M., Riese, H., Ormel, J., Verhulst, F. and Oldehinkel, A. J. (2009). Stressful life events and depressive symptoms in young adolescents: Modulation by respiratory sinus arrhythmia? The TRAILS study. *Biological Psychology, 81*, 40–7.

Boscolo, L., Cecchin, G., Hoffman, L. and Penn, P. (1987). *Milan systemic family therapy: Conversations in theory and practice*. New York: Basic Books.

Bostwick, J. M. and Pankratz, V. S. (2000). Affective disorders and suicide risk: A reexamination. *The American Journal of Psychiatry, 157*, 1925–32.

Botella, C., Garcia-Palacios, A., Banos, R. M. and Quero, S. (2009). Cybertherapy: Advantages, limitations, and ethical issues. *Psychology Journal, 7*, 77–100.

Botticello, A. L. (2009). A multilevel analysis of gender differences in psychological distress over time. *Journal of Research on Adolescence, 19*, 217–47.

Botvinick, M., Nystrom, L. E., Fissell, K., Carter, C. S. and Cohen, J. D. (1999). Conflict monitoring versus selection-for-action in anterior cingulate cortex. *Nature, 402*, 179–81.

Bouchard, S. (2011). Could virtual reality be effective in treating children with phobias? *Expert Review of Neurotherapeutics, 11*, 207–13.

Bowen, R. C., Offord, D. R. and Boyle, M. H. (1990). The prevalence of overanxious disorder and separation anxiety disorder: Results from the Ontario Child Health Study. *Journal of the American Academy of Child and Adolescent Psychiatry, 29*, 753–8.

Bowlby, J. (1969). Disruption of affectional bonds and its effects on behavior. *Canada's Mental Health Supplement, 59*, 12.

Bowlby, J. (1973). *Attachment and loss. Volume II: Separation: Anxiety and anger*. New York: Basic Books.

Bowlby, J. (1977). The making and breaking of affectional bonds: Aetiology and psychopathology in the light of attachment theory. *British Journal of Psychiatry, 130,* 201–10.

Boyce, W. T., Quas, J., Alkon, A., Smider, N. A., Essex, M. J., Kupfer, D. J. et al. (2001). Autonomic reactivity and psychopathology in middle childhood. *British Journal of Psychiatry, 179,* 144–50.

Boylan, K., Vaillancourt, T., Boyle, M. and Szatmari, P. (2007). Comorbidity of internalizing disorders in children with oppositional defiant disorder. *European Child and Adolescent Psychiatry, 16,* 484–94.

Boyle, C. L., Sanders, M. R., Lutzker, J. R., Prinz, R. J., Shapiro, C. and Whitaker, D. J. (2010). An analysis of training, generalization, and maintenance effects of Primary Care Triple P for parents of preschool-aged children with disruptive behaviour. *Child Psychiatry and Human Development, 41,* 114–31.

Bracken, P. and Thomas, P. (2010). From Szasz to Foucault: On the role of critical psychiatry. *Philosophy, Psychiatry and Psychology, 17,* 219–28.

Bradley, C. (1937). Definition of childhood in psychiatric literature. *American Journal of Psychiatry, 94,* 33–6.

Bradley, K. (2008). Juvenile delinquency, the juvenile courts and the Settlement Movement 1908–1950: Basil Henriques and Toynbee Hall. *Twentieth Century British History, 19.*

Bradley, M. M. (2000). Emotion and motivation. In J. T. Cacioppo, L. G. Tassinary and G. G. Berntson (Eds.), *Handbook of psychophysiology* (2nd edn., pp. 602–42). New York: Cambridge University Press.

Brady, E. U. and Kendall, P. C. (1992). Comorbidity of anxiety and depression in children and adolescents. *Psychological Bulletin, 111,* 244–55.

Bramble, D. (2003). Annotation: The use of psychotropic medications in children: A British view. *Journal of Child Psychology and Psychiatry, 44,* 169–79.

Branje, S. J. T., van Lieshout, C. F. M., van Aken, M. A. G. and Haselager, G. J. T. (2004). Perceived support in sibling relationships and adolescent adjustment. *Journal of Child Psychology and Psychiatry, 45,* 1385–96.

Brassett-Harknett, A. and Butler, N. (2007). Attention-deficit/hyperactivity disorder: An overview of the etiology and a review of the literature relating to the correlates and lifecourse outcomes for men and women. *Clinical Psychology Review, 27,* 188–210.

Bratus, B. S. and Davis, H. (Eds.) (1990). *Anomalies of personality: From the deviant to the norm.* Orlando, FL: Paul M. Deutsch Press.

Bravo, M., Ribera, J., Rubio-Stipec, M., Canino, G., Shrout, P., Ramirez, R.,…Martinez-Taboas, A. (2001). Test–retest reliability of the Spanish version of the Diagnostic Interview Schedule for Children (DISC-IV). *Journal of Abnormal Child Psychology, 29,* 433–44.

Breiter, H. C., Etcoff, N. L., Whalen, P. J., Kennedy, W. A., Rauch, S. L., Buckner, R. L. et al. (1996). Response and habituation of the human amygdala during visual processing of facial expression. *Neuron, 17*(5), 875–87.

Breiter, H. C., Aharon, I., Kahneman, D., Dale, A. and Shizgal, P. (2001). Functional imaging of neural responses to expectancy and experience of monetary gains and losses. *Neuron, 30,* 619–39.

Breivik, K., Olweus, D. and Endresen, I. (2009). Does the quality of parent–child relationships mediate the increased risk of antisocial behavior and substance use in adolescents in single mother and single father families? *Journal of Divorce and Remarriage, 50,* 400–26.

Breland-Noble, A. M., Bell, C. and Nicolas, G. (2006). Family First: The development of an evidence-based family intervention for increasing participation in psychiatric clinical care and research in depressed African American adolescents. *Family Process, 45,* 153–69.

Brendgen, M. (2012). Genetics and peer relations: A review. *Journal of Research on Adolescence, 22,* 419–37.

Brendgen, M., Vitaro, F. and Bukowski, W. M. (2000). Deviant friends and early adolescents' emotional and behavioral adjustment. *Journal of Research on Adolescence, 10,* 173–89.

Brendgen, M., Wanner, B., Morin, A. J. S. and Vitaro, F. (2005). Relations with parents and with peers, temperament, and trajectories of depressed mood during early adolescence. *Journal of Abnormal Child Psychology, 33,* 579–94.

Brendgen, M. and Boivin, M. (2008). Genetic factors in children's peer relations. In K. H. Rubin, W. M. Bukowski and B. Laursen (Eds.), *Peer interactions, relationships, and groups* (pp. 455–72). Cambridge: Cambridge University Press.

Brendgen, M., Boivin, M., Vitaro, F., Bukowski, W. M., Dionne, G., Tremblay, R. E. et al. (2008). Linkages between children's and their friends' social and physical aggression: Evidence for a gene–environment interaction? *Child Development, 79,* 13–29.

Brendgen, M., Vitaro, F., Boivin, M., Girard, A., Bukowski, W. M., Dionne, G. et al. (2009). Gene–environment linkages between peer rejection and depressive symptoms in children. *Journal of Child Psychology and Psychiatry, 50,* 1009–17.

Brendgen, M., Boivin, M., Barker, E. D., Girard, A., Vitaro, F., Dionne, G., Tremblay, R. E. and Pérusse, D. (2011). Gene–environment processes linking aggression, peer victimization, and the teacher-child relationship. *Child Development, 82,* 2021–36.

Brennan, L. M. and Shaw, D. S. (2013). Revisiting data related to the age of onset and developmental course of female conduct problems. *Clinical Child and Family Review, 16,* 35–8.

Brendgen, M., Vitaro, F., Barker, E. D., Girard, A., Dionne, G., Tremblay, R. E. and Boivin, M. (in press). Do other peoples' plights matter? A genetically informed twin study of the role of social context in the link between peer victimization and children's aggression and depression symptoms. *Developmental Psychology*.

Breslau, N., Davis, G. C., Andreski, P. and Peterson, E. (1991). Traumatic events and posttraumatic stress disorder in an urban population of young adults. *Archives of General Psychiatry, 48*, 216–22.

Bretherton, I. (1990). Open communication and internal working models: Their role in the development of attachment relationships. In R. A. Thompson (Ed.), *Nebraska Symposium on Motivation, 1988: Socioemotional development* (pp. 57–113). Lincoln, NE: University of Nebraska Press.

Bretherton, I., Golby, B. and Cho, E. (1997). Attachment and the transmission of values. In J. E. Grusec and L. Kuczynski (Eds.), *Parenting and children's internalization of values: A handbook of contemporary theory* (pp. 103–34). Hoboken, NJ: John Wiley and Sons.

Bretherton, I., Lambert, J. D. and Golby, B. (2005). Involved fathers of preschool children as seen by themselves and their wives: Accounts of attachment, socialization, and companionship. *Attachment and Human Development, 7*, 229–51.

Brett, E. A. (1996). The classification of posttraumatic stress disorder. In B. A. van der Kolk, A. C. McFarlane and L. Weisaeth (Eds.), *Traumatic stress: The effects of overwhelming experience on mind, body, and society* (pp. 117–28). New York: Guilford Press.

Briesch, A. M., Chafouleas, S. M. and Riley-Tillman, T. C. (2010). Generalizability and dependability of behaviour assessment methods to estimate academic engagement: A comparison of systematic direct observation and direct behavior rating. *School Psychology Review, 39*, 408–21.

Bright, C. L., Decker, S. H. and Burch, A. M. (2007). Gender and justice in the progressive era: An investigation of Saint Louis Juvenile Court cases, 1909–1912. *Justice Quarterly, 24*, 657–78.

Brock, R. L. and Lawrence, E. (2009). Too much of a good thing: Underprovision versus overprovision of partner support. *Journal of Family Psychology, 23*, 181–92.

Broderick, C. B. and Shrader, S. S. (1981). The history of professional marriage and family therapy. In A. S. Gurman and D. P. Kniskern (Eds.), *Handbook of family therapy* (pp. 5–35). New York: Brunner/Mazel.

Brody, G. H. (1998). Sibling relationship quality: Its causes and consequences. *Annual Review of Psychology, 49*, 1–24.

Brody, H. and Waters, D. B. (1980). Diagnosis is treatment. *The Journal of Family Practice, 10*, 445–9.

Brody, L. R. and Hall, J. A. (1993). Gender and emotion. In M. Lewis and J. M. Haviland (Eds.). *Handbook of emotions* (pp. 447–60). New York: Guilford Press.

Broidy, L. M., Nagin, D. S., Tremblay, R. E., Bates, J. E., Brame, B., Dodge, K. A.,…Vitaro, F. (2003). Developmental trajectories of childhood disruptive behaviours and adolescent delinquency: A six-site, cross-national study. *Developmental Psychology, 39*, 222–45.

Bronfenbrenner, U. (1979). *The ecology of human development: Experiments by nature and design.* Cambridge, MA: Harvard University Press.

Bronfenbrenner, U. (1986). Ecology of the family as a context for human development: Research perspectives. *Developmental Psychology, 22*, 723–42.

Brookmeyer, K. A., Henrich, C. C., Cohen, G. and Shahar, G. (2011). Israeli adolescents exposed to community and terror violence: The protective role of social support. *The Journal of Early Adolescence, 31*, 577–603.

Brooks-Gunn, J. and Johnson, A. D. (2006). G. Stanley Hall's contribution to science, practice and policy. *History of Psychology, 9*, 247–58.

Brown, B. B. and Mounts, N. S. (2007). Linking parents and family to adolescent peer relations: Ethnic and cultural considerations. *New Directions in Child and Adolescent Development* (Vol. 116, pp. 1–15). San Francisco: Jossey-Bass.

Brown, B. B., Bakken, J. P., Ameringer, S. W. and Mahon, S. D. (2008). A comprehensive conceptualization of the peer influence process in adolescence. In M. J. Prinstein and K. A. Dodge (Eds.), *Understanding peer influence in children and adolescents* (pp. 17–44). New York: Guilford Press.

Brown, C. H. and Liao, J. (1999). Principles for designing randomized preventive trials in mental health: An emerging developmental epidemiology paradigm. *American Journal of Community Psychology, 27*, 673–710.

Brown, J. B., Winzelberg, A. J., Abascal, L. B. and Taylor, C. B. (2004). An evaluation of an internet-delivered eating disorder prevention program for adolescents and their parents. *Journal of Adolescent Health, 35*, 290–6.

Brown, L. S. (1991a). Diagnosis and dialogue. *Canadian Psychology, 32*, 142–4.

Brown, L. S. (1991b). Not outside the range: One feminist perspective on psychic trauma. *American Imago, 48*, 119–33.

Brown, R. T. and Pacini, J. N. (1989). Perceived family functioning, marital status, and depression in parents of boys with attention deficit disorder. *Journal of Learning Disabilities, 22*, 581–7.

Brown, S. A. and D'Amico, E. J. (2003). Outcomes of alcohol treatment for adolescents. In M. Galanter

(Ed.), *Recent developments in alcoholism, Volume XVI: Research on alcoholism treatment* (pp. 289–312). New York: Kluwer Academic/Plenum Publishers.

Brownley, K. A., Hurwitz, B. E. and Schneiderman, N. (2000). Cardiovascular psychophysiology. In J. T. Cacioppo, L. G. Tassinary and G. G. Berntson (Eds.), *Handbook of psychophysiology* (pp. 224–64). New York: Cambridge.

Bruder, C. E. G., Piotrowski, A., Gijsbers, A. A., Andersson, R., Erickson, S., Diaz de Ståhl, T. et al. (2008). Phenotypically concordant and discordant monozygotic twins display different DNA copy-number-variation profiles. *The American Journal of Human Genetics, 82,* 763–71.

Brumariu, L. E. and Kerns, K. A. (2008). Mother–child attachment and social anxiety symptoms in middle childhood. *Journal of Applied Developmental Psychology, 29,* 393–402.

Brumariu, L. E. and Kerns, K. A. (2010). Mother–child attachment patterns and different types of anxiety symptoms: Is there specificity of relations? *Child Psychiatry and Human Development, 41,* 663–74.

Brunstein Klomek, A., Sourander, A., Kumpulainen. K., Piha, J., Tuula, T., Irma, M., Almqvist, F. and Gould, M. S. (2008). Childhood bullying as a risk for later depression and suicidal ideation among Finnish males. *Journal of Affective Disorders, 109,* 47–55.

Bryant-Waugh, R. J., Cooper, P. J., Taylor, C. L. and Lask, B. D. (1996). The use of the eating disorder examination with children: A pilot study. *International Journal of Eating Disorders, 19,* 391–7.

Bubier, J. L. and Drabick, D. A. (2008). Affective decision-making and externalizing behaviors: The role of autonomic activity. *Journal of Abnormal Child Psychology, 36,* 941–53.

Buchan, T. and Gregory, L. D. (1984). Anorexia nervosa in a Black Zimbabwean. *British Journal of Psychiatry, 145,* 326–30.

Buchanan, R. L. and Bowen, G. L. (2008). In the context of adult support: The influence of peer support on the psychological well-being of middle-school students. *Child and Adolescent Social Work Journal, 25,* 397–407.

Buchholz, A., Mack, H., McVey, G., Feder, S. and Barrowman, N. (2008). BodySense: An evaluation of a positive body image intervention on sport climate for female athletes. *Eating Disorders, 16,* 308–21.

Buckalew, L. W. and Coffield, K. E. (1982). Drug expectations associated with perceptual characteristics: Ethnic factors. *Perceptual and Motor Skills, 55,* 915–18.

Buckley, L., Sheehan, M. and Chapman, R. (2009). Adolescent protective behavior to reduce drug and alcohol use, alcohol-related harm and interpersonal violence. *Journal of Drug Education, 39*(3), 289–301.

Buhrmester, D. and Furman, W. (1990). Perceptions of sibling relationships during middle childhood and adolescence. *Child Development, 61,* 1387–98.

Buhs, E. S. and Ladd, G. W. (2001). Peer rejection as antecedent of young children's school adjustment: An examination of mediating processes. *Developmental Psychology, 37,* 550–60.

Buitelaar, J. K., van Andel, H., Duyx, J. H. M. and van Strien, D. C. (1994). Depressive and anxiety disorders in adolescence: A follow-up of adolescents with school refusal. *Acta Paedopsychiatrica: International Journal of Child and Adolescent Psychiatry, 56*(4), 249–53.

Buitelaar, J. K., Barton, J., Danckaerts, M., Friedrichs, E., Gillberg, C., Hazell, P. L., … Zuddas, A. (2006). A comparison of North American versus non-North American ADHD study populations. *European Child and Adolescent Psychiatry, 15,* 177–81.

Bukowski, W. M. and Adams, R. (2005). Peer relations and psychopathology: Markers, mechanisms, mediators, moderators, and meanings. *Journal of Clinical Child and Adolescent Psychology, 34,* 3–10.

Bukowksi, W. M., Newcomb, A. and Hartup, W. W. (1996). *The company they keep: Friendships in children and adolescence.* New York: Cambridge University Press.

Bukowski, W. M., Laursen, B. and Hoza, B. (2010). The snowball effect: Friendship moderates escalations in depressed affect among avoidant and excluded children. *Development and Psychopathology, 22,* 749–57.

Bukstein, O. G. (2000). Disruptive behavior disorder and substance use disorders in adolescents. *Journal of Psychoactive Drugs, 32,* 67–79.

Bulik, C. M., Sullivan, P. F., Wade, T. D. and Kendler, K. S. (2000). Twin studies of eating disorders: A review. *International Journal of Eating Disorders, 27,* 2–20.

Burke, J. D., Loeber, R. and Birmaher, B. (2002). Oppositional defiant disorder and conduct disorder: A review of the past 10 years, part II. *Journal of the Academy of Child and Adolescent Psychiatry, 41,* 1275–93.

Burke, J. D., Loeber, R. and Lahey, B. B. (2007). Adolescent conduct disorder and interpersonal callousness as predictors of psychopathy in young adults. *Journal of Clinical Child and Adolescent Psychology, 36,* 334–46.

Burke, W. and Diekema, D. S. (2006). Ethical issues arising from the participation of children in genetic research. *The Journal of Pediatrics, 149,* S34–S38.

Burns, G. L., Walsh, J. A., Patterson, D. R., Holte, C. S., Sommersflanagan, R. and Parker, C. M. (1997). Internal validity of the disruptive behaviour disorder symptoms – implications from parent ratings for a dimensional approach to symptom validity. *Journal of Abnormal Child Psychology*, 25, 307–19.

Burns, S., Cross, D. and Maycock, B. (2010). "That could be me squishing chip on someone's car." How friends can positively influence bullying behaviors. *The Journal of Primary Prevention*, 31, 209–222.

Burt, S. A. (2009a). A mechanistic explanation of popularity: Genes, rule breaking, and evocative gene-environment correlations. *Journal of Personality and Social Psychology*, 96, 783–94.

Burt, S. A. (2009b). Rethinking environmental contributions to child and adolescent psychopathology: A meta-analysis of shared environmental influences. *Psychological Bulletin*, 135, 608–37.

Burt, S. A. (2008a). Gene-environment interactions and their impact on the development of personality traits. *Psychiatry*, 7, 507–10.

Burt, S. A. (2008b). Genes and popularity: Evidence of an evocative gene-environment correlation. *Psychological Science*, 19, 112–13.

Bush, G., Luu, P. and Posner, M. I. (2000). Cognitive and emotional influences in anterior cingulate cortex. *Trends in Cognitive Sciences*, 4, 215–22.

Bush, G., Valera, E. M. and Seidman, L. J. (2005). Functional neuroimaging of attention-deficit/ hyperactivity disorder: A review and suggested future directions. *Biological Psychiatry*, 57(11), 1273–84.

Bushman, B. J. (2002). Does venting anger feed or extinguish the flame? Catharsis, rumination, distraction, anger and aggressive responding. *Personality and Social Psychology Bulletin*, 28, 724–31.

Buss, D. (2004). *Evolutionary psychology: The new science of the mind* (2nd edn.). Boston, MA: Allyn & Bacon.

Buss, K. A. and Goldsmith, H. H. (1998). Fear and anger regulation in infancy: Effects on the temporal dynamics of affective expression. *Child Development*, 69, 359–74.

Buss, K. A., Davidson, R. J., Kalin, N. H. and Goldsmith, H. H. (2004). Context-specific freezing and associated physiological reactivity as a dysregulated fear response. *Developmental Psychology*, 40, 583–94.

Bussing, R., Gary, F. A., Mason, D. M., Leon, C. E., Sinha, K. and Garvan, C. W. (2003). Child temperament, ADHD, and caregiver strain: Exploring relationships in an epidemiological sample. *Journal of the American Academy of Child and Adolescent Psychiatry*, 42, 184–92.

Butnik, S. M. (2005). Neurofeedback in adolescents and adults with attention deficit hyperactivity disorder. *Journal of Clinical Psychology*, 61, 621–5.

Butterfield, J. (2003). *Collins English dictionary: Complete and unabridged*. Glasgow: HarperCollins.

Buysse, V., Goldman, B. D. and Skinner, M. L. (2002). Setting effects on friendship formation among young children with and without disabilities. *Exceptional Children*, 68, 503–17.

Bylund, D. B. and Reed, A. L. (2007). Childhood and adolescent depression: Why do children and adults respond differently to antidepressant drugs? *Neurochemistry International*, 51, 246–53.

Cadoret, R. J., Troughton, E., O'Gorman, T.W. and Heywood, E. (1986). An adoption study of genetic and environmental factors in drug abuse. *Archives of General Psychiatry*, 43, 1131–6.

Cairns, R., Xie, H. and Leung, M. C. (1998). The popularity of friendship and the neglect of social networks: Toward a new balance. In W. M. Bukowski and A. H. Cillessen (Eds.), *Sociometry then and now: Building on six decades of measuring children's experiences with the peer group* (pp. 25–53). San Francisco, CA: Jossey-Bass.

Cairns., R. B., Cairns, B. D., Neckerman, H. J., Gest, S. D. and Gariepy, J. L. (1988). Peer networks and aggressive behavior: Social support or social rejection? *Developmental Psychology*, 24, 815–23.

Cairns, R. B. and Cairns, B. D. (2006). The making of developmental psychology. In R. M. Lerner (Ed.), *Handbook of child psychology, 6th Edition, Volume I* (pp. 89–186). New York: Wiley.

Calear, A. L., Christensen, H., Mackinnon, A., Griffiths, K. M. and O'Kearney, R. (2009). The YouthMood Project: A cluster randomized controlled trial of an online cognitive behavioral program with adolescents. *Journal of Consulting and Clinical Psychology*, 77, 1021–32.

Calkins, S. D. and Keane, S. P. (2004). Cardiac vagal regulation across the preschool period: Stability, continuity, and implications for childhood adjustment. *Developmental Psychobiology*, 45, 101–12.

Calkins, S. D., Graziano, P. A. and Keane, S. P. (2007). Cardiac vagal regulation differentiates among children at risk for behavior problems. *Biological Psychiatry*, 74, 144–53.

Callahan, C. L. and Eyberg, S. M. (2010). Relations between parenting behavior and SES in a clinical sample: Validity of SES measures. *Child and Family Behavior Therapy*, 32, 125–38.

Callahan, E. H., Gillis, J. M., Romanczyk, R. G. and Mattson, R. E. (2011). The behavioral assessment of social interactions in young children: An examination of convergent and incremental validity. *Research in Autism Spectrum Disorders*, 5, 768–74.

Callicott, J. H., Bertolino, A., Egan, M. F., Mattay, V. S., Langheim, F. J. and Weinberger, D. R. (2000). Selective relationship between prefrontal N-acetylaspartate measures and negative symptoms in schizophrenia. *American Journal of Psychiatry, 157,* 1646–51.

Cameron, N. M., Champagne, F. A., Parent, C., Fish, E. W., Ozaki-Kuroda, K. and Meaney, M. J. (2005). The programming of individual differences in defensive responses and reproductive strategies in the rat through variations in maternal care. *Neuroscience and Biobehavioral Reviews, 29,* 843–65.

Campbell, S. B. (1994). Hard-to-manage preschool boys: Externalizing behavior, social competence, and family context at two-year followup. *Journal of Abnormal Child Psychology, 22,* 147–66.

Campbell, S. B. (2000). Attention-deficit/hyperactivity disorder: A developmental view. In A. J. Sameroff, M. Lewis and S. M. Miller (Eds.), *Handbook of developmental psychopathology* (pp. 383–401). Dordrecht, Netherlands: Kluwer Academic Publishers.

Campbell, S. B. and Ewing, L. J. (1990). Follow-up of hard-to-manage preschoolers: Adjustment at age 9 and predictors of continuing symptoms. *Journal of Child Psychology and Psychiatry, 31,* 871–89.

Campbell, S. B., Shaw, D. S. and Gilliom, M. (2000). Early externalizing behavior problems: Toddlers and preschoolers at risk for later maladjustment. *Development and Psychopathology, 12,* 467–88.

Canadian Broadcasting Corporation (2006, July 7). Court: Ontario can stop autism funding once children turn 6. Retrieved from www.cbc.ca/news/canada/ story/2006/07/07/autism-ontario.html

Canino, G., Shrout, P. E., Rubio-Stipec, M., Bird, H. R., Bravo, M., Ramirez, R.,…Martinez-Taboas, A. (2004). The DSM-IV rates of child and adolescent disorders in Puerto Rico. *Archives of General Psychiatry, 61,* 85–93.

Canino, G. and Alegria, M. (2008). Psychiatric diagnosis – is it universal or relative to culture?*Journal of Child Psychology and Psychiatry, 49,* 237–50.

Cantwell, D. P., Baker, L., Rutter, M. and Mawhood, L. (1989). Infantile autism and developmental receptive dysphasia: A comparative follow-up into middle childhood. *Journal of Autism and Developmental Disorders, 19,* 19–31.

Cappadocia, M. C., Desrocher, M., Pepler, D. and Schroeder, J. H. (2009). Contextualizing the neurobiology of conduct disorder in an emotion dysregulation framework. *Clinical Psychology Review, 29,* 506–18.

Caplan, G. (1964). *Principles of preventive psychiatry.* New York: Basic Books.

Caplan, P. J. (1992). Gender issues in the diagnosis of mental disorders. *Women and Therapy, 12,* 71–82.

Caplan, P. J. (1995). *They say you're crazy: How the world's most powerful psychiatrists decide who's normal.* Jackson, MI: De Capo.

Caplan, P. J. and Hall-McCorquodale, I. (1985). Mother-blaming in major clinical journals. *American Journal of Orthopsychiatry, 55,* 345–53.

Card, N. A. and Little, T. D. (2006). Proactive and reactive aggression in childhood and adolescence: A meta-analysis of differential relations with psychosocial adjustment. *International Journal of Behavioral Development, 30,* 466–80.

Cardemil, E., Reivich, K. J., Beevers, C. G., Seligman, M. E. P. and James, J. (2007). The prevention of depressive symptoms in low-income, minority children: Two-year follow-up. *Behaviour Research and Therapy, 45,* 313–27.

Carey, W. B. (2002). Is ADHD a valid disorder? In P. S. Jensen and J. R. Cooper (Eds.), *Attention deficit hyperactivity disorder: State of the science-best practices.* Kingston, NJ: Civic Research Institute.

Carlson, G. A. and Cantwell, D. P. (1980). Unmasking masked depression in children and adolescents. *American Journal of Psychiatry, 137,* 445–9.

Carney, J. V., Hazler, R. J., Oh, I., Hibel, L. C. and Granger, D. A. (2010). The relations between bullying exposures in middle childhood, anxiety, and adrenocortical activity. *Journal of School Violence, 9,* 194–211.

Caron, C. and Rutter, M. (1991). Comorbidity in child psychopathology: Concepts, issues and research strategies. *Journal of Child Psychology and Psychiatry, 32,* 1063–80.

Carpenter, W. T. (2009). Anticipating DSM-V: Should psychosis risk become a diagnostic class? *Schizophrenia Bulletin, 35,* 841–3.

Carr, A. (1991). Milan systemic family therapy: A review of ten empirical investigations. *Journal of Family Therapy, 13,* 237–63.

Carrey, N. (2008). Guest editorial: Classification in child psychiatry. *Journal of the Canadian Academy of Child and Adolescent Psychiatry, 17,* 49.

Carrey, N. (2010). Antipsychotics for children: Can we do better? *Journal of the Canadian Academy of Child and Adolescent Psychiatry, 19,* 70–1.

Carrey, N. and Gregson, J. (2008). A context for classification in child psychiatry. *Journal of the Canadian Academy of Child and Adolescent Psychiatry, 17,* 50–7.

Carter, C. S., Macdonald, A. M., Botvinick, M., Ross, L. L., Stenger, V. A., Noll, D. and Cohen, J. D. (2000). Parsing executive processes: Strategic vs. evaluative functions of the anterior cingulate cortex. *Proceedings of the National Academy of Sciences of the United States of America, 97,* 1944–8.

Carter, E. W., Sisco, L. G., Brown, L., Brickham, D. and Al-Khabbaz, Z. A. (2008). Peer interactions and academic engagement of youth with developmental disabilities in inclusive middle- and high-school classrooms. *American Journal on Mental Retardation, 113*, 479–94.

Carter, J. C., Stewart, D. A., Dunn, V. J. and Fairburn, C. G. (1997). Primary prevention of eating disorders: Might it do more harm than good? *International Journal of Eating Disorders, 22*, 167–72.

Cartledge, G. (2005). Learning disabilities and social skills: Reflections. *Learning Disability Quarterly, 28*, 179–81.

Cartledge, G. and Milburn, J. F. (1994). *Teaching social skills to children and youth: Innovative approaches.* Boston, MA: Allyn & Bacon.

Cartwright-Hatton, S., Roberts, C., Chitsabesan, P., Fothergill, C. and Harrington, R. (2004). Systematic review of the efficacy of cognitive behaviour therapies for childhood and adolescent anxiety disorders. *British Journal of Clinical Psychology, 43*, 421–36.

Cartwright-Hatton, S., McNally, D., Field, A. P., Rust, S., Laskey, B., Dixon, C.,…Woodham, A. (2011). A new parenting-based group intervention for young anxious children: Results of a randomized controlled trial. *Journal of the American Academy of Child and Adolescent Psychiatry, 50*, 242–51.

Casey, B. J., Trainor, R., Giedd, J., Vauss, Y., Vaituzis, C. K., Hamburger, S. et al. (1997). The role of the anterior cingulate in automatic and controlled processes: A developmental neuroanatomical study. *Developmental Psychobiology, 30*, 61–9.

Casey, B. J., Giedd, J. N. and Thomas, K. M. (2000). Structural and functional brain development and its relation to cognitive development. *Biological Psychology, 54*(1–3), 241–57.

Casey, R. J. and Berman, J. S. (1985). The outcome of psychotherapy with children. *Psychological Bulletin, 98*, 388–400.

Caspi, A., McClay, J., Moffitt, T. E., Mill, J., Martin, J., Craig, I. W and Poulton, R. (2002). Role of genotype in the cycle of violence in maltreated children. *Science, 297*, 851–4.

Caspi, A., Sugden, K., Moffitt, T. E., Taylor, A., Craig, I. W., Harrington, H., McClay, J., Mill, J., Martin, J., Braithwaite, A. and Poulton, R. (2003). Influence of life stress on depression: Moderation by a polymorphism in the 5-HTT gene. *Science, 301*, 386–9.

Castellanos, F. X., Giedd, J. N., Marsh, W. L., Hamburger, S. D., Vaituzis, A. C., Dickstein, D. P.,…Rapoport, J. L. (1996). Quantitative brain magnetic resonance imaging in attention-deficit hyperactivity disorder. *Archives of General Psychiatry, 53*, 607–16.

Castellanos, F. X. and Tannock, R. (2002). Neuroscience of attention-deficit/hyperactivity disorder: The search for endophenotypes. *Nature Reviews: Neuroscience, 3*, 617–28.

Catron, T. F. and Masters, J. C. (1993). Mothers' and children's conceptualizations of corporal punishment. *Child Development, 64*, 1815–28.

Cefai, J., Smith, D. and Pushak, R. E. (2010). Parenting wisely: Parent training via CD-ROM with an Australian sample. *Child and Family Behavior Therapy, 32*, 17–33.

Chakrabarti, B., Kent, L., Suckling, J., Bullmore, E. and Baron-Cohen, S. (2006). Variations in the human cannabinoid receptor (CNR1) gene modulate striatal responses to happy faces. *European Journal of Neuroscience, 23*, 1944–8.

Chakrabarti, S. and Fombonne, E. (2001). Pervasive developmental disorders in preschool children. *Journal of the American Medical Association, 285*, 3093–9.

Chamberlain, B., Kasari, C. and Rotheram-Fuller, E. (2007). Involvement or isolation? The social networks of children with autism in regular classrooms. *Journal of Autism and Developmental Disorders, 37*, 230–42.

Chamberlain, P. and Rosicky, J. G. (1995). The effectiveness of family therapy in the treatment of adolescents with conduct disorders and delinquency. *Journal of Marital and Family Therapy, 21*, 441–59.

Champagne, F. A. (2012) *Interplay between social experiences and the genome: Epigenetic consequences for behavior, 77*, 33–57.

Champagne, F. A., Chretien, P., Stevenson, C. W., Zhang, T. Y., Gratton, A. and Meaney, M. J. (2004). Variations in nucleus accumbens dopamine associated with individual differences in maternal behavior in the rat. *The Journal of Neuroscience, 24*, 4113–23.

Champagne, F. A., Weaver, I. C., Diorio, J., Dymov, S., Szyf, M. and Meaney, M. J. (2006). Maternal care associated with methylation of the estrogen receptor-alpha 1b promoter and estrogen receptor-alpha expression in the medial preoptic area of female offspring. *Endocrinology, 147*, 2909–15.

Champagne, F. A. and Meaney, M. J. (2007). Transgenerational effects of social environment on variations in maternal care and behavioral response to novelty. *Behavioral Neuroscience, 121*, 1353–63.

Chao, R. K. (1994). Beyond parental control and authoritarian parenting style: Understanding Chinese parenting through the cultural notion of training. *Child Development, 65*, 1111–19.

Charlesworth, W. R. (1992). Darwin and developmental psychology: Past and present. *Developmental Psychology, 28*, 5–16.

Charman, T. and Pervova, I. (1996). Self-reported depressed mood in Russian and UK schoolchildren: A research note. *Journal of Child Psychology and Psychiatry, 37*, 879–83.

Charmandari, E., Tsigos, C. and Chrousos, G. (2005). Endocrinology of the stress response. *Annual Review of Physiology, 67*, 259–84.

Chassin, L., Presson, C. C., Rose, J. S. and Sherman, S. J. (2001). From adolescence to adulthood: Age-related changes in beliefs about cigarette smoking in a Midwestern community sample. *Health Psychology, 20*, 377–86.

Chatters, L. M., Taylor, R. J. and Jayakody, R. (1994). Fictive kinship relations in Black extended families. *Journal of Comparative Family Studies, 25*, 297–312.

Chawla, N. and Marlatt, G. A. (2006). The varieties of Buddhism. In E. T. Dowd and S. L. Nielsen (Eds.), *The psychologies in religion: Working with the religious client* (pp. 271–86). New York: Springer Publishing.

Chen, C., Visootsak, J., Dills, S. and Graham, J. M. (2007). Prader-Willi syndrome: An update and review for the primary paediatrician, *Clinical Pediatrics, 46*, 580–91.

Chen, X., Hastings, P., Rubin, K. H., Chen, H., Cen, G. and Stewart, S. L. (1998). Childrearing attitudes and behavioral inhibition in Chinese and Canadian toddlers: A cross-cultural study. *Developmental Psychology, 34*, 677–86.

Chen, X., Cen, G., Li, D. and He, Y. (2005). Social functioning and adjustment in Chinese children: The imprint of historical time. *Child Development, 76*, 182–95.

Cheng, Y., Chiang, H.-C., Ye, J. and Cheng, L. (2010). Enhancing empathy instruction using a collaborative virtual learning environment for children with autistic spectrum conditions. *Computers and Education, 55*, 1449–58.

Chesney-Lind, M. and Jones, N. (2010). *Fighting for girls: New perspectives on gender and violence.* Albany, NY: State University of New York Press.

Chess, S. and Thomas, A. (1996). *Temperament: theory and practice.* New York: Brunner Mazel.

Chess, S. and Thomas, A. (1999). *Goodness of fit: Clinical applications from infancy through adult life.* Philadelphia, PA: Brunner/Mazel.

Chida, Y. and Steptoe, A. (2009). Cortisol awakening response and psychosocial factors: A systematic review and meta-analysis. *Biological Psychology, 80*, 265–78.

Chisuwa, N. and O'Dea, J. A. (2010). Body image and eating disorders amongst Japanese adolescents. A review of the literature. *Appetite, 54*, 5–15.

Chorpita, B. F., and Barlow, D. H. (1998). The development of anxiety: The role of control in the early environment. *Psychological Bulletin, 124*, 3–21.

Chorpita, B. F., Albano, A. M. and Barlow, D. H. (1998). The structure of negative emotions in a clinical sample of children and adolescents. *Journal of Abnormal Psychology, 107*, 74–85.

Chorpita, B. F. and Daleiden, E. L. (2002). Tripartite dimensions of emotion in a child clinical sample: Measurement strategies and implications for clinical utility. *Journal of Consulting and Clinical Psychology, 70*, 1150–60.

Christ, A. E., Adler, A. G., Isacoff, M. and Gershansky, I. S. (1981). Depression: Symptoms versus diagnosis in 10,412 hospitalized children and adolescents (1957–1977). *American Journal of Psychotherapy, 35*, 400–12.

Chronis, A. M., Fabiano, G. A., Gnagy, E. M., Wymbs, B. T., Burrows-MacLean, L. and Pelham, W. E. (2001). Comprehensive, sustained behavioral and pharmacological treatment for attention-deficit/hyperactivity disorder: A case study. *Cognitive and Behavioral Practice, 8*, 346–58.

Chronis, A. M., Jones, H. A. and Raggi, V. L. (2006). Evidence-based psychosocial treatments for children and adolescents with attention-deficit/hyperactivity disorder. *Clinical Psychology Review, 26*, 486–502.

Chronis-Tuscano, A., Degnan, K. A., Pine, D. S., Perez-Edgar, K., Henderson, H. A., Diaz, Y. et al. (2009). Stable early maternal report of behavioral inhibition predicts lifetime social anxiety disorder in adolescence. *Journal of the American Academy of Child and Adolescent Psychiatry, 48*, 928–35.

Chun, C., Enomoto, K. and Sue, S. (1996). Health care issues among Asian Americans: Implications of somatisation. In P. M. Kato and T. Mann (Eds.), *Handbook of diversity issues in health psychology* (pp. 347–66). New York: Plenum.

Chung, T. (2008). Adolescent substance use, abuse, and dependence: Prevalence, course and outcomes. In Y. Kaminer and O. G. Bukstein (Eds.), *Adolescent substance abuse: Psychiatric comorbidity and high-risk behaviors* (pp. 5–27). New York: Routledge/Taylor & Francis Group.

Chung, T. and Martin, C. S. (2005). What were they thinking? Adolescents' interpretations of DSM-IV alcohol dependence symptom queries and implications for diagnostic validity. *Drug and Alcohol Dependence, 80*, 191–200.

Cicchetti, D. (2006). Development and psychopathology. In D. Cicchetti and D. J. Cohen (Eds.), *Developmental psychopathology* (Vol. I, pp. 1–23). Hoboken, NJ: John Wiley and Sons.

Cicchetti, D. and Rogosch, F. A. (1996). Equifinality and multifinality in developmental psychopathology. *Development and Psychopathology, 8*, 597–600.

Cicchetti, D. and Toth, S. L. (2005). Child maltreatment. *Annual Review of Clinical Psychology, 1*, 409–38.

Cicchetti, D. and Posner, M. I. (2005). Cognitive and affective neuroscience and developmental psychopathology. *Development and Psychopathology, 17*, 569–75.

Cicchetti, D., Rogosch, F. A. and Sturge-Apple, M. L. (2007). Interactions of child maltreatment and serotonin transporter and monoamine oxidase A polymorphisms: Depressive symptomatology among adolescents from low socioeconomic status backgrounds. *Development and Psychopathology, 19*, 1161–80.

Cicchetti, D. and Curtis, W. J. (2007). Multilevel perspectives on pathways to resilient functioning. *Development and Psychopathology, 19*, 627–9.

Cicchetti, D. and Gunnar, M. R. (2008). Integrating biological measures into the design and evaluation of preventive interventions. *Development and Psychopathology, 20*, 737–43.

Cicchetti, D., Toth, S. I. and Rogosch, F. A. (2008). Toddler–parent psychotherapy for depressed mothers and their offspring: Implications for attachment theory. In L. Atkinson and S. Goldberg (Eds.), *Attachment issues in psychopathology and intervention* (pp. 229–76). Mahwah, NJ: Lawrence Erlbaum Associates.

Cicchetti, D. and Rogosch, F. A. (2012). Neuroendocrine regulation and emotional adaptation in the context of child maltreatment. *Monographs of the Society for Research in Child Development, 77*, 87–95.

Cillessen, A. H. N. (2008). Sociometric methods. In K. H. Rubin, W. M. Bukowski and B. Laursen (Eds.), *Handbook of peer interactions, relationships, and groups* (pp. 82–99). New York: Guilford Press.

Cillessen, A. H. N. and Mayeux, L. (2004). From censure to reinforcement: Developmental changes in the association between aggression and social status. *Child Development, 75*, 147–63.

Clapp, E. J. (1998). *Mothers of all children: Women reformers and the rise of juvenile courts in progressive-era America.* University Park, PA: Pennsylvania State University Press.

Clark, D. A. and Beck, A. T. (1999). *Scientific foundations of cognitive theory and therapy of depression.* New York: Wiley.

Clarke, G. N., Hawkins, W., Murphy, M. and Sheeber, L. (1993). School-based primary prevention of depressive symptomatology in adolescents: Findings from two studies. *Journal of Adolescent Research, 8*, 183–204.

Clark, L. A. and Watson, D. (1999). Personality, disorder, and personality disorder: Towards a more rational conceptualization. *Journal of Personality Disorders, 13*, 142–51.

Clasen, D. R., and Brown, B. B. (1985). The multidimensionality of peer pressure in adolescence. *Journal of Youth and Adolescence, 14*, 451–68.

Cloninger, C. R., Bohman, M., Sigvardsson, S. and von Knorring, A. L. (1985). Psychopathology in adopted-out children of alcoholics: The Stockholm Adoption Study. In M. Galanter (Ed.) *Recent Developments in Alcoholism* (Vol. III, pp. 37–51). New York: Plenum.

Coates, S. (1992). The etiology of boyhood gender identity disorder: An integrative model. In J. W. Barron, M. N. Eagle and D. L. Wolitzky (Eds.), *Interface of psychoanalysis and psychology* (pp. 245–65). Washington, DC: American Psychological Association.

Coates, S. W. (2004). Bowlby and Mahler: Their lives and theories. *Journal of the American Psychoanalytic Association, 52*, 571–601.

Cobb, S. (1976). Social support as a moderator of life stress. *Psychosomatic Medicine, 38*, 300–14.

Cochran, S. V. and Rabinowitz, F. E. (2000). *Men and depression: Clinical and empirical perspectives.* San Diego, CA: Academic Press.

Coghill, D. and Sonuga-Barke, E. J. S. (2012). Annual Research Review: Categories versus dimensions in the classification and conceptualisation of child and adolescent mental disorders – implications of recent empirical study. *Journal of Child Psychology and Psychiatry, 53*, 469–89.

Coghill, D. R., Rhodes, S. M. and Matthews, K. (2007). The neuropsychological effects of chronic methylphenidate on drug-naive boys with attention-deficit/hyperactivity disorder. *Biological Psychiatry, 62*, 954–62.

Cohen, D., Deniau, E., Maturana, A., Tanguy, M., Bodeau, N., Labelle, R., … Guile, J. (2008). Are child and adolescent responses to placebo higher in major depression than in anxiety disorders? A systematic review of placebo-controlled trials. *PLoS ONE, 3*, e2632.

Cohen, D., Consoli, A., Bodeaua, N., Purper-Ouakil, D., Deniau, E., Guile, J. and Donnelly, C. (2010). Predictors of placebo response in randomized controlled trials of psychotropic drugs for children and adolescents with internalizing disorders. *Journal of Child and Adolescent Psychopharmacology, 20*, 39–47.

Cohen, G. L. and Prinstein, M. J. (2006). Peer contagion of aggression and health risk behavior among adolescent males: An experimental investigation of effects on public conduct and private attitudes. *Child Development, 77*, 967–83.

Cohen, J. (1992). A power primer. *Psychological Bulletin, 112*, 155–9.

Cohen, J. (1988). *Statistical power analysis for the behavioral sciences* (2nd edn.). New Jersey: Lawrence Erlbaum.

Cohen, J. A. (2008). Helping adolescents affected by war, trauma, and displacement. *Journal of the American Academy of Child and Adolescent Psychiatry, 47*, 981–2.

Cohen, J. A., Berliner, L. and Mannarino, A. (2010). Trauma focused CBT for children with co-occurring trauma and behavior problems. *Child Abuse and Neglect, 34*, 215–24.

Cohen, J. A. and Mannarino, A. P. (1996). Factors that mediate treatment outcome of sexually abused preschool children. *Journal of the American Academy of Child and Adolescent Psychiatry, 35*, 1402–10.

Cohen, J. A., Deblinger, E., Mannarino, A. P. and Steer, R. A. (2004). A multisite, randomized controlled trial for children with sexual abuse-related PTSD symptoms. *Journal of the American Academy of Child and Adolescent Psychiatry, 43*, 393–402.

Cohen, J. A., Mannarino, A. P. and Deblinger, E. (2006). *Treating trauma and traumatic grief in children and adolescents.* New York: Guilford Press.

Cohen, J. A., Mannarino, A. P., Perel, J. M. and Staron, V. (2007). A pilot randomized controlled trial of combined trauma-focused CBT and setraline for childhood PTSD symptoms. *Journal of the American Academy of Child and Adolescent Psychiatry, 46*, 811–19.

Cohen, J. A., Bukstein, O., Walter, H., Benson, R. S., Chrisman, A., Farchione, T. A.,…Stock, S. (2010). Practice parameter for the assessment and treatment of children and adolescents with posttraumatic stress disorder. *Journal of the American Academy of Child and Adolescent Psychiatry, 49*, 414–30.

Cohen, P. and Flory, M. (1998). Issues in the disruptive behavior disorders: Attention deficit disorder without hyperactivity and the differential validity of oppositional defiant and conduct disorders. In T. Widiger (Ed.), *DSM-IV sourcebook* (Vol. IV, pp. 455–63). Washington, DC: American Psychiatric Press.

Cohen-Bendahan, C., van de Beek, C. and Berenbaum, S. (2005). Prenatal sex hormone effects on child and adult sex-typed behavior: Methods and findings. *Neuroscience and Biobehavioral Reviews, 29*, 353–84.

Cohen-Kettenis, P. T. and Pfafflin, F. (2010). The DSM diagnostic criteria for gender identity disorder in adolescents and adults. *Archives of Sexual Behavior, 39*, 499–513.

Coie, J. (1985). Fitting social skills interventions to the target group. In B. H. Schneider, K. H. Rubin and J. E. Ledingham (Eds.), *Children's peer relations: Issues in assessment and intervention* (pp. 141–56). New York: Springer-Verlag.

Colby, S. M. and Murrell, W. (1998). Child welfare and substance abuse services: From barriers to collaboration. In R. L. Hampton, V. Senatore and T. P. Gullotta (Eds.), *Substance abuse, family violence, and child welfare: Bridging perspectives* (pp. 188–219). Thousand Oaks, CA: Sage Publications.

Cole, J., Ball, H. A., Martin, N. C., Scourfield, J. and McGuffin, P. (2009). Genetic overlap between measures of hyperactivity/inattention and mood in children and adolescents. *Journal of the American Academy of Child and Adolescent Psychiatry, 48*, 1094–101.

Cole, P. M., Michel, M. K. and Teti, L. O. (1994). The development of emotion regulation and dysregulation: A clinical perspective. *Monographs of the Society for Research in Child Development, 59*, 73–100, 250–83.

Cole, P. M., Martin, S. E. and Dennis, T. A. (2004). Emotion regulation as a scientific construct: Methodological challenges and directions for child development research. *Child Development, 75*, 317–33.

Coley, R. L. (2001). (In)visible men: Emerging research on low-income, unmarried, and minority fathers. *American Psychology, 56*, 743–53.

Collear, M. and Hines, M. (1995). Human behavioural sex differences: A role for gonadal hormones during early development? *Psychological Bulletin, 118*, 55–107.

Collins, F. S., Morgan, M. and Patrinos, A. (2004). The Human Genome Project: Lessons from large-scale biology. *Science, 300*, 286–90.

Colman, A. M. (2009). *A dictionary of psychology.* Oxford: Oxford University Press.

Colonnesi, C. et al. (2011). The relation between attachment and child anxiety: A meta-analytic review. *Journal of Clinical Child and Adolescent Psychology, 40*, 630–45.

Comer, R. J. (2006). *Abnormal psychology* (6th edn.). New York: Worth Publishers.

Compton, M. T. (2010). Applying prevention practices to schizophrenia and other psychotic disorders. In M. T. Compton (Ed.), *Clinical manual of prevention in mental health* (pp. 125–64). Arlington, VA: American Psychiatric Publishing, Inc.

Compton, M. T. (2010). *Clinical manual of prevention in mental health.* Washington, DC: American Psychiatric Publishing.

Condas, J. (1980). Personal reflections on the Larry P. trial and its aftermath. *School Psychology Review, 9*, 154–8.

Conduct Problems Prevention Research Group. (2002a). Evaluation of the first three years of the FAST Track Prevention Trial with children at high risk for adolescent conduct problems. *Journal of Abnormal Child Psychology, 30*, 19–35.

Conduct Problems Prevention Research Group. (2002b). Implementation of the FAST Track Program: An example of a large-scale prevention science efficacy trial. *Journal of Abnormal Child Psychology, 30*, 1–17.

Conduct Problems Prevention Research Group. (2002c). Predictor variables associated with positive FAST Track outcomes at the end of the third grade. *Journal of Abnormal Child Psychology, 30,* 37–52.

Conduct Problems Prevention Research Group. (2011). The effects of the FAST Track preventive intervention on the development of conduct disorder across childhood. *Child Development, 82,* 331–45.

Connell, A. M. and Goodman, S. H. (2002). The association between psychopathology in fathers versus mothers and children's internalizing and externalizing behavior problems: A meta-analysis. *Psychological Bulletin, 128,* 746–73.

Conners, C. K. (2000). Attention-deficit/hyperactivity disorder – historical development and overview. *Journal of Attention Disorders, 3,* 173–91.

Conners, C. K. (2008). *Conners 3rd edition: Manual.* Toronto, ON: Multi-Health Systems.

Connor, D. F., Edwards, G., Fletcher, K. E., Baird, J., Barkley, R. A. and Steingard, R. J. (2003). Correlates of comorbid psychopathology in children with ADHD. *Journal of the American Academy of Child and Adolescent Psychiatry, 42,* 193–200.

Conrad, P. (1975). The discovery of hyperkinesis: Notes on the medicalization of deviant behavior. *Social Problems, 23,* 12–21.

Coo, H., Ouellette-Kuntz, H., Lloyd, J. E. V., Kasmara, L., Holden, J. J. A. and Lewis, M. E. S. (2008). Trends in autism prevalence: Diagnostic substitution revisited. *Journal of Autism and Developmental Disorders, 38,* 1036–46.

Cook, G. (2012, November 29). The Autism Advantage. The *New York Times.* Retrieved from www.nytimes.com/2012/12/02/magazine/the-autism-advantage.html

Cooke, M. B., Ford, J., Levine, J., Bourke, C., Newell, L. and Lapidus, G. (2007). The effects of city-wide implementation of "Second Step" on elementary school students' prosocial and aggressive behaviors. *The Journal of Primary Prevention, 28,* 93–115.

Coolidge, F. L., Thede, L. L. and Young, S. E. (2002). The heritability of gender identity disorder in a child and adolescent twin sample. *Behavior Genetics, 32,* 251–7.

Cooper, B. (1990). Epidemiology and prevention in the mental health field. *Social Psychiatry and Psychiatric Epidemiology, 25,* 9–15.

Cooper, H. (2010). *Research synthesis and meta-analysis: A step-by-step approach* (3rd edn.). Thousand Oaks, CA: Sage.

Cooper, M., Rowland, N., McArthur, K., Pattison, S., Cromarty, K. and Richards, K. (2010). Randomized controlled trial of school-based humanistic counselling for emotional distress in young people: Feasibility study and preliminary indications of efficacy. *Child and Adolescent Psychiatry and Mental Health, 4.*

Cooper, Z., Fairburn, C. G. and Hawker, D. M. (2003). *Cognitive-behavioral treatment of obesity: A clinician's guide.* New York: Guilford Press.

Copeland, W., Shanahan, L., Costello, E. J. and Angold, A. (2009). Configurations of common childhood psychosocial risk factors. *Journal of Child Psychology and Psychiatry, 50,* 451–9.

Coplan, R., Findlay, L. C. and Schneider, B. H. (2010). Where do anxious children "fit" best? Childcare and the emergence of anxiety in early childhood. *Canadian Journal of Behavioural Science, 42,* 185–93.

Corcoran, J. and Dattalo, P. (2006). Parent involvement in treatment for ADHD: A meta-analysis of the published studies. *Research on Social Work Practice, 16,* 561–70.

Cornelius, J. R. and Clark, D. B. (2008). Depressive disorders and adolescent substance use disorders. In Y. Kaminer and O. G. Bukstein (Eds.), *Adolescent substance abuse: Psychiatric comorbidity and high-risk behaviors* (pp. 5–27). New York: Routledge/Taylor & Francis Group.

Costanzo, P. R. (1970). Conformity development as a function of self-blame. *Journal of Personality and Social Psychology, 14,* 366–74.

Costanzo, P. R. and Shaw, M. E. (1966). Conformity as a function of age level. *Child Development, 37,* 967–75.

Costello, E. J., Angold, A., Burns, B. J., Stangl, D. K., Tweed, D. L., Erkanli, A. and Worthman, C. M. (1996). The Great Smoky Mountains Study of youth: Goals, design, methods, and the prevalence of DSM-III-R disorders. *Archives of General Psychiatry, 53,* 1129–36.

Costello, E. J., Erkanli, A., Federman, E. and Angold, A. (1999). Development of psychiatric comorbidity with substance abuse in adolescents: Effects of timing and sex. *Journal of Clinical Child Psychology, 28,* 298–311.

Costello, E. J. and Angold, A. (2000). Developmental psychopathology and mental health: Past, present and future. *Development and Psychopathology, 12,* 599–618.

Costello, E. J., Erkanli, A., Fairbank, J. A. and Angold, A. (2002). The prevalence of potentially traumatic events in childhood and adolescence. *Journal of Traumatic Stress, 15,* 99–112.

Costello, E. J., Mustillo, S., Erkanli, A., Keeler, G. and Angold, A. (2003). Prevalence and development of psychiatric disorders in childhood and adolescence. *Archives of General Psychiatry, 60,* 837–44.

Costello, E. J., Compton, S. N., Keeler, G. and Angold, A. (2003). Relationships between poverty and psychopathology: A natural experiment. *Journal of the American Medical Association, 290,* 2023–9.

Costello, E. J., Erkanli, A. and Angold, A. (2006). Is there an epidemic of child or adolescent depression? *Journal of Child Psychology and Psychiatry, 47,* 1263–71.

Cotrufo, P., Gnisci, A. and Caputo, I. (2005). Brief report: Psychological characteristics of less severe forms of eating disorders: An epidemiological study among 259 female adolescents. *Journal of Adolescence, 28,* 147–54.

Cottrell, D. and Boston, P. (2002). Practitioner review: The effectiveness of systemic family therapy for children and adolescents. *Journal of Child Psychology and Psychiatry, 43,* 573–86.

Courchesne, E. (2004). Brain development in autism: Early overgrowth followed by premature arrest of growth. *Mental Retardation and Developmental Disabilities Research Reviews, 10,* 106–11.

Coutinho, M. J. and Oswald, D. P. (2005). State variation in gender disproportionality in special education: Findings and recommendations. *Remedial and Special Education, 26,* 7–15.

Cowen, E. L. (1996). The ontogenesis of primary prevention: Lengthy strides and stubbed toes. *American Journal of Community Psychology, 24,* 235–49.

Cox, A., Rutter, M. and Holbrook, D. (1981). Psychiatric interviewing techniques v. experimental study: Eliciting factual information. *British Journal of Psychiatry, 139,* 29–37.

Cox, R. B., Blow, A. J., Maier, K. S. and Parra Cardona, J. R. (2010). Covariates of substance use initiation for Venezuelan youth: Using a multilevel approach to guide prevention programs. *Journal of Studies on Alcohol and Drugs, 71,* 424–33.

Coyne, J. (1976). Depression and the response of others. *Journal of Abnormal Psychology, 85,* 186–93.

Cozzi, F. and Ostuzzi, R. (2007). Relational competence and eating disorders. *Eating and Weight Disorders, 12,* 101–7.

Craske, M. G. (1999). *Anxiety disorders: Psychological approaches to theory and treatment.* Boulder, CO: Westview Press.

Cravens, H. (2006). The historical context of G. Stanley Hall's *Adolescence* (1904). *History of Psychology, 9,* 172–85.

Crawley, S. A., Beidas, R. S., Benjamin, C. L., Martin, E. and Kendall, P. C. (2008). Treating socially phobic youth with CBT: Differential outcomes and treatment considerations. *Behavioural and Cognitive Psychotherapy, 36,* 379–89.

Creswell, C. and Cartwright-Hatton, S. (2007). Family treatment of child anxiety: Outcomes, limitations and future directions. *Clinical Child and Family Psychology Review, 10,* 232–52.

Crick, N. R., Casas, J. F. and Mosher, M. (1997). Relational and overt aggression in preschool. *Developmental Psychology, 33,* 579–88.

Crick, N. R., Murray-Close, D., Marks, P. E. L. and Mohajeri-Nelson, N. (2009). Aggression and peer relationship in school-age children: Relational and physical aggression in group and dyadic contexts. In K. H. Rubin, W. M. Bukowski and B. Laursen (Eds.), *Handbook of peer interactions, relationships, and groups* (pp. 287–302). New York: Guilford Press.

Crijnen, A. A. M., Achenbach, T. M. and Verhulst, F. C. (1997). Comparisons of problems reported by parents of children in 12 cultures: Total problems, externalizing, and internalizing. *Journal of the American Academy of Child and Adolescent Psychiatry, 36,* 1269–77.

Crisp, A. H. (1983). Anorexia nervosa. *British Medical Journal, 287,* 855–8.

Critchley, H. D., Mathias, C. J., Josephs, O., O'Doherty, J., Zanini, S., Dewar, B. K.,…Raymond, J. D. (2003). Human cingulate cortex and autonomic control: Converging neuroimaging and clinical evidence. *Brain, 126,* 2139–52.

Critchley, H. D., Wiens, S., Rotshtein, P., Öhman, A. and Dolan, R. J. (2004). Neural systems supporting interoceptive awareness. *Nature Neuroscience, 7,* 189–95.

Crockett, L., Losoff, M. and Petersen, A. C. (1984). Perceptions of the peer group and friendship in early adolescence. *The Journal of Early Adolescence, 4,* 155–81.

Crone, E. A., Wendelken, C., Donohue, S., van Leijenhorst, L. and Bunge, S. A. (2006). Neurocognitive development of the ability to manipulate information in working memory. *Proceedings of the National Academy of Sciences of the United States of America, 103,* 9315–20.

Cross, W. and Wyman, P. A. (2006). Training and motivational factors as predictors of job satisfaction and anticipated job retention among implementers of a school-based prevention program. *The Journal of Primary Prevention, 27,* 195–215.

Crowell, S. E., Beauchaine, T. P., Gatzke-Kopp, L., Sylvers, P., Mead, H. and Chipman-Chacon, J. (2006). Autonomic correlates of attention-deficit/hyperactivity disorder and oppositional defiant disorder in preschool children. *Journal of Abnormal Psychology, 115,* 174–8.

Crowther, J. H., and Sherwood, N. E. (1997). Assessment. In D. M. Garner and P. E. Garfinkel (Eds.), *Handbook of treatment for eating disorders* (2nd edn.) (pp. 34–49). New York: Guilford Press.

Cruickshank, W. M. (1975). Perceptual and learning disability: A definition and projection. *Educational Leadership, 32,* 499–502.

Cuckle, P. and Wilson, J. (2002). Social relationships and friendships among young people with Down's syndrome in secondary schools. *British Journal of Special Education, 29,* 66–71.

Cummings, E. M., El-Sheikh, M., Kouros, C. D., Keller, P. S. Children's skin conductance reactivity as a mechanism of risk in the context of parental depressive symptoms. *Journal of Child Psychology and Psychiatry*, *48*, 436–45.

Cummings, M. E., Papp, L. M. and Kouros, C. D. (2009). Regulatory processes in children's coping with exposure to marital conflict. In S. L. Olson and A. J. Sameroff (Eds.), *Biopsychosocial regulatory processes in the development of childhood behavioral problems* (pp. 212–37). New York: Cambridge University Press.

Cunningham, C. E., Cunningham, L. J., Martorelli, V., Tran, A., Young, J. and Zacharias, R. (1998). The effects of primary division, student-mediated conflict resolution programs on playground aggression. *Journal of Child Psychology and Psychiatry*, *39*, 653–62.

Cunningham, M. G., Bhattacharyya, S. and Benes, F. M. (2002). Amygdalo-cortical sprouting continues into early adulthood: Implications for the development of normal and abnormal function during adolescence. *Journal of Comparative Neurology*, *453*, 116–30.

Cunningham, M. J., Wuthrich, V. M., Rapee, R. M., Lyneham, H. J., Schniering, C. A. and Hudson, J. L. (2009). The Cool Teens CD-ROM for anxiety disorders in adolescents: A pilot case series. *European Child and Adolescent Psychiatry*, *18*, 125–9.

Curren, R. (Ed.) (2007). *Philosophy of education: An Anthology*. Malden, MA: Blackwell.

Curry, J. F. (2009). Research psychotherapy: Aspirin or music? *Clinical Psychology: Science and Practice*, *16*, 318–22.

Curry, J. F. and Reinecke, M. A. (2003). Modular therapy for adolescents with major depression. In M. A. Reinecke, F. M. Dattilio and A. Freeman (Eds.) *Cognitive therapy with children and adolescents: A casebook for clinical practice* (pp. 95–128). New York: Guilford Press.

Curtis, L. T. and Patel, K. (2008). Nutritional and environmental approaches to preventing and treating autism and attention deficit hyperactivity disorder (ADHD): A review. *The Journal of Alternative and Complementary Medicine*, *14*, 79–85.

Cushman, P. (2002). How psychology erodes personhood. *Journal of Theoretical and Philosophical Psychology*, *22*, 103–13.

Cutting, A. L. and Dunn, J. (2006). Conversations with siblings and with friends: Links between relationship quality and social understanding. *British Journal of Developmental Psychology*, *24*, 73–87.

Cyranowski, J. M., Frank, E., Young, E. and Shear, K. (2000). Adolescent onset of the gender difference in lifetime rates of major depression. *Archives of General Psychiatry*, *57*, 21–7.

Dadds, M. and Hawes, D. (2006). *Integrated family intervention for child conduct problems: A behaviour-attachment-systems intervention for parents*. Bowen Hills, QLD: Australian Academic Press.

Dain, M. (1980). *Clifford W. Beers, advocate for the insane*. Pittsburgh: University of Pittsburgh Press.

Daley, D., Jones, K., Hutchings, J. and Thompson, M. (2009). Attention deficit hyperactivity disorder in pre-school children: Current findings, recommended interventions and future directions. *Child Care, Health and Development*, *35*, 754–66.

Dalgleish, T., Taghavi, R., Neshat-Doost, H., Moradi, A., Canterbury, R. and Yule, W. (2003). Patterns of processing bias for emotional information across clinical disorders: A comparison of attention, memory, and prospective cognition in children and adolescents with depression, generalized anxiety, and posttraumatic stress disorder. *Journal of Clinical Child and Adolescent Psychology*, *32*, 10–21.

Dalrymple, A. J. and Feldman, M. A. (1992). Effects of reinforced directed rehearsal on expressive sign language learning by persons with mental retardation. *Journal of Behavioral Education*, *2*, 1–16.

Dalton, K. M., Nacewicz, B. M., Johnstone, T., Schaefer, H. S., Gernsbacher, M. A., Goldsmith, H. H....Davidson, R. J. (2005). Gaze fixation and the neural circuitry of face processing in autism. *Nature Neuroscience*, *8*, 519–26.

Damasio, A. R. (2000). A neural basis for sociopathy. *Archives of General Psychiatry*, *57*, 128–9.

Damasio, A. R., Grabowski, T. J., Bechara, A., Damasio, H., Ponto, L. L. B., Parvizi, J. et al. (2000). Subcortical and cortical brain activity during the feeling of self-generated emotions. *Neuroscience*, *3*(10), 1049–56.

Damasio, H., Grabowski, T., Frank, R., Galaburda, A. M. and Damasio, A. R. (1994). The return of Phineas Gage: Clues about the brain from the skull of a famous patient. *Science*, *264*, 1102–5.

Damen, L. (1987). *Culture learning: The fifth dimension on the language classroom*. Reading, MA: Addison-Wesley.

Dane, A. and Schneider, B. H. (1998). Integrity in primary prevention programs: Are implementation effects out of control? *Clinical Psychology Review*, *18*, 23–45.

Danforth, J. S., Harvey, E., Ulaszek, W. R. and McKee, T. E. (2006). The outcome of group parent training for families of children with attention-deficit/hyperactivity disorder and defiant/aggressive behavior. *Journal of Behavior Therapy and Experimental Psychiatry*, *37*, 188–205.

Daniel, L. S. and Billingsley, B. S. (2010). What boys with an autism spectrum disorder say about establishing and maintaining friendships. *Focus on Autism and Other Developmental Disabilities*, *25*, 220–9.

D'Antonio, M. (2004). *The state boys rebellion.* New York: Simon & Schuster.

Daugherty, T. K., Quay, H. C. and Ramos, L. (1993). Response perseveration, inhibitory control, and central dopaminergic activity in childhood behavior disorders. *Journal of Genetic Psychology, 154,* 177–88.

Davidson, G. (1999). Cultural competence as an ethical precept in psychology. In P. R. Martin and W. Noble (Eds.), *Psychology and society* (pp. 162–74). Brisbane: Australian Academic Press.

Davidson, R. J. (2000). Affective style, psychopathology, and resilience: Brain mechanisms and plasticity. *American Psychologist, 55*(11), 1196–214.

Davidson, R. J., Scherer, K. R. and Goldsmith, H. (2003). *Handbook of affective sciences.* Oxford: Oxford University Press.

Daviss, W. B., Diler, R. S. and Birmaher, B. (2009). Associations of lifetime depression with trauma exposure, other environmental adversities, and impairment in adolescents with ADHD. *Journal of Abnormal Child Psychology, 37,* 857–71.

Dawson, G. (2013). Dramatic increase in autism parallels explosion of research into its biology and causes. *JAMA Psychiatry, 70,* 9–10.

Dawson, G., Rogers, S., Munson, J., Smith, M., Winter, J., Greenson, J., Donaldson, A. and Varley, J. (2010). Randomized, controlled trial of an intervention for toddlers with autism: The Early Start Denver Model. *Pediatrics, 125,* 17–23.

Dawson, M. E., Schell, A. M. and Filion, D. L. (2007). The electrodermal system. In J. T. Cacioppo, L. G. Tassinary and G. G. Berntson (Eds.), *Handbook of psychophysiology* (pp. 159–81). New York: Cambridge University Press.

Deary, I., Johnson, W. and Houlihan, L. (2009). Genetic foundations of human intelligence. *Human Genetics, 126,* 215–32.

Deater-Deckard, K. and Dodge, K. A. (1997). Spare the rod, spoil the authors: Emerging themes in research on parenting and child development. *Psychological Inquiry, 8,* 230–35.

Deater-Deckard, K. (2005). Parenting stress and children's development: Introduction to the special issue. *Infant and Child Development, 14*(2), 111–15.

Deater-Deckard, K., Dodge, K. A., Bates, J. E. and Pettit, G. S. (1996). Physical discipline among African American and European American mothers: Links to children's externalizing behaviours. *Developmental Psychology, 32,* 1065–72.

De Bellis, M. D., Hooper, S. R., Spratt, E. G. and Woolley, D. P. (2009). Neuropsychological findings in childhood neglect and their relationships to pediatric PTSD.

Journal of the International Neuropsychological Society, 15, 868–78.

De Bellis, M. D., Hooper, S. R., Woolley, D. P. and Shenk, C. E. (2010). Demographic, maltreatment, and neurobiological correlates of PTSD. *Journal of Pediatric Psychology, 35,* 570–7.

De Boo, G. M. and Prins, P. J. M. (2007). Social incompetence in children with ADHD: Possible moderators and mediators in social skills training. *Clinical Psychology Review, 27,* 78–97.

De Brito, S. A., Mechelli, A., Wilke, M., Laurens, K. R., Jones, A. P., Barker, G. J. et al. (2009). Size matters: increased grey matter in boys with conduct problems and callous-unemotional traits. *Brain, 132* (Pt. 4), 843–52.

De Cuypere, G., Knudson, G. and Bockting, W. (2011). Second response of the World Professional Association for Transgendered Health to the proposed revision of the diagnosis of gender dysphoria in DSM-5. *International Journal of Transgenderism, 13,* 51–3.

De Graaf, I., Speetjens, P., Smit, F., de Wolff, M. and Tavecchio, L. (2008). Effectiveness of the Triple P positive parenting program on behavioral problems in children: A meta-analysis. *Behavior Modification, 32,* 714–35.

De Graaf, I., Speetjens, P., Smit, F., de Wolff, M. and Tavecchio, L. (2008). Effectiveness of the Triple P Positive Parenting Program on parenting: A meta-analysis. *Family Relations, 57,* 553–66.

De Los Reyes, A. and Kazdin, A. E. (2005) Informant discrepancies in the assessment of childhood psychopathology. *Psychological Bulletin, 131,* 483–509.

de Mause, L. (1974). *The history of childhood.* New York: Psychohistory Press.

de Schipper, J. C., Tavecchio, L. W. C., van IJzendoorn, M. H. and van Zeijl, J. (2004). Goodness-of-fit in center day care: Relations of temperament, stability, and quality of care with the child's adjustment. *Early Childhood Research Quarterly, 19,* 257–72.

DeBoard-Lucas, R. L., Fosco, G. M., Raynor, S. R. and Grych, J. H. (2010). Interparental conflict in context: Exploring relations between parenting processes and children's conflict appraisals. *Journal of Clinical Child and Adolescent Psychology, 39,* 163–75.

Decety, J., Michalska, K. J., Akitsuki, Y. and Lahey, B. B. (2009). Atypical empathic responses in adolescents with aggressive conduct disorder: A functional MRI investigation. *Biological Psychology, 80,* 203–11.

DeSantis, T., Brodie, E. L., Moberg, J., Zubieta, I., Piceno, Y. and Andersen, G. (2007). High-density universal 16S rRNA microarray analysis reveals broader diversity than typical clone library when sampling the environment. *Microbiological Ecology, 53,* 371–83.

Deci, E. L. and Ryan, R. M. (1985). The general causality orientations scale: Self-determination in personality. *Journal of Research in Personality, 19*, 109–34.

Degnan, K. A., Almas, A. N. and Fox, N. A. (2010). Temperament and the environment in the etiology of childhood anxiety. *Journal of Child Psychology and Psychiatry, 51*, 497–517.

DeGrandpre, R. (1999). *Ritalin nation*. New York: Norton.

DeKlyen, M., Speltz, M. L. and Greenberg, M. T. (1998). Fathering and early onset conduct problems: Positive and negative parenting, father–son attachment, and the marital context. *Clinical Child and Family Psychology Review, 1*, 3–21.

DelBello, M. P., Adler, C. M. and Strakowski, S. M. (2006). The neurophysiology of child and adolescent bipolar disorder. *CNS Spectrums, 11*, 298–311.

DelBello, M. P., Hanseman, D., Adler, C. M., Fleck, D. E. and Strakowski, S. M. (2007). Twelve-month outcome of adolescents with bipolar disorder following first hospitalization for a manic or mixed episode. *American Journal of Psychiatry, 164*, 582–90.

Dell, P. F. and O'Neill, J. (Eds.) (2009). *Dissociation and the dissociative Disorders: DSM-V and beyond*. New York: Routledge.

Dembo, R. and Muck, R. D. (2009). Adolescent outpatient treatment. In C. Leukefeld, T. P. Gullotta, M. Staton-Tindall (Eds.), *Adolescent substance abuse: Evidence-based approaches to prevention and treatment* (Vol. IX, pp. 97–117). New York: Springer.

Dempsey, T. and Matson, J. L. (2009). General methods of treatment. In J. L. Matson (Ed.), *Social behavior and skills in children* (pp. 77–95). New York: Springer Science and Business Media.

Department for Education (2010). *Statistical release: Children in need in England, including their characteristics and further information on children who were the subject of a child protection plan (children in need census – final) year ending 31 March 2010*. London, UK: author. Retrieved from www.education.gov.uk/rsgateway/DB/STR/d000970/osr28-2010v3.pdf

Derks, E. M., Dolan, C. V., Hudziak, J. J., Neale, M. C. and Boomsma, D. I. (2006). Assessment and etiology of attention deficit hyperactivity disorder and oppositional defiant disorder in boys and girls. *Behavior Genetics, 37*, 559–66.

Derks, E. M., Hudziak, J. J. and Boomsma, D. I. (2007). Why more boys than girls with ADHD receive treatment: A study of Dutch twins. *Twin Research and Human Genetics, 10*, 765–70.

Dershowitz, A. M. (1994). *The abuse excuse: And other cop-outs, sob stories, and evasions of responsibility*. Little, Brown and Company.

Descuret, J. B. F. (1841). *Médecine de passions*. Paris: Béchet and Labé.

DesLauriers, A. M. and Carlson, C. F. (1969). *Your child is asleep: Early infantile autism: Etiology, treatment, and parental influences*. Homewood, IL: Dorsey Press.

Despert, L. (1965). *The emotionally disturbed child, then and now*. New York: Brunner.

Deter, H. C., Schellberg, D., Kopp, W., Friederich, H. C. and Herzog, W. (2005). Predictability of a favorable outcome in anorexia nervosa. *European Psychiatry, 20*, 165–72.

Deutsch, M. and Gerard, H. B. (1955). A study of normative and informational social influences upon individual judgement. *The Journal of Abnormal and Social Psychology, 51*, 629–36.

DeVylder, J. E. (2013). The fall and rise of Adolf Meyer's psychogenic etiology of dementia praecox (schizophrenia): 1903–1910 and beyond. *Smith College Studies in Social Work, 83*, 2–73.

Diamond, M. (2002). Sex and gender are different: Sexual identity and gender identity are different. *Clinical Child Psychology and Psychiatry, 7*, 320–34.

DiBartolo, P. M. and Helt, M. (2007). Theoretical models of affectionate versus affectionless control in anxious families: A critical examination based on observations of parent–child interactions. *Clinical Child and Family Psychology Review, 10*, 253–74.

Dick, D. M. (2007). Identification of genes influencing a spectrum of externalizing psychopathology. *Current Directions in Psychological Science, 16*, 331–5.

Dick, D. M., Agrawal, A., Schuckit, M. A., Bierut, L., Hinrichs, A., Fox, L. et al. (2006). Marital status, alcohol dependence, and GABRA2: Evidence for gene–environment correlation and interaction. *Journal of Studies on Alcohol, 67*, 185–94.

Dick, D. M., Pagan, J. L., Viken, R., Purcell, S., Kaprio, J., Pulkinnen, L. et al. (2007). Changing environmental influences on substance use across development. *Twin Research and Human Genetics, 10*, 315–26.

Dick, D. M., Aliev, F., Wang, J. C., Grucza, R. A., Schuckit, M., Kuperman, S....Goate, A. (2008). Using dimensional models of externalizing psychopathology to aid in gene identification. *Archives of General Psychiatry, 65*, 310–18.

Dick, D. M., Latendresse, S. J., Lansford, J. E., Budde, J. P., Goate, A., Dodge, K. A....Bates, J. E. (2009). Role of GABRA2 in trajectories of externalizing behavior across development and evidence of moderation by parental monitoring. *Archives of General Psychiatry, 66*, 649–57.

Dickstein, D. P., Rich, B. A., Binstock, A. B., Pradella, A. G., Towbin, K. E., Pine, D. S. and Leibenluft, E. (2005). Comorbid anxiety in phenotypes of pediatric bipolar disorder. *Journal of Child and Adolescent Psychopharmacology, 15*, 534–48.

Didden, R., Scholte, R. H. J., Korzilius, H., de Moor, J. M. H., Vermeulen, A., O'Reilly, M., Lang, R. and Lancioni, G. E. (2009). Cyberbullying among students with intellectual and developmental disability in special educational settings. *Developmental Neurorehabilitation, 12*, 146–51.

Dienes, K. A., Hammen, C., Henry, R. M., Cohen, A. N. and Daley, S. E. (2006). The stress sensitization hypothesis: Understanding the course of bipolar disorder. *Journal of Affective Disorders, 95*, 43–9.

Dietrich, A., Riese, H., Sondeijker, F. E. P. L., Greaves-Lord, K., Van roon, A. M., Ormel, J....Rosmalen, J. G. M. (2007). Externalizing and internalizing problems in relation to autonomic function: A population-based study in preadolescents. *Journal of the American Academy of Child and Adolescent Psychiatry, 46*, 378–86.

Dikotter, F. (1998). Race culture: Recent perspectives on the history of eugenics. *American Historical Review, 103*, 467–79.

Dill, E. J., Vernberg, E. M., Fonagy, P., Twemlow, S. W. and Gamm, B. K. (2004). Negative affect in victimized children: The roles of social withdrawal, peer rejection, and attitudes toward bullying. *Journal of Abnormal Child Psychology, 32*, 159–73.

Diller, L. H. (1998). *Running on Ritalin*. New York: Norton.

DiLorenzo, T. M. (1988). Operant and classical conditioning. In J. L. Matson (Ed.), *Handbook of treatment approaches in childhood psychopathology* (pp. 65–77). New York: Plenum.

Dishion, T. J., McCord, J. and Poulin, F. (1999). When interventions harm: Peer groups and problem behavior. *American Psychologist, 54*, 755–64.

Dishion, T. J., Nelson, S. E., Winter, C. E. and Bullock, B. M. (2004). Adolescent friendship as a dynamic system: Entropy and deviance in the etiology and course of male antisocial behaviour. *Journal of Abnormal Child Psychology, 32*, 651–63.

Dishion, T. J. and Granic, I. (2004). Naturalistic observation of relationship processes. In S. N. Haynes and E. M. Heiby (Eds.), *Comprehensive handbook of psychological assessment*, Vol. III: *Behavioral assessment* (pp. 143–161). Hoboken, NJ: John Wiley and Sons Inc.

Dishion, T. J. and McMahon, R. H. (1998). Parental monitoring and the prevention of child and adolescent problem behavior: A conceptual and empirical formulation. *Clinical Child and Family Psychology Review, 1*, 61–75.

Dishion, T. J. and Patterson, S. (2006). *Parenting young children with love, encouragement, and limits*. New York: Research Press.

Dishion, T. J., Piehler, T. F. and Myers, M. W. (2008). Dynamics and ecology of adolescent peer influence. In M. J. Prinstein and K. A. Dodge (Eds.), *Understanding peer influence in children and adolescents* (pp. 72–93). New York: Guilford Press.

Dishion, T. J. and Stormshak, E. A. (2007). *Intervening in children's lives: An ecological, family-centered approach to mental health care*. Washington, DC: American Psychological Association.

Dixon, A., Howie, P. and Starling, J. (2005). Trauma exposure, posttraumatic stress, and psychiatric comorbidity in female juvenile offenders. *Journal of the American Academy of Child and Adolescent Psychiatry, 44*, 798–806.

Dodge, K. (1985). Facets of social interaction and the assessment of social competence in children. In B. H. Schneider, K. H. Rubin and J. E. Ledingham (Eds.), *Children's peer relations: Issues in assessment and intervention*. New York: Springer-Verlag.

Dodge, K., Coie, J. and Lynam, D. (2006). Aggression and antisocial behaviour in youth. In N. Eisenberg (Ed.), *Handbook of child psychology: Social, emotional and personality development*, (Vol. III, pp. 719–85). New York: Wiley.

Dodge, K. A. and Newman, J. P. (1981). Biased decision-making processes in aggressive boys. *Journal of Abnormal Psychology, 90*, 375–9.

Dodge, K. A. and Frame, C. L. (1982). Social cognitive biases and deficits in aggressive boys. *Child Development, 53*, 620–35.

Dodge, K. A. and Pettit, G. S. (2003). A biopsychosocial model of the development of chronic conduct problems in adolescence. *Developmental Psychology, 39*, 349–71.

Dodge, K. A., and Sherrill, M. R. (2007). The interaction of nature and nurture in antisocial behavior. In D. J. Flannery, A. T. Vazsonyi and I. D. Waldman (Eds.), *The Cambridge handbook of violent behavior and aggression* (pp. 215–42). New York: Cambridge University Press.

Dodge, K. A., Malone, P. S., Lansford, J. E., Miller, S., Pettit, G. S. and Bates, J. E. (2009). A dynamic cascade model of the development of substance-use onset. *Monographs of the Society for Research in Child Development, 74*, vii–103.

Doi, Y., Roberts, R. E., Takeuchi, K. and Suzuki, S. (2001). Multiethnic comparison of adolescent major depression based on the DSM – IV criteria in a U.S.-Japan study. *Journal of the American Academy of Child and Adolescent Psychiatry, 40*, 1308–15.

Domenech Rodriguez, M. M., Donovick, M. R. and Crowley, S. L. (2009). Parenting styles in a cultural context: Observations of "protective parenting" in first-generation Latinos. *Family Process, 48*, 195–210.

Dominus, S. (2011, April 20). The crash and burn of an autism guru. The *New York Times*. Retrieved from www.nytimes.com/2011/04/24/magazine/mag-24Autism-t.html?_r=3

Donlan, W., Lee, J. and Paz, J. (2009) Corazon de Aztlan: Culturally competent substance abuse prevention. *Journal of Social Work Practice in the Addictions, 9*, 215–32.

Donvan, C. and Zucker, C. (2010). Autism's first child. The *Atlantic*. Retrieved February 11, 2013 from www.theatlantic.com/magazine/archive/2010/10/autisms-first-child/308227/

Dopfner, M., Breuer, D., Schurmann, S., Metternich, T. W., Rademacher, C. and Lehmkuhl, G. (2004). Effectiveness of an adaptive multimodal treatment in children with attention-deficit hyperactivity disorder – global outcome. *European Child and Adolescent Psychiatry, 13*, 117–29.

Dorland, W. A. N. (2007). *Dorland's medical dictionary for health consumers*, Philadelphia: Saunders.

Dosen, A. (1994). The European scene. In N. Bourras (Ed.), *Mental health in mental retardation* (pp. 375–8). Cambridge: Cambridge University Press.

Double, D. B. (2007). Eclecticism and Adolf Meyer's functional understanding of mental illness. *Philosophy, Psychiatry, and Psychology, 14*, 356–8.

Douglas, V. I. (1972). Stop, look and listen: The problem of sustained attention and impulse control in hyperactive and normal children. *Canadian Journal of Behavioral Science/Revue canadienne des sciences du comportement, 4*(4), 259–82.

Dowell, K. A. and Ogles, B. M. (2010). The effects of parent participation on child psychotherapy outcome: A meta-analytic review. *Journal of Clinical Child and Adolescent Psychology, 39*, 151–62.

Downey, G. and Coyne, J. C. (1990). Children of depressed parents: An integrative review. *Psychological Bulletin, 108*, 50–76.

Downey, G., Lebolt, A., Rincon, C. and Freitas, A. L. (1998). Rejection sensitivity and children's interpersonal difficulties. *Child Development, 69*, 1074–91.

Drabick, D. A. G. (2009). Can a developmental psychopathology perspective facilitate a paradigm shift toward a mixed categorical-dimensional classification system? *Clinical Psychology: Science and Practice, 16*, 41–9.

Dragowski, E. A., Scharron-del Rio, M. R. and Sandigorsky, A. L. (2011). Childhood gender identity . . . disorder?

Developmental, cultural, and diagnostic concerns. *Journal of Counseling and Development, 89*, 360–6.

Drescher, J. (2010). Queer diagnoses: Parallels and contrasts in the history of homosexuality, gender variance, and the Diagnostic and Statistical Manual. *Archives of Sexual Behavior, 39*, 427–60.

Dretzke, J., Davenport, C., Frew, E., Barlow, J., Stewart-Brown, S., Bayliss, S.,...Hyde, C. (2009). The clinical effectiveness of different parenting programmes for children with conduct problems: A systematic review of randomised controlled trials. *Child and Adolescent Psychiatry and Mental Health, 3*.

Drotar, D. (1999). The diagnostic and statistical manual for primary care (DSM-PC), child and adolescent version: What pediatric psychologists need to know. *Journal of Pediatric Psychology, 24*, 369–80.

Ducharme, J. M. (2008). Errorless remediation: A success-focused and noncoercive model for managing severe problem behaviour in children. *Infants and Young Children, 21*, 296–305.

Ducharme, J. M., di Padova, T. and Ashworth, M. (2010). Errorless compliance training to reduce extreme conduct problems and intrusive control strategies in home and school settings. *Clinical Case Studies, 9*, 167–80.

Duemm, I., Adams, G. R. and Keating, R. (2003). The addition of sociotropy to the dual pathway model of bulimia. *Canadian Journal of Behavioral Sciences, 35*, 281–91.

Duffy, A. (2009). The early course of bipolar disorder in youth at familial risk. *Journal of the Canadian Academy of Child and Adolescent Psychiatry, 18*, 200–5.

Duffy, J. C. (1976). Special article in honor of the bicentennial year 1976–1996. *Child Psychiatry and Human Development, 6*, 189–97.

Duhl, F. S., Kantor, D. and Duhl, B. S. (1973). Learning space and action in family therapy: A primer of sculpting. In D. Bloch (Ed.), *Techniques of family psychotherapy: A primer*. New York: Grune and Stratton.

Dumenci, L., Achenbach, T. M. and Windle, M. (2011). Measuring context-specific and cross-contextual components of hierarchical constructs. *Journal of Psychopathology and Behavioral Assessment, 33*, 3–10.

Duncan, D. F. (1994). The prevention of primary prevention, 1960–1994: Notes towards a case study. The *Journal of Primary Prevention, 15*, 73–9.

Dunn, J. and Plomin, R. (1990). *Separate lives: Why siblings are so different*. New York: Basic Books.

Dunn, J., Stocker, C. and Plomin, R. (1990). Nonshared experiences within the family: Correlates of behavior problems in middle childhood. *Development and Psychopathology, 2*, 113–26.

Dunn, J., Slomkowski, C. and Beardsall, L. (1994). Sibling relationships from the preschool period through middle childhood and early adolescence. *Developmental Psychology, 30*, 315–24.

DuPaul, G. J. and Eckert, T. L. (1997). The effects of school-based interventions for Attention Deficit Hyperactivity Disorder: A meta-analysis. *School Psychology Review, 26*, 5–27.

DuPaul, G. J., McGoey, K. E., Eckert, T. L. and VanBrakle, J. (2001). Preschool children with attention-deficit/hyperactivity disorder: Impairments in behavioral, social, and school functioning. *Journal of the American Academy of Child and Adolescent Psychiatry, 40*, 508–15.

DuPaul, G. J., Jitendra, A. K., Tresco, K. E., Junod, R. E., Volpe, R. J. and Lutz, J. G. (2006). Children with attention deficit hyperactivity disorder: Are there gender differences in school functioning? *School Psychology Review, 35*, 292–308.

Dura-Vila, G., Dein, S. and Hodes, M. (2010). Children with intellectual disability: A gain not a loss: Parental beliefs and family life. *Clinical Child Psychology and Psychiatry, 15*, 171–84.

Durlak, J. A. and Wells, A. M. (1997). Primary prevention mental health programs for children and adolescents: A meta-analytic review. *American Journal of Community Psychology, 25*, 115–52.

Durston, S. (2008). Converging methods in studying attention-deficit/hyperactivity disorder: What can we learn from neuroimaging and genetics? *Development and Psychopathology, 20*(4), 1133–43.

Durston, S., Mulder, M., Casey, B. J., Ziermans, T. and van Engeland, H. (2006). Activation in ventral prefrontal cortex is sensitive to genetic vulnerability for attention-deficit hyperactivity disorder. *Biological Psychiatry, 60*(10), 1062–70.

Durston, S., Tottenham, N. T., Thomas, K. M., Davidson, M. C., Eigsti, I. M., Yang, Y. et al. (2003). Differential patterns of striatal activation in young children with and without ADHD. *Biological Psychiatry, 53*(10), 871–8.

Dwairy, M. A. (2008). Parental inconsistency versus parental authoritarianism: Associations with symptoms of psychological disorders. *Journal of Youth and Adolescence, 37*, 616–26.

Dwivedi, K. N. (2006). An Eastern perspective on change. *Clinical Child Psychology and Psychiatry, 11*, 205–12.

Dykman, R. A., Ackerman, P. T. and Oglesby, D. M. (1992). Heart rate reactivity in attention deficit disorder subgroups. *Integrative Physiological and Behavioral Science, 27*, 228–45.

Dyregrov, A. and Yule, W. (2006). A review of PTSD in children. *Child and Adolescent Mental Health, 11*, 176–84.

Dyson, L. (1996). The experiences of families of children with learning disabilities: Parental stress, family functioning, and sibling self-concept. *Journal of Learning Disabilities, 29*, 280–6.

Dyson, L. (2010). Unanticipated effects of children with learning disabilities on their families. *Learning Disability Quarterly, 33*, 43–55.

Earls, F. and Mezzacappa, E. (2002). Conduct and oppositional disorders. In M. Rutter and E. Taylor (Eds.), *Child and adolescent psychiatry* (pp. 419–30). London: Blackwell Science.

Eaves, L., Silberg, J. and Erkanli, A. (2003). Resolving multiple epigenetic pathways to adolescent depression. *Journal of Child Psychology and Psychiatry, 44*, 1006–14.

ebrary, Inc. (2005). *The Hutchinson pocket dictionary of biology.* Abingdon: Helicon Publishing.

Eder, D. (1995). *School talk: Gender and adolescent culture.* New Brunswick, NJ: Rutgers University Press.

Edwards, A. C., Dodge, K. A., Latendresse, S. J., Lansford, J. E., Bates, J. E., Pettit, G. S.…Dick, D. M. (2010). MAOA-uVNTR and early physical discipline interact to influence delinquent behaviour. *Journal of Child Psychology and Psychiatry, 51*, 679–87.

Edwards, V. J., Holden, G. W., Felitti, V. J. and Anda, R. F. (2003). Relationship between multiple forms of childhood maltreatment and adult mental health in community respondents: Results from the Adverse Childhood Experiences study. *American Journal of Psychiatry, 160*, 1453–60.

Egger, H. L. and Angold, A. (2006). Common emotional and behavioural disorders in preschool children: Presentation, nosology, and epidemiology. *Journal of Child Psychology and Psychiatry, 47*, 313–37.

Egger, H. L., Costello, E. J. and Angold, A. (2003). School refusal and psychiatric disorders: A community study. *American Academy of Child and Adolescent Psychiatry, 42*, 797–807.

Einfeld, S. and Emerson, E. (2010). Intellectual disability. In M. Rutter, D. Bishop, D. Pine, S. Scott, J. Stevenson, E. Taylor and A. Thapar (Eds.), *Rutter's child and adolescent psychiatry* (5th edn., pp. 820–40). Oxford: Blackwell.

Eisen, M. L., Goodman, G. S., Qin, J., Davis, S. and Crayton, J. (2007). Maltreated children's memory: Accuracy, suggestibility, and psychopathology. *Developmental Psychology, 43*, 1275–94.

Eisenberg, L. (1986). Mindlessness and brainlessness in psychiatry. *British Journal of Psychiatry, 148*, 497–508.

Eisenberg, L. (2007). Commentary with a historical perspective by a child psychiatrist: When "ADHD" was the "brain-damaged child." *Journal of Child and Adolescent Psychopharmacology, 17*, 279–83.

Eisenberg, N., Cumberland, A., Spinrad, T. L., Fabes, R. A., Shepard, S. A., Reiser, M.,...Guthrie, I. K. (2001). The relations of regulation and emotionality to children's externalizing and internalizing problem behaviour. *Child Development*, *72*, 1112–34.

Eisenberg, N. and Fabes, R. A. (1994). Mothers' reactions to children's negative emotions: Relations to children's temperament and anger behavior. *Merrill-Palmer Quarterly*, *40*, 138–56.

Eisenberger, N. I., Way, B. M., Taylor, S. E., Welch, W. T. and Lieberman, M. D. (2007). Understanding genetic risk for aggression: Clues from the brain's response to social exclusion. *Biological Psychiatry*, *61*, 1100–8.

Eisler, I., Simic, M., Russell, G. F. M. and Dare, C. (2007). A randomised controlled treatment trial of two forms of family therapy in adolescent anorexia nervosa: A five-year follow-up. *Journal of Child Psychology and Psychiatry*, *48*, 552–60.

Eley, T. C., Lichtenstein, P. and Moffitt, T. E. (2003). A longitudinal behavioural genetic analysis of the etiology of aggressive and nonaggressive antisocial behaviour. *Development and Psychopathology*, *15*, 383–402.

Eley, T. C., Stirling, L., Ehlers, A., Gregory, A. M. and Clark, D. M. (2004). Heart-beat perception, panic/somatic symptoms and anxiety sensitivity in children. *Behaviour Research and Therapy*, *42*, 439–48.

Eley, T. C. and Rijsdijk, F. (2005). Introductory guide to the statistics of molecular genetics. *Journal of Child Psychology and Psychiatry*, *46*, 1042–4.

Eley, T. C., Gregory, A. M., Clark, D. M. and Ehlers, A. (2007). Feeling anxious: A twin study of panic/somatic ratings, anxiety sensitivity and heartbeat perception in children. *Journal of Child Psychology and Psychiatry*, *48*, 1184–91.

Eley, T. C., Hudson, J. L., Creswell, C., Tropeano, M., Lester, K. J., Cooper, P.,...Collier, D. A. (2012). Therapygenetics: The 5HTTLPR and response to psychological therapy. *Molecular Psychiatry*, *17*, 236–7.

Elia, J., Arcos-Burgos, M., Bolton, K. L., Ambrosini, P. J., Berrettini, W. and Muenke, M. (2009). ADHD latent class clusters: DSM-IV subtypes and comorbidity. *Psychiatry Research*, *170*, 192–8.

El-Islam, M. F. (2008). Arab culture and mental health care. *Transcultural Psychiatry*, *45*, 671–82.

Elkind, D. (1988). *The hurried child: Growing up too fast too soon*. Reading, MA: Perseus Publishing.

Elkins, D. N. (2009). The medical model in psychotherapy: Its limitations and failures. *Journal of Humanistic Psychology*, *49*, 66–84.

Elliott, D. S., Huizinga, D. and Menard, S. (1989). *Multiple problem youth: Delinquency, substance use, and mental health problems*. New York: Springer-Verlag Publishing.

Elliott, S. A. and Brown, J. S. L. (2002). What are we doing to waiting list controls? *Behavior Research and Therapy*, *40*, 1047–52.

Ellis, B. H., Lincoln, A. K., Charney, M. E., Ford-Paz, R., Benson, M. and Strunin, L. (2010). Mental health service utilization of Somali adolescents: Religion, community, and school as gateways to healing. *Transcultural Psychiatry*, *47*, 789–811.

Ellis, B. H., Miller, A. B., Abdi, S., Barrett, C., Blood, E. A. and Betancourt, T. S. (2013). Multi-tier mental health program for refugee youth. *Journal of Consulting and Clinical Psychology*, *81*, 129–40.

Ellis, B. J., Boyce, W. T., Belsky, J., Bakersman-Kranenburg, M. J. and van IJzendoorn, M. H. (2011). Differential susceptibility to the environment: An evolutionary-neurodevelopmental theory. *Development and Psychopathology*, *23*, 7–28.

Ellis, H. and Symonds, J. A. (2008). *Sexual inversion: A critical edition*. Houndmills: Palgrave Macmillan.

El-Sheikh, M. (2001). Parental drinking problems and children's adjustment: Vagal regulation and emotional reactivity as pathways and moderators of risk. *Journal of Abnormal Psychology*, *110*, 499–515.

El-Sheikh, M. (2005). Stability of respiratory sinus arrhythmia in children and young adolescents: A longitudinal examination. *Developmental Psychobiology*, *46*, 66–74.

El-Sheikh, M. and Harger, J. (2001). Appraisals of marital conflict and children's adjustment, health, and physiological reactivity. *Developmental Psychology*, *37*, 875–85.

El-Sheikh, M., Harger, J. and Whitson, S. M. (2001). Exposure to interparental conflict and children's adjustment and physical health: The moderating role of vagal tone. *Child Development*, *72*, 1617–36.

El-Sheikh, M. and Elmore-Staton, L. (2004). The link between marital conflict and child adjustment: Parent–child conflict and perceived attachments as mediators, potentiators, and mitigators of risk. *Development and Psychopathology*, *16*, 631–48.

El-Sheikh, M. and Whitson, S. A. (2006). Longitudinal relations between marital conflict and child adjustment: Vagal regulation as a protective factor. *Journal of Family Psychology*, *20*, 30–9.

El-Sheikh, M., Erath, S. A., Buckhalt, J. A., Granger, D. A. and Mize, J. (2008). Cortisol and children's adjustment: The moderating role of sympathetic nervous system activity. *Journal of Abnormal Child Psychology*, *36*, 601–11.

El-Sheikh, M., Kouros, C. D., Erath, S., Cummings, E. M., Keller, P. and Staton, L. (2009). Marital conflict and children's externalizing behavior: interactions between parasympathetic and sympathetic nervous system activity. *Monographs of the Society for Research in Child Development, 74*(1), vii–79.

Eme, R. F. (2007). Sex differences in child-onset, life-course-persistent conduct disorder. A review of biological influences. *Clinical Psychology Review, 27*, 607–27.

Emerson, A., Grayson, A. and Griffiths, A. (2001). Can't or won't? Evidence relating to authorship in facilitated communication. *International Journal of Language and Communication Disorders, 36*, 98–103.

Emerson, E., Shahtahmasebi, S., Lancaster, G. and Berridge, D. (2010). Poverty transitions among families supporting a child with intellectual disability. *Journal of Intellectual and Developmental Disability, 35*, 224–34.

Engfer, A. and Schneewind, K. A. (1982). Causes and consequences of harsh parental punishment: An empirical investigation in a representative sample of 570 German families. *Child Abuse and Neglect, 6*, 129–39.

Epstein, J. N., Delbello, M. P., Adler, C. M., Altaye, M., Kramer, M., Mills, N. P. et al. (2009). Differential patterns of brain activation over time in adolescents with and without attention deficit hyperactivity disorder (ADHD) during performance of a sustained attention task. *Neuropediatrics, 40*(1), 1–5.

Epstein, J. N., Casey, B. J., Tonev, S. T., Davidson, M. C., Reiss, A. L., Garrett, A. et al. (2007). ADHD- and medication-related brain activation effects in concordantly affected parent–child dyads with ADHD. *Journal Child Psychology and Psychiatry, 48*(9), 899–913.

Ennett, S. T., Tobler, N. S., Ringwalt, C. L. and Flewelling, R. L. (1994). How effective is drug abuse resistance education? A meta-analysis of Project DARE outcome evaluations. *American Journal of Public Health, 84*, 1394–401.

Enoch, M. A. (2011). The role of early life stress as a predictor for alcohol and drug dependence. *Psychopharmacology, 214*, 17–31.

Erath, S. A., Flanagan, K. S., Bierman, K. L. and Tu, K. M. (2010). Friendships moderate psychosocial maladjustment in socially anxious early adolescents. *Journal of Applied Developmental Psychology, 31*, 15–26.

Ericsson, K. (1985). The principle of normalization: History and experiences in Scandinavian countries. Presented at ILSMH Congress, Hamburg, Department of Education, Uppsala University.

Eriksen, K. and Kress, V. E. (2005). *Beyond the DSM story: Ethical quandaries, challenges, and best practices.* Thousand Oaks, CA: Sage Publications, Inc.

Erikson, E. H. (1950). *Childhood and society.* New York: Norton.

Ernst, M., Zametkin, A. J., Matochik, J. A., Jons, P. H. and Cohen, R. M. (1998). DOPA decarboxylase activity in attention deficit hyperactivity disorder adults. A [fluorine-18]fluorodopa positron emission tomographic study. *The Journal of Neuroscience, 18*(15), 5901–7.

Eslea, M., Menesini, E., Morita, Y., O'Moore, M., Mora-Merchan, J. A., Pereira, B. and Smith, P. K. (2004). Friendship and loneliness among bullies and victims: Data from seven countries. *Aggressive Behavior, 30*, 71–83.

Esposito-Smythers, C., Goldstein, T., Birmaher, B., Goldstein, B., Hunt, J., Ryan, N., Axelson, D., Strober, M., Gill, M., Hanley, A. and Keller, M. (2010). Clinical and psychosocial correlates of nonsuicidal self-injury in a sample of children and adolescents with bipolar disorder. *Journal of Affective Disorders, 125*, 89–97.

Essau, C. A., Conradt, J. and Petermann, F. (2000). Frequency, comorbidity, and psychosocial impairment of anxiety disorders in German adolescents. *Journal of Anxiety Disorders, 14*, 263–79.

Essau, C. A., Sakano, Y., Ishikawa, S. and Sasagawa, S. (2004). Anxiety symptoms in Japanese and in German children. *Behaviour Research and Therapy, 42*, 601–12.

Essau, C. A., Leung, P. W. L., Koydcmir, S., Sasagawa, S., O'Callaghan, J. and Bray, D. (2012). The impact of self-construals and perceived social norms on social anxiety in young adults: A cross-cultural comparison. *International Journal of Culture and Mental Health, 5*, 109–20.

Essex, M. J., Klein, M. H., Slattery, M. J., Goldsmith, H. H. and Kalin, N. H. (2010). Early risk factors and developmental pathways to chronic high inhibition and social anxiety disorder in adolescence. *American Journal of Psychiatry, 167*, 40–6.

Estell, D. B., Jones, M. H., Pearl, R., van Acker, R., Farmer, T. W. and Rodkin, P. C. (2008). Peer groups, popularity, and social preference: Trajectories of social functioning among students with and without learning disabilities. *Journal of Learning Disabilities, 41*, 5–14.

Etkin, A., Egner, T. and Kalisch, R. (2011). Emotional processing in anterior cingulate and medial prefrontal cortex. *Trends in Cognitive Sciences, 15*, 85–93.

Evans, F. B. III (1996). *Harry Stack Sullivan: Interpersonal theory and psychotherapy.* New York: Routledge.

Evers, A. W., Verhoeven, E. W., Kraaimaat, F. W., de Jong, E. M. et al. (2010). How stress gets under the skin: Cortisol and stress reactivity in psoriasis. *British Journal of Dermatology, 163*, 986–91.

Eyberg, S. M., Nelson, M. M. and Boggs, S. R. (2008). Evidence-based psychosocial treatments for children and adolescents with disruptive behaviour. *Journal of Clinical Child and Adolescent Psychology, 37*, 215–37.

Eysenck, H. J. (1952). The effects of psychotherapy: An evaluation. *Journal of Consulting Psychology, 16,* 319–24.

Eysenck, H. J. (1978). An exercise in mega-silliness. *American Psychologist, 33,* 517.

Fabiano, G. A. and Pelham, W. E. (2003). Improving the effectiveness of behavioral classroom interventions for attention-deficit/hyperactivity disorder: A case study. *Journal of Emotional and Behavioral Disorders, 11,* 124–30.

Fabiano, G. A., Pelham, W. E., Coles, E. K., Gnagy, E. M., Chronis-Tuscano, A. and O'Connor, B. C. (2009). A meta-analysis of behavioral treatments for attention-deficit/hyperactivity disorder. *Clinical Psychology Review, 29,* 129–40.

Fairburn, C. G. and Cooper, Z. (1993). The eating disorder examination (12th edn.). In C. G. Fairburn and G. T. Wilson (Eds.), *Binge eating: Nature, assessment, and treatment* (pp. 317–60). New York: Guilford Press.

Fairburn, C. G., Cooper, Z., Doll, H. A., Norman, P. and O'Connor, M. (2000). The natural course of bulimia nervosa and binge eating disorder in young women. *Archives of General Psychiatry, 57,* 659–65.

Fairburn, C. G., Cooper, Z. and Shafran, R. (2003). Cognitive behaviour therapy for eating disorders: A "transdiagnostic" theory and treatment. *Behaviour Research and Therapy, 41,* 509–28.

Fairburn, C. G. and Gowers, S. G. (2010). Eating disorders. In M. Rutter, D. Bishop, D. Pine, S. Scott, J. Stevenson, E. Taylor and A. Thapar. (Eds.), *Rutter's child and adolescent psychiatry* (pp. 670–85). Oxford: Blackwell.

Fairchild, G., van Goozen, S. H. M., Stollery, S. J., Brown, J., Gardiner, J., Herbert, J. and Goodyer, I. M. (2008). Cortisol diurnal rhythm and stress reactivity in male adolescents with early-onset or adolescence-onset conduct disorder. *Biological Psychiatry, 64,* 599–606.

Faith, M. S., Berkowitz, R. I., Stallings, V. A., Kerns, J., Storey, M. and Stunkard, A. J. (2004). Parental feeding attitudes and styles and child body mass index: Prospective analysis of a gene–environment interaction. *Pediatrics, 114,* 429–36.

Falconer, D. S. (1960). *Introduction to quantitative genetics.* Edinburgh/London: Oliver and Boyd.

Faller, K. (2007). Mother blaming the son. *Journal of Child Sexual Abuse: Research, Treatment, and Program Innovations for Victims, Survivors, and Offenders, 16*(1), 129–36.

Fang, L., Schinke, S. P. and Cole, K. C. A. (2010). Preventing substance use among early Asian-American adolescent girls: Initial evaluation of a web-based, mother–daughter program. *Journal of Adolescent Health, 47,* 529–32.

Faraone, S. V. (1997). Familial transmission of attention-deficit/hyperactivity disorder and comorbidities. Presented at the Annual meeting of the American Academy of Child and Adolescent Psychiatry, Toronto, Canada.

Faraone, S. V., Biederman, J., Weber, W. and Russell, R. L. (1998). Psychiatric, neuropsychological, and psychological features of DSM-IV subtypes of attention-deficit/hyperactivity disorder: Results from a clinically referred sample. *Journal of the American Academy of Child and Adolescent Psychiatry, 37,* 185–93.

Faraone, S. V., Biederman, J. and Monuteaux, M. C. (2000). Attention-deficit disorder and conduct disorder in girls: Evidence for a familial subtype. *Biological Psychiatry, 48,* 21–9.

Faraone, S. V., Biederman, J., Mick, E., Williamson, S., Wilens, T., Spencer, T.,…Zallen, B. (2000). Family study of girls with attention deficit hyperactivity disorder. *The American Journal of Psychiatry, 157,* 1077–83.

Faraone, S. V. and Doyle, A. E. (2000). Genetic influences on attention deficit hyperactivity disorder. *Current Psychiatry Reports, 2,* 143–6.

Faraone, S. V. and Biederman, J. (2000). Nature, nurture, and attention deficit hyperactivity disorder. *Developmental Review, 20,* 568–81.

Faraone, S. V., Sergeant, J., Gillberg, C. and Biederman, J. (2003). The worldwide prevalence of ADHD: Is it an American condition? *World Psychiatry, 2,* 104–13.

Faraone, S. V., Perlis, R. H., Doyle, A. E., Smoller, J. W., Goralnick, J. J., Holmgren, M. A. and Sklar, P. (2005). Molecular genetics of attention-deficit/hyperactivity disorder. *Biological Psychiatry, 57,* 1313–23.

Faravelli, C., Sauro, C. L., Castellini, G., Ricca, V. and Pallanti, S. (2009). Prevalence and correlates of mental disorders in a school-survey sample. *Clinical Practice and Epidemiology in Mental Health, 5,* 1–8.

Farley, S. E., Adams, J. S., Lutton, M. E. and Scoville, C. (2005). What are effective treatments for oppositional and defiant behaviours in preadolescents? *The Journal of Family Practice, 54,* 162–5.

Farnham-Diggory, S. (1992). *The learning-disabled child.* Cambridge, MA: Harvard University Press.

Farrington, D. P. (1995). The development of offending and antisocial behaviour from childhood: Key findings from the Cambridge study in delinquent development. *Journal of Child Psychology and Psychiatry, 36,* 929–64.

Farrington, D. P. and Hawkins, J. D. (1991). Predicting participation, early onset and later persistence in officially recorded offending. *Criminal Behavior and Mental Health, 1,* 1–33.

Fayyad, J. A., Farah, L., Cassir, Y., Salamoun, M. M. and Karam, E. G. (2010). Dissemination of an evidence-based intervention to parents of children with behavioral problems in a developing country. *European Child and Adolescent Psychiatry*, *19*, 629–36.

Feather, J. S. and Ronan, K. R. (2006). Trauma-focused cognitive-behavioural therapy for abused children with posttraumatic stress disorder: A pilot study. *New Zealand Journal of Psychology*, *35*, 132–45.

Federman, D. (2006). The biology of human sex differences. *New England Journal of Medicine*, *354*, 1507–14.

Fein, D. (2013). Optimal outcome in individuals with a history of autism. *Journal of Child Psychology and Psychiatry*, *54*, 195–205.

Feindler, E. L. (2006). *Anger related disorders: A practitioner's guide to comparative treatments*. New York: Spring Publishing.

Feingold, B. F. (1975a). Hyperkinesis and learning disabilities linked to artificial food flavours and colors. *American Journal of Nursing*, *75*, 797–803.

Feingold, B. F. (1975b). *Why Your Child is Hyperactive*. New York: Random House.

Feinstein, A. R. (1970). The pre-therapeutic classification of co-morbidity in chronic disease. *Journal of Chronic Diseases*, *23*, 455–68.

Ferdinand, R. F., Dieleman, G., Ormel, J. and Verhulst, F. C. (2007). Homotypic versus heterotypic continuity of anxiety symptoms in young adolescents: Evidence for distinctions between DSM-IV subtypes. *Journal of Abnormal Child Psychology*, *35*, 325–33.

Ferguson, C. J. (2010). Genetic contributions to antisocial personality and behavior: A meta-analytic review from an evolutionary perspective. *Journal of Social Psychology*, *150*, 160–80.

Ferguson, C. J. and Kilburn, J. (2010). Much ado about nothing: The misestimation and overinterpretation of violent video game effects in Eastern and Western nations: Comment on Anderson et al. (2010). *Psychological Bulletin*, *136*, 174–8.

Fergusson, D. M. and Horwood, L. J. (2002). Male and female offending trajectories. *Development and Psychopathology*, *14*, 159–77.

Fernando, S. (2005). Multicultural mental health services: Projects for minority ethnic communities in England. *Transcultural Psychiatry*, *42*, 420–36.

Feuerstein, R., Rand, Y. and Rynders, J. (1997). *Don't accept me as I am: Helping "retarded" people to excel*. Arlington Heights, IL: Skylight.

Fichter, M. M., Quadflieg, N., Georgopoulou, E., Xepapadakos, F. and Fthenakis, E. W. (2005). *International Journal of Eating Disorders*, *38*, 310–22.

Field, A. E., Camargo, C. A., Taylor, C. B., Berkey, C. S., Roberts, S. B. and Colditz, G. A. (2001). Peer, parent, and media influences of weight concerns and frequent dieting among preadolescent and adolescent girls and boys. *Pediatrics*, *107*, 54–60.

Field, T., Pickens, J., Fox, N. A., Nawrocki, T. and Gonzalez, J. (1995). Vagal tone in infants of depressed mothers. *Development and Psychopathology*, *7*, 227–31.

Field, T. M., Hossain, Z. and Malphurs, J. (1999). Depressed? Fathers' interactions with their infants. *Infant Mental Health Journal*, *20*, 322–32.

Fields, A. J. (2010). Multicultural research and practice: Theoretical issues and maximizing cultural exchange. *Professional Psychology: Research and Practice*, *4*, 196–201.

Findlay, L. C. and Coplan, R. J. (2008). Come out and play: Shyness in childhood and the benefits of organized sports participation. *Canadian Journal of Behavioural Science*, *40*, 153–61.

Fingeret, M. C., Warren, C. S., Cepeda-Benito, A. and Gleaves, D. H. (2006). Eating disorder prevention research: A meta-analysis. *Eating Disorders: The Journal of Treatment and Prevention*, *14*, 191–213.

Finn, S. (2007). *In our client's shoes: Theory and techniques of therapeutic assessment*. Mahwah, NJ: Lawrence Erlbaum.

Finkelhor, D., Mitchell, K. J. and Wolak, J. (2011). Second Youth Internet Safety Survey (YISS-2) [Dataset]. Available from National Data Archive on Child Abuse and Neglect. Retrieved from www.ndacan.cornell.edu

First, M. B. (2009). Harmonisation of ICD-11 and DSM-V: Opportunities and challenges. *British Journal of Psychiatry*, *195*, 382–90.

Firth, N., Greaves, D. and Frydenberg, E. (2010). Coping styles and strategies: A comparison of adolescent students with and without learning disabilities. *Journal of Learning Disabilities*, *43*, 77–85.

Fisher, J. O., Sinton, M. M. and Birch, L. L. (2009). Early parental influence and risk for the emergence of disordered eating. In L. Smolak and J. K. Thompson (Eds.), *Body image, eating disorders, and obesity in youth: Assessment, prevention, and treatment* (2nd edn., pp. 17–33). Washington, DC: American Psychological Association.

Fisher, M., Schneider, M., Burns, J., Symons, H. and Mandel, F. S. (2001). Differences between adolescents and young adults at presentation to an eating disorders program. *Journal of Adolescent Health*, *28*, 222–7.

FitzPatrick, J. F. and Bringmann, G. (1995). William Preyer and Charles Darwin. In S. Jaeger, I. Staeuble, L. Sprung and H.-P. Brauns, *Psychologie im soziokulturellenWandel – Kontinuitäten und Diskontinuitäten* (pp. 238–44). Frankfurt: Peter Lang.

Fivush, R., Pipe, M.-E., Murachver, T. and Reese, E. (1997). Events spoken and unspoken: Implications of language and memory development for the recovered memory debate. In M. Conway (Ed.), *False and recovered memories* (pp. 34–62). London: Oxford University Press.

Flannery, K. A., Liederman, J., Daly, L. and Schultz, J. (2000). Male prevalence for reading disability is found in large sample of black and white children free from ascertainment bias. *Journal of the International Neuropsychological Society, 6,* 433–42.

Flaskas, C. (1992). A reframe by any other name: On the process of reframing in strategic, Milan and analytic therapy. *Journal of Family Therapy, 14,* 145–61.

Flavell, J. (1976). Metacognitive aspects of problem-solving. In L. B. Resnick (Ed.), *The nature of intelligence* (pp. 231–6). Hillsdale, NJ: Erlbaum.

Fletcher, A., Bonell, C. and Hargreaves, J. (2008). School effects on young people's drug use: A systematic review of intervention and observational studies. *Journal of Adolescent Health, 42,* 209–20.

Fletcher, J. M. (2009a). Childhood mistreatment and adolescent and young adult depression. *Social Science and Medicine, 68,* 799–806.

Fletcher, J. M. (2009b). Dyslexia: The evolution of a scientific concept. *Journal of the International Neuropsychological Society, 15,* 501–8.

Fletcher, J. M., Lyon, G. R., Fuchs, L. S. and Barnes, M. A. (2007). *Learning disabilities: From identification to intervention.* New York: Guilford Press.

Flouri, E. (2008). Temperament influences on parenting and child psychopathology: Socio-economic disadvantage as moderator. *Child Psychiatry and Human Development, 39,* 369–79.

Flynn, C. P. (1998). To spank or not to spank: The effect of situation and age of child on support for corporal punishment. *Journal of Family Violence, 13,* 21–37.

Fombonne, E. (2005). The changing epidemiology of autism. *Journal of Applied Research in Intellectual Disabilities, 18,* 281–94.

Fombonne, E., Wostear, E., Cooper, V., Harrington, R. and Rutter, M. (2001a). The Maudsley long-term follow-up of child and adolescent depression: 1. Psychiatric outcomes in adulthood. *British Journal of Psychiatry, 179,* 201–17.

Fombonne, E., Wostear, E., Cooper. V. Harrington, R. and Rutter, M. (2001b). The Maudsley long-term follow-up of child and adolescent depression: 2. Suicidality, criminality and social dysfunction in adulthood. *British Journal of Psychiatry, 179,* 218–23.

Fombonne, E. and Zinck, S. (2008). Psychopharma-cological treatment of depression in children and adolescents. In J. R. Z. Abela and B. L. Hankin (Eds.) *Handbook of depression in children and adolescents* (pp. 207–23). New York: Guilford Press.

Forbes, E. E., Fox, N. A., Cohn, J. F., Galles, S. F. and Kovacs, M. (2006). Children's affect regulation during a disappointment: Psychophysiological responses and relation to parent history of depression. *Biological Psychology, 71,* 264–77.

Ford T., Goodman, R. and Meltze, H. (2003). The British Child and Adolescent Mental Health Survey 1999: The prevalence of DSM-IV disorders. *Journal of the American Academy of Child and Adolescent Psychiatry, 42,* 1203–11.

Fordham, K., and Stevenson-Hinde, J. (1999). Shyness, friendship quality, and adjustment during middle childhood. *Journal of Child Psychology and Psychiatry, 40,* 757–68.

Fordham, M. (1989). Some historical reflections. *The Journal of Analytical Psychology, 34,* 213–24.

Forehand, R., Middlebrook, J., Rogers, T. and Steffe, M. (1983). Dropping out of parent training. *Behaviour Research and Therapy, 21,* 663–8.

Forness, S. R. and Kavale, K. A. (1996). Treating social skill deficits in children with learning disabilities: A meta-analysis of the research. *Learning Disabilities Quarterly, 19,* 2–13.

Forrest, B. J. (2004). The utility of math difficulties, internalized psychopathology, and visual-spatial deficits to identify children with the nonverbal learning disability syndrome: Evidence for a visual-spatial disability. *Child Neuropsychology, 10,* 129–46.

Forsyth, R. J. (2004). Voices from the past: Feuerstein, R., Rand, Y., Hoffman, M. et al.: Cognitive modifiability in retarded adolescents: Effects of instrumental enrichment. *Pediatric Rehabilitation, 7,* 17–29.

Foschi, R. and Cicciola, E. (2006) Politics and naturalism in the 20th century psychology of Alfred Binet. *History of Psychology, 9,* 267–89.

Foster, E. M., Olchowski, A. E. and Webster-Stratton, C. H. (2007). Is stacking intervention components cost-effective? An analysis of the Incredible Years program. *Journal of the American Academy of Child and Adolescent Psychiatry, 46,* 1414–24.

Foster, H., Brooks-Gunn, J. and Martin, A. (2007). Poverty/socioeconomic status and exposure to violence in the lives of children and adolescents. In D. J. Flannery, A. T. Vazsonyi and I. D. Waldman (Eds.), *The Cambridge handbook of violent behavior and aggression* (pp. 664–87). New York: Cambridge University Press.

Foster, S. (1988). Cognitive and social-learning theories. In J. L. Matson (Ed.), *Handbook of treatment approaches in childhood psychopathology* (pp. 79–17). New York: Plenum.

Foucault, M. (2006). *The history of madness.* Abingdon: Routledge.

Fowles, D. C. (1988). Psychophysiology and psychopathology: A motivational approach. *Psychophysiology, 25,* 373–91.

Fox, N. A., Henderson, H. A., Marshall, P. J., Nichols, K. E. and Ghera, M. M. (2005). Behavioral inhibition: Linking biology and behavior within a developmental framework. *Annual Review of Psychology, 56,* 235–62.

Fraga, M. F., Ballestar, E., Paz, M. F., Ropero, S., Setien, F., Ballestar, M. L....Esteller, M. (2005). Epigenetic differences arise during the lifetime of monozygotic twins. *Proceedings of the National Academy of Sciences of the United States of America, 102,* 10604–9.

Frances, A. J. (1994). Preface. In J. Z. Sadler, O. P. Wiggins and M. A. Schwartz (Eds.), *Philosophical perspectives on psychiatric diagnosis and classification* (pp. i–iv). Baltimore: Johns Hopkins University Press.

Frankel, F., Myatt, R., Sugar, C., Whitham, C., Gorospe, C. M. and Laugeson, E. (2010). A randomized controlled study of parent-assisted children's friendship training with children having autism spectrum disorders. *Journal of Autism and Developmental Disorders, 40,* 827–42.

Fredricks, J. A. and Eccles, J. S. (2008). Participation in extracurricular activities in the middle school years: Are there developmental benefits for African American and European American youth? *Journal of Youth and Adolescence, 37,* 1029–43.

Fredrickson, B. L., and Roberts, T.-A. (1997). Objectification theory: Toward understanding women's lived experiences and mental health risks. *Psychology of Women Quarterly, 21,* 173–206.

The Free Dictionary, by Farlex (n.d.). Retrieved from www.thefreedictionary.com/

Freedman, J. L. (1984). Effect of television violence on aggressiveness. *Psychological Bulletin, 96,* 227–46.

Freeman, H. and Brown, B. B. (2001). Primary attachment to parents and peers during adolescence: Differences by attachment style. *Journal of Youth and Adolescence, 30,* 653–74.

Freeman, H., Newland, L. A. and Coyl, D. D. (2010). New directions in father attachment. *Early Child Development and Care, 180,* 1–8.

Freeman, S. and Kasari, C. (2013). Parent–child interactions in autism: Characteristics of play. *Autism, 17,* 147–61.

Freitag, C. M., Hanig, S., Palmason, H., Meyer, J., Wust, S. and Seitz, C. (2009). Cortisol awakening response in healthy children and children with ADHD: Impact of comorbid disorders and psychosocial risk factors. *Psychoneuroendocrinology, 34,* 1019–28.

French, D. C., Pidada, S. and Victor, A. (2005). Friendships of Indonesian and United States youth. *International Journal of Behavioral Development, 29,* 304–13.

French, V. (1977). History of the child's influence: Ancient Mediterranean civilizations. In R. Bell and L. Harper (Eds.), *Child effects on adults* (pp. 3–29). Hillsdale, NJ: Erlbaum.

Freud, A. and Burlingame, D. T. (1943). *War and children.* Oxford: Medical War Books.

Freud, S. (1951). Historical notes: A letter from Freud. *The American Journal of Psychiatry, 107,* 786–7.

Friars, P. and Mellor, D. (2009). Drop-out from parenting training programmes: A retrospective study. *Journal of Child and Adolescent Mental Health, 21,* 29–38.

Frick, P. J. and Dickens, C. (2006). Current perspectives on conduct disorder. *Current Psychiatry Reports, 8,* 59–72.

Frick, P. J., Barry, C. T. and Kamphaus, R. W. (2010). *Clinical assessment of child and adolescent personality and behavior.* New York: Springer Science and Business Media.

Friedman, N., Sadhu, J. and Jelinek, M. (2012). DSM5: Implications for pediatric mental health care. *Journal of Developmental and Behavioral Pediatrics, 35,* 163–77.

Frijda, N. H. (1994). Emotion and Adaptation – Lazarus, R. S. *Cognition and Emotion, 8,* 473–82.

Fristad, M. A. (2006). Psychoeducational treatment for school-aged children with bipolar disorder. *Development and Psychopathology, 18,* 1289–306.

Fristad, M. A., Verducci, J. S., Walters, K. and Young, M. E. (2009). Impact of multifamily psychoeducational psychotherapy in treating children aged 8 to 12 years with mood disorders. *Archives of General Psychiatry, 66,* 1013–21.

Frith, U. (2003). *Autism: Explaining the enigma.* Malden, MA: Blackwell Publishing.

Frodl, T., Reinhold, E., Koutsouleris, N., Donohoe, G., Bondy, B., Maximilian Reiser, M., Möller, H. J. and Meisenzahl, E. M. (2010). Childhood stress, serotonin transporter gene and brain structures in major depression. *Neuropsychopharmacology, 35,* 1383–90.

Fry, D. P. (1988). Intercommunity differences in aggression among Zapotec children. *Child Development, 59,* 1008–19.

Fryxell, D. and Kennedy, C. H. (1995). Placement along the continuum of services and its impact on students' social relationships. *Journal of the Association for Persons with Severe Handicaps, 20,* 259–69.

Fuchs, D. and Deshler, D. D. (2007). What we need to know about responsiveness to intervention (and shouldn't be afraid to ask). *Learning Disabilities Research and Practice, 22*, 129–36.

Fuller, T. (1992). Masked depression in maladaptive Black adolescents. *School Counselor, 40*, 24–31.

Furnham, A. and Gibbs, M. (1984). School children's attitudes towards the handicapped. *Journal of Adolescence, 7*, 99–117.

Furnham, A. and Malik, R. (1994). Cross-cultural beliefs about "depression." *International Journal of Social Psychiatry, 40*, 106–23.

Gadow, K. D., Nolan, E. E., Litcher, L., Carlson, G. A., Panina, N., Golovakha, E.,…Bromet, E. J. (2000). Comparison of attention-deficit/hyperactivity disorder symptoms subtypes in Ukrainian schoolchildren. *Journal of the American Academy of Child and Adolescent Psychiatry, 39*, 1520–27.

Gadow, K. D. and Nolan, E. E. (2002). Differences between preschool children with ODD, ADHD and ODD+ADHD symptoms. *Journal of Child Psychology and Psychiatry, 43*, 191–201.

Gaillard, W. D., Hertz-Pannier, L., Mott, S. H., Barnett, A. S., LeBihan, D. and Theodore, W. H. (2000). Functional anatomy of cognitive development: fMRI of verbal fluency in children and adults. *Neurology, 54*, 180–5.

Galloway, A. T., Fiorito, L. M., Francis, L. A. and Birch, L. L. (2006). "Finish your soup": Counterproductive effects of pressuring children to eat on intake and affect. *Appetite, 46*, 318–23.

Galway, T. M. and Metsala, J. L. (2011). Social cognition and its relation to psychosocial adjustment in children with nonverbal learning disabilities. *Journal of Learning Disabilities, 44*, 33–49.

Garb, H. N., Wood, J. M., Lilienfeld, S. O. and Nezworski, M. T. (2002). Effective use of projective techniques in clinical practice: Let the data help with selection and interpretation. *Professional Psychology: Research and Practice, 33*, 454–63.

Garavan, H., Ross, T. J., Murphy, K., Roche, R. A. and Stein, E. A. (2002). Dissociable executive functions in the dynamic control of behavior: Inhibition, error detection, and correction. *Neuroimage, 17*(4), 1820–9.

Garcia-Coll, C., Akerman, A. and Cicchetti, D. (2000). Cultural influences on developmental processes and outcomes: Implications for the study of development and psychopathology. *Development and Psychopathology, 12*, 333–56.

Gard, M. C. E. and Freeman, C. P. (1996). The dismantling of a myth: A review of eating disorders and socioeconomic status. *International Journal of Eating Disorders, 20*, 1–12.

Gardner, H. (1993) *Multiple intelligences: The theory in practice*. New York: Basic Books.

Gardener, H., Spiegelman, D. and Buka, S. L. (2009). Prenatal risk factors for autism: Comprehensive meta-analysis. *British Journal of Psychiatry, 195*, 7–14.

Gardner, M., Barajas, R. G. and Brooks-Gunn, J. (2010). Neighborhood influences on substance use etiology: Is where you live important? In L. Scheier (Ed.) *Handbook of drug use etiology: Theory, methods, and empirical findings* (pp. 423–41). Washington, DC: American Psychological Association.

Garmezy, N. (1991). Resilience and vulnerability to adverse developmental outcomes associated with poverty. *American Behavioral Scientist, 34*, 416–30.

Gazelle, H. and Ladd, G. W. (2003). Anxious solitude and peer exclusion: A diathesis-stress model of internalizing trajectories in childhood. *Child Development, 74*, 257–78.

Gazelle, H. and Druhen, M. J. (2009). Anxious solitude and peer exclusion predict social helplessness, upset affect, and vagal regulation in response to behavioral rejection by a friend. *Developmental Psychology, 45*, 1077–96.

Gazelle, H., Workman, J. O. and Allan, W. (2010). Anxious solitude and clinical disorder in middle childhood: Bridging developmental and clinical approaches to childhood social anxiety. *Journal of Abnormal Child Psychology, 38*, 1–17.

Geary, D. (1998). *Male, female: The evolution of human sex differences*. Washington, DC: APA Press.

Gelfand, D. M. and Peterson, L. (1985). *Child development and psychopathology*. Beverly Hills, CA: Sage.

Gelhorn, H. L., Stallings, M. C., Young, S. E., Corley, R. P., Rhee, S. H. and Hewitt, J. K. (2005). Genetic and environmental influences on conduct disorder: Symptom, domain and full-scale analyses. *Journal of Child Psychology and Psychiatry, 46*, 580–91.

Geller, B. et al. (2000). Psychosocial functioning in a prepubertal and early adolescent bipolar disorder phenotype. *Journal of the American Academy of Child and Adolescent Psychiatry, 39*, 1543–8.

Gelso, C. and Fretz, B. (2001). *Counseling psychology*. Fort Worth: Harcourt College Publishers.

Gentzler, A. L., Santucci, A. K., Kovacs, M. and Fox, N. A. (2009). Respiratory sinus arrhythmia reactivity predicts emotion regulation and depressive symptoms in at-risk and control children. *Biological Psychology, 82*, 156–63.

Georgaca, E. (2013). Social constructionist contributions to critiques of psychiatric diagnosis and classification. *Feminism and Psychology, 23*, 56–62.

George, J. B. E. and Franko, D. L. (2010). Cultural issues in eating pathology and body image among children and adolescents. *Journal of Pediatric Psychology, 35*, 231–42.

Gershoff, E. T. (2002). Corporal punishment by parents and associated child behaviours and experiences: A meta-analytic and theoretical review. *Psychological Bulletin, 128*, 539–79.

Geurts, C. M., Linsen, C. M., ten Brink, P. W. and van Lieshout, C. F. (1987). Socio-emotional relations of adolescents in special education assessed by teachers and peers. *Pedagogische Studien, 64*, 104–14.

Ghaziuddin, M. (2010). Brief report: Should the DSM-V drop Asperger syndrome? *Journal of Autism and Developmental Disorders, 40*, 1146–8.

Ghaziuddin, N., King, C. A., Welch, K. B., Zaccagnini, J., Weidmer-Mikhail, E., Mellow, A. M., Ghaziuddin, M. and Greden, J. F. (2000). Serotonin dysregulation in adolescents with major depression: Hormone response to meta-chlorophenylpiperazine (mCPP) infusion. *Psychiatry Research, 96*, 183–94.

Gheyara, S., Klump, K. L., McGue, M., Iacono, W. G. and Burt, S. A. (2011). The death(s) of close friends and family moderate genetic influences on symptoms of major depressive disorder in adolescents. *Psychological Medicine, 41*, 721–9.

Gibbons, F. X., Pomery, E. A. and Gerrard, M. (2008). Cognitive social influence: Moderation, mediation, modification, and the media. In M. J. Prinstein and K. A. Dodge (Eds.), *Understanding peer influence in children and adolescents* (pp. 45–71). New York: Guilford Press.

Gibson, B. S., Gondoll, D. M., Johnson, A. C., Steeger, C. M., Dobrzenski, B. A., Morrissey, R. A. (2011). Component analysis of verbal versus spatial working memory training in adolescents with ADHD: A randomized, controlled trial. *Child Neuropsychology, 17*, 546–63.

Gibson, E. L., Checkley, S., Papadopoulos, A., Poon, L., Daley, S. and Wardle, J. (1999). Increased salivary cortisol reliably induced by a protein-rich midday meal. *Psychosomatic Medicine, 61*, 214–24.

Giedd, J. N. and Rapoport, J. L. (2010). Structural MRI of pediatric brain development: What have we learned and where are we going? *Neuron, 67*, 728–34.

Gillberg, C. (2003). Deficits in attention, motor control, and perception: A brief review. *Archives of Disease in Childhood, 88*, 904–10.

Gillis, H. D., Gass, M. A. and Russell, K. C. (2008). The effectiveness of project adventure's behaviour management programs for male offenders in residential treatment. *Residential Treatment for Children and Youth, 25*, 227–47.

Ginsburg, G. S. and Silverman, W. K. (1996). Phobic and anxiety disorders in Hispanic and Caucasian youth. *Journal of Anxiety Disorders, 10*, 517–28.

Ginsburg, G. S. and Kingery, J. N. (2007). Evidence-based practice for childhood anxiety disorders. *Journal of Contemporary Psychotherapy, 37*, 123–32.

Glaser, B., Shelton, K. H. and van den Bree, M. (2010). The moderating role of close friends in the relationship between conduct problems and adolescent substance use. *Journal of Adolescent Health, 47*, 35–42.

Glassberg, L. A., Hooper, S. R. and Mattison, R. E. (1999). Prevalence of learning disabilities at enrolment in special education students with behavioral disorders. *Behavioral Disorders, 25*, 9–21.

Gleaves, D. H., Latner, J. D. and Ambwani, S. (2009). Eating disorders. In J. L. Matson, F. Andrasik and M. L. Matson (Eds.), *Treating childhood psychopathology and developmental disabilities* (pp. 403–34). New York: Spring Science and Business Media.

Godlee, F., Smith, J. and Marcovitch, H. (2011). Wakefield's article linking MMR vaccine and autism was fraudulent. *British Medical Journal, 342*, c7452.

Goldberg, D., Kendler, K. S., Sirovatka, P. J. and Regier, D. A. (2010). *Diagnostic issues in depression and generalized anxiety disorder: Refining the research agenda for DSM-V*. Washington, DC: American Psychiatric Association.

Goldman-Rakic, P. S. (1996). The prefrontal landscape: Implications of functional architecture for understanding human mentation and the central executive. *Philosophical Transactions of the Royal Society B: Biological Sciences, 351*(1346), 1445–53.

Goldsmith, H. H. and Davidson, R. J. (2004). Disambiguating the components of emotion regulation. *Child Development, 75*, 361–5.

Goldstein, A. P., Glick, B. and Gibbs, J. C. (1998). *Replacement training: A comprehensive intervention for aggressive youth* (3rd edn.). Champaign, IL: Research Press.

Goldstein, J. (1987). *Console and classify: The French psychiatric profession in the nineteenth century*. Cambridge: Cambridge University Press.

Goldstein, R. B., Olfson, M., Wickramaratne, P. and Wolk, S. I. (2006). Use of outpatient mental health services by depressed and anxious children as they grow up. *Psychiatric Services, 57*, 966–75.

Goldstein, S. and Schwebach, A. (2009). Neuropsychological basis of learning disabilities. In C. R. Reynolds and E. Fletcher-Janzen (Eds.), *Handbook of clinical child neuropsychology* (3rd edn., pp. 187–202). New York: Springer Science and Business Media.

Goldstein, T. R., et al. (2009). Psychosocial functioning among bipolar youth. *Journal of Affective Disorders, 114*, 174–83.

Gomez, R., Burns, G. L. and Walsh, J. A. (2008). Parent ratings of the oppositional defiant disorder symptoms:

Item response theory analyses of cross-national and cross-racial invariance. *Journal of Psychopathology and Behavioral Assessment, 30*, 10–19.

Gonda, X., Fountoulakis, K. N., Harro, J., Pompili, M., Akiskal, H. S., Bagdy, G. and Rihmer, Z. (2011). The possible contributory role of the S allele of 5-HTTLPR in the emergence of suicidality. *Journal of Psychopharmacology, 25*, 857–66.

Gonzales, N. and Dodge, K. A. (2009). Family and peer influences on adolescent behavior and risk-taking. Paper presented at IOM Committee on the Science of Adolescence Workshop, Washington, DC. Retrieved from http://iom.edu/~/media/Files/Activity%20Files/Children/AdolescenceWS/Commissioned%20Papers/dodge_gonzales_paper.pdf

Goodlin-Jones, B. L., Waters, S. and Anders, T. F. (2009). Objective sleep measurement in typically and atypically developing preschool children with ADHD-like profiles. *Child Psychiatry and Human Development, 40*, 257–68.

Goodman, R., Slobodskaya, H. and Knyazev, G. (2005) Russian child mental health – a cross-sectional study of prevalence and risk factors. *European Child and Adolescent Psychiatry, 14*(1), 28–33.

Goodman, S. H. and Gotlib, I. (1999). Risk for psychopathology in the children of depressed mothers: A developmental model for understanding the mechanisms of transmission. *Psychological Review, 106*, 458–90.

Goodman, S. H. and Tully, E. (2008). Children of depressed mothers. In J. R. Z. Abela and B. L. Hankin (Eds.). *Handbook of depression in children* (pp. 415–40). New York: Guilford Press.

Goodyer, I. M. (2008). Emanuel Miller lecture: Early onset depressions – meanings, mechanisms and processes. *Journal of Child Psychology and Psychiatry, 49*, 1239–56.

Goodyer, I. M., Herbert, J. and Tamplin, A. (2003). Psychoendocrine antecedents of persistent first-episode major depression in adolescents: A community-based longitudinal enquiry. *Psychological Medicine, 33*, 601–10.

Gordis, E. B., Feres, N., Olezeski, C. L., Rabkin, A. N. and Trickett, P. K. (2010). Skin conductance reactivity and respiratory sinus arrhythmia among maltreated and comparison youth: Relations with aggressive behavior. *Journal of Pediatric Psychology, 35*, 547–58.

Gordon, M., Antshel, K., Faraone, S. V., Barkley, R., Lewandowski, I., Hudziak, J,…Cunningham, C. (2005). Symptoms versus impairment: The case for respecting DSM-IV's criterion D. *ADHD Report, 13*, 1–9.

Gordon, R. S. (1983). An operational classification of disease prevention. *Public Health Reports, 98*, 107–9.

Gottesman, I. I. and Gould, T. D. (2003). The endophenotype concept in psychiatry: Etymology and strategic intentions. *American Journal of Psychiatry, 160*, 636–45.

Gottlieb, J. S. and Howell, R. W. (1957). The concepts of "prevention" and "creative development" as applied to mental health. In R. H. Ojemann (Ed.), *Four basic aspects of preventive psychiatry: Report of the first institute on preventive psychiatry*. Iowa City, IA: State University of Iowa Department of Publications.

Gould, S. J. (1981). *The mismeasure of man*. New York: Norton and Co.

Gowers, S., Claxton, M., Rowlands, L., Inbasagaran, A., Wood, D., Yi, I.,…Ayton, A. (2010). Drug prescribing in child and adolescent eating disorder services. *Child and Adolescent Mental Health, 15*, 18–22.

Grand, N. (Ed.). (2008). *A comprehensive dictionary of biology*. Chandigarh, India: Abhishek Publications.

Granger, D. A., Weisz, J. R., McCracken, J. T., Kauneckis, D. and Ikeda, S. (1994). Testosterone and conduct problems. *Journal of the American Academy of Child and Adolescent Psychiatry, 33*, 908.

Granger, D. A., Weisz, J. R., McCracken, J. T., Ikeda, S. C. and Douglas, P. (1996). Reciprocal influences among adrenocortical activation, psychosocial processes, and the behavioral adjustment of clinic-referred children. *Child Development, 67*, 3250–62.

Granic, I. and Dishion, T. J. (2003). Deviant talk in adolescent friendships: A step toward measuring a pathogenic attractor process. *Social Development, 12*, 314–34.

Grasso, D. J., Joselow, B., Marquez, Y. and Webb, C. (2011). Trauma-focused cognitive behavioral therapy of a child with posttraumatic stress disorder. *Psychotherapy, 48*, 188–97.

Gray, J. A. (1970). The psychophysiological basis of introversion–extraversion. *Behavior Research and Therapy, 8*, 249–66.

Gray, J. A. (1982). *The neuropsychology of anxiety: An enquiry into the functions of the septohippocampal system*. Oxford: Oxford University Press.

Gray, J. A. and McNaughton, N. (1996). The neuropsychology of anxiety: reprise. *Nebraska Symposium on Motivation, 43*, 61–134.

Gray, K. M. and Tonge, B. J. (2001). Are there early features of autism in infants and preschool children? *Journal of Paediatrics and Child Health, 37*, 221–6.

Gray, S. E. O., Carter, A. S. and Levitt, H. (2012). A critical review of assumptions about gender variant children in psychological research. *Journal of Gay and Lesbian Mental Health, 16*, 4–30.

Graziano, A. M. (Ed.) (1975). *Behavior therapy with children II*. Chicago: Aldine.

Greaves-Lord, K., Ferdinand, R. F., Sondeijker, F. E. P. L., Dietrich, A., Oldehinkel, A. J., Rosmalen, J. G. M., et al. (2007). Testing the tripartite model in young adolescents: Is hyperarousal specific for anxiety and not depression? *Journal of Affective Disorders, 102,* 55–63.

Greaves-Lord, K., Huizink, A. C., Oldehinkel, A. J., Ormel, J., Verhulst, F. C. and Ferdinand, R. F. (2009). Baseline cortisol measures and developmental pathways of anxiety in early adolescence. *Acta Psychiatrica Scandinavica, 120,* 178–86.

Greco, L. A. and Morris, T. L. (2002). Paternal child-rearing style and child social anxiety: Investigation of child perceptions and actual father behavior. *Journal of Psychopathology and Behavioral Assessment, 24,* 259–67.

Greco, L. A. and Morris, T. L. (2005). Factors influencing the link between social anxiety and peer acceptance: Contributions of social skills and close friendships during middle childhood. *Behavior Therapy, 36,* 197–205.

Green, B. L., Grace, M. C., Vary, M. G., Kramer, T. L., Gleser, G. C. and Leonard, A. C. (1994). Children of disaster in the second decade: A 17-year follow-up of Buffalo Creek survivors. *Journal of the American Academy of Child and Adolescent Psychiatry, 33,* 71–9.

Green, G. H. (1922). *Psychoanalysis in the classroom.* New York: Putnam.

Green, G. H. (1947) The psychological significance of some children's comic papers. *Egyptian Journal of Psychology, 3,* 303–38.

Green, J., Charman, T., McConachie, H., Aldred, C., Slonims, V., Howlin, V.,…Pickles, A. (2010). Parent-mediated communication-focused treatment in children with autism (PACT): A randomised controlled trial. The *Lancet, 375,* 2152–60.

Green, R. (1976). One-hundred ten feminine and masculine boys: Behavioral contrasts and demographic similarities. *Archives of Sexual Behavior, 5,* 425–46.

Green, R. (1987). *The sissy boy syndrome: The developmental of homosexuality.* New Haven, CT: Yale University Press.

Green, R. (2009). Darwinian theory, functionalism, and the first American psychological revolution. *American Psychologist, 64,* 75–83.

Green, S. E. (2004). Attitudes toward control in uncontrollable situations: The multidimensional impact of health locus of control on the well-being of mothers of children with disabilities. *Sociological Inquiry, 74,* 20–49.

Greenberg, M. T. (1999). Attachment and psychopathology in childhood. In J. Cassidy and P. R. Shaver (Eds.), *Handbook of attachment: Theory, research, and clinical applications.* New York: Guilford Press.

Greenberg, M. T., Speltz, M. L., DeKlyen, M. and Jones, K. (2001). Correlates of clinic referral for early conduct problems: Variable- and person-oriented approaches. *Development and Psychopathology, 13,* 255–76.

Greenberg, M. T., Riggs, N. R. and Blair, C. (2007). The role of preventive interventions in enhancing neurocognitive functioning and promoting competence in adolescence. In D. Romer and E. E. Walker (Eds.), *Adolescent psychopathology and the developing brain: Integrating brain and prevention science*: Oxford: Oxford University Press.

Greene, R. W., Biederman, J., Faraone, S. V., Monuteaux, M. C., Mick, E., DuPre, E. P.,…Goring, J. G. (2001). Social impairment in girls with ADHD: Patterns, gender comparisons, and correlates. *Journal of the American Academy of Child and Adolescent Psychiatry, 40,* 704–10.

Greenman, P. S., Schneider, B. H. and Tomada, G. (2009). Stability and change in patterns of peer rejection: Implications for children's academic performance over time. *School Psychology International, 30,* 163–83.

Greenwood, M. (1948). *Medical statistics from Graunt to Farr.* Cambridge: Cambridge University Press.

Gresham, F. M. (1995). Best practices in social skills training. In A. Thomas, and J. Grimes (Eds.), *Best practices in school psychology* (pp. 1021–30). Washington, DC: NASP.

Gresham, F. M. (1997). Social competence and student with behavior disorders: Where we've been, where we are, and where we should go. *Education and Treatment of Children, 20,* 233–49.

Gresham, F. M. and Elliott, S. N. (1989). Social skills deficits as a primary learning disability. *Journal of Learning Disabilities, 22,* 120–4.

Gresham, F. M., MacMillan, D. L., Bocian, K. M., Ward, S. L. and Forness, S. R. (1998). Comorbidity of hyperactivity-impulsivity-inattention and conduct problems: Risk factors in social, affective, and academic domains. *Journal of Abnormal Child Psychology, 26,* 393–406.

Gresham, F. M., Cook, C. R., Crews, S. D. and Kern, L. (2004). Social skills training for children and youth with emotional and behavioral disorders: Validity considerations and future directions. *Behavioral Disorders, 30,* 32–46.

Gresham, F. M. and Vellutino, F. R. (2010). What is the role of intelligence in the identification of specific learning disabilities? Issues and clarifications. *Learning Disabilities Research and Practice, 25,* 194–206.

Griffin, D. and Steen, S. (2010). School–family–community partnerships: Applying Epstein's theory of the six types of involvement to school counselor practice. *Professional School Counseling, 13,* 218–26.

Griffiths, P. J. and Hutter, R. (2005). *Reason and the reasons of faith.* Edinburgh: T&T Clark.

Groesz, L. M., Levine, M. P. and Murnen, S. K. (2002). The effect of experimental presentation of thin media images on body satisfaction: A meta-analytic review. *International Journal of Eating Disorders*, *31*, 1–16.

Gross, D., Fogg, L. and Conrad, B. (1993). Designing interventions in psychosocial research. *Archives of Psychiatric Nursing*, *7*, 259–64.

Gross, E. F. (2004). Adolescent internet use: What we expect, what teens report. *Journal of Applied Developmental Psychology*, *25*, 633–49.

Grove, W. M. et al. (1990). Heritability of substance abuse and antisocial behavior: A study of monozygotic twins reared apart. *Biological Psychiatry*, *27*(12), 1293–304.

Grusec, J. E. and Lytton, H. (1988). *Social development: History, theory, and research.* New York: Springer-Verlag Publishing.

Grusec, J. E. and Goodnow, J. J. (1994). Impact of parental discipline methods on the child's internalization of values: A reconceptualization of current points of view. *Developmental Psychology*, *30*, 4–19.

Guillec, G. (2000). Comment écrire l'histoire de la psychologie? Réflections à propos du débat idéologique sur les "enfants abnormaux" en France. [How should the history of psychology be written? Reflections about the ideological debate about "abnormal children" in France]. *Canadian Psychology*, *41*, 94–103.

Gump, B. B. and Matthews, K. A. (1999). Do background stressors influence reactivity to and recovery from acute stressors? *Journal of Applied Social Psychology*, *29*, 469–94.

Gunnar, M. R. (2001). The role of glucocorticoids in anxiety disorders: A critical analysis. In M. W. Vasey and M. R. Dadds (Eds.), *The developmental psychopathology of anxiety* (pp. 143–59). New York: Oxford University Press.

Gunnar, M. R. and Talge, N. M. (2006). Neuroendocrine measures in developmental research. In L. A. Schmidt and S. J. Segalowitz (Eds.), *Developmental psychophysiology: Theory, systems, and methods* (pp. 343–66). New York: Cambridge University Press.

Gunnar, M. R. and Quevedo, K. (2007). The neurobiology of stress and development. *Annual Review of Psychology*, *58*, 145–73.

Gunnar, M. R., Talge, N. M. and Herrera, A. (2009). Stressor paradigms in developmental studies: What does and does not work to produce mean increases in salivary cortisol. *Psychoneuroendocrinology*, *34*, 953–67.

Gunnar, M. R., Kryzer, E., van Ryzin, M. J. and Phillips, D. A. (2010). The rise in cortisol in family day care: Associations with aspects of care quality, child behavior, and child sex. *Child Development*, *81*, 851–69.

Gunnar, M. R. and Adam, E. K. (2012). The hypothalamic-pituitary-adrenocortical system and emotion: Current

wisdom and future directions. *Monographs of the Society for Research in Child Development*, *77*, 109–19.

Guralnick, M. J. and Groom, J. M. (1987). The peer relations of mildly delayed and nonhandicapped preschool children in mainstreamed playgroups. *Child Development*, *58*, 1556–72.

Gurguis, G. N. M., Meadorwoodruff, J. H., Haskett, R. F. and Greden, J. F. (1990). Multiplicity of depressive episodes – Phenomenological and neuroendocrine correlates. *Biological Psychiatry*, *27*, 1156–64.

Gutierrez-Maldonado, J., Magallon-Neri, E., Rus-Calafell, M. and Penaloza-Salazar, C. (2009). Virtual reality exposure therapy for school phobia. *Anuario de Psicologia*, *40*, 223–36.

Guyer, A. E., Lau, J. Y., McClure-Tone, E. B., Parrish, J., Shiffrin, N. D., Reynolds, R. C. et al. (2008). Amygdala and ventrolateral prefrontal cortex function during anticipated peer evaluation in pediatric social anxiety. *Archives of General Psychiatry*, *65*, 1303–12.

Guyer, A. E., McClure-Tone, E. B., Shiffrin, N. D., Pine, D. S. and Nelson, E. E. (2009). Probing the neural correlates of anticipated peer evaluation in adolescence. *Child Development*, *80*, 1000–15.

Guyer, A. E., Choate, V. R., Pine, D. S. and Nelson, E. E. (2012). Neural circuitry underlying affective response to peer feedback in adolescence. *Social Cognitive and Affective Neuroscience*, *7*, 81–92.

Haas, M., Karcher, K. and Pandina, G. J. (2008). Treating disruptive behaviour disorders with risperidone: A 1-year, open-label safety study in children and adolescents. *Journal of Child and Adolescent Psychopharmacology*, *18*, 337–46.

Hage, S. M., Romano, J. L., Conyne, R. K., Kenny, M., Matthews, C., Schwartz, J. P. and Waldo, M. (2007). Best practice guidelines on prevention practice, research, training, and social advocacy for psychologists. *The Counseling Psychologist*, *35*, 493–566.

Hage, S. and Romano, J. (2010). History of prevention and prevention groups: Legacy for the 21st century. *Ground Dynamics: Theory, Research and Practice*, *14*, 199–210.

Hagerman, R. J. and Hagerman, P. J. (2002). *Fragile X syndrome: Diagnosis, treatment, and research.* Baltimore, MD: Johns Hopkins University Press.

Hains, A. A. and Ellmann, S. W. (1994). Stress inoculation training as a preventative intervention for high school youths. *Journal of Cognitive Psychotherapy*, *8*, 219–232.

Haley, J. (1973). *Uncommon therapy: The psychiatric techniques of Milton Erikson, M.D.* New York: Norton.

Halit, H., de Haam, M. and Johnson, M. H. (2003). Cortical specialization for face processing: Face-sensitive event-related potential components in 3- and 12-month-old infants. *Neuroimage*, *19*, 1180–93.

Halligan, S. L., Herbert, J., Goodyer, I. M. and Murray, L. (2004). Exposure to postnatal depression predicts elevated cortisol in adolescent offspring. *Biological Psychiatry*, *55*, 376–81.

Hallowell, A. I. (1934). Culture and mental disorder. *The Journal of Abnormal and Social Psychology*, *29*, 1–9.

Halverson, C. F., Havill, V. L., Deal, J., Baker, S. R., Victor, J. B., Pavlopoulous, V., Besevegis, E. and Wen, L. (2003). Personality structure as derived from parental ratings of free descriptions of children: The inventory of child individual differences. *Journal of Personality*, *71*, 995–1026.

Hammond, C. (2009). The pseudo-patient study. In *Mind Changers* (series 4) [radio show]. BBC Radio 4. Retrieved from www.bbc.co.uk/programmes/b00lny48

Hampton, T. (2004). Suicide caution stamped on antidepressants. *Journal of the American Medical Association*, *291*, 2060–1.

Handler, M. W. and DuPaul, G. J. (2005). Assessment of ADHD: Differences across psychology specialty areas. *Journal of Attention Disorders*, *9*, 402–12.

Hankin, B. L. and Abela, J. R. Z. (2005). *Development of psychopathology: A vulnerability-stress perspective*. Thousand Oaks, CA: Sage Publications.

Hankin, B. L., Wetter, E. and Cheely, C. (2008). Sex differences in child and adolescent depression: A developmental psychopathological approach. In J. R. Z. Abela and B. L. Hankin (Eds.) *Handbook of depression in children and adolescents* (pp. 35–78). New York: Guilford Press.

Hare, T. A., Tottenham, N., Davidson, M. C., Glover, G. H. and Casey, B. J. (2005). Contributions of amygdala and striatal activity in emotion regulation. *Biological Psychiatry*, *57*, 624–32.

Haring, T. (1991). Social relationships. In L. H. Meyer, C. A. Peck and L. Brown (Eds.), *Critical issues in the lives of people with severe disabilities* (pp. 195–217). Baltimore, MD: Brookes.

Harkness, K. L., Bruce, A. E. and Lumley, M. N. (2006). The role of childhood abuse and neglect in the sensitization to stressful life events in adolescent depression. *American Journal of Abnormal Psychology*, *115*, 730–41.

Harmon, H., Langley, A. and Ginsburg, G. S. (2006). The role of gender and culture in treating youth with anxiety disorders. *Journal of Cognitive Psychotherapy*, *20*, 301–10.

Harold, G., Shelton, K., Goeke-Morey, M. and Cummings, E. (2004). Marital conflict, child emotional security about family relationships, and child adjustment. *Social Development*, *13*, 350–76.

Harper, J. and Kelly, E. M. (1985). Anti social behaviour as a mask for depression in year 5 and 6 boys. *Mental Health in Australia*, *1*, 14–19.

Harrington, R., Bredenkamp, D., Groothues, C. and Rutter, M., et al. (1994). Adult outcomes of childhood and adolescent depression: III. Links with suicidal behaviours. *Journal of Child Psychology and Psychiatry*, *35*, 1309–19.

Harris, J. R. (1995). Where is the child's environment? A group socialization theory of development. *Psychological Review*, *102*, 458–89.

Harris, J. R. (1998). *The nurture assumption: Why children turn out the way they do*. New York: Free Press.

Hart, E. L., Lahey, B. B., Loeber, R., Applegate, B., Green, S. M. and Frick, P. J. (1995). Developmental change in attention-deficit hyperactivity disorder in boys: A four-year longitudinal study. *Journal of Abnormal Child Psychology*, *23*, 729–49.

Hart, N., Grand, N. and Riley, K. (2006). Making the grade: The gender gap, ADHD and the medicalization of boyhood. In D. Rosenfeld and C. Faircloth (Eds.), *Medicalized masculinities*. Philadelphia, PA: Temple University Press.

Hartman, C. A., Hox, J., Mellenberg, G. J., Boyle, M. H., Offord, D. R., Racine, Y.,…Sergeant, J. A. (2001). DSM-IV internal construct validity: When a taxonomy meets data. *Journal of Child Psychology and Psychiatry*, *42*, 817–36.

Harvey, E. A., Youngwirth, S. D., Thakar, D. A. and Errazuriz, P. A. (2009). Predicting attention-deficit/ hyperactivity disorder and oppositional defiant disorder from preschool diagnostic assessments. *Journal of Consulting and Clinical Psychology*, *77*, 349–54.

Harvey, N. A. (1918). *Imaginary companions and other mental phenomena of children*. Ypsilanti, MI: State Normal College.

Harvey, S. T. and Taylor, J. E. (2010). A meta-analysis of the effects of psychotherapy with sexually abused children and adolescents. *Clinical Psychology Review*, *30*, 517–35.

Haselager, G. J. T., Hartup, W. W., van Lieshout, C. F. M. and Riksen-Walraven, J. M. A. (1998). Similarities between friends and nonfriends in middle childhood. *Child Development*, *69*, 1198–208.

Hastings, P. D., Nuselovici, J. N., Utendale, W. T., Coutya, J., McShane, K. E. and Sullivan, C. (2008). Applying the polyvagal theory to children's emotion regulation: Social context, socialization, and adjustment. *Biological Psychology*, *79*, 299–306.

Hastings, P. D., Sullivan, C., McShane, K. E., Coplan, R. J., Utendale, W. T. and Vyncke, J. D. (2008). Parental socialization, vagal regulation, and preschoolers' anxious difficulties: Direct mothers and moderated fathers. *Child Development*, *79*, 45–64.

Hastings, P. D., Fortier, I., Utendale, W. T., Simard, L. R. and Robaey, P. (2009). Adrenocortical functioning in boys with Attention-Deficit/Hyperactivity Disorder: Examining subtypes of ADHD and associated comorbid conditions. *Journal of Abnormal Child Psychology, 37,* 565–78.

Hastings, P. D., Ruttle, P., Serbin, L. A., Mills, R. S. L., Stack, D. M. and Schwartzman, A. E. (2011). Adrenocortical stress reactivity and regulation in preschoolers: Relations with parenting, temperament, and psychopathology. *Developmental Psychobiology, 53,* 694–710.

Hastings, P. D., Buss, K. A. and Dennis, T. A. (2012) Socialization and environmental factors in the physiology of emotion. *Monographs of the Society for Research in Child Development, 77,* 39–41.

Hastings, R. P. and Beck, A. (2004). Practitioner review: Stress intervention for parents of children with intellectual disabilities. *Journal of Child Psychology and Psychiatry, 45,* 1338–49.

Hathaway, W. L., Scott, S. Y. and Garver, S. A. (2004). Assessing religious/spiritual functioning: A neglected domain in clinical practice? *Professional Psychology: Research and Practice, 35,* 97–104.

Hattie, J., Marsh, H. W., Neill, J. T. and Richards, G. E. (1997). Adventure education and outward bound: Out-of-class experiences that make a lasting difference. *Review of Educational Research, 67,* 43–87.

Hatzinger, M., Brand, S., Perren, S., von Wyl, A., von Klitzing, K. and Holsboer-Trachsler, E. (2007). Hypothalamic-pituitary-adrenocortical (HPA) activity in kindergarten children: Importance of gender and associations with behavioral/emotional difficulties. *Journal of Psychiatric Research, 41,* 861–70.

Hauch, E. F. (1946). *Gottfried Keller as a democratic idealist.* New York: Columbia University Press.

Hawker, D. S. J. and Boulton, M. J. (2000). Twenty years' research on peer victimization and psychosocial maladjustment: A meta-analytic review of cross-sectional studies. *Journal of Child Psychology and Psychiatry, 41,* 441–55.

Hawkins, D. F. and Kempf-Leonard, K. (2005). *Our children, their children: Confronting racial and ethnic differences in American juvenile justice.* Chicago, IL: University of Chicago Press.

Hay, T. and Jones, L. (1994). Societal interventions to prevent child abuse and neglect. *Child Welfare: Journal of Policy, Practice, and Program, 73,* 379–403.

Hayatbakhsh, M. R., McGee, T. R., Bor, W., Najman, J. M. et al. (2008). Child and adolescent externalizing behavior and cannabis use disorders in early adulthood: An Australian prospective birth cohort study. *Addictive Behaviors, 33,* 422–38.

Haynes, S. N. and Yoshioka, D. T. (2007). Clinical assessment applications of ambulatory biosensors. *Psychological Assessment, 19,* 44–57.

Hazen, N. L., McFarland, L., Jacobvitz, D. and Boyd-Soisson, E. (2010). Fathers' frightening behaviours and sensitivity with infants: Relations with fathers' attachment representations, father–infant attachment, and children's later outcomes. *Early Child Development and Care, 180,* 51–69.

Healey, D. M., Miller, C. J., Castelli, K. L., Marks, D. J. and Halperin, J. M. (2008). The impact of impairment criteria on rates of ADHD diagnoses in preschoolers. *Journal of Abnormal Child Psychology, 36,* 771–8.

Heatherton, T. F. and Baumeister, R. F. (1991). Binge eating as escape from self-awareness. *Psychological Bulletin, 110,* 86–108.

Hecht, D. B., Inderbitzen, H. M. and Bukowski, A. L. (1998). The relationship between peer status and depressive symptoms in children and adolescents. *Journal of Abnormal Child Psychology, 26,* 153–60.

Heiman, T. and Berger, O. (2008). Parents of children with Asperger syndrome or with learning disabilities: Family environment and social support. *Research in Developmental Disabilities, 29,* 289–300.

Heiman, T., Zinck, L. C. and Heath, N. L. (2008). Parents and youth with learning disabilities: Perceptions of relationships and communication. *Journal of Learning Disabilities, 41,* 524–34.

Hein, L. C. and Berger, K. C. (2013). Gender dysphoria in children: Let's think this through. *Journal of Child and Adolescent Psychiatric Nursing, 25,* 237–40.

Heinrichs, N., Rapee, R. M., Alden, L. A., Bögels, S., Hofmann, S. G., Oh, K. J. and Sakano, Y. (2006). Cultural differences in perceived social norms and social anxiety. *Behaviour Research and Therapy, 44,* 1187–197.

Heitmann, D., Schmuhl, M., Reinisch, A. and Bauer, U. (2012). Primary prevention for children of mentally ill parents: The Kanu-program. *Journal of Public Health, 20,* 125–30.

Hektner, J. M., Schmidt, J. A. and Csikszentmihalyi, M. (2007). *Experience sampling method: Measuring the quality of everyday life.* Thousand Oaks, CA: Sage Publications.

Helt, M., Kelley, E., Kinsbourne, M., Pandey, J., Boorstein, H., Herbert, M. and Fein, D. (2008). Can children with autism recover? If so, how? *Neuropsychology Review, 18,* 339–66.

Helzer, J. E., Wittchen, H., Krueger, R. F., Kraemer, H. C. (2008). Dimensional options for DSM-V: The way forward. In J. E. Helzer, H. C. Kraemer, R. F. Krueger, H. Wittchen, P. J. Sirovatka and D. A. Regier (Eds.),

Dimensional approaches in diagnostic classification: Refining the research agenda for DSM-V (pp. 115–27). Washington, DC: American Psychiatric Association.

Hendggeler, S. W., Melton, G. B., Brondino, M. J., Scherer, D. G. and Hanley, J. H. (1997). Multisystemic therapy with violent and chronic juvenile offenders and their families: The role of treatment fidelity in successful dissemination. *Journal of Consulting and Clinical Psychology, 65*, 821–33.

Henrich, C. C. and Shahar, G. (2008). Social support buffers the effects of terrorism on adolescent depression: Findings from Sderot, Israel. *Journal of the American Academy of Child and Adolescent Psychiatry, 47*, 1073–6.

Hermens, D. F., Kohn, M. R., Clarke, S. D., Gordon, E. and Williams, L. M. (2005). Sex differences in adolescent ADHD: Findings from concurrent EEG and EDA. *Clinical Neurophysiology, 116*, 1455–63.

Hettema, J. M., Neale, M. and Kendler, K. (1995). Physical similarity and the equal-environment assumption in twin studies of psychiatric disorders. *Behavior Genetics, 25*, 327–35.

Hettema, J. M., Neale, M. C. and Kendler, K. S. (2001). A review and meta-analysis of the genetic epidemiology of anxiety disorders. *American Journal of Psychiatry, 158*, 1568–78.

Hettema, J. M., Prescott, C. A., Myers, J. M., Neale, M. C. and Kendler, K. S. (2005). The structure of genetic and environmental risk factors for anxiety disorders in men and women. *Archives of General Psychiatry, 62*, 182–9.

Hetzel-Riggin, M. D., Brausch, A. M. and Montgomery, B. S. (2007). A meta-analytic investigation of therapy modality outcomes for sexually abused children and adolescents: An exploratory study. *Child Abuse and Neglect, 31*, 125–41.

Hewitt, P. L. and Flett, G. L. (2007). Diagnosing the perfectionistic personality. *Current Psychiatry, 6*, 53–64.

Heydon, R. M. (2008). The case of special education and pathologizing. In R. Heydon and L. Iannacci (Eds.), *Early childhood curricula and the de-pathologizing of childhood* (pp. 82–99). Toronto: University of Toronto Press Inc.

Heyne, D., Sauter F. M., van Widenfelt, B. M., Vermeiren, R., Westenberg, P. M. (2011). School refusal and anxiety in adolescence: Non-randomized trial of a developmentally sensitive cognitive behavioral therapy. *Journal of Anxiety Disorders, 25*, 870–8.

Hickey, P. (1998). DSM and behavior therapy. *The Behavior Therapist, 21*, 43–6.

Hicks, B. M., Krueger, R. F., Iacono, W. G., McGue, M. and Patrick, C. J. (2004). Family transmission and heritability of externalizing disorders: A twin-family study. *Archives of General Psychiatry, 61*, 922–8.

Hicks, B. M., South, S. C., DiRago, A. C., Iacono, W. G. and McGue, M. (2009). Environmental adversity and increasing genetic risk for externalizing disorders. *Archives of General Psychiatry, 66*, 640–8.

Hill, C. L., and Ridley, C. R. (2001). Diagnostic decision making: Do counsellors delay final judgements? *Journal of Counseling and Development, 79*, 98–118.

Hill, D. B., Rozanski, C., Carfagnini, J. and Willoughby, B. (2007). Gender identity disorders in childhood and adolescence. *International Journal of Sexual Health, 19*, 57–75.

Hill, J. P. and Lynch, M. E. (1983). The intensification of gender-related role expectations during early adolescence. In J. Brooks-Gunn and A. Petersen (Eds.), *Girls at puberty: Biological and psychosocial perspectives* (pp. 201–28). New York: Plenum.

Hilt, L. M., Sander, L. C., Nolen-Hoeksema, S. and Simen, A. A. (2007). The BDNF Val66Met polymorphism predicts rumination and depression differently in young adolescent girls and their mothers. *Neuroscience Letters, 429*, 12–16.

Hine, E. and Martin, R. (2008). *A dictionary of biology.* Oxford Reference Online. Oxford: Oxford University Press.

Hines, M. (2004). *Brain gender.* Oxford: Oxford University Press.

Hinshaw, S. P. (2006). Treatment for children and adolescents with attention-deficit/hyperactivity disorder. In P. C. Kendall (Ed.), *Child and adolescent therapy: Cognitive-behavioral procedures* (pp. 82–113). New York: Guilford Press.

Hirshfeld-Becker, D. R. (2010). Familial and temperamental risk factors for social anxiety disorder. In H. Gazelle and K. H. Rubin (Eds.), *Social anxiety in childhood: Bridging developmental and clinical perspectives* (pp. 51–66). San Francisco, CA: Wiley Subscription Services.

Hirshoren, A. and Kavale, K. (1976). Profile analysis of the WISC-R: A continuing malpractice. *Exceptional Child, 23*, 83–7.

Ho, T. P., Leung, P. W. L., Luk, E. S. L., Taylor, E., Bacon-Shone, J. and Mak, F. L. (1996). Establishing the constructs of childhood behavioral disturbances in a Chinese population: A questionnaire study. *Journal of Abnormal Child Psychology, 24*, 417–31.

Hoag, M. and Burlingame, G. M. (1997). Child and adolescent group psychotherapy: A narrative review of effectiveness and the case for meta-analysis. *Journal of Child and Adolescent Group Therapy, 7*, 51–68.

Hodapp, R. M. and Dykens, E. M. (1991). Toward an etiology-specific strategy of early intervention with handicapped children. In K. Marfo (Ed.), *Early intervention in transition: Current perspectives on programs for handicapped children* (pp. 41–60). New York: Praeger.

Hodges, E. V. E., Boivin, M., Vitaro, F. and Bukowski, W. M. (1999). The power of friendship: Protection against an escalating cycle of peer victimization. *Developmental Psychology, 35,* 94–101.

Hoek, H. W. (2006). Incidence, prevalence and mortality of anorexia nervosa and other eating disorders. *Current Opinion in Psychiatry, 19,* 389–94.

Hoffman, C. D., Sweeney, D. P., Hodge, D., Lopez-Wagner, M. C. and Looney, L. (2009). Parenting stress and closeness: Mothers of typically developing children and mothers of children with autism. *Focus on Autism and Other Developmental Disabilities, 24,* 178–87.

Hoffman, K. T., Marvin, R. S., Cooper, G. and Powell, B. (2006). Changing toddlers' and preschoolers' attachment classifications: The circle of security intervention. *Journal of Consulting and Clinical Psychology, 74,* 1017–26.

Hoffman, M. L. (1983). Affective and cognitive processes in moral internalization: An information processing approach. In E. T. Higgins, D. Ruble and W. Hartup (Eds.), *Social cognition and social development: A socio-cultural perspective* (pp. 236–74). Cambridge: Cambridge University Press.

Hoffman, M. L. (1988). Moral development. In M. Bornstein, M. Sorrentino and E. T. Higgins (Eds.), *Handbook of motivation and cognition: Foundations of social behavior* (pp. 244–80). New York: Guilford Press.

Hofmann, S. G., Asnaani, A. and Hinton, D. E. (2010). Cultural aspects in social anxiety and social anxiety disorder. *Depression and Anxiety, 27,* 1117–27.

Hofstede, G. (1984). National cultures and corporate cultures. In L. A. Samovar, and R. E. Porter (Eds.), *Communication between cultures.* Belmont, CA: Wadsworth.

Hofstede, G. (2003). *Culture's consequences: Comparing values, behaviors, institutions and organization across nations* (2nd edn.). Thousand Oaks, CA: Sage Publications.

Hojnoski, R. L., Morrison, R., Brown, M. and Matthews, W. J. (2006). Projective test use among school psychologists: A survey and critique. *Journal of Psychoeducational Assessment, 24,* 145–59.

Holden, C. (2004). An everlasting gender gap? *Science, 305,* 639–40.

Holmbeck, G. N., Devine, K. A. and Bruno, E. F. (2010). Developmental issues and considerations in research and practice. In J. R. Weisz and A. E. Kazdin (Eds.), *Evidence-based psychotherapies for children and adolescents* (2nd edn., pp. 28–39). New York: Guilford Press.

Honda, H., Shimizu, Y. and Rutter, M. (2005). No effect of MMR withdrawal on the incidence of autism: A total population study. *Journal of Child Psychology and Psychiatry, 46,* 572–9.

Hooker, E. (1957). The adjustment of the male overt homosexual. *Journal of Projective Techniques, 21,* 18–31.

Hooley, J. M., Maher, W. B. and Maher, B. A. (2013). Abnormal psychology. In D. K. Freedheim and I. B. Wiener (Eds.), *Handbook of psychology: History of psychology* (pp. 340–76). Hoboken, NJ: Wiley.

Hope, T. and McMillan, J. (2004). Challenge studies of human volunteers: Ethical issues. *Journal of Medical Ethics, 30,* 110–16.

Horn, M. (1989). *Before it's too late: The child guidance movement in the United States, 1922–1945.* Philadelphia: Temple University Press.

Horowitz, J. L., Garber, J., Ciesla, J. A., Young, J. F. and Mufson, L. (2007). Prevention of depressive symptoms in adolescents: A randomized trial of cognitive-behavioral and interpersonal prevention programs. *Journal of Consulting and Clinical Psychology, 75,* 693–706.

Hosman, C. M. H. (1992). Primary prevention of mental disorders and mental health promotion in Europe: Developments and possibilities for innovation. In G. W. Albee, L. A. Bond and T. V. C. Monsey (Eds.), *Improving children's lives: Global perspectives on prevention* (pp. 151–66). Newbury Park, CA: Sage Publications.

Hosp, J. L. and Reschly, D. J. (2004). Disproportionate representation of minority students in special education: Academic, demographic, and economic predictors. *Exceptional Children, 70,* 185–99.

Hourmanesh, N. (2007). Early comprehensive interventions for children with autism: A meta-analysis. *Dissertation Abstracts International Section A: Humanities and Social Sciences, 67,* 2463.

Houts, A. C. (2002). Discovery, invention, and the expansion of the modern Diagnostic and Statistical Manuals of Mental Disorders. In L. E. Beutler and M. L. Malik (Eds.), *Rethinking the DSM: A psychological perspective* (pp. 17–65). Washington, DC: American Psychological Association.

Hoven, C. W., Duarte, C. S., Lucas, C. P., Wu, P., Mandell, D. J., Goodwin, R. D.,…Susser, E. (2005). Psychopathology among New York City public school children 6 months after September 11. *Archives of General Psychiatry, 62,* 545–52.

Howe, N., Aquan-Assee, J. and Bukowski, W. M. (1995). Self-disclosure and the sibling relationship: What did Romulus tell Remus? In K. J. Rotenberg (Ed.), *Disclosure processes in children and adolescents* (pp. 78–99). New York: Cambridge University Press.

Howes, C. (1983). Patterns of friendship. *Child Development, 54*, 1041–53.

Howlin, P. and Jones, D. P. H. (1996). An assessment approach to abuse allegations made through facilitated communication. *Child Abuse and Neglect, 20*, 103–10.

Howlin, P., Magiati, I. and Charman, T. (2009). Systematic review of early intensive behavioral interventions for children with autism. *American Journal on Intellectual and Developmental Disabilities, 114*, 23–41.

Hoza, B., Mrug, S., Gerdes, A. C., Hinshaw, S. P., Bukowski, W. M., Gold, J. A.,…Arnold, L. E. (2005). What aspects of peer relationships are impaired in children with attention-deficit/hyperactivity disorder? *Journal of Consulting and Clinical Psychology, 73*, 411–23.

Hudson, J. L. (2005). Efficacy of cognitive-behavioural therapy for children and adolescents with anxiety disorders. *Behaviour Change, 22*, 55–70.

Hudson, J. L. and Kendall, P. C. (2002). Showing you can do it: Homework in therapy for children and adolescents with anxiety disorders. *Journal of Clinical Psychology, 58*, 525–34.

Hudson, J. L., Rapee, R. M., Deveney, C., Schniering, C. A., Lyneham, H. J. and Bovopoulos, N. (2009). Cognitive-behavioral treatment versus an active control for children and adolescents with anxiety disorders: A randomized trial. *Journal of the American Academy of Child and Adolescent Psychiatry, 48*, 533–44.

Hudziak, J. J., Derks, E. M., Althoff, R. R., Copeland, W. and Boomsma, D. I. (2005). The genetic and environmental contributions to oppositional defiant behavior: A multi-informant twin study. *Journal of the American Academy of Child and Adolescent Psychiatry, 44*, 907–14.

Hudziak, J. J., Achenbach, T. M., Althoff, R. R. and Pine, D. S. (2008). A dimensional approach to developmental psychopathology. In J. E. Helzer, H. C. Kraemer, R. F. Krueger, H. Wittchen, P. J. Sirovatka and D. A. Regier (Eds.), *Dimensional approaches in diagnostic classification: Refining the research agenda for DSM-V* (pp. 101–13). Washington, DC: American Psychiatric Association.

Humphries, T. W. and Bauman, E. (1980). Maternal child rearing attitudes associated with learning disabilities. *Journal of Learning Disabilities, 13*, 459–62.

Hunsley, J. (2002). Psychological testing and psychological assessment: A closer examination. *American Psychologist, 57*, 139–40.

Huntemann, N. N. (2000). *Game over: Gender, race and violence in video games.* Northampton, MA: Media Education Foundation.

Hurley, R. S. E., Losh, M., Parlier, M., Reznick, J. S. and Piven, J. (2007). The Broad Autism Phenotype Questionnaire. *Journal of Autism and Developmental Disorders, 37*, 1679–90.

Hutchinson, A. D., Mathias, J. L. and Banich, M. T. (2008). Corpus callosum morphology in children and adolescents with attention deficit hyperactivity disorder: A meta-analytic review. *Neuropsychology, 22*, 341–9.

Hutschemaekers, G. J. M., Tiemens, B. G. and de Winter, M. (2007). Effects and side-effects of integrating care: The case of mental health care in the Netherlands. *International Journal of Integrated Care, 7*.

Hwang, S. K. and Charnley, H. (2010). Making the familiar strange and making the strange familiar: Understanding Korean children's experiences of living with an autistic sibling. *Disability and Society, 25*, 579–92.

Hwang, W., Myers, H. F., Abe-Kim, J. and Ting, J. Y. (2008). A conceptual paradigm for understanding culture's impact on mental health: The cultural influences on mental health (CIMH) model. *Clinical Psychology Review, 28*, 211–27.

Hyde, J. S. (2005). The gender similarities hypothesis. *American Psychologist, 60*, 581–92.

Hyde, J. S., Mezulis, A. H. and Abramson, L. Y. (2008). The ABCs of depression: Integrating affective, biological, and cognitive models to explain the emergence of the gender difference in depression. *Psychological Review, 115*, 291–313.

Iaboni, F., Douglas, V. I. and Ditto, B. (1997). Psychophysiological response of ADHD children to reward and extinction. *Psychophysiology, 34*, 116–123.

Inderbitzen, H. M., Walters, K. S. and Bukowski, A. L. (1997). The role of social anxiety in adolescent peer relations: Differences among sociometric status groups and rejected subgroups. *Journal of Clinical Child Psychology, 26*, 338–48.

Inderbitzen-Nolan, H., Davies, C. A. and McKeon, N. D. (2004). Investigating the construct validity of the SPAI-C: Comparing the sensitivity and specificity of the SPAI-C and the SAS-A. *Journal of Anxiety Disorders, 18*, 547–60.

Ingram, R. E. and Price, J. M. (2010). *Vulnerability to psychopathology: Risk across the lifespan.* New York: Guilford Press.

Inoue, K., Tanii, H., Nishimura, Y., Masaki, M., Nishida, A., Kajiki, N.,…Ono, Y. (2008). Current state of refusal to attend school in Japan. *Psychiatry and Clinical Neurosciences, 62*, 622.

Iscoe, I. (2007). George Albee, exemplar of primary prevention. *The Journal of Primary Prevention, 28*, 29.

Ishikawa, S., Sato, H. and Sasagawa, S. (2009). Anxiety disorder symptoms in Japanese children and adolescents. *Journal of Anxiety Disorders, 23*, 104–11.

Isley, S., O'Neil, R. and Parke, R. D. (1996). The relation of parental affect and control behaviors to children's classroom acceptance: A concurrent and predictive analysis. *Early Education and Development, 7*, 7–23.

Itard, J. (1962). *The wild boy of Aveyron* (C. Humphrey and M. Humphrey, trans.). New York: Appleton-Century Crofts (originally published 1806).

Iwawaki, S., Sumida, K., Okuno, S. and Cowen, E. L. (1967). Manifest anxiety in Japanese, French, and United States children. *Child Development, 38*, 713–22.

Izutsu, T., Shimotsu, S., Matsumoto, T., Okada, T., Kikuchi, A., Kojimoto, M., Noguchi, H. and Yoshikawa, K. (2006). Deliberate self-harm and childhood hyperactivity in junior high school students. *European Child and Adolescent Psychiatry, 15*, 172–6.

Jablensky, A. (1999). The conflict of the nosologists: Views on schizophrenia and manic-depressive illness in the early part of the 20th century. *Schizophrenia Research, 39*, 95–100.

Jackowski, A. P., de Araujo, C. M., de Lacerda, A. L. T., de Jesus Mari, J. and Kaufman, J. (2009). Neurostructural imaging findings in children with post-traumatic stress disorder: Brief review. *Psychiatry and Clinical Neurosciences, 63*, 1–8.

Jackson, D. A. and King, A. R. (2004). Gender differences in the effects of oppositional behavior on teacher ratings of ADHD symptoms. *Journal of Abnormal Child Psychology, 32*, 215–24.

Jackson, G. (2010). Test of time: Dibs: In search of self. *Clinical Child Psychology and Psychiatry, 15*, 121–8.

Jackson, S. W. (1986). *Melancholia and depression from Hippocratic times to modern times*. New Haven: Yale University Press.

Jacob, T. et al. (2003). Genetic and environmental effects on offspring alcoholism: New insights using an offspring-of-twins design. *Archives of General Psychiatry, 60*(12), 1265–72.

Jacobs, B. W. and Isaacs, S. (1986). Pre-pubertal anorexia nervosa: A retrospective controlled study. *Journal of Child Psychology and Psychiatry, 27*, 237–50.

Jaffee, S. R., Caspi, A., Moffitt, T. E., Dodge, K. A., Rutter, M., Taylor, A. and Tully, L. A. (2005). Nature x nurture: Genetic vulnerabilities interact with physical maltreatment to promote conduct problems. *Development and Psychopathology, 17*, 67–84.

Jaffee, S. R. and Price, T. S. (2007). Gene–environment correlations: A review of the evidence and implications for prevention of mental illness. *Molecular Psychiatry, 12*, 432–42.

Jaffee, W. B., Chu, J. A., Woody, G. E., (2009). Trauma, dissociation, and substance dependence in an adolescent male. *Harvard Review of Psychiatry, 17*, 60–7.

Jaffee, S. R. and Price, T. S. (2012). The implications of genotype–environment correlation for establishing causal processes in psychopathology. *Development and Psychopathology, 24*, 1253–64.

James, I. (2006). *Asperger's syndrome and high achievement: Some very remarkable people*. London: Jessica Kingsley Publishers.

James, W. (1981). *The principles of psychology*. Cambridge, MA: Harvard University Press.

Janet, P. (1929). *L'évolution psychologique de la personnalité*. Paris: Chahine.

Jang, K. L. (2005). *The behavioral genetics of psychopathology: A clinical guide*. Mahwah, NJ: Lawrence Erlbaum Associates.

Jansen, L. M., Gispen-de Wied, C. C., Jansen, M. A., van der Gaag, R. J., Matthys, W. and van Engeland, H. (1999). Pituitary-adrenal reactivity in a child psychiatric population: Salivary cortisol response to stressors. *European Neuropsychopharmacology, 9*, 67–75.

Jenkins, J. R., Odom, S. L. and Speltz, M. L. (1989). Effects of social integration on preschool children with handicaps. *Exceptional Children, 55*, 420–8.

Jenkins, M. M., Youngstrom, E. A., Washburn, J. J. and Youngstrom, J. K. (2011). Evidence-based strategies improve assessment of pediatric bipolar disorder by community practitioners. *Professional Psychology, Research and Practice, 42*, 121–9.

Jennings, J. R., van der Molen, M. W., Pelham, W., Debski, K. B. and Hoza, B. (1997). Inhibition in boys with attention deficit hyperactivity disorder as indexed by heart rate change. *Developmental Psychology, 33*, 308–18.

Jensen, P. S. and Hoagwood, K. (1997). The book of names: DSM-IV in context. *Development and Psychopathology, 9*, 231–49.

Jensen, P. S., Hoagwood, K. and Zitner, L. (2006). What's in a name? Problems versus prospects in current diagnostic approaches. In D. Cicchetti and D. J. Cohen (Eds.), *Developmental psychopathology: Theory and method* (pp. 24–40). Hoboken, NJ: John Wiley and Sons Inc.

Jensen, P. S., Arnold, L. E., Swanson, J. M., Vitiello, B., Abikoff, H. B., Greenhill, L. L.,...Hur, K. (2007). 3-year follow-up of the NIMH MTA study. *Journal of the American Academy of Child and Adolescent Psychiatry, 46*, 989–1002.

Jick, H., Kaye, J. A. and Black, C. (2004). Incidence and prevalence of drug-treated attention deficit disorder among boys in the UK. *British Journal of General Practice, 54*, 345–7.

Jiménez Chafey, M. I., Bernal, G. and Rosselló, J. (2009). Clinical case study: CBT for depression in a Puerto Rican adolescent: Challenges and variability in treatment response. *Depression and Anxiety, 26*, 98–103.

Jimenez, J. E. and Garcia de la Cadena, C. (2007). Learning disabilities in Guatemala and Spain: A cross-national study of the prevalence and cognitive processes associated with reading and spelling disabilities. *Learning Disabilities Research and Practice, 22*, 161–9.

Johnson, D. J. and Myklebust, H. R. (1967). *Learning disabilities: Educational principles and practices.* New York: Grune and Stratton.

Johnson, M. (1980). Mental illness and psychiatric treatment among women: *A response. Psychology of Women Quarterly, 4*, 363–71.

Johnson, M. H., Griffin, R., Csibra, G., Halit, H., Farroni, T., de Haan, M.,…Richards, J. (2005). The emergence of the social brain network: Evidence from typical and atypical development. *Development and Psychopathology, 17*, 599–619.

Johnson-Laird, P. N. and Oatley, K. (1992). Basic emotions, rationality, and folk theory. *Cognition and Emotion, 6*, 201–23.

Johnston, C. and Mash, E. J. (2001). Families of children with Attention-Deficit/Hyperactivity Disorder: Review and recommendations for future research. *Clinical Child and Family Psychology Review, 4*, 183–207.

Johnston, C. and Murray, C. (2003). Incremental validity in the psychological assessment of children and adolescents. *Psychological Assessment, 15*, 496–507.

Joiner, T. E., Metalsky, G. I., Katz, J. and Beach, S. R. H. (1999). Depression and excessive reassurance-seeking. *Psychological Inquiry, 10*, 269–78.

Jonas, W. B. (2005). *Mosby's dictionary of complementary and alternative medicine.* St. Louis, MO: Elsevier-Mosby.

Jones, K. (1999). *Taming the troublesome child: American families, child guidance, and the limits of psychiatric authority.* Cambridge: Harvard University Press.

Jones, K., Evans, C., Byrd, R. and Campbell, K. (2000). Gender equity training and teaching behavior. *Journal of Instructional Psychology, 27*, 173–8.

Jones, K. W. (2002). *Taming the troublesome child: American families, child guidance, and the limits of psychiatric authority.* Cambridge, MA: Harvard University Press.

Jones, M. C. (1924). A laboratory study of fear: The case of Peter. *Pedagogical Seminar, 31*, 308.

Jones, R. (2009). Extracting, storing and distributing DNA for a birth cohort study. *Paediatric and Perinatal Epidemiology, 23*, 127–33.

Juang, L. P., Syed, M. and Takagi, M. (2007). Intergenerational discrepancies of parental control among Chinese American families: Links to family conflict and adolescent depressive symptoms. *Journal of Adolescence, 30*, 965–75.

Juarascio, A., Shaw, J., Forman, E., Timko, C. A., Herbert, J., Butryn, M.,…Lowe, M. (2013). Acceptance and commitment therapy as a novel treatment for eating disorders: An initial test of efficacy and mediation. *Behavior Modification, 37*, 459–89.

Juffer, F., Bakermans-Kranenburg, M. J. and van IJzendoorn, M. H. (2008). Methods of the video-feedback to promote positive parenting alone, with sensitive discipline, and with representational attachment discussions. In F. Juffer, M. J. Bakermans-Kranenburg and M. H. van IJzendoorn (Eds.), *Promoting positive parenting: An attachment-based intervention* (pp. 22–36). London: Lawrence Erlbaum Associates.

Kagan, J. (2005). Temperament. In R. E. Tremblay, R. G. Barr and R. DeV. Peters (Eds.), *Encyclopedia on early childhood development.* Montreal, PQ: Centre of Excellence for Early Childhood Development. Retrieved from www.child-encyclopedia.com/documents/KaganANGxp.pdf

Kagan, J., Reznick, J. S. and Snidman, N. (1988). Biological bases of childhood shyness. *Science, 240*, 167–71.

Kagan, J., Reznick, J. S. and Gibbons, J. (1989). Inhibited and uninhibited types of children. *Child Development, 60*, 838–45.

Kagan, J. and Snideman, N. (1991). Temperamental factors in human development. *American Psychologist, 46(8)*, 856–62.

Kahlbaum, K. and Berrios, G. E. (2007). The clinico-diagnostic perspective in psychopathology. *History of Psychiatry, 18*, 231–45.

Kahn, E. and Cohen, L. H. (1934). Organic driveness: A brain stem syndrome and an experience. *New England Journal of Medicine, 210*, 748–56.

Kahr, B. (1996). Donald Winnicott and the foundations of child psychotherapy. *Journal of Child Psychotherapy, 22*, 327–42.

Kalinauskiene, L., Cekuoliene, D., van IJzendoorn, M. H., Bakermans-Kranenburg, M. J., Juffer, F. and Kusakovaskaja, I. (2009). Supporting insensitive mothers: The Vilnius randomized control trial of video-feedback intervention to promote maternal sensitivity and infant attachment security. *Child Care, Health and Development, 35*, 613–23.

Kaltas, G. A. and Chrousos, G. P. (2007). The neuroendocrinology of stress. In J. T. Cacioppo, L. G. Tassinary and G. G. Berntson (Eds.), *Handbook of psychophysiology* (3rd edn., pp. 303–18). New York: Cambridge University Press.

Kamens, S. (2010). Controversial issues for the future: DSM-V. *Society for Humanistic Psychology Newsletter.* Retrieved from www.apadivisions.org/division-32/publications/newsletters/humanistic/2010/01/dsm-v.aspx

Kandel, D. B. (1978). Homophily, selection, and socialization in adolescent friendships. *American Journal of Sociology, 84,* 427–36.

Kanner, L. (1943). Autistic disturbances of affective contact. *Nervous Child, 2,* 217–50.

Kanner, L. (1962). Emotionally disturbed children: A historical review. *Child Development, 33,* 97–102.

Kanner, L. (1971). Follow-up study of eleven autistic children originally reported in 1943. *Journal of Autism and Childhood Schizophrenia, 1,* 119–45.

Kanner, L. (1973). Historical perspective on developmental deviations. *Journal of Autism and Childhood Schizophrenia, 3,* 187–98.

Kar, N. and Bastia, B. K. (2006). Post-traumatic stress disorder, depression and generalised anxiety disorder in adolescents after a natural disaster: A study of comorbidity. *Clinical Practice and Epidemiology in Mental Health, 2,* 17.

Karcher, M. J., Brown, B. B. and Elliott, D. W. (2004). Enlisting peers in developmental interventions: Principles and practices. In S. F. Hamilton and M. A. Hamilton (Eds.), *The youth development handbook: Coming of age in American communities* (pp. 193–215). Thousand Oaks, CA: Sage Publications Inc.

Karg, K., Burmeister, M., Shedden, K. and Sen, S. (2011). The serotonin transporter promoter variant (5-HTTLPR), stress, and depression meta-analysis revisited: Evidence of genetic moderation. *Archives of General Psychiatry, 68,* 444–54.

Karna, A., Voeten, M., Little, T. D., Poskiparta, E., Kaljonen, A. and Salmivalli, C. (2011). A large-scale evaluation of the KiVa antibullying program: Grades 4–6. *Child Development, 82,* 311–30.

Karver, M. S., Handelsman, J. B., Fields, S. and Bickman, L. (2006). Meta-analysis of therapeutic relationship variables in youth and family therapy: The evidence for different relationship variables in the child and adolescent treatment outcome literature. *Clinical Psychology Review, 26,* 50–65.

Kataoka, S., Langley, A., Stein, B., Jaycox, L., Shang, L., Sanchez, N. and Wong, M. (2009). Violence exposure and PTSD: The role of English language fluency in Latino youth. *Journal of Child and Family Studies, 18,* 334–41.

Katz, L. F. (2007). Domestic violence and vagal reactivity to peer provocation. *Biological Psychology, 74,* 154–64.

Katz, M. (1976). *History of compulsory education laws.* Bloomington, IN: Phi Delta Kappa.

Katz, S. N., Schroeder, W. A. and Sidman, L. R. (1973). Emancipating our children – coming of legal age in America. *Family Law Quarterly, 7,* 211–41.

Kaufman, J., Yang, B. Z., Douglas-Palumberi, H., Grasso, D., Lipschitz, D., Houshyar, S., Krystal, J. H. and Gelernter, J. (2006). Brain-derived neurotrophic factor-5-HTTLPR gene interactions and environmental modifiers of depression in children. *Biological Psychiatry, 59,* 673–80.

Kavale, K. (1982). Psycholinguistic training programs: Are there differential treatment effects? *Exceptional Child, 29,* 21–30.

Kavale, K. A. and Forness, S. R. (1983). Hyperactivity and diet treatment: A meta-analysis of the Feingold hypothesis. *Journal of Learning Disabilities, 16,* 324–30.

Kavale, K. A. and Forness, S. R. (1985). Learning disability and the history of science: Paradigm or paradox? *Remedial and Special Education, 6,* 12–24.

Kavale, K. A. and Forness, S. R. (1996). Social skill deficits and learning disabilities: A meta-analysis. *Journal of Learning Disabilities, 29,* 226–37.

Kavale, K. A. and Forness, S. R. (1998). The politics of learning disabilities. *Learning Disability Quarterly, 21,* 245–73.

Kavale, K. and Forness, S. (1999). Effectiveness of special education. In C. Reynolds and T. Gutkin (Eds.), *Handbook of school psychology* (3rd edn., pp. 984–1024) New York: Wiley.

Kavale, K. A. and Mostert, M. P. (2004). *The positive side of special education: A history of fads, fancies, and follies.* Lanham, MD: Scarecrow Press.

Kaye, W. (2008). Neurobiology of anorexia and bulimia nervosa. *Physiology and Behavior, 94,* 121–35.

Kazdin, A. (1984). *Behavior modification in applied settings.* Homewood, IL: Dorsey Press.

Kazdin, A. E., Siegel, T. C. and Bass, D. (1992). Cognitive problem-solving skills training and parent management training in the treatment of antisocial behavior in children. *Journal of Consulting and Clinical Psychology, 60,* 733–47.

Kazdin, A. E. (2000). Perceived barriers to treatment participation and treatment acceptability among antisocial children and their families. *Journal of Child and Family Studies, 9,* 157–74.

Kazdin, A. E. (2005). Evidence-based assessment for children and adolescents: Issues in measurement development and clinical application. *Journal of Clinical Child and Adolescent Psychology, 34,* 548–58.

Kearney, C. A. (2005). *Social anxiety and social phobia in youth: Characteristics, assessment, and psychological treatment.* New York: Springer Publishing.

Kearney, C. A. (2008). School absenteeism and school refusal behavior in youth: A contemporary review. *Clinical Psychology Review, 28*, 451–71.

Kearney, C. A. and Hugelshofer, D. (2000). Systemic and clinical strategies for preventing school refusal behavior in youth. *Journal of Cognitive Psychotherapy, 14*, 51–65.

Kearney, C. A. and Albano, A. M. (2004). The functional profiles of school refusal behavior: Diagnostic aspects. *Behavior Modification, 28*, 147–61.

Kearney, C. A., Wechsler, A., Kaur, H. and Lemos-Miller, A. (2010). Posttraumatic stress disorder in maltreated youth: A review of contemporary research and thought. *Clinical Child and Family Psychology Review, 13*, 46–76.

Keel, P. K., Klump, K. L., Leon, G. R. and Fulkerson, J. A. (1998). Disordered eating in adolescent males from a school-based sample. *International Journal of Eating Disorders, 23*, 125–32.

Keen, D. V., Reid, F. D. and Arnone, D. (2010). Autism, ethnicity and maternal immigration. *British Journal of Psychiatry, 196*, 274–81.

Keenan, K. and Shaw, D. (1997). Developmental and social influences on young girls' early problem behavior. *Psychological Bulletin, 12*, 95–113.

Keenan, K. and Shaw, D. (2003). Starting at the beginning: Exploring the etiology of antisocial behaviour in the first years of life. In B. Lahey, T. Moffitt and A. Caspi (Eds.), *Causes of conduct disorder and juvenile delinquency* (pp. 153–81). New York: Guilford Press.

Keery, H., van den Berg, P. and Thompson, J. K. (2004). An evaluation of the Tripartite Influence Model of body dissatisfaction and eating disturbance with adolescent girls. *Body Image: An International Journal of Research, 1*, 237–51.

Keiley, M. K. (2002). Attachment and affect regulation: A framework for family treatment of conduct disorder. *Family Process, 41*, 477–93.

Kellam, S. G. and van Horn, Y. V. (1997). Life course development, community epidemiology and preventive trials: A scientific structure for prevention research. *American Journal of Community Psychology, 23*, 177–88.

Keller, M. C. and Coventry, W. L. (2005). Quantifying and addressing parameter indeterminacy in the classical twin design. *Twin Research and Human Genetics, 8*, 201–13.

Keller, M. C., Medland, S. E., Duncan, L. E., Hatemi, P. K., Neale, M. C., Maes, H. H. M. et al. (2009). Modeling extended twin family data I: Description of the cascade model. *Twin Research and Human Genetics, 12*, 8–18.

Kelley, B. T., Loeber, R., Keenan, K. and DeLamatre, M. (1997). *Developmental pathways in boys' disruptive and delinquent behavior*. Washington, DC: Office of Juvenile Justice and Delinquency Prevention, US Department of Justice.

Kelly, C. M. and Jorm, A. F. (2007). Adolescents' intentions to offer assistance to friends with depression or conduct disorder: Associations with psychopathology and psychosocial characteristics. *Early Intervention in Psychiatry, 1*, 150–6.

Kelsoe, J. R. (2003). Arguments for the genetic basis of the bipolar spectrum. *Journal of Affective Disorders, 73*, 183–97.

Kendall, P. C. (1985). Toward a cognitive-behavioral model of child psychopathology and a critique of relevant interventions. *Journal of Abnormal Child Psychology, 13*, 357–72.

Kendall, P. C. (1994). Treating anxiety disorders in children: Results of a randomized clinical trial. *Journal of Consulting and Clinical Psychology, 62*, 100–10.

Kendall, P. C. and Braswell, L. (1982). Cognitive-behavioral self-control therapy for children: A component analysis. *Journal of Consulting and Clinical Psychology, 50*, 672–89.

Kendall, P. C., Safford, S., Flannery-Schroeder, E. and Webb, A. (2004). Child anxiety treatment: Outcomes in adolescence and impact on substance use and depression at 7.4-year follow-up. *Journal of Consulting and Clinical Psychology, 72*, 276–87.

Kendall, P. C. and Hedtke, K. A. (2006). *Coping cat workbook*. Ardmore: Workbook Publishing Inc.

Kendall, P. C. and Beidas, R. S. (2007). Smoothing the trail for dissemination of evidence-based practices for youth: Flexibility within fidelity. *Professional Psychology: Research and Practice, 38*, 13–20.

Kendall, P. C., Khanna, M. S., Edson, A., Cummings, C. and Harris, M. S. (2011). Computers and psychosocial treatment for child anxiety: Recent advances and ongoing efforts. *Depression and Anxiety, 28*, 58–66.

Kendell, R. and Jablensky, A. (2003). Distinguishing between the validity and utility of psychiatric diagnoses. *The American Journal of Psychiatry, 160*, 4–12.

Kendler, K. S. (2005). "A gene for…": The nature of gene action in psychiatric disorders. *American Journal of Psychiatry, 162*, 1243–52.

Kendler, K. S., Kuhn, J. and Prescott, C. A. (2004). The interrelationship of neuroticism, sex, and stressful life events in the prediction of episodes of major depression. *American Journal of Psychiatry, 161*, 631–6.

Kendler, K. S., Neale, M. C., Kessler, R. C., Heath, A. C. and Eaves, L. J. (1993). A test of the equal-environment assumption in twin studies of psychiatric illness. *Behavior Genetics, 23*, 21–7.

Kennard, B. D., Silva, S. G., Tonev, S., Hughes, J. L., Kratochvil, C. J., Emslie, G.J., March, J. et al. (2009). Remission and recovery in the Treatment for Adolescents With Depression Study (TADS): Acute and long-term outcomes. *Journal of the American Academy of Child and Adolescent Psychiatry, 48*, 186–95.

Kent. M. (2000). *The Oxford dictionary of sports science and medicine* (2nd edn.). Oxford: Oxford University Press.

Kephart, N. C. (1940). Influencing the rate of mental growth in retarded children through environmental stimulation. In G. M. Whipple (Ed.), *The thirty-ninth yearbook of the National Society for the Study of Education: Intelligence: Its nature and nurture, Part II, Original studies and experiments* (pp. 223–30). Bloomington, IN: Public School Publishing.

Kerns, C. M., Read, K. L., Klugman, J. and Kendall, P. C. (2013). Cognitive behavioral therapy for youth with social anxiety: Differential short and long-term treatment outcomes. *Journal of Anxiety Disorders, 27*, 210–15.

Kerr, M. A. and Schneider, B. H. (2008). Anger expression in children and adolescents: A review of the empirical literature. *Clinical Psychology Review, 28*, 559–77.

Kerremans, A., Claes, L. and Bijttebier, P. (2010). Disordered eating in adolescent males and females: Association with temperament, emotional and behavioral problems and perceived self-competence. *Personality and Individual Differences, 49*, 955–60.

Kessler, R., Sonnega, A., Bromet, E., Hughes, M. and Nelson, C. (1995). Posttraumatic stress disorder in the National Comorbidity Survey. *Archives of General Psychiatry, 52*, 1048–60.

Kessler, R., Berglund, P., Demler, O., Jin, R., Merikangas, K. R. and Walters, E. E. (2005). Lifetime prevalence and age-of-onset distributions of DSM-IV disorders in the National Comorbidity Survey Replication. *Archives of General Psychiatry, 62*, 593–602.

Kestler, L. P. and Lewis, M. (2009). Cortisol response to inoculation in 4-year-old children. *Psychoneuroendocrinology, 34*, 743–51.

Khan, A. (Director). (2007). Taare zameen par [motion picture]. India: Aamir Khan Productions.

Kiesner, J. (2002). Depressive symptoms in early adolescence: Their relations with classroom problem behavior and peer status. *Journal of Research on Adolescence, 12*, 463–78.

Killgore, W. D. and Yurgelun-Todd, D. A. (2005). Social anxiety predicts amygdala activation in adolescents viewing fearful faces. *Neuroreport, 16*, 1671–5.

Kilpatrick, D. G., Ruggiero, K. J., Acierno, R., Saunders, B. E., Resnick, H. S. and Best, C. L. (2003). Violence and risk of PTSD, major depression, substance abuse/ dependence, and comorbidity: Results from the National Survey of Adolescents. *Journal of Consulting and Clinical Psychology, 71*, 692–700.

Kim, J., Rapee, R. M. and Gaston, J. E. (2008). Symptoms of offensive type Taijin-Kyomsho among Australian social phobics. *Depression and Anxiety, 25*, 601–8.

Kim, U. and Choi, S.-H. (1994). Individualism, collectivism, and child development: A Korean perspective. In P. M. Greenfield and R. R. Cocking (Eds.), *Cross-cultural roots of minority child development* (pp. 227–57). Hillsdale, NJ: Lawrence Erlbaum Associates.

Kim-Cohen, J. (2003). Prior juvenile diagnoses in adults with mental disorder: Developmental follow-back of a prospective-longitudinal cohort. *Archives of General Psychiatry, 60*(7), 709–17.

Kim-Cohen, J., Arseneault, L., Caspi, A., Polo Tomas, M., Taylor, A. and Moffitt, T. E. (2005). Validity of DSM-IV conduct disorder in 4 ½–5-year-old children: A longitudinal epidemiological study. *American Journal of Psychiatry, 162*, 1108–17.

Kind, J. R., Ross-Toledo, K., John, S., Hall, J. L., Ross, L., Freeland, L.,...Lee, C. (2010). Promoting healing and restoring trust: Policy recommendations for improving behavioral health care for American Indian/Alaska native adolescents. *American Journal of Community Psychology, 46*, 386–94.

Kindermann, T. (1998). Children's development within peer groups: Using composite social maps to identify peer networks and to study their influences. In W. M. Bukowski and A. H. Cillessen (Eds.), *Sociometry then and now: Building on six decades of measuring children's experiences with the peer group* (pp. 55–82). San Francisco, CA: Jossey-Bass.

King, N., Tonge, B. J., Heyne, D. and Ollendick, T. H. (2000). Research on the cognitive-behavioral treatment of school refusal: A review and recommendations. *Clinical Psychology Review, 20*, 495–507.

King, N., Heyne, D., Tonge, B., Gullone, E. and Ollendick, T. H. (2001). School refusal: Categorical diagnoses, functional analysis and treatment planning. *Clinical Psychology and Psychotherapy, 8*, 352–60.

King, S., Waschbusch, D. A., Pelham, W. E., Frankland, B. W., Andrade, B. F., Jacques, S. and Corkum, P. V. (2009). Social information processing in elementary-school aged children with ADHD: Medication effects and comparisons with typical children. *Journal of Abnormal Child Psychology, 37*, 579–89.

Kirillova, G. P., Vanyukov, M. M., Kirisci, L. and Reynolds, M. (2008). Physical maturation, peer environment, and the ontogenesis of substance use disorders. *Psychiatry Research, 158*, 43–53.

Kirk, S. A. (2004). Are children's DSM diagnoses accurate? *Brief Treatment and Crisis Intervention, 4,* 255–70.

Kirk, S. A., McCarthy, J. J. and Kirk, W. D. (1961). *Illinois Test of Psycholinguistic Abilities (Experimental edn.).* Urbana, IL: University of Illinois Press.

Kirk, S. A. and Kirk, W. D. (2001). *Psycholinguistic learning disabilities: Diagnosis and remediation.* Urbana, IL: University of Illinois Press.

Kirk, S. A. and Hsieh, D. K. (2004). Diagnostic consistency in assessing conduct disorder: An experiment on the effect of social context. *American Journal of Orthopsychiatry, 74,* 43–55.

Kiser, L. J., Ackerman, B. J., Brown, E., Edwards, N. B., McColgan, E., Pugh, R. and Pruitt, D. B. (1988). Posttraumatic stress disorder in young children: A reaction to purported sexual abuse. *Journal of the American Academy of Child and Adolescent Psychiatry, 27,* 645–9.

Kistner, J. A., David-Ferdon, C. F., Repper, K. K. and Joiner, T. E. (2006). Bias and accuracy of children's perceptions of peer acceptance: Prospective associations with depressive symptoms. *Journal of Abnormal Child Psychology, 34,* 349–61.

Kleinman, A. M. (1977). Depression, somatization, and the "new cross-cultural psychiatry." *Social Sciences and Medicine, 11,* 3–10.

Klerman, G. L., Vaillant, G. E., Spitzer, R. L. and Michels, R. (1984). A debate on DSM-III. *American Journal of Psychiatry, 141,* 539–53.

Klimes-Dougan, B., Hastings, P. D., Granger, D. A., Usher, B. A. and Zahn-Waxler, C. (2001a). Adrenocortical activity in at-risk and normally developing adolescents: individual differences in salivary cortisol basal levels, diurnal variation, and responses to social challenges. *Developmental Psychopathology, 13*(3), 695–719.

Klimes-Dougan, B., Hastings, P. D., Granger, D. A., Usher, B. A. and Zahn-Waxler, C. (2001b). Adrenocortical activity in at-risk and normally developing adolescents: Individual differences in salivary cortisol basal levels, diurnal variation, and responses to social challenges. *Developmental and Psychopathology, 13,* 695–719.

Klinger, E., Bouchard, S., Legeron, P., Roy, S., Lauer, F., Chemin, I. and Nugues, P. (2005). Virtual reality therapy versus cognitive behavior therapy for social phobia: A preliminary controlled study. *CyberPsychology and Behavior, 8,* 76–88.

Klomek, A. B., Marrocco, F., Kleinman, M., Schonfeld, I. S. and Gould, M. S. (2007). Bullying, depression and suicidality in adolescents. *Journal of the American Academy of Child and Adolescent Psychiatry, 46,* 40–9.

Kluckhohn, C. and Kelly, W. H. (1945). The concept of culture. In R. Linton (Ed.), *The science of man in the world crisis* (pp. 78–105). New York: Columbia University Press.

Klump, K. L., McGue, M. and Iacono, W. G. (2003). Differential heritability of eating attitudes and behaviors in prepubertal versus pubertal twins. *International Journal of Eating Disorders, 33,* 287–92.

Klump, K. L., Strober, M., Bulik, C. M., Thornton, L., Johnson, C., Devlin, W.,…Kaye, W. H. (2004). Personality characteristics of women before and after recovery from an eating disorder. *Psychological Medicine, 34,* 1407–18.

Klump, K. L., Suisman, J. L., Burt, S. A., McGue, M. and Iacono, W. G. (2009). Genetic and environmental influences on disordered eating: An adoption study. *Journal of Abnormal Psychology, 118,* 797–805.

Knecht, A., Snijders, T. A. B., Baerveldt, C., Steglich, C. E. G. and Raub, W. (2010). Friendship and delinquency: Selection and influence processes in early adolescence. *Social Development, 19,* 494–514.

Knight, G., Guthrie, I., Page, M. and Fabes, R. (2002). Emotional arousal and gender differences in aggression: A meta-analysis. *Aggressive Behavior, 28,* 366–93.

Kog, E., Vertommen, H. and Vandereycken, W. (1987). Minuchin's psychosomatic family model revised: A concept-validation study using a multitrait-multimethod approach. *Family Process, 26,* 235–53.

Kohlberg, L., LaCrosse, J. and Ricks, D. (1972). The predictability of adult mental health from childhood behaviour. In B. B. Wolman (Ed.) *Manual of child psychopathology* (pp. 1217–84). New York: McGraw-Hill.

Kohler, F. W., Strain, P. S. and Goldstein, H. (2005). The effectiveness of peer-mediated intervention for young children with autism. In E. Hibbs and P. Jenson (Eds.), *Psychosocial treatments for child and adolescent disorders* (pp. 659–88). Washington, DC: American Psychological Association.

Kolko, D. J., Baumann, B. L., Bukstein, O. G. and Brown, E. J. (2007). Internalizing symptoms and affective reactivity in relation to the severity of aggression in clinically referred, behavior-disordered children. *Journal of Child and Family Studies, 16,* 745–59.

Kollins, S. H. and Greenhill, L. L. (2006). Evidence base for the use of stimulant medication in preschool children with ADHD. *Infants and Young Children, 19,* 132–41.

Kollins, S. H. and March, J. S. (2007). Advances in the pharmacotherapy of attention-deficit/hyperactivity disorder. *Biological Psychiatry, 62,* 951–53.

Koltko, M. E. (1990). How religious beliefs affect psychotherapy: The example of Mormonism. *Psychotherapy, 27,* 132–41.

Kolvin, I., Berney, T. P. and Bhate, S. R. (1984). Classification and diagnosis of depression in school phobia. *British Journal of Psychiatry, 145*, 347–57.

Koob, G. F. and Le Moal, M. (2001). Drug addiction, dysregulation of reward, and allostasis. *Neuropsychopharmacology, 24*, 97–129.

Koopmans, M. (2001). From double bind to N-Bind: Toward a new theory of schizophrenia and family interaction. *Nonlinear Dynamics, Psychology, and Life Sciences, 5*, 289–323.

Koretz, D. S. (1991). Prevention-centered science in mental health. *American Journal of Community Psychology, 19*, 453–8.

Korhonen, T., Latvala, A., Dick, D. M., Pulkkinen, L., Rose, R. J., Kaprio, J. and Huizink, A. C. (2012). Genetic and environmental influences underlying externalizing behaviors, cigarette smoking and illicit drug use across adolescence. *Behavior Genetics, 42*, 614–25.

Kovacs, M., Goldston, D. and Gatsonis, C. (1993). Suicidal behaviors and childhood-onset depressive disorders: A longitudinal investigation. *Journal of the American Academy of Child and Adolescent Psychiatry, 32*, 8–20.

Kovas, Y., Haworth, C. M. A., Dale, P. S., Plomin, R., Weinberg, R. A., Thomson, J. M. and Fischer, K. W. (2007). The genetic and environmental origins of learning abilities and disabilities in the early school years. *Monographs of the Society for Research in Child Development, 72*, 1–123.

Kowatch, R. A., Devous, M. D. Sr., Harvey, D. C., Mayes, T.L., Trivedi, M. H., Emslie, G. J. and Weinberg, W. A. (1999). A SPECT HMPAO study of regional cerebral blood flow in depressed adolescents and normal controls. *Progress in Neuropsychopharmacology and Biological Psychiatry, 23*, 643–56.

Kowatch, R. A., Fristad, M., Birmaher, B., Wagner, K. D., Findling, R. L. and Hellander, M. (2005). Treatment guidelines for children and adolescents with bipolar disorder. *Journal of the American Academy of Child and Adolescent Psychiatry, 44*, 213–35.

Kraemer, H. C. (2008). DSM categories and dimensions in clinical and research contexts. In J. E. Helzer, H. C. Kraemer, R. F. Krueger, H. Wittchen, P. J. Sirovatka and D. A. Regier (Eds.), *Dimensional approaches in diagnostic classification: Refining the research agenda for DSM-V* (pp. 5–17). Washington, DC: American Psychiatric Association.

Kratzer, L. and Hodgins, S. (1997). Adult outcomes of child conduct problems: A cohort study. *Journal of Abnormal Psychology, 25*, 65–81.

Kraut, R., Patterson, M., Lundmark, V., Kiesler, S., Mukopadhyay, T. and Scherlis, W. (1998). Internet paradox: A social technology that reduces social involvement and psychological well-being? *American Psychologist, 53*, 1017–31.

Kroeber, A. L. and Kluckhohn, C. (1952). *Culture: A critical review of concepts and definitions*, Vol. XLVII. Cambridge, MA: Harvard University Peabody Museum of American Archeology and Ethnology.

Kroll, J. (1973). The reappraisal of psychopathology in the Middle Ages. *Archives of General Psychiatry, 29*, 276–83.

Krueger, R. F. and Markon, K. E. (2006). Reinterpreting comorbidity: A model-based approach to understanding and classifying psychopathology. *Annual Review of Clinical Psychology, 2*, 111–33.

Kruesi, M. J., Hibbs, E. D., Zahn, T. P., Keysor, C. S., Hamburger, M. S., Bartko, J. J. and Rapoport, J. L. (1992). A 2-year prospective follow-up study of children and adolescents with disruptive behaviour disorders. *Archives of General Psychiatry, 49*, 429–35.

Kung, E. M. and Farrell, A. D. (2000). The role of parents and peers in early adolescent substance use: An examination of mediating and moderating effects. *Journal of Child and Family Studies, 9*, 509–28.

Kuntsche, E. and Jordan, M. D. (2006). Adolescent alcohol and cannabis use in relation to peer and school factors: Results of multilevel analyses. *Drug and Alcohol Dependence, 84*, 167–74.

Kuntsi, J. and Stevenson, J. (2000). Hyperactivity in children: A focus on genetic research and psychological theories. *Clinical Child and Family Psychology Review, 3*, 1–23.

Kuriyan, A. B., Pelham Jr., W. E. P., Molina, B. S. G., Waschbusch, D. A., Gnagy, E. M., Sibley, M. H.,...Kent, K. M. (2013). Young adult educational and vocational outcomes of children diagnosed with ADHD. *Journal of Abnormal Child Psychology, 41*, 27–41.

Kusche, C. A. and Greenberg, M. T. (1995). *The PATHS curriculum*. Seattle, WA: Developmental Research and Programs.

Kutcher, S., Aman, M., Brooks, S. J., Buitelaar, J., van Daalen, E., Fegert, J.,...Tyano, S. (2004). International consensus statement on attention-deficit/hyperactivity disorder (ADHD) and disruptive behaviour disorders (DBDs): Clinical implications and treatment practice suggestions. *European Neuropsychopharmacology, 14*, 11–28.

Kwon, H., Reiss, A. L. and Menon, V. (2002). Neural basis of protracted developmental changes in visuo-spatial working memory. *Proceedings of the National Academy of Sciences U.S.A., 99*, 13336–41.

Kwon, K. and Lease, A. M. (2007). Clique membership and social adjustment in children's same-gender cliques: The contribution of the type of clique to children's self-reported adjustment. *Merrill-Palmer Quarterly: Journal of Developmental Psychology, 53*, 216–42.

Ladd, G. W. and Hart, C. H. (1992). Creating informal play opportunities: Are parents' and preschoolers' initiations related to children's competence with peers? *Developmental Psychology, 28*, 1179–87.

Lahey, B. B., Hart, E. L., Pliszka, S., Applegate, B. and McBurnett, K. (1993). Neurophysiological correlates of conduct disorder: A rationale and a review of research. *Journal of Clinical Child Psychology, 22*, 141–53.

Lahey, B. B., Applegate, B., McBurnett, K., Biederman, J., Greenhill, L., Hynd, G. W.,…Richters, J. (1994). DSM-IV field trials for attention deficit hyperactivity disorder in children and adolescents. *The American Journal of Psychiatry, 151*, 1673–85.

Lahey, B. B., Loeber, R., Hart, E. L., Frick, P. J., Applegate, B., Zhang, Q.,…Russo, M. F. (1995). Four year longitudinal study of conduct disorder in boys: Patterns and predictors of persistence. *Journal of Abnormal Psychology, 104*, 83–93.

Lahey, B. B., Loeber, R., Quay, H. C., Applegate, B., Shaffer, D., Waldman, I.,…Bird, H. R. (1998). Validity of DSM-IV subtypes of conduct disorder based on age of onset. *Journal of the American Academy of Child and Adolescent Psychiatry, 37*, 435–42.

Lahey, B. B., Pelham, W. E., Loney, J., Lee, S. S. and Willcutt, E. (2005). Instability of the DSM-IV Subtypes of ADHD from preschool through elementary school. *Archives of General Psychiatry, 62*, 896–902.

Lahey, B. B., van Hulle, C. A., Waldman, I. D., Rodgers, J. L., D'Onofrio, B. M., Pedlow, S.,…Keenan, K. (2006). Testing descriptive hypotheses regarding sex differences in the development of conduct problems and delinquency. *Journal of Abnormal Child Psychology, 34*, 737–55.

Lahey, B. B., Hartung, C. M., Loney, J., Pelham, W. E., Chronis, A. M. and Lee, S. S. (2007). Are there sex differences in the predictive validity of DSM-IV ADHD among younger children? *Journal of Clinical Child and Adolescent Psychology, 36*, 113–26.

Lai, B. S., La Greca, A. M., Auslander, B. A. and Short, M. B. (2013). Children's symptoms of posttraumatic stress and depression after a natural disaster: Comorbidity and risk factors. *Journal of Affective Disorders, 146*, 71–8.

Laing, R. D. (1960). *The divided self: An existential study in sanity and madness.* London: Tavistock.

Laird, R. D., Pettit, G. S., Bates, J. E. and Dodge, K. A. (2003). Parents' monitoring-relevant knowledge and adolescents' delinquent behaviour: Evidence of correlated developmental changes and reciprocal influences. *Child Development, 74*, 752–68.

Laitila, A., Aaltonen, J., Piilinen, H.-O. and Rasanen, E. H. (1996). Dealing with negative connotations in family therapeutic treatment of an enmeshed family: A case study. *Contemporary Family Therapy: An International Journal, 18*, 331–43.

Lakdawalla, Z., Hankin, B. L. and Mermelstein, R. (2007). Cognitive theories of depression in children and adolescents: A conceptual and quantitative review. *Clinical Child and Family Psychology Review, 10*, 1–24.

Lam, C. B., Solmeyer, A. R. and McHale, S. M. (2012). Sibling differences in parent–child conflict and risky behavior: A three-wave longitudinal study. *Journal of Family Psychology, 26*, 523–31.

Lam, K. S. L., Bodfish, J. W. and Piven, J. (2008). Evidence for three subtypes of repetitive behavior in autism that differ in familiality and association with other symptoms. *Journal of Child Psychology and Psychiatry, 49*, 1193–1200.

Lambert, M. C., Weisz, J. R. and Knight, F. (1989). Over- and undercontrolled clinic referral problems of Jamaican and American children and adolescents: The culture general and the culture specific. *Journal of Consulting and Clinical Psychology, 57*, 467–72.

Lambert, M. C., Weisz, J. R., Knight, F., Desrosiers, M.-F., Overly, K. and Thesiger, C. (1992). Jamaican and American adult perspectives on child psychopathology: Further exploration of the threshold model. *Journal of Consulting and Clinical Psychology, 60*, 146–9.

Lane, C. (2007). *Shyness: How normal behavior became a sickness.* New Haven, CT: Yale University Press.

Lane, J. and Addis, M. E. (2005). Male gender role conflict and patterns of help seeking in Costa Rica and the United States. *Psychology of Men and Masculinity, 6*, 155–68.

Langberg, J. M., Epstein, J. N., Urbanowicz, C. M., Simon, J. O. and Graham, A. J. (2008). Efficacy of an organization skills intervention to improve the academic functioning of students with attention-deficit/hyperactivity disorder. *School Psychology Quarterly, 23*, 407–17.

Langberg, J. M., Epstein, J. N., Altaye, M., Molina, B. S. G., Arnold, L. E. and Vitiello, B. (2008). The transition to middle school is associated with changes in the developmental trajectory of ADHD symptomatology in young adolescents with ADHD. *Journal of Clinical Child and Adolescent Psychology, 37*, 651–63.

Lansford, J. E., Deater-Deckard, K., Dodge, K. A., Bates, J. E. and Pettit, G. S. (2004). Ethnic differences in the link between physical discipline and later adolescent externalizing behaviours. *Journal of Child Psychology and Psychiatry, 45*, 801–12.

Lansford, J. E., Chang, L., Dodge, K. A., Malone, P. S., Oburu, P., Palmerus, K.,…Quinn, N. (2005). *Child Development, 76*, 1234–46.

Lansford, J. E., Criss, M. M., Dodge, K. A., Shaw, D. S., Pettit, G. S. and Bates, J. E. (2009). Trajectories of physical discipline: Early childhood antecedents and developmental outcomes. *Child Development, 80,* 1385–402.

Laor, N., Wolmer, L., Mayes, L. C., Avner, G., Weizman, R. and Cohen, D. J. (1997). Israeli preschool children under scuds: A 30-month follow-up. *Journal of the American Academy of Child and Adolescent Psychiatry, 36,* 349–56.

Lara, C., Fayyad, J., de Graaf, R., Kessler, R. C., Aguilar-Gaxiola, S., Angermeyer, R.,…Sampson, N. (2009). Childhood predictors of adult attention-deficit/hyperactivity disorder: Results from the World Health Organization World Mental Health Survey initiative. *Biological Psychiatry, 65,* 46–54.

Lardieri, L. A., Blacher, J. and Swanson, H. L. (2000). Sibling relationships and parent stress in families of children with and without learning disabilities. *Learning Disability Quarterly, 23,* 105–16.

Larsen, S. C., Parker, R. M. and Hammill, D. D. (1982). Effectiveness of psycholinguistic training: A response to Kavale. *Exceptional Children, 49,* 60–6.

Last, C. G. and Strauss, C. C. (1990). School refusal in anxiety-disordered children and adolescents. *Journal of the American Academy of Child and Adolescent Psychiatry, 29,* 31–5.

Laszloffy, T. A. (2002). Rethinking family development theory: Teaching with the Systemic Family Development (SFD) models. *Family Relations, 51,* 206–15.

Lau, J. Y. F., Gregory, A. M., Goldwin, M. A., Pine, D. S. and Eley, T. C. (2007). Assessing gene–environment interactions on anxiety symptom subtypes across childhood and adolescence. *Development and Psychopathology, 19,* 1129–46.

Lau, J. Y. F. and Eley, T. C. (2008). New behavioral genetic approaches to depression in childhood and adolescence. In J. R. Z. Abela and B. L. Hankin (Eds.), *Handbook of childhood depression* (pp. 124–48). New York: Guilford.

Laursen, B., Furman, W. and Mooney, K. S. (2006). Predicting interpersonal competence and self-worth from adolescent relationships and relationship networks: Variable-centered and person-centered perspectives. *Merrill-Palmer Quarterly: Journal of Developmental Psychology, 52,* 572–600.

Lavigne, J. V., LeBailly, S. A., Hopkins, J., Gouze, K. R. and Binns, H. J. (2009). The prevalence of ADHD, ODD, depression, and anxiety in a community sample of 4-year-olds. *Journal of Clinical Child and Adolescent Psychology, 38,* 315–28.

Lazarsfeld, P. F. and Merton, R. K. (1954). Friendship as social process: A substantive and methodological analysis. In M. Berger, T. Abel and C. H. Page (Eds.), *Freedom and control in modern society* (pp. 18–66). New York: Van Nostrand.

Lazarus, R. S. (1991). *Emotion and adaptation.* New York: Oxford University Press.

Le Couteur, A. and Gardner, F. (2010). Use of structured interviews and observational methods in clinical settings. In M. Rutter, D. Bishop, D. S. Pine, S. Scott, J. S. Stevenson, E. A. Taylor and A. Thapar (Eds.), *Rutter's child and adolescent psychiatry* (pp. 271–88). Oxford: Blackwell.

Le Grange, D. (1999). Family therapy for adolescent anorexia nervosa. *Journal of Clinical Psychology, 55,* 727–39.

Le Grange, D., Crosby, R. D. and Lock, J. (2008). Predictors and moderators of outcome in family-based treatment for adolescent bulimia nervosa. *Journal of the American Academy of Child and Adolescent Psychiatry, 47,* 464–70.

LeBlanc, L. A. and Matson, J. L. (1995). A social skills training program for preschoolers with developmental delays: Generalization and social validity. *Behavior Modification, 19,* 234–46.

Lederach, J. P. (1995). *Preparing for peace: Conflict transformation across cultures.* Syracuse, NY: Syracuse University Press.

LeDoux, J. (1994). Emotion, memory and the brain. *Scientific American, 270,* 50–7.

LeDoux, J. (2000). Emotion circuits in the brain. *Annual Review of Neurosciences, 23,* 155–84.

Lee, C. M. and Hunsley, J. (2003). Evidence-based assessment of childhood mood disorders: Comment on McClure, Kubiszyn and Kaslow (2002). *Professional Psychology: Research and Practice, 34,* 112–13.

Lee, S. S., Lahey, B. B., Owens, E. B. and Hinshaw, S. P. (2008). Few preschool boys and girls with ADHD are well-adjusted during adolescence. *Journal of Abnormal Child Psychology, 36,* 373–83.

Leffler, J. M., Fristad, M. A. and Klaus, N. M. (2010). Psychoeducational psychotherapy (PEP) for children with bipolar disorder: Two case studies. *Journal of Family Psychotherapy, 21,* 269–86.

LeGoff, D. B. (2004). Use of LEGO© as a therapeutic medium for improving social competence. *Journal of Autism and Developmental Disorders, 34,* 557–71.

Legrand, L. N., Keyes, M., McGue, M., Iacono, W. G. and Krueger, R. F. (2008). Rural environments reduce the genetic influence on adolescent substance use and rulebreaking behavior. *Psychological Medicine, 38,* 1341–50.

Leit, R. A., Pope, H. G. and Gray, J. J. (2001). Cultural expectations of muscularity in men: The evolution of *Playgirl* centerfolds. *International Journal of Eating Disorders, 29,* 90–3.

Lempers, J. D. and Clark-Lempers, D. S. (1992). Young, middle, and late adolescents' comparisons of the functional importance of five significant relationships. *Journal of Youth and Adolescence, 21*, 53–96.

Leonard, A. L. (1920). A parent's study of children's lies. *Pedagogical Seminary, 27*, 123–4.

Leung, K., Lau, S. and Lam, W.-L. (1998). Parenting styles and academic achievement: A cross-cultural study. *Merrill-Palmer Quarterly: Journal of Developmental Psychology, 44*, 157–72.

Leung, P. W. L., Hung, S., Ho, T., Lee, C., Liu, W., Tang, C. and Kwong, S. (2008). Prevalence of DSM-IV disorders in Chinese adolescents and the effects of an impairment criterion: A pilot community study in Hong Kong. *European Child and Adolescent Psychiatry, 17*, 452–61.

Lev, A. (2006). Disordering gender identity: Gender Identity Disorder in the *DSM-IV-TR. Journal of Psychology and Human Sexuality, 17*, 35–69.

Levitt, E. E. (1957). The results of psychotherapy with children: An evaluation. *Journal of Consulting Psychology, 21*, 189–96.

Levitt, E. E. (1963). Psychotherapy with children: A further evaluation. *Behaviour Research and Therapy, 1*, 45–51.

Levy, F., Hay, D. A., Bennett, K. S. and McStephen, M. (2005). Gender differences in ADHD subtype comorbidity. *Journal of the American Academy of Child and Adolescent Psychiatry, 44*, 368–76.

Lewinsohn, P. M., Klein, D. N. and Seeley, J. R. (1995). Bipolar disorders in a community sample of older adolescents: Prevalence, phenomenology, comorbidity, and course. *Journal of the American Academy of Child and Adolescent Psychiatry, 34*, 454–63.

Lewinsohn, P. M. and Clarke, G. N. (1999). Psychosocial treatments for adolescent depression. *Clinical Psychology Review, 19*, 329–42.

Lewis, C., Watson, M. and Schaps, E. (2003). Building community in school: The child development project. In M. J. Elias, H. Arnold and C. S. Hussey (Eds.), *EQ+ IQ = Best leadership practices for caring and successful schools* (pp. 100–8). Thousand Oaks, CA: Corwin Press.

Lewis, J. (1993). Integration in Victorian schools: Radical social policy or old wine? In R. Slee (Ed.) *Is there a desk with my name on it?* (pp. 1–25). London: Routledge.

Lewis, K. (1993). Family functioning as perceived by parents of boys with attention deficit disorder. *Issues in Mental Health Nursing, 13*, 369–86.

Lewis, M., Haviland-Jones, J. M. and Barrett, L. F. (2008). *Handbook of Emotions* (3rd edn.). New York: Guilford Press.

Lewis-Fernandez, R., Guarnaccia, P. J., Martinez, I. E., Salman, E., Schmidt, A. and Liebowitz, M. (2002). Comparative phenomenology of ataques de nervios,

panic attacks, and panic disorder. *Culture, Medicine and Psychiatry, 26*, 199–223.

Libby, A. M., Brent, D. A., Morrato, E. H., Orton, H. D., Allen, R. and Valuck, R. J. (2007). Decline in treatment of pediatric depression after FDA advisory on risk of suicidality with SSRIs. *American Journal of Psychiatry, 164*, 884–91.

Liberman, A. F., van Horn, P. and Ippen, C. G. (2005). Toward evidence-based treatment: Child–parent psychotherapy with preschoolers exposed to marital violence. *Journal of the American Academy of Child and Adolescent Psychiatry, 44*, 1241–8.

Liechti, M. D., Valko, L., Müller, U. C., Döhnert, M., Drechsler, R., Steinhausen, H.-C. and Brandeis, D. (2013). Diagnostic value of resting electroencephalogram in Attention-Deficit/Hyperactivity Disorder across the lifespan. *Brain Topography, 26*, 135–51.

Light, R. J. and Pillemer, D. B. (1984). *Summing up: The science of reviewing research*. Cambridge, MA: Harvard University Press.

Lilenfeld, L. R., Walter, H. K., Greeno, C. G., Merikangas, K. R., Plotnicov, K., Pollice, C.,…Nagy, L. (1998). A controlled family study of anorexia nervosa and bulimia nervosa: Psychiatric disorders in first-degree relatives and effects of proband comorbidity. *Archives of General Psychiatry, 55*, 603–10.

Lim, A. (2011, February 24). Aspies, you are not alone. The *New York Times*. Retrieved from www.nytimes.com/2011/02/25/opinion/25iht-edlim25.html?_r=2&scp=4&sq=Gates%20asperger&st=cse

Lin, F., Downs, J., Li, J., Ba, X. O. and Leonard, H. (2013). Caring for a child with severe intellectual disability in China: The example of Rett syndrome. *Disability and Retardation, 35*, 343–51.

Lin, K., Smith, M. W. and Ortiz, V. (2001). Culture and psychopharmacology. *Psychiatric Clinics of North America, 24*, 523–38.

Lindgren, S. D., de Renzi, E. and Richman, L. C. (1985). Cross-national comparisons of developmental dyslexia in Italy and the United States. *Child Development, 56*, 1404–17.

Lindt, H. (1950). Mental hygiene clinics. In M. J. Shore (Ed.), *Twentieth century mental hygiene: New directions in mental health*. New York: Social Science Publishers.

Lingely-Pottie, P. and McGrath, P. J. (2006). A therapeutic alliance can exist without face-to-face contact. *Journal of Telemedicine and Telecare, 12*, 396–9.

Linton, R. (1945). *The cultural background of personality*. New York: Appleton-Century-Crofts.

Liu, C., Conn, K., Sarkar, N. and Stone, W. (2008). Physiology-based affect recognition for computer-assisted intervention of children with Autism Spectrum

Disorder. *International Journal of Human-Computer Studies, 66,* 662–77.

Liu, R. T. (2010). Early life stressors and genetic influences on the development of bipolar disorder: The roles of childhood abuse and brain-derived neurotrophic factor. *Child Abuse and Neglect, 34,* 516–22.

Locascio, G., Mahone, E. M., Eason, S. H. and Cutting, L. E. (2010). Executive dysfunction among children with reading comprehension deficits. *Journal of Learning Disabilities, 43,* 441–54.

Lochman, J. E., Lampron, L. B., Gemmer, T. C., Harris, S. R. and Wyckoff, G. M. (1989). Teacher consultation and cognitive-behavioral interventions with aggressive boys. *Psychology in the Schools, 26,* 179–88.

Lochman, J. E. and Wells, K. C. (2004). The coping power program for preadolescent aggressive boys and their parents: Outcome effects at the 1-year follow-up. *Journal of Consulting and Clinical Psychology, 72,* 571–8.

Lock, J. and Fitzpatrick, K. K. (2009). Advances in psychotherapy for children and adolescents with eating disorders. *American Journal of Psychotherapy, 63,* 287–303.

Lock, J., Le Grange, D., Agras, W. S. and Dare, C. (2001). *Treatment manual for anorexia nervosa: A family-based approach.* New York: Guilford Press.

Lock, J., Le Grange, D., Agras, W. S., Moye, A., Bryson, S. W. and Jo, B. (2010). Randomized clinical trial comparing family-based treatment with adolescent-focused individual therapy for adolescents with anorexia nervosa. *Archives of General Psychiatry, 67,* 1025–32.

Locurto, C. (1991). Beyond IQ in preschool programs? *Intelligence, 15,* 295–312.

Loeb, K. L., Hirsch, A. M., Greif, R. and Hildebrandt, T. B. (2009). Family-based treatment of a 17-year-old twin presenting with emerging anorexia nervosa: A case study using the "Maudsley Method." *Journal of Clinical Child and Adolescent Psychology, 38,* 176–83.

Loeber, R., Keenan, K., Lahey, B. B., Green, S. M. and Thomas, C. (1993). Evidence for developmentally based diagnoses of oppositional defiant disorder and conduct disorder. *Journal of Abnormal Child Psychology, 21,* 377–410.

Loeber, R., Keenan, K. and Zhang, Q. (1997). Boys' experimentation and persistence in developmental pathways toward serious delinquency. *Journal of Child and Family Studies, 6,* 321–57.

Loeber, R., DeLamatre, M. S., Keenan, K. and Zhang, Q. (1998). A prospective replication of developmental pathways in disruptive and delinquent behavior. In R. B. Cairns, L. R. Bergman and J. Kagan (Eds.), *Methods and models for studying the individual* (pp. 185–216). Thousand Oaks, CA: Sage.

Loeber, R., Burke, J. D., Lahey, B. B., Winters, A. and Zera, M. (2000). Oppositional defiant and conduct disorder: A review of the past 10 years, part 1. *Journal of the American Academy of Child and Adolescent Psychiatry, 39,* 1468–84.

Loeber, R., Burke, J. and Pardini, D. A. (2009). Perspectives on oppositional defiant disorder, conduct disorder, and psychopathic features. *Journal of Child Psychology and Psychiatry, 50,* 133–42.

Logan, A. (2005). A suitable person for suitable cases: The gendering of juvenile courts in England c.1910–39, *20th Century British History, 16,* 129–45.

Lombardo, M. V. and Baron-Cohen, S. (2011). The role of the self in mindblindness in autism. *Consciousness and Cognition, 20,* 130–40.

Loncan, A. (2009). Neglected children: From destructive impulses to creativity. *Le Divan Familial, 23,* 59–73.

Loney, B. R., Taylor, J., Butler, M. A. and Iacono, W. G. (2007). Adolescent psychopathy features: 6-year temporal stability and the prediction of externalizing symptoms during the transition to adulthood. *Aggressive Behavior, 33,* 242–52.

Lopata, C., Thomeer, M. L., Volker, M. A. and Nida, R. E. (2006). Effectiveness of a cognitive-behavioral treatment on the social behaviors of children with Asperger Disorder. *Focus on Autism and Other Developmental Disabilities, 21,* 237–44.

Lopez-Duran, N. L., Kovacs, M. and George, C. J. (2009). Hypothalamic-pituitary-adrenal axis dysregulation in depressed children and adolescents: A meta-analysis. *Psychoneuroendocrinology, 34,* 1272–83.

Lopez, I., Rivera, F., Ramirez, R., Guarnaccia, P. J., Canino, G. and Bird, H. R. (2009). Ataques de nervios and their psychiatric correlates in Puerto Rican children from two different contexts. *Journal of Nervous and Mental Disease, 197,* 923–9.

Lopez, S. R. and Guarnaccia, P. J. J. (2000). Cultural psychopathology: Uncovering the social world of mental illness. *Annual Review of Psychology, 51,* 571–98.

Lorber, M. F. (2004). Psychophysiology of aggression, psychopathy, and conduct problems: A meta-analysis. *Psychological Bulletin, 130,* 531–52.

Lorusso, M. L., Facoetti, A. and Bakker, D. J. (2011). Neuropsychological treatment of dyslexia: Does type of treatment matter? *Journal of Learning Disabilities, 44,* 136–49.

Losel, F. and Beelmann, A. (2003). Effects of child skills training in preventing antisocial behavior: A systematic review of randomized evaluations. *Annals of the American Academy of Political and Social Science, 587,* 84–109.

Losh, M. and Capps, L. (2006). Understanding of emotional experience in autism: Insights from the personal accounts of high-functioning children with autism. *Developmental Psychology*, *42*, 809–18.

Lovaas, O. I. (1987). Behavioral treatment and normal educational and intellectual functioning in young autistic children. *Journal of Consulting and Clinical Psychology*, *55*, 3–9.

Lovaas, O. I. (1989). Concerns about misinterpretation and placement of blame. *American Psychologist*, *44*, 1243–4.

Lovejoy, M. C., Graczyk, P. A., O'Hare, E. and Neuman, G. (2000). Maternal depression and parenting behavior: A meta-analytic review. *Clinical Psychology Review*, *20*, 561–92.

Lowry-Webster, H., Barrett, P. M. and Dadds, M. R. (2001). A universal prevention trial of anxiety and depressive symptomotology in childhood: Preliminary data from an Australian study. *Behaviour Change*, *18*, 36–50.

Lubke, G. H., Hudziak, J. J., Derks, E. M., van Bijsterveldt, T. C. E. M. and Boomsma, D. I. (2009). Maternal ratings of attention problems in ADHD: Evidence for the existence of a continuum. *Journal of the American Academy of Child and Adolescent Psychiatry*, *48*, 1085–93.

Luby, J. L., Heffelfinger, A., Mrakotsky, C., Brown, K., Hessler, M. and Spitznagel, E. (2003). Alterations in stress cortisol reactivity in depressed preschoolers relative to psychiatric and no-disorder comparison groups. *Archives of General Psychiatry*, *60*, 1248–55.

Luby, J. L., Mrakotsky, C., Heffelfinger, A., Brown, K. and Spitznagel, E. (2004). Characteristics of depressed preschoolers with and without anhedonia: Evidence for a melancholic depressive subtype in young children. *American Journal of Psychiatry*, *161*, 1998–2004.

Lucassen, N. et al. (2011). The association between paternal sensitivity and infant–father attachment security: A meta-analysis of three decades of research. *Journal of Family Psychology*, *25*(6), 986–92.

Luciano, S. and Savage, R. S. (2007). Bullying risk in children with learning difficulties in inclusive educational settings. *Canadian Journal of School Psychology*, *22*, 14–31.

Luckasson, R., Borthwick-Duffy, S., Buntinx, W. H. E., Coulter, D. L., Craig, E. M., Reeve, A.,…Tasse, M. J. (2002). *Mental retardation: Definition, classification, and systems of supports* (10th edn.). Washington, DC: American Association on Mental Retardation.

Lui, L. L., Lau, A. S., Chen, A. C., Dinh, K. T. and Kim, S. Y. (2009). The influence of maternal acculturation, neighbourhood disadvantage, and parenting on Chinese American adolescents' conduct problems: Testing the segmented assimilation hypothesis. *Journal of Youth and Adolescence*, *38*, 691–702.

Luis, T. M., Varela, R. E. and Moore, K. W. (2008). Parenting practices and childhood anxiety reporting in Mexican, Mexican American, and European American families. *Journal of Anxiety Disorders*, *22*, 1011–20.

Luna, B. and Sweeney, J. A. (2004). The emergence of collaborative brain function: fMRI studies of the development of response inhibition. *Annals of the New York Academy of Sciences*, *1021*, 296–309.

Lundahl, B., Risser, H. J. and Lovejoy, M. C. (2006). A meta-analysis of parent training: Moderators and follow-up effects. *Clinical Psychology Review*, *26*, 86–104.

Luu, P., Collins, P. and Tucker, D. M. (2000). Mood, personality, and self-monitoring: Negative affect and emotionality in relation to frontal lobe mechanisms of error monitoring. *Journal of Experimental Psychology: General*, *129*, 43–60.

Luzzatto, M. H. (1997). *The Way of God*. New York: Feldheim.

Lynskey, M. T., Agrawal, A. and Heath, A. C. (2010). Genetically informative research on adolescent substance use: Methods, findings, and challenges. *Journal of the American Academy of Child and Adolescent Psychiatry*, *49*, 1202–14.

Lyon, A. R. and Cotler, S. (2009). Multi-systemic intervention for school refusal behavior: Integrating approaches across disciplines. *Advances in School Mental Health Promotion*, *2*, 20–34.

Lyons, V. and Fitzgerald, M. (2005). *Asperger Syndrome: A gift or a curse?* New York: Nova Science Publishers.

Lyons-Ruth, K. (1996). Attachment relationships among children with aggressive behavior problems: The role of disorganized early attachment patterns. *Journal of Consulting and Clinical Psychology*, *64*, 64–73.

Lyons-Ruth, K., Alpern, L. and Repacholi, B. (1993). Disorganized infant attachment classification and maternal psychosocial problems as predictors of hostile-aggressive behavior in the preschool classroom. *Child Development*, *64*, 572–85.

Lyytinen, P., Rasku-Puttonen, H., Poikkeus, A., Laakso, M. and Ahonen, T. (1994). Mother–child teaching strategies and learning disabilities. *Journal of Learning Disabilities*, *27*, 186–92.

Maccoby, E. (1990). Gender and relationships: A developmental account. *American Psychologist*, *45*, 513–20.

Maccoby, E. (1998). *The two sexes growing up apart, coming together*. Cambridge, MA: The Belknap Press of Harvard University Press.

Maccoby, E. D. and Martin, J. A. (1983). Socialization in the context of the family: Parent–child interaction. In P. H. Mussen (Series Ed.) and E. M. Hetherington

(Vol. Ed.), *Handbook of child psychology:* Vol. IV. *Socialization, personality, and social development* (4th edn.). New York: Wiley.

MacDonald, E. E. and Hastings, R. P. (2010). Mindful parenting and care involvement of fathers of children with intellectual disabilities. *Journal of Child and Family Studies, 19,* 236–40.

Machado, L. A. (1980). *The right to be intelligent.* New York: Pergamon Press.

MacLean, P. D. (1990). A reinterpretation of memorative functions of the limbic system. In E. Goldberg (Ed.), *Contemporary neuropsychology and the legacy of Luria* (pp. 127–54). Hillsdale, NJ: Lawrence Erlbaum Associates.

MacMillan, D. L. and Siperstein, G. N. (2002). Learning disabilities as operationally defined as schools. In R. Bradley, L. Danielson and D. P. Hallahan (Eds.), *Identification of learning disabilities: Research to practice* (pp. 287–333). Mahwah, NJ: Lawrence Erlbaum Associates.

MacMillan, D. L., Siperstein, G. N. and Leffert, J. S. (2006). Children with mild mental retardation: A challenge for classification practices – revised. In H. N. Switzky and S. Greenspan (Eds.), *What is mental retardation: Ideas for an evolving disability in the 21st century* (pp. 197–220). Washington, DC: American Association on Mental Retardation.

Magaña, S., Schwartz, S. J., Rubert, M. P. and Szapocznik, J. (2006). Hispanic caregivers of adults with mental retardation: Importance of family functioning. *American Journal on Mental Retardation, 111,* 250–62.

Maher, C. A. (1984). Handicapped adolescents as cross-age tutors: Program description and evaluation. *Exceptional Children, 51,* 56–63.

Maheu, F. S., Dozier, M., Guyer, A. E., Mandell, D., Peloso, E., Poeth, K. et al. (2010). A preliminary study of medial temporal lobe function in youths with a history of caregiver deprivation and emotional neglect. *Cognitive, Affective, and Behavioral Neuroscience, 10,* 34–49.

Maikovich, A. K., Jaffee, S. R., Odgers, C. L. and Gallop, R. (2008). Effects of family violence on psychopathology symptoms in children previously exposed to maltreatment. *Child Development, 79,* 1498–512.

Maimonides, M. (1956). *The guide for the perplexed.* New York: Dover. (Original work published in the twelfth century A.D.)

Main, M. and Hesse, E. (1990). Parents' unresolved traumatic experiences are related to infant disorganized attachment status: Is frightened and/or frightening parental behaviour the linking mechanism? In M. T. Greenberg, D. Cicchetti and M. E. Cummings (Eds.), *Attachment in the preschool years: Theory, research,*

and intervention (pp. 161–82). Chicago, IL: University of Chicago Press.

Main, M. and Solomon, J. (1990). Procedures for identifying infants as disorganized/disoriented during the Ainsworth strange situation. In M. T. Greenberg, D. Cicchetti and M. Cummings (Eds.), *Attachment in the preschool years: Theory, research, and intervention* (pp. 121–60). Chicago: The University of Chicago Press.

Manassis, K. (2001). Child–parent relations: Attachment and anxiety disorders. In W. K. Silverman and P. D. A. Treffers (Eds.), *Anxiety disorders in children and adolescents: Research, assessment and intervention* (pp. 255–72). New York: Cambridge University Press.

Mandler, G. (1979). Emotion. In E. Hearst (Ed.), *The first century of experimental psychology* (pp. 375–91). Hilldale, NJ: Erlbaum.

Manetti, M., Schneider, B. H. and Siperstein, G. (2001). Social acceptance of children with mental retardation: Testing the contact hypothesis with an Italian sample. *International Journal of Behavioral Development, 25,* 279–86.

Maniadaki, K., Sonuga-Barke, E. and Kakouros, E. (2005). Parents' causal attributions about attention deficit/hyperactivity disorder: The effect of child and parent sex. *Child: Care, Health and Development, 31,* 331–40.

Manners, P. J. (2009). Gender identity disorder in adolescence: A review of the literature. *Child and Adolescent Mental Health, 14,* 62–8.

Mannie, Z. N., Harmer, C. J. and Cowen, P. J. (2007). Increased waking salivary cortisol levels in young people at familial risk of depression. *American Journal of Psychiatry,164,* 617–21.

March, S., Spence, S. H. and Donovan, C. L. (2009). The efficacy of an Internet-based cognitive-behavioral therapy intervention for child anxiety disorders. *Journal of Pediatric Psychology, 34,* 474–87.

Marchand, E., Stice, E., Rohde, P. and Becker, C. B. (2011). Moving from efficacy to effectiveness trials in prevention research. *Behaviour Research and Therapy, 49,* 32–41.

Marchand, W. R., Wirth, L. and Simon, C. (2006). Delayed diagnosis of pediatric bipolar disorder in a community mental health setting. *Journal of Psychiatric Practice, 12,* 128–33.

Marcus, R. F. and Betzer, P. D. S. (1996). Attachment and antisocial behavior in early adolescence. *The Journal of Early Adolescence, 16,* 229–48.

Marecek, J. (1993). Disappearances, silences, and anxious rhetoric: Gender in abnormal psychology textbooks. *Journal of Theoretical and Philosophical Psychology, 13,* 114–23.

Margalit, M. and Al-Yagon, M. (2002). The loneliness experience of children with learning disabilities. In

B. Y. L. Wong and M. L. Donahue (Eds.), *The social dimensions of learning disabilities: Essays in honor of Tanis Bryan* (pp. 53–75). Mahwah, NJ: Lawrence Erlbaum Associates.

Margalit, M. and Heiman, T. (1986). Family climate and anxiety in families with learning disabled boys. *Journal of the American Academy of Child Psychiatry, 25,* 841–6.

Margolin, G. and Vickerman, K. A. (2007). Posttraumatic stress in children and adolescents exposed to family violence: I. Overview and issues. *Professional Psychology: Research and Practice, 38,* 613–19.

Mariano, K. A. and Harton, H. C. (2005). Similarities in aggression, inattention/hyperactivity, depression, and anxiety in middle childhood friendships. *Journal of Social and Clinical Psychology, 24,* 471–96.

Marineau, R. F. (1989). *Jacob Levy Moreno, 1889–1974: Father of psychodrama, sociometry, and group psychotherapy.* London: Routledge.

Marini, Z. A., Dane, A. V. and Bosacki, S. L. (2006). Direct and indirect bully-victims: Differential psychosocial risk factors associated with adolescents involved in bullying and victimization. *Aggressive Behavior, 32,* 551–69.

Markus, H. R. and Kitayama, S. (1991). Culture and the self: Implications for cognition, emotion, and motivation. *Psychological Review, 98,* 224–53.

Marsh, P., Beauchaine, T. P. and Williams, B. (2008b). Dissociation of sad facial expressions and autonomic nervous system responding in boys with disruptive behavior disorders. *Psychophysiology, 45,* 100–10.

Martin, C. S. et al. (1995), Patterns of DSM-IV alcohol abuse and dependence symptoms in adolescent drinkers. *Journal of Studies on Alcohol, 56*(6), 672–80.

Martin, E. A. (2010). *Concise Medical Dictionary* (8th edn.). Oxford: Oxford University Press.

Marvin, R., Cooper, G., Hoffman, K. and Powell, B. (2002). The circle of security project: Attachment-based intervention with caregiver-pre-school child dyads. *Attachment and Human Development, 4,* 107–24.

Mascres, C. and Strobel, M. (2000). Relations between depressive mood and somatization: Recension of the writings around the portrait targets of the somatisator. *Canadian Psychology, 41,* 52–60.

Maser, J. D., Norman, S. B., Zissok, S., Everall, I. P., Stein, M. B., Schettler, P. J. and Judd, L. L. (2009). Psychiatric nosology is ready for a paradigm shift in DSM-V. *Clinical Psychology: Science and Practice, 16,* 24–40.

Mash, E. J. and Johnston, C. (1982). A comparison of mother–child interactions of younger and older hyperactive and normal children. *Child Development, 53,* 1371–81.

Mash, E. J. and Barkley, R. A. (2002). *Child psychopathology.* New York: Guilford Press.

Mash, E. J. and Hunsley, J. (2005). Evidence-based assessment of child and adolescent disorders: Issues and challenges. *Journal of Clinical Child and Adolescent Psychology, 34,* 362–79.

Mason, M. J., Schmidt, C., Abraham, A., Walker, L. and Tercyak, K. (2009). Adolescents' social environment and depression: Social networks, extracurricular activity, and family relationship influences. *Journal of Clinical Psychology in Medical Settings, 16,* 346 54.

Masten, A. S. and Curtis, W. J. (2000). Integrating competence and psychopathology: Pathways toward a comprehensive science of adaptation in development. *Development and Psychopathology, 12,* 529–50.

Masten, A. S. (2005). Peer relationships and psychopathology in developmental perspective: Reflections on progress and promise. *Journal of Clinical Child and Adolescent Psychology, 34,* 87–92.

Masten, A. S. (2011). Resilience in children threatened by extreme adversity: Frameworks for research, practice, and translational synergy. *Development and Psychopathology, 23,* 493–506.

Masterpasqua, F. (2009). Psychology and epigenetics. *Review of General Psychology, 13,* 194–201.

Matheson, C., Olsen, R. J. and Weisner, T. (2007). A good friend is hard to find: Friendship among adolescents with disabilities. *American Journal on Mental Retardation, 112,* 319–29.

Mathew, S. J., Coplan, J. D., Goetz, R. R., Feder, A., Greenwald, S., Dahl, R. E. et al. (2003). Differentiating depressed adolescent 24 h cortisol secretion in light of their adult clinical outcome. *Neuropsychopharmacology, 28,* 1336–43.

Matos, M., Bauermeister, J. J. and Bernal, G. (2009). Parent–child interaction therapy for Puerto Rican preschool children with ADHD and behavior problems: A pilot efficacy study. *Family Process, 48,* 232–52.

Matsumoto, D. (Ed.) (2009). *The Cambridge dictionary of psychology.* Cambridge: Cambridge University Press.

Mattick, J. S. (2005). The functional genomics of noncoding RNA. *Science, 309,* 1527–8.

Maughan, B. and Rutter, M. (2001). Antisocial children grown up. In J. Hill and B. Maughan (Eds.), *Conduct disorders in childhood and adolescence* (pp. 507–52). Cambridge: Cambridge University Press.

Maughan, B., Rowe, R., Messer, J., Goodman, R. and Meltzer, H. (2004). Conduct disorder and oppositional defiant disorder in a national sample: Developmental epidemiology. *Journal of Child Psychology and Psychiatry, 45,* 609–21.

Maughan, B., Iervolino, A. C. and Collishaw, S.(2005) Time trends in child and adolescent mental disorders. *Current Opinion in Psychiatry*, *18*(4), 381–5.

Maughan, B., Messer, J., Collishaw, S., Pickles, A., Snowling, M., Yule, W. and Rutter, M. (2009). Persistence of literacy problems: Spelling in adolescence and at mid-life. *Journal of Child Psychology and Psychiatry*, *50*, 893–901.

Maulik, P. K., Mascarenhas, M. N., Mathers, C. D., Dua, T. and Saxena, S. (2011). Prevalence of intellectual disability: A meta-analysis of population-based studies. *Research in Developmental Disabilities*, *32*, 419–36.

Maurice, C., Green, G. and Foxx, R. M. (2001). *Making a difference: Behavioral intervention for autism*. Austin, TX: Pro-Ed.

Maxwell, M. A. and Cole, D. A. (2009). Weight change and appetite disturbance as symptoms of adolescent depression: Toward an integrative biopsychosocial model. *Clinical Psychology Review*, *29*, 260–73.

Mayes, R. and Horwitz, A. V. (2005). DSM-III and the revolution in the classification of mental illness. *Journal of the History of the Behavioral Sciences*, *41*, 249–67.

Mayes, R. and Rafalovich, A. (2007). Suffer the restless children: The evolution of ADHD and paediatric stimulant use, 1900–80. *History of Psychiatry*, *18*, 435–57.

Mayes, S. D., Calhoun, S. L., Chase, G. A., Mink, D. M. and Stagg, R. E. (2009). ADHD subtypes and co-occurring anxiety, depression, and oppositional-defiant disorder: Differences in Gordon Diagnostic System and Wechsler Working Memory and Processing Speed Index scores. *Journal of Attention Disorders*, *12*, 540–50.

Mazurek, M. O. and Kanne, S. M. (2010). Friendship and internalizing symptoms among children and adolescents with ASD. *Journal of Autism and Developmental Disorders*, *40*, 1512–20.

Mazzeo, S. E., Landt, M. C. T., van Furth, E. F. and Bulik, C. M. (2006). Genetics of eating disorders. In S. Wonderlich, J. E. Mitchell, M. de Zwaan and H. Steiger (Eds.), *Annual review of eating disorders: Part 2* (pp. 17–33). Abingdon: Radcliffe Publishing.

McAdams, T., Rowe, R., Rijsdijk, F., Maughan, B. and Eley, T. C. (2012). The covariation of antisocial behavior and substance use in adolescence: A behavioral genetic perspective. *Journal of Research on Adolescence*, *22*, 100–12.

McBurnett, K., Lahey, B. B., Rathouz, P. J. and Loeber, R. (2000). Low salivary cortisol and persistent aggression in boys referred for disruptive behavior. *Archives of General Psychiatry*, *57*, 38–43.

McBurnett, K., Raine, A., Stouthamer-Loeber, M., Loeber, R., Kumar, A. M., Kumar, M. et al. (2005). Mood and hormone responses to psychological challenge in adolescent males with conduct problems. *Biological Psychiatry*, *57*, 1109–16.

McCabe, K. M., Lucchini, S. E., Hough, R. L., Yeh, M. and Hazen, A. (2005). The relation between violence exposure and conduct problems among adolescents: A prospective study. *American Journal of Orthopsychiatry*, *75*, 575–84.

McCabe, M. P. and Ricciardelli, L. A. (2003). Body image and strategies to lose weight and increase muscle among boys and girls. *Health Psychology*, *22*, 39–46.

McCabe, R. and Priebe, S. (2004). Explanatory models of illness in schizophrenia: Comparison of four ethnic groups. *British Journal of Psychiatry*, *185*, 25–30.

McCain, A. P. and Kelley, M. L. (1993). Managing the classroom behavior of an ADHD preschooler: The efficacy of a school–home note intervention. *Child and Family Behavior Therapy*, *15*, 33–44.

McCarthy, D. M., Tomlinson, K. L., Anderson, K. G., Marlatt, G. A. and Brown, S. A. (2005). Relapse in Alcohol- and Drug-Disordered Adolescents With Comorbid Psychopathology: Changes in Psychiatric Symptoms. *Psychology of Addictive Behaviors*, *19*, 28–34.

McClure, E. B., Kubiszyn, T. and Kaslow, N. J. (2002). Advances in the diagnoses and treatment of childhood disorders. *Professional Psychology: Research and Practice*, *33*, 125–34.

McClure, E. B., Monk, C. S., Nelson, E. E., Parrish, J. M., Adler, A., Blair, R. J. et al. (2007). Abnormal attention modulation of fear circuit function in pediatric generalized anxiety disorder. *Archives of General Psychiatry*, *64*, 97–106.

McCord, J. (1992). The Cambridge-Somerville Study: A pioneering longitudinal experimental study of delinquency prevention. In J. McCord and R. E. Tremblay (Eds.), *Preventing antisocial behavior: Interventions from birth through adolescence* (pp. 196–206). New York: Guilford Press.

McCready, K. F. (1986). The Medical Metaphor: A Better Model? *Health Alliance for Life and Longevity*. Retrieved from www.medsfree.com/Metaphor.htm

McCune, N. and Hynes, J. (2005). Ten year follow-up of children with school refusal. *Irish Journal of Psychological Medicine*, *22*, 56–8.

McDermott, P. A. (1996). A nationwide study of developmental and gender prevalence for psychopathology in childhood and adolescence. *Journal of Abnormal Child Psychology*, *24*, 53–66.

McDowell, D. J. and Parke, R. D. (2009). Parental correlates of children's peer relations: An empirical test of a tripartite model. *Developmental Psychology*, *45*, 224–35.

McDowell, J. J. (1988). Matching theory in natural human environments. *The Behavior Analyst, 11*, 95–109.

McFall, R. M. (2005). Theory and utility-key themes in evidence-based assessment: Comment on the special section. *Psychological Assessment, 17*, 312–23.

McEwen, B. S. (2012). Brain on stress: How the social environment gets under the skin. *PNAS, 109*, 17180–5.

McGowan, P. O., Sasaki, A., D'Alessio, A. C., Dymov, S., Labonte, B., Szyf, M. et al. (2009). Epigenetic regulation of the glucocorticoid receptor in human brain associates with childhood abuse. *Nature Neuroscience, 12*, 342–8.

McGraw-Hill dictionary of scientific and technical terms (6th edn.) (2003). New York: McGraw-Hill.

McHale, S. and Crouter, A. C. (2000). The social contexts of activities in preadolescence: Links with psychosocial adjustment. Paper presented at the Society for Research on Adolescence, Chicago, IL.

McIntosh, K., Chard, D. J., Boland, J. B. and Horner, R. H. (2006). Demonstration of combined efforts in school-wide academic and behavioral systems and incidence of reading and behavior challenges in early elementary grades. *Journal of Positive Behavior Interventions, 8*, 146–54.

McKenzie, R. G. (2009). Obscuring vital distinctions: The oversimplification of learning disabilities within RTI. *Learning Disability Quarterly, 32*, 203–15.

McKinley, N. M. (1999). Women and objectified body consciousness: Mothers' and daughters' body experience in cultural, developmental, and familial context. *Developmental Psychology, 35*, 760–9.

McKinley, N. M. and Hyde, J. S. (1996). The objectified body consciousness scale: Development and validation. *Psychology of Women Quarterly, 20*, 181–215.

McKinney, C. and Renk, K. (2011). Atypical antipsychotic medications in the management of disruptive behaviors in children: Safety guidelines and recommendations. *Clinical Psychology Review, 31*, 465–71.

McLeod, B. D., Weisz, J. R. and Wood, J. J. (2007). Examining the association between parenting and childhood depression: A meta-analysis. *Clinical Psychology Review, 27*, 986–1003.

McMahon, C. M., Wacker, D. P., Sasso, G. P., Berg, W. K. and Newton, S. M. (1996). Analysis of frequency and type of interactions in a peer-mediated social skills intervention: instructional vs. social interactions. *Education and Training in Mental Retardation and Developmental Disabilities, 31*, 339–52.

McMahon, R. J. and Kotler, J. S. (2008). Evidence-based therapies for oppositional behaviour in young children. In R. G. Steele, T. D. Elkin and M. C. Roberts (Eds.), *Handbook of evidence-based therapies for children and adolescents: Bridging science and practice* (pp. 221–40). New York: Springer Science and Business Media.

McMillan, D. W. and Chavis, D. M. (1986). Sense of community: A definition and theory. *Journal of Community Psychology, 14*, 6–23.

McNamara, J., Vervaeke, S. and Willoughby, T. (2008). Learning disabilities and risk-taking behavior in adolescents: A comparison of those with and without comorbid attention-deficit/hyperactivity disorder. *Journal of Learning Disabilities, 41*, 561–74.

McNamara, J. K., Willoughby, T., Chalmers, H. and YLC-CURA. (2005). Psychosocial status of adolescents with learning disabilities with and without comorbid attention deficit hyperactivity disorder. *Learning Disabilities Research and Practice, 20*, 234–44.

McNamara, R. K., Nandagopal, J. J., Strakowski, S. M. and DelBello, M. P. (2010). Preventative strategies for early-onset bipolar disorder: Towards a clinical staging model. *CNS Drugs, 24*, 983–96.

McNaughton, N. and Corr, P. J. (2004). A two-dimensional neuropsychology of defense: Fear/anxiety and defensive distance. *Neuroscience and Biobehavioral Reviews, 28*, 285–305.

McNeely, C. A. and Barber, B. K. (2010). How do parents make adolescents feel loved? Perspectives on supportive parenting from adolescents in 12 cultures. *Journal of Adolescent Research, 25*, 601–31.

McNeil, D. W. (2001). Evolution of terminology and constructs in social anxiety and its disorders. In S. G. Hofmann and P. M. DiBartolo (Eds.), *Social anxiety: Clinical, developmental, and social perspectives* (pp. 3–23). London: Academic Press.

McShane, G., Walter, G. and Rey, J. M. (2004). Functional outcome of adolescents with "school refusal." *Clinical Child Psychology and Psychiatry, 9*, 53–60.

McShane, K. E. and Hastings, P. D. (2009). The new friends vignettes: Measuring parental psychological control that confers risk for anxious adjustment in preschoolers. *International Journal of Behavioral Development, 33*, 481–95.

McVey, G. and Davis, R. (2002). A program to promote positive body image: A 1-year follow-up evaluation. *The Journal of Early Adolescence, 22*, 96–108.

Mealey, L. (2005). Evolutionary psychopathology and abnormal development. In R. L. Burgess and K. MacDonald (Eds.), *Evolutionary perspectives on human development* (pp. 381–406). Thousand Oaks, CA: Sage Publications.

Mead, G. E., Morley, W., Campbell, P., Greig, C. A., McMurdo, M. and Lawlor, D. A. (2008). Exercise for depression. *Cochrane Database of Systematic Reviews*, Oct. 8; (4):CD004366.

Measelle, J. R., Stice, E. and Hogansen, J. M. (2006). Developmental trajectories of co-occurring depressive, eating, antisocial, and substance abuse problems in female adolescents. *Journal of Abnormal Psychology*, *115*, 524–38.

Meehl, P. (1960). The cognitive activity of the clinician. *American Psychologist*, *15*, 19–27.

Meehl, P. E. (1973). *Psychodiagnosis: Selected papers*. Oxford: Oxford University Press.

Meehl, P. E. (1992). Factors and taxa, traits and types, differences of degree and differences in kind. *Journal of Personality*, *60*, 117–74.

Meehl, P. E. (1995). Bootstraps taximetrics: Solving the classification problem in psychopathology. *American Psychologist*, *50*, 266–75.

Meichenbaum, D. (1977). *Cognitive-behavior modification: An integrative approach*. New York: Plenum.

Meiser-Stedman, R. (2002). Toward a cognitive-behavioral model of PTSD in children and adolescents. *Clinical Child and Family Psychology Review*, *5*, 217–32.

Mejia, A., Calam, R. and Sanders, M. R. (2012). A review of parenting programs in developing countries: Opportunities and challenges for preventing emotional and behavioral difficulties in children. *Clinical Child and Family Psychology Review*, *15*, 163–75.

Melekian, B. A. (1990). Family characteristics of children with dyslexia. *Journal of Learning Disabilities*, *23*, 386–91.

Menninger, K., Mayman, M. and Pruyser, P. (1963). *The vital balance: The life process in mental health and illness*. New York: Viking Press.

Menvielle, E. J. and Tuerk, C. (2002). A support group for parents of gender-nonconforming boys. *Journal of the American Academy of Child and Adolescent Psychiatry*, *41*, 1010–13.

Merikangas, K. R., Dierker, L. C. and Szatmari, P. (1998). Psychopathology among offspring of parents with substance abuse and/or anxiety disorders: A high-risk study. *Journal of Child Psychology and Psychiatry*, *39*, 711–20.

Merikangas, K. R., Avenevoli, S., Dierker, L. and Grillon, C. (1999). Vulnerability factors among children at risk for anxiety disorders. *Biological Psychiatry*, *46*, 1523–35.

Merwin, R. M., Zucker, N. L., Lacy, J. L. and Elliott, C. A. (2010). Interoceptive awareness in eating disorders: Distinguishing lack of clarity from nonacceptance of internal experience. *Cognition and Emotion*, *24*, 892–902.

Mesmen, E., Nolen, W. A., Reichart, C. G., Wais, M. and Hillegers, M. H. J. (2013). The Dutch bipolar offspring study: 12-year follow-up. *The American Journal of Psychiatry*, *170*, 542–9.

Mesman, J., Stolk, M. N., van Zeijl, J., Alink, L. R. A., Juffer, F., Bakermans-Kranenburg, M. J., van IJzendoorn, M. H. and Koot, H. M. (2008). Extending the video-feedback intervention to sensitive discipline: The early prevention of antisocial behavior. In F. Juffer, M. J. Bakermans-Kranenburg and M. H. van IJzendoorn (Eds.), *Promoting positive parenting: An attachment-based intervention* (pp. 171–91). New York: Lawrence Erlbaum/Taylor & Francis.

Meunier, J. C., Bisceglia, R. and Jenkins, J. M. (2012). Differential parenting and children's behavioral problems: Curvilinear associations and mother–father combined effects. *Developmental Psychology*, *48*, 987–1002.

Meyer, J. S. and Quenzer, L. F. (2005). *Psychopharmacology: Drugs, the brain, and behavior*. Sunderland, MA: Sinauer Associates.

Meyer-Bahlburg, H. F. L. (2002). Gender identity disorder in young boys: A parent- and peer-based treatment protocol. *Clinical Child Psychology and Psychiatry*, *7*, 360–76.

Meyer-Bahlburg, H. F. L. (2010). From mental disorder to iatrogenic hypogonadism: Dilemmas in conceptualizing gender identity variants as psychiatric conditions. *Archives of Sexual Behavior*, *39*, 461–76.

Meyler, A., Keller, T. A., Cherkassky, V. L., Gabrieli, J. D. E. and Just, M. A. (2008). Modifying the brain activation of poor readers during sentence comprehension with extended remedial instruction: A longitudinal study of neuroplasticity. *Neuropsychologia*, *46*, 2580–92.

Mezulis, A. H., Abramson, L. Y., Hyde, J. S. and Hankin, B. L. (2004). Is there a universal positivity bias in attributions? A meat-analytic review of individual, developmental and cultural differences in the self-serving attributional bias. *Psychological Bulletin*, *30*, 711–47.

Mezulis, A. H., Hyde, J. S. and Abramson, L. Y. (2006). The developmental origins of cognitive vulnerability to depression: Temperament, parenting, and negative life events in childhood as contributors to negative cognitive style. *Developmental Psychology*, *42*, 1012–25.

Mezzacappa, E., Tremblay, R. E., Kindlon, D., Saul, J. P., Arseneault, L., Seguin, J. et al. (1997). Anxiety, antisocial behavior, and heart rate regulation in adolescent males. *Journal of Child Psychology and Psychiatry*, *38*, 457–69.

Mezzich, J. E., Kirmayer, L. J., Kleinman, A., Fabrega, H., Parron, D. L., Good, B. J., Lin, K.-M. and Spero, M. (1999). The place of culture in DSM-IV. *Journal of Nervous and Mental Disease*, *187*, 457–64.

Michaud, I. and Boivin, J. (2009). When attachment disorder presents with symptoms of gender identity disorder: Case discussion. *Journal of the Canadian Academy of Child and Adolescent Psychiatry, 18,* 136–7.

Middeldorp, C. M., Cath, D. C., van Dyck, R. and Boomsma, D. I. (2005). The co-morbidity of anxiety and depression in the perspective of genetic epidemiology: A review of twin and family studies. *Psychological Medicine, 35,* 611–24.

Miers, A. C., Blöte, A. W. and Westenberg, P. M. (2010). Peer perceptions of social skills in socially anxious and nonanxious adolescents. *Journal of Abnormal Child Psychology, 38,* 33–41.

Miklowitz, D. J. (2004). The role of family systems in severe and recurrent psychiatric disorders: A developmental psychopathology view. *Development and Psychopathology, 16,* 667–88.

Miklowitz, D. J. and Chang, K. D. (2008). Prevention of bipolar disorder in at-risk children: Theoretical assumptions and empirical foundations. *Development and Psychopathology, 20,* 881–97.

Miklowitz, D. J., Schneck, C. D., Singh, M. K., Taylor, D. O., George, E. L., Cosgrove, V. E., Howe, M.,...Chang, K. D. (2013). Early intervention for symptomatic youth at risk for bipolar disorder: A randomized trial of family-focused therapy. *The Journal of the American Academy of Child Psychiatry, 52,* 121–31.

Milan, S., Zona, K., Acker, J. and Turcios-Cotto, V. (2013). Prospective risk factors for adolescent PTSD: Sources of differential exposure and differential vulnerability. *Journal of Abnormal Child Psychology, 41,* 339–53.

Milich, R. and Landau, S. (1982). Socialization and peer relations in hyperactive children. *Advances in Learning and Behavioral Disabilities, 1,* 283–339.

Milich, R. and Dodge, K. A. (1984). Social information processing in child psychiatric populations. *Journal of Abnormal Child Psychology, 12,* 471–89.

Milich, R. and Pelham, W. E. (1986). Effects of sugar ingestion on the classroom and playgroup behavior of attention deficit disordered boys. *Journal of Consulting and Clinical Psychology, 54,* 714–18.

Mill, J., Tang, T., Kaminsky, Z., Khare, T., Yazdanpanah, S., Bouchard, L. et al. (2008). Epigenomic profiling reveals DNA-methylation changes associated with major psychosis. *The American Journal of Human Genetics, 82,* 696–711.

Miller, A., Lee, S., Raina, A., Klassen, A., Zupancic, J. and Olsen, L. (1998). *A review of therapies for attention-deficit/hyperactivity disorder.* Ottawa: Canadian Coordinating Office for Health Technology Assessment.

Miller, G. A., Elbert, T., Sutton, B. P. and Heller, W. (2007). Innovative clinical assessment techniques: Challenges and opportunities in neuroimaging. *Psychological Assessment, 19,* 58–73.

Miller, G. M. and Tompkins, S. (1977). *Kidnapped! At Chowchilla.* Plainfield, NJ: Logos International.

Miller, H. C. (1923). *The new psychology and the parent.* London: Jarrolds.

Miller, L. and Kelley, B. (2006). Spiritually oriented psychotherapy with youth: A child-centered approach. In E. C. Roehlkepartain, P. E. King, L. Wagener and P. L. King (Eds.), *The handbook of spiritual development in childhood and adolescence* (pp. 421–34). Thousand Oaks, CA: Sage Publications.

Millon, T., Grossman, S. D. and Meagher, S. E. (2004). *Masters of the mind: Exploring the story of mental illness from ancient times to the new millennium.* Hoboken, NJ: Wiley.

Mills, C., Guerin, S., Lynch, F., Daly, I. and Fitzpatrick, C. (2004). The relationship between bullying, depression and suicidal thoughts/behaviour in Irish adolescents. *Irish Journal of Psychological Medicine, 21,* 112–16.

Minuchin, P. (1985). Families and individual development: Provocations from the field of family therapy. *Child Development, 56,* 289–302.

Minuchin, S. (1974). *Families and family therapy.* Cambridge, MA: Harvard University Press.

Minuchin, S., Rosman, B. L. and Baker, L. (1978). *Psychosomatic families: Anorexia nervosa in context.* Oxford: Harvard University Press.

Miranda, A. and Presentacion, M. J. (2000). Efficacy of cognitive-behavioral therapy in the treatment of children with ADHD, with and without aggressiveness. *Psychology in the Schools, 37,* 169–82.

Mirowsky, J. and Ross, C. E. (1989). Psychiatric diagnosis as reified measurement. *Journal of Health and Social Behavior, 30,* 11–25.

Mischel, W. (1968). *Personality and assessment.* Hoboken, NJ: John Wiley and Sons, Inc.

Miyaki, K. and Yamazaki, K. (1995). Self-conscious emotions, child rearing, and child psychopathology in Japanese culture. In J. P. Tangney and K. W. Fischer (Eds.), *Self-conscious emotions: The psychology of shame, guilt, embarrassment, and pride* (pp. 488–504). New York: Guilford Press.

Moffitt, T. (2005). The new look of behavioral genetics in developmental psychopathology: Gene–environment interplay in antisocial behaviors. *Psychological Bulletin, 131,* 533–54.

Moffitt, T. (2006). Life-course-persistent versus adolescent-limited antisocial behavior. In D. Cicchetti and D. Cohen (Eds.), *Developmental psychopathology* (Vol. III, pp. 570–98). New York: John Wiley and Sons, Inc.

Moffitt, T., Caspi, A., Rutter, M. and Silva, P. (2001). *Sex differences in antisocial behaviour: Conduct disorder, delinquency and violence in the Dunedin longitudinal study.* New York: Cambridge University Press.

Moffitt, T. E. (1993). Adolescence-limited and life-course-persistent antisocial behaviour: A developmental taxonomy. *Psychological Review, 100,* 674–701.

Moffitt, T. E. (2003). Life-course persistent and adolescent-limited antisocial behavior: A 10-year research review and a research agenda. In B. Lahey, T. E. Moffitt and A. Caspi (Eds.), *The causes of conduct disorder and serious juvenile delinquency* (pp. 49–75). New York: Guilford.

Mogg, K. and Bradley, B. P. (1998). A cognitive-motivational analysis of anxiety. *Behaviour Research and Therapy, 36,* 809–848.

Mogg, K., Millar, N. and Bradley, B. P. (2000). Biases in eye movements to threatening facial expressions in generalized anxiety disorder and depressive disorder. *Journal of Abnormal Psychology, 109,* 695–704.

Molina, B. S. G. and Pelham, W. E. (2003). Childhood predictors of adolescent substance use in a longitudinal study of children with ADHD. *Journal of Abnormal Psychology, 112,* 497–507.

Molina, B. S. G., Hinshaw, S. P., Swanson, J. M., Arnold, L. E., Vitiello, B., Jensen, P. S.,...Houck, P. R. (2009). The MTA at 8 years: Prospective follow-up of children treated for combined-type ADHD in a multisite study. *Journal of the American Academy of Child and Adolescent Psychiatry, 48,* 484–500.

Molinuevo, B., Bonillo, A., Pardo, Y., Doval, E. and Torrubia, R. (2010). Participation in extracurricular activities and emotional and behavioral adjustment in middle childhood in Spanish boys and girls. *Journal of Community Psychology, 38,* 842–57.

Molnar, B. E., Buka, S. L. and Kessler, R. C. (2001). Child sexual abuse and subsequent psychopathology: Results from the National Comorbidity Survey. *American Journal of Public Health, 91,* 753–60.

Monastra, V. J. (2004). *Parenting children with ADHD.* Washington, DC: American Psychological Association.

Monk, C. S., Nelson, E. E., Woldehawariat, G., Montgomery, L. A., Zarahn, E., McClure, E. B. et al. (2004). Experience-dependent plasticity for attention to threat: Behavioral and neurophysiological evidence in humans. *Biological Psychiatry, 56,* 607–10.

Monk, C. S., Telzer, E. H., Mogg, K., Bradley, B. P., Mai, X., Louro, H. M. et al. (2008). Amygdala and ventrolateral prefrontal cortex activation to masked angry faces in children and adolescents with generalized anxiety disorder. *Archives of General Psychiatry, 65,* 568–76.

Mora, G. (2008). Mental disturbances, unusual mental states and their interpretation in the Middle Ages. In E. R. Wallace and J. Gach (Eds.). *History of psychiatry and medical psychology.* New York: Springer.

Moradi, B. (2011). Objectification theory: Areas of promise and refinement. *The Counseling Psychologist, 39,* 153–63.

Morawska, A., Stallman, H. M., Sanders, M. R. and Ralph, A. (2005). Self-directed behavioural family intervention: Do therapists matter? *Child and Family Behavior Therapy, 27,* 51–72.

Moreland, A. D. and Dumas, J. E. (2009). Categorical and dimensional approaches to the measurement of disruptive behavior in the preschool years: A meta-analysis. *Clinical Psychology Review, 28,* 1059–70.

Morelen, D., Jacob, M. L., Suveg, C., Jones, A. and Thomassin, K. (2013). Family emotion expressivity, emotion regulation, and the link to psychopathology: Examination across race. *British Journal of Psychology, 104,* 149–66.

Moreno, C., Laje, G., Blanco, C., Jiang, H., Schmidt, A. B. and Olfson, M. (2007). National trends in the outpatient diagnosis and treatment of bipolar disorder in youth. *Archives of General Psychiatry, 64,* 1032–9.

Moreno, J. L. (1947). *The theater of spontaneity.* New York: Beacon.

Moreno, J. L. (1953). *Who shall survive?* New York: Beacon.

Morgan, P. L., Farkas, G., Tufis, P. A. and Sperling, R. A. (2008). Are reading and behavior problems risk factors for each other? *Journal of Learning Disabilities, 41,* 417–36.

Morgan, P. L., Farkas, G. and Wu, Q. (2009). Kindergarten predictors of recurring externalizing and internalizing psychopathology in the third and fifth grades. *Journal of Emotional and Behavioral Disorders, 17,* 67–79.

Morral, A. R., McCaffrey, D. F. and Ridgeway, G. (2004). Adolescent substance abuse treatment: A review of evidence-based research. *Psychology of Addictive Behavior, 18,* 267–8.

Morris, J. S., Frith, C. D., Perrett, D. I., Rowland, D., Young, A. W., Calder, A. J. et al. (1996). A differential neural response in the human amygdala to fearful and happy facial expressions. *Nature, 383,* 812–15.

Morris, T. L. and Masia, C. L. (1998). Psychometric evaluation of the Social Phobia and Anxiety Inventory for Children: Concurrent validity and normative data. *Journal of Clinical Child Psychology, 27,* 452–8.

Morris, W. (2000). *American heritage dictionary of the English language.* Boston: Houghton-Mifflin.

Morrison, G. M. and Zetlin, A. (1992). Family profiles of adaptability, cohesion, and communication for learning handicapped and nonhandicapped adolescents. *Journal of Youth and Adolescence, 21,* 225–40.

Moser, R. P. and Jacob, T. (2002). Parental and sibling effects in adolescent outcomes. *Psychological Reports, 91,* 463–79.

Moss, E., Smolla, N., Cyr, C., Dubois-Comtois, K., Mazzarello, T. and Berthiaume, C. (2006). Attachment and behavior problems in middle childhood as reported by adult and child informants. *Development and Psychopathology, 18*, 425–44.

Mostert, M. P. (2010). Facilitated communication and its legitimacy – twenty-first century developments. *Exceptionality, 18*, 31–41.

Mowlds, W., Shannon, C., McCusker, C. G., Meenagh, C., Robinson, D., Wilson, A. and Mulholland, C. (2010). Autobiographical memory specificity, depression, and trauma in bipolar disorder. *British Journal of Clinical Psychology, 49*, 217–33.

Mrazek, P. J. and Haggerty, R. J. (1994). *Reducing risks for mental disorders: Frontiers for preventive intervention research.* Washington, DC: National Academy Press.

Mrug, S., Gaines, J., Su, W. and Windle, M. (2010). School-level substance use: Effects on early adolescents' alcohol, tobacco, and marijuana use. *Journal of Studies on Alcohol and Drugs, 71*, 488–95.

Mrug, S., Hoza, B. and Gerdes, A. C. (2001). Children with attention-deficit/hyperactivity disorder: Peer relationships and peer-oriented interventions. In D. W. Nangle and C. A. Erdley (Eds.), *The role of friendship in psychological adjustment* (pp. 51–77). San Francisco, CA: Jossey-Bass.

Mrug, S., Hoza, B., Gerdes, A. C., Hinshaw, S., Arnold, L. E., Hechtman, L. and Pelham, W. E. (2009). Discriminating between children with ADHD and classmates using peer variables. *Journal of Attention Disorders, 12*, 372–80.

MTA Cooperative Group. (1999a). A 14-month randomized clinical trial of treatment strategies for attention-deficit hyperactivity disorder. *Archives of General Psychiatry, 56*, 1073–86.

MTA Cooperative Group. (1999b). Moderators and mediators of treatment response for children with attention-deficit/hyperactivity disorder: The Multimodal Treatment Study of children with attention-deficit/hyperactivity disorder. *Archives of General Psychiatry, 56*, 1088–96.

MTA Cooperative Group. (2004). National institute of mental health multimodal treatment study of ADHD follow-up: 24-month outcomes of treatment strategies for attention-deficit/hyperactivity disorder. *Pediatrics, 113*, 754–61.

Mufson, L., Dorta, K. P., Wickramaratne, P., Nomura, Y., Olfson, M. and Weissman, M. M. (2004). A randomized effectiveness trial of interpersonal psychotherapy for depressed adolescents. *Archives of General Psychiatry, 61*, 577–84.

Mufson, L., Pollack Dorta, K., Olfson, M., Weissman, M. M., Hoagwood, K., Mufson, L., Dorta, K. P., Olfson, M., Weissman, M. M. and Hoagwood, K. (2004).

Effectiveness research: Transporting interpersonal psychotherapy for depressed adolescents (IPT-A) from the lab to school-based health clinics. *Clinical Child and Family Psychology Review, 7*, 251–61.

Mulder, E. J., Anderson, G. M., Kema, I. P., de Bildt, A., van Lang, N. D. J., den Boer, J. A. and Minderaa, R. B. (2004). Platelet serotonin levels in pervasive developmental disorders and mental retardation: Diagnostic group differences, within-group distribution, and behavioral correlates. *Journal of the American Academy of Child and Adolescent Psychiatry, 43*, 491–9.

Muller, C. (2003). Paul Dubois, pionnier de la psychothérapie. *Psychothérapies, 23*, 49–52.

Munoz, L. C. and Frick, P. J. (2007). The reliability, stability, and predictive utility of the self-report version of the Antisocial Process Screening Device. *Scandinavian Journal of Psychology, 48*, 299–312.

Munro, J. D. (2011). Couple therapy for people with intellectual disabilities: A positive treatment model. In R. J. Fletcher (Ed.), *Psychotherapy for individuals with intellectual disability* (pp. 235–61). Kingston, NY: NADD Press.

Murphy, K. R. and Barkley, R. A. (1996). Parents of children with attention-deficit/hyperactivity disorder: Psychological and attentional impairment. *American Journal of Orthopsychiatry, 66*, 93–102.

Murray-Seegert, C. (1989). *Nasty girls, thugs, and humans like us: Social relations between severely disabled and non-disabled students in high school.* Baltimore, MD: Paul H. Brookes.

Na, J. and Kitayama, S. (2011). Spontaneous trait inference is culture-specific behavioral and neural evidence. *Psychological Science, 22*, 1025–32.

Nabuzoka, D. and Ronning, J. A. (1997). Social acceptance of children with intellectual disabilities in an integrated school setting in Zambia: A pilot study. *International Journal of Disability, Development and Education, 44*, 105–15.

Nagin, D. S., Farrington, D. P. and Moffitt, T. E. (1995). Life-course trajectories of different types of offenders. *Criminology, 29*, 163–90.

Naithani, A. (2008, April 14). Taare Zameen Par could change the face of education in India. The *Economic Times.* Retrieved from http://articles.economictimes.indiatimes.com/2008-04-14/news/27724495_1_dyslexic-students-special-children-government-teachers

Nakhaie, M. R., Silverman, R. A. and LeGrange, T. C., (2000). Self-control and resistance to school. *Canadian Review of Sociology and Anthropology. 37*(4), 443–60.

Nangle, D. W., Hansen, D. J., Erdley, C. A. and Norton, P. J. (Eds.) (2010). *Practitioner's guide to empirically based measures of social skills.* New York: Springer.

Nantel-Vivier, A. and Pihl, R. O. (2008). Biological vulnerability to depression. In J. R. Z. Abela and B. L. Hankin (Eds.) *Handbook of depression in children and adolescents* (pp. 103–23). New York: Guilford Press.

Nasser, M., Katzman, M. A. and Gordon, R. A. (2001). *Eating disorders and cultures in transition*. New York: Taylor & Francis, Inc.

Nater, U. M., Rohleder, N., Gaab, J., Berger, S., Jud, A., Kirschbaum, C. et al. (2005). Human salivary alpha-amylase reactivity in a psychosocial stress paradigm. *International Journal of Psychophysiology*, *55*, 333–42.

Nation, M., Crusto, C., Wandersman, A., Kumpfer, K. L., Seybolt, D., Morrissey-Kane, E. and Davino, K. (2003). What works in prevention: Principles of effective prevention programs. *American Psychologist*, *58*, 449–56.

Naumova, O. Y., Lee, M., Koposov, R., Szyf, M., Dozier, M. and Grigorenko, E. L. (2012). Differential patterns of whole-genome DNA methylation in institutionalized children and children raised by their biological parents. *Development and Psychopathology*, *24*, 143–55.

Neale, M. C. (2009). Biometrical models in behavioral genetics. In Y.-K. Kim (Ed.), *Handbook of behavior genetics* (pp. 15–33). New York: Springer.

Neale, M. C. and Cardon, L. R. (1992). *Methodology for genetic studies of twins and families*. Dordrecht, Netherlands: Kluwer Academic.

Neece, C. L., Baker, B. L., Crnic, K. and Blacher, J. (2013). Examining the validity of ADHD as a diagnosis for adolescents with intellectual disabilities: Clinical presentation. *Journal of Abnormal Child Psychology*, *41*, 597–612.

Neiderhiser, J. M., Reiss, D., Pedersen, N. L., Lichtenstein, P., Spotts, E. L., Hansson, K.,…Elthammer, O. (2004). Genetic and environmental influences on mothering of adolescents: A comparison of two samples. *Developmental Psychology*, *40*, 335–51.

Neiderhiser, J. M., Reiss, D., Lichtenstein, P., Spotts, E. L. and Ganiban, J. (2007). Father–adolescent relationships and the role of genotype-environment correlation. *Journal of Family Psychology*, *21*, 560–71.

Neil, A. L. and Christensen, H. (2009). Efficacy and effectiveness of school-based prevention and early intervention programs for anxiety. *Clinical Psychology Review*, *29*, 208–15.

Nelson, D. A. and Coyne, S. M. (2009). Children's intent attributions and feelings of distress: Associations with maternal and paternal parenting practices. *Journal of Abnormal Child Psychology*, *37*, 223–37.

Nelson, E. C., Heath, A. C., Madden, P. A., Cooper, L., Dinwiddie, S. H., Bucholz, K. K.,…Martin, N. G. (2002). Association between self-reported childhood sexual abuse and adverse psychosocial outcomes: Results from a twin study. *Archives of General Psychiatry*, *59*, 139–45.

Nelson, E. E., Leibenluft, E., McClure, E. B. and Pine, D. S. (2005). The social re-orientation of adolescence: A neuroscience perspective on the process and its relation to psychopathology. *Psychological Medicine*, *35*, 163–74.

Nelson, E. E. and Guyer, A. E. (2011). The development of the ventral prefrontal cortex and social flexibility. *Developmental Cognitive Neuroscience*, *1*, 233–45.

Nelson, J. M. and Harwood, H. (2011). Learning disabilities and anxiety: A meta-analysis. *Journal of Learning Disabilities*, *44*, 3–17.

Nelson, T. E. (2009). *Handbook of prejudice, stereotyping and discrimination*. London: Psychology Press.

Nemeroff, C. B. and Owens, M. J. (2009). The role of serotonin in the pathophysiology of depression: As important as ever. *Clinical Chemistry*, *55*, 1578–9.

Nemeroff, C. B. and Goldschmidt-Clermont, P. J. (2011). In the aftermath of tragedy: Medical and psychiatric consequences. *Academic Psychiatry*, *35*, 4–7.

Nestler, E. J., Barrot, M., DiLeone, R. J., Eisch, A. J., Gold, S. J. and Monteggia, L. M. (2002). Neurobiology of depression. *Neuron*, *34*, 13–25.

Nestler, E. J. and Carlezon, W. A., Jr. (2006). The mesolimbic dopamine reward circuit in depression. *Biological Psychiatry*, *59*, 1151–9.

Neugebauer, R. (1979). Medieval and early modern theories of mental illness. *Archives of General Psychiatry*, *36*, 477–83.

Neugebauer, R. (1989). Diagnosis, guardianship, and residential care of the mentally ill in medieval and modern England. *American Journal of Psychiatry*, *146*, 1580–3.

Neumark-Sztainer, D. (2005). Can we simultaneously work toward the prevention of obesity and eating disorders in children and adolescents? *International Journal of Eating Disorders*, *38*, 220–7.

Newcomb, A. F. and Bagwell, C. L. (1995). Children's friendship relations: A meta-analytic review. *Psychological Bulletin*, *117*, 306–47.

Newland, L. A. and Coyl, D. D. (2010). Fathers' role as attachment figures: An interview with Sir Richard Bowlby. *Early Child Development and Care*, *180*, 25–32.

Newman, K. M. (1996). Winnicott goes to the movies: The false self in Ordinary People. *The Psychoanalytic Quarterly*, *65*, 787–807.

Newman, L. K. (2002). Sex, gender and culture: Issues in the definition, assessment and treatment of gender identity disorder. *Clinical Child Psychology and Psychiatry, 7*, 352–9.

New Oxford American dictionary (3rd edn.). (2010). Oxford: Oxford University Press.

Nicholls, D., Chater, R. and Lask, B. (2000). Children into DSM don't go: A comparison of classification systems for eating disorders in childhood and early adolescence. *International Journal of Eating Disorders, 28*, 317–24.

Nichols, W. C. and Schwartz, R. C. (1991). *Family therapy: Concepts and methods* (2nd edn.). Boston: Allyn & Bacon.

Nigg, J. T. (2006). *What causes ADHD? Understanding what goes wrong and why*. New York: Guilford Publications, Inc.

Nigg, J. T., Goldsmith, H. H. and Sachek, J. (2004). Temperament and attention deficit hyperactivity disorder: The development of a multiple pathway model. *Journal of Clinical Child and Adolescent Psychology, 1*, 42–53.

Nikapota, A. and Rutter, M. (2010). Sociocultural/ethnic groups and psychopathology. In M. Rutter, D. Bishop, D. Pine, S. Scott, J. Stevenson, E. Taylor and A. Thapar. (Eds.) *Rutter's child and adolescent psychiatry* (pp. 199–211). Oxford: Blackwell.

Nikolas, M. A. and Burt, S. A. (2010). Genetic and environmental influences on ADHD symptom dimensions of inattention and hyperactivity: A meta-analysis. *Journal of Abnormal Psychology, 119*, 1–17.

Nirje, B. (1969). The normalization principle and its human management implications. In R. Kugel and W. Wolfensberger (Eds.), *Changing patterns in residential services for the mentally retarded* (pp. 181–95). Washington, DC: President's Committee on Mental Retardation.

Nobakht, M. and Dezhkam, M. (2000). An epidemiological study of eating disorders in Iran. *International Journal of Eating Disorders, 28*, 265–71.

Nobile, M., Rusconi, M., Bellina, M., Marino, C., Giorda, R., Carlet, O., Vanzin, L. et al. (2009). The influence of family structure, the TPH2 G-703T and the 5-HTTLPR serotonergic genes upon affective problems in children aged 10–14 years. *Journal of Child Psychology and Psychiatry, 50*, 317–25.

Nock, M. K. and Kurtz, S. M. S. (2005). Direct behavioral observation in school settings: Bringing science to practice. *Cognitive and Behavioral Practice, 12*, 359–70.

Nock, M. K., Kazdin, A. E., Hiripi, E. and Kessler, R. C. (2007). Lifetime prevalence, correlates, and persistence of oppositional defiant disorder: Results from the National Comorbidity Survey Replication. *Journal of Child Psychology and Psychiatry, 48*, 703–13.

Nolan, E. E., Gadow, K. D. and Sprafkin, J. (2001). Teacher reports of DSM-IV ADHD, ODD, and CD symptoms in schoolchildren. *Journal of the American Academy of Child and Adolescent Psychiatry, 40*, 241–49.

Nolan, S. A., Flynn, C. and Garber J. (2003). Prospective relations between depression and rejection in young adolescents. *Journal of Personality and Social Psychology, 68*, 664–70.

Nolen-Hoeksema, S., Girgus, J. S. and Seligman, M. E. P. (1986). Learned helplessness in children: A longitudinal study of depression, achievement and attributional style. *Journal of Personality and Social Psychology, 51*, 435–42.

Nolen-Hoeksema, S. and Girgus, J. S. (1994). The emergence of gender differences in depression during adolescence. *Psychological Bulletin, 115*, 424–43.

Norman, D. A. and Shallice, T. (2000). Attention to action: Willed and automatic control of behaviour. In M. S. Gazzaniga (Ed.), *Cognitive neuroscience: A reader* (pp. 376–90). Oxford: Blackwell.

Normand, S., Schneider, B. H. and Robaey, P. (2007). Attention-deficit/hyperactivity disorder and the challenges of close friendship. *Journal of the Canadian Academy of Child and Adolescent Psychiatry, 16*, 67–73.

Normand, S., Schneider, B. H., Lee, M. D., Maisonneuve, M. F., Kuehn, S, and Robaey, P. (2011). How do children with ADHD (mis)manage their real-life dyadic friendships? A multi-method investigation. *Journal of Abnormal Child Psychology, 39*, 293–305.

Nottelmann, E. D. and Jensen, P. S. (1995). Comorbidity of disorders in children and adolescents: Developmental perspectives. In T. H. Ollendick and R. J. Prinz (Eds.), *Advances in clinical child psychology* (Vol. XVII, pp. 109–55). New York: Plenum.

NSPCC (2011). *Child cruelty in the UK 2011: An NSPCC study into childhood abuse and neglect over the past 30 years*. Retrieved from www.nspcc.org.uk/news-and-views/our-news/nspcc-news/11-02-15-report-launch/child-abuse-leaflet_wdf80825.pdf

Nuehring, E. M., Abrams, H. A., Fike, D. F. and Ostrowsky, E. F. (1983). Evaluating the impact of prevention programs aimed at children. *Social Work Research and Abstracts, 19*, 11–18.

Nuffield, E. J. (1988). Psychotherapy. In J. L. Matson (Ed.), *Handbook of treatment approaches in childhood psychopathology* (pp. 135–60). New York: Plenum.

Oberlander, T. F., Weinberg, J., Papsdorf, M., Grunau, R., Misri, S. and Devlin, A. M. (2008). Prenatal exposure to maternal depression, neonatal methylation of human glucocorticoid receptor gene (NR3C1) and infant cortisol stress responses. *Epigenetics, 3*, 97–106.

Obradović, J. and Boyce, W. T. (2012). Developmental psychophysiology of emotion process. *Monographs of the Society for Research in Child Development, 77*, 120–8.

Obradović, J., Bush, N. R., Stamperdahl, J., Adler, N. E. and Boyce, W. T. (2010). Biological sensitivity to context: The interactive effects of stress reactivity and family adversity on socioemotional behavior and school readiness. *Child Development, 81*, 270–89.

Ochsner, K. N. and Schacter, D. L. (2000). A social cognitive neuroscience approach to emotion and memory. In J. C. Borod (Ed.), *The neurobiology of emotion* (pp. 163–93). New York: Oxford University Press.

Ochsner, K. N., Bunge, S. A., Gross, J. J. and Gabrieli, J. D. (2002). Rethinking feelings: An fMRI study of the cognitive regulation of emotion. *Journal of Cognitive Neuroscience, 14*, 1215–29.

O'Connell, M. E., Boat, T. and Warner, K. E. (2009). *Preventing mental, emotional, and behavioral disorders among young people: Progress and possibilities.* Washington, DC: National Academies Press.

Odgers, C., Caspi, A., Poulton, R., Harrington, H. L., Thomson, M., Broadbent, A.,…Moffitt, T. E. (2007). Conduct problem subtypes predict differential adult health burden. *Archives of General Psychiatry, 64*, 476–84.

Odgers, C. L., Caspi, A., Nagin, D. S., Piquero, A. R., Slutske, W. S., Milne, B. J.,…Moffitt, T. E. (2008). Is it important to prevent early exposure to drugs and alcohol among adolescents? *Psychological Science, 19*, 1037–44.

Odom, S. L. and McEvoy, M. A. (1988). Integration of young handicapped children and normally developing children. In S. L. Odom and M. K. Barnes (Eds.), *Early interventions for infants and children with handicaps: An empirical base* (pp. 241–67). Baltimore, MD: Brookes.

Office for National Statistics. (1999). *The mental health of children and adolescents in Great Britain.* London: Author.

Offord, D. R., Boyle, M. H., Racine, Y. A., Fleming, J. E., Cadman, D. T., Blum, M. H.,…Woodward, C. A. (1992). Outcome, prognosis, and risk in a longitudinal follow-up study. *Journal of the American Academy of Child and Adolescent Psychiatry, 31*, 916–23.

Ogilvie, L. and Prior, M. (1982). Behaviour modification and the overjustification effect. *Behavioural Psychotherapy, 10*, 26–39.

O'Hara, J. and Bouras, N. (2007). Intellectual disabilities across cultures. In D. Bhugra and K. Bhui (Eds.), *Textbook of cultural psychiatry* (pp. 461–70). Cambridge: Cambridge University Press.

O'Kearney, R., Kang, K., Christensen, H. and Griffiths, K. (2009). A controlled trial of a school-based Internet program for reducing depressive symptoms in adolescent girls. *Depression and Anxiety, 26*, 65–72.

Oldehinkel, A. J., Rosmalen, J. G. M, Veenstra, R., Dijkstra, J. K. and Ormel, J. (2007). Being admired or being liked: Classroom social status and depressive problems in early adolescent girls and boys. *Journal of Abnormal Child Psychology, 35*, 417–27.

O'Leary, K. D. and O'Leary, S. G. (1972). *Classroom management: The successful use of behavioral modification.* New York: Pergamon.

Oliver, B. R. and Plomin, R. (2007). Twins' early development study (TEDS): A multivariate, longitudinal genetic investigation of language, cognition and behavior problems from childhood through adolescence. *Twin Research and Human Genetics, 10*, 96–105.

Ollendick, T. H., Matson, J. L. and Helsel, W. J. (1985). Fears in children and adolescents: Normative data. *Behaviour Research and Therapy, 23*, 465–7.

Ollendick, T. H. and Hersen, M. (1993). Child and adolescent behavioral assessment. In T. H. Ollendick and M. Hersen (Eds.), *Handbook of child and adolescent assessment* (pp. 3–14). Needham Heights, MA: Allyn & Bacon.

Ollendick, T. H., Yang, B., King, N. J., Dong, Q. and Akande, A. (1996). Fears in American, Australian, Chinese, and Nigerian children and adolescents: A cross-cultural study. *Journal of Child Psychology and Psychiatry, 37*, 213–20.

Ollendick, T. H., Jarrett, M. A., Grills-Taquechel, A. E., Hovey, L. D. and Wolff, J. C. (2008). Comorbidity as a predictor and moderator of treatment outcome in youth with anxiety, affective, attention deficit/hyperactivity disorder, and oppositional/conduct disorders. *Clinical Psychology Review, 28*, 1447–71.

Olsson, K. A., Kenardy, J. A., de Young, A. C. and Spence, S. H. (2008). Predicting children's post-traumatic stress symptoms following hospitalization for accidental injury: Combining the Child Trauma Screening Questionnaire and heart rate. *Journal of Anxiety Disorders, 22*, 1447–53.

Ono, Y., Yoshimura, K., Yamauchi, K., Asai, M., Young, J., Fujuhara, S. and Kitamura, T. (2001). Taijin kyofusho in a Japanese community population. *Transcultural Psychiatry, 38*, 506–14.

Opp, G. (2007). Inclusion of students with disabilities in German schools. *Educational and Child Psychology, 24*, 8–17.

Ornstein, P. A., Manning, E. L. and Pelphrey, K. A. (1999). Children's memory for pain. *Journal of Developmental and Behavior Pediatrics, 20*, 262–77.

Ortiz, J. and Raine, A. (2004). Heart rate level and antisocial behaviour in children and adolescents: A meta-analysis. *Journal of the American Academy of Child and Adolescent Psychiatry, 43*, 154–62.

Orvaschel, H., Lewinsohn, P. M. and Seeley, J. R. (1995). Continuity of psychopathology in a community sample of adolescents. *Journal of the American Academy of Child and Adolescent Psychiatry, 34*, 1525–35.

Osterling, J. and Dawson, G. (1994). Early recognition of children with autism: A study of first birthday home videotapes. *Journal of Autism and Developmental Disorders, 24*, 247–57.

Otero-Ojeda, A. A. (2002). Third Cuban Glossary of Psychiatry (GC-3): Key features and contributions. *Psychopathology, 35*, 181–4.

Ottman, R. (1994). Epidemiologic analysis of gene–environment interaction in twins. *Genetic Epidemiology, 11*, 75–86.

Owen, A. M. (2000). The role of the lateral frontal cortex in mnemonic processing: The contribution of functional neuroimaging. *Experimental Brain Research, 133*, 33–43.

Oyserman, D. and Lee, S. W. S. (2008). Does culture influence what and how we think? Effects of priming individualism and collectivism. *Psychological Bulletin, 134*, 311–42.

Ozonoff, S. (2013). Editorial: Recovery from autism spectrum disorder (ASD) and the science of hope. *Journal of Child Psychology and Psychiatry, 54*, 113–14.

Palazzoli Selvini, M. Boscolo, L., Cecchin, G. and Prata, C. (1978). *Paradox and counterparadox: A new model in the therapy of the family in schizophrenic transaction.* New York: Aronson.

Panagiotopoulos, C., Ronsley, R., Elbe, D., Davidson, J. and Smith, D. H. (2010). First do no harm: Promoting an evidence-based approach to atypical antipsychotic use in children and adolescents. *Journal of the Canadian Academy of Child and Adolescent Psychiatry, 19*, 124–37.

Papageorgiou, V., Georgiades, S. and Mavreas, V. (2008). Brief report: Cross-cultural evidence for the heterogeneity of the restricted, repetitive behaviours and interests domain of autism: A Greek study. *Journal of Autism and Developmental Disorders, 38*, 558–61.

Pappadopulos, E., Jensen, P. S., Chait, A. R., Arnold, L. E., Swanson, J. M., Greenhill, L. L.,...Newcorn, J. H. (2009). Medication adherence in the MTA: Saliva methylphenidate samples versus parent report and mediating effect of concomitant behavioral treatment. *Journal of the American Academy of Child and Adolescent Psychiatry, 48*, 501–10.

Paquette, D. and Bigras, M. (2010). The risky situation: A procedure for assessing the father–child activation relationship. *Early Child Development and Care, 180*, 33–50.

Pardini, D. A., Frick, P. J. and Moffitt, T. E. (2010). Building an evidence base for DSM-5 conceptualizations of oppositional defiant disorder and conduct disorder. *Journal of Abnormal Psychology, 119*, 683–88.

Parker, G., Graham, R., Synnott, H. and Anderson, J. (2014). Is the DSM-5 duration criterion valid for the definition of hypomania? *Journal of Affective Disorders, 156*, 87–91.

Parker, J. G. and Asher, S. R. (1987). Peer relations and later personal adjustment: Are low-accepted children at risk? *Psychological Bulletin, 102*, 357–89.

Parker, J. G. and Asher, S. R. (1993). Friendship and friendship quality in middle childhood: Links with peer group acceptance and feelings of loneliness and social dissatisfaction. *Developmental Psychology, 29*, 611–21.

Parry-Jones, B. and Parry-Jones, W. L. (1991). Bulimia: An archival review of its history in psychosomatic medicine. *International Journal of Eating Disorders, 10*, 129–43.

Parry-Jones, W. L. (1989). Annotation: The history of child and adolescent psychiatry: Its present day relevance. *Journal of Child Psychology and Psychiatry, 30*, 3–11.

Parry-Jones, W. L. (2006). Historical aspects of mood and its disorders in young people. In I. M. Goodyer (Ed.), *The depressed child and adolescent* (2nd edn.). Cambridge: Cambridge University Press.

Parry-Jones, W. L. L. (2001). Historical aspects of mood and its disorders in young people. In I. M. Goodyear (Ed.), The depressed child and adolescent (2nd edn.; pp. 1–23). Cambridge: Cambridge University Press.

Parson, T. (1949). *Essays in sociological theory.* New York: Free Press.

Patel, D. R., Pratt, H. D. and Greydanus, D. E. (2003). Treatment of adolescents with anorexia nervosa. *Journal of Adolescent Research, 18*, 244–60.

Paternite, C. E., Loney, J. and Roberts, M. A. (1996). A preliminary validation of subtypes of DSM-IV attention-deficit/hyperactivity disorder. *Journal of Attention Disorders, 1*, 70–86.

Patterson, C. J. and Chan, R. W. (1999). Families headed by lesbian and gay parents. In M. E. Lamb (Ed.), *Parenting and child development in "non-traditional" families* (pp. 191–219). Mahwah, NJ: Lawrence Erlbaum Associates Publishers.

Patterson, G. R. (1982). *Coercive family process.* Eugene, OR: Castalia.

Patterson, G. R. and Guillion, M. E. (1971). *Living with children: New methods of parents and teachers.* Champaign, IL: Research Press.

Patterson, G. R. and Capaldi, D. M. (1990). A mediational model for boys' depressed mood. In J. Rolf, A. S. Masten, D. Cicchetti, K. H. Nuechterlein and S. Weintraub (Eds.), *Risk and protective factors in the development of psychopathology* (pp. 141–63). New York: Cambridge University Press.

Patterson, S. T. (2009). The effects of teacher–student small talk on out-of-seat behavior. *Education and Treatment of Children, 32,* 167–74.

Paule, M. G., Rowland, A. S., Ferguson, S. A., Chelonis, J. J., Tannock, R., Swanson, J. M. and Castellanos, F. X. (2000). Attention deficit/hyperactivity disorder: Characteristics, interventions and models. *Neurotoxicology and Teratology, 22,* 631–51.

Pauli-Pott, U. and Beckmann, D. (2007). On the association of interparental conflict with developing behavioral inhibition and behavior problems in early childhood. *Journal of Family Psychology, 21,* 529–32.

Pavuluri, M. N., Graczyk, P. A., Henry, D. B., Carbray, J. A., Heidenreich, J. and Miklowitz, D. J. (2004). Child- and family-focused cognitive-behavioral therapy for pediatric bipolar disorder: Development and preliminary results. *Journal of the American Academy of Child and Adolescent Psychiatry, 43,* 528–37.

Payne, J. P. (1900). *Thomas Sydenham.* London: T. F. Unwin.

Pearl, R. and Cosden, M. (1982). Sizing up a situation: LD children's understanding of social interactions. *Learning Disability Quarterly, 5,* 371–3.

Peirce, G. R., Lakey, B., Sarason, I. G., Sarason, B. R. and Joseph, H. J. (1997). Personality and social support processes: A conceptual overview. In G. R. Pierce, B. Lakey, I. G. Sarason and B. R. Sarason (Eds.), *Sourcebook of social support and personality* (pp. 3–18). New York: Plenum Press.

Pelham, W. E. and Bender, M. E. (1982). Peer relationships in hyperactive children: Description and treatment. In K. Gadow and I. Bialer (Eds.), *Advances in learning and behavioral disabilities* (pp. 366–436). Greenwich, CT: JAI.

Pelham, W. E., and Hoza, B. (1996). Intensive treatment: A summer treatment program for children with ADHD. In E. D. Hibbs, and P. S. Jensen (Eds.), *Psychosocial treatments for child and adolescent disorders: Empirically based strategies for clinical practice* (pp. 311–40). Washington, DC: American Psychological Association.

Pelham, W. E., Fabiano, G. A. and Massetti, G. M. (2005). Evidence-based assessment of attention deficit hyperactivity disorder in children and adolescents. *Journal of Clinical Child and Adolescent Psychology, 34,* 449–76.

Pelham, W. E. and Fabiano, G. A. (2008). Evidence-based psychosocial treatments for attention-deficit/hyperactivity disorder. *Journal of Clinical Child and Adolescent Psychology, 37,* 184–214.

Pellegrini, D. W. (2007). School non-attendance: Definitions, meanings, responses, interventions. *Educational Psychology in Practice, 23,* 63–77.

Peltonen, K., Qouta, S., El Sarraj, E. and Punamaki, R.-L. (2010). Military trauma and social development: The moderating and mediating roles of peer and sibling relations in mental health. *International Journal of Behavioral Development, 34,* 554–63.

Pena, E. D. (2007). Lost in translation: Methodological considerations in cross-cultural research. *Child Development, 78,* 1255–64.

Pennington, B. F. and Ozonoff, S. Executive function and developmental psychopathology. *Journal of Child Psychology and Psychiatry, 37,* 51–87.

Perera, A., Gupta, P., Samuel, R. and Berg, B. (2007). A survey of anti-depressant prescribing practice and the provision of psychological therapies in a South London CAMHS from 2003–2006. *Child and Adolescent Metal Health, 12,* 70–2.

Perera, H., Wickramasinghe, V., Wanigasinghe, K. and Perera, G. (2002). Anorexia nervosa in early adolescence in Sri Lanka. *Annals of Tropical Paediatrics, 22,* 173–7.

Perez-Edgar, K. and Fox, N. A. (2005). A behavioral and electrophysiological study of children's selective attention under neutral and affective conditions. *Journal of Cognition and Development, 6,* 89–118.

Perez-Edgar, K., Roberson-Nay, R., Hardin, M. G., Poeth, K., Guyer, A. E., Nelson, E. E. et al. (2007). Attention alters neural responses to evocative faces in behaviorally inhibited adolescents. *Neuroimage, 35,* 1538–46.

Perret, P. and Faure, S. (2006). The foundations of developmental psychopathology. *Enfance, 58,* 317–33.

Perron, A., Brendgen, M., Vitaro, F., Côté, S. M., Tremblay, R. E. and Boivin, M. (2010). Moderating effects of team sports participation on the link between peer victimization and mental health problems. *Mental Health and Physical Activity, 5,* 107–15.

Perry, A., Harris, K. and Minnes, P. (2004). Family environments and family harmony: An exploration across severity, age, and type of DD. *Journal on Developmental Disabilities, 11,* 17–29.

Perry, A., Cummings, A., Geier, J. D., Freeman, N. L., Hughes, S., LaRose, L.,…Williams, J. (2008). Effectiveness of intensive behavioral intervention in a large, community-based program. *Research in Autism Spectrum Disorders, 2,* 621–42.

Perry, H. (1982). *Psychiatrist of America: The Life of Harry Stack Sullivan.* Cambridge, MA: Belknap Press.

Perry, N. W. and Millimet, C. R. (1977). Child-rearing antecedents of low and high anxiety eighth-grade children. In C. D. Spielberger and I. G. Sarason (Eds.), *Stress and anxiety: IV* (pp. 189–204). Oxford: Hemisphere Press.

Perry, R., Cohen, I. and DeCarlo, R. (1995). Case study: Deterioration, autism, and recovery in two siblings. *Journal of the American Academy of Child and Adolescent Psychiatry, 34,* 232–7.

Perske, R. (2004). Nirje's eight planks. *Mental Retardation, 42,* 147–50.

Persons, J. B. and Silberschatz, G. (1998). Are results of randomized controlled trials useful to psychotherapists? *Journal of Consulting and Clinical Psychology, 66,* 126–35.

Pervanidou, P. (2008). Biology of post-traumatic stress disorder in childhood and adolescence. *Journal of Neuroendocrinology, 20,* 632–8.

Perron, A., Brendgen, M., Vitaro, F., Cote, S., Tremblay, R. E. and Boivin, M. (2012). Moderating effects of team sports participation on the link between peer victimization and mental health problems. *Mental Health and Physical Activity, 5,* 107–15.

Peter Collin (Ed.) (2007). *Dictionary of nursing.* London: A. & C. Black.

Peterson, L. and Burbach, D. J. (1988). Historical trends. In J. L. Matson (Ed.), *Handbook of treatment approaches in childhood psychopathology* (pp. 3–28). New York: Plenum.

Petti, V. L., Voelker, S. L., Shore, D. L. and Hayman-Abello, S. E. (2003). Perception of nonverbal emotion cues by children with nonverbal learning disabilities. *Journal of Developmental and Physical Disabilities, 15,* 23–36.

Pettit, G. S. and Harrist, A. W. (1993). *Children's aggressive and socially unskilled playground behavior with peers: Origins in early family relations.* Albany, NY: State University of New York Press.

Pfefferbaum, B., Stuber, J., Galea, S. and Fairbrother, G. (2006). Panic reactions to terrorist attacks and probable posttraumatic stress disorders in adolescents. *Journal of Traumatic Stress, 19,* 217–28.

Pfeiffer, J. C., Kowatch, R. A. and DelBello, M. P. (2010). Pharmacotherapy of bipolar disorder in children and adolescents. *CNS Drugs, 24,* 575–93.

Pfiffner, L. J. and McBurnett, K. (1997). Social skills training with parent generalization: Treatment effects for children with attention deficit disorder. *Journal of Consulting and Clinical Psychology, 65,* 749–57.

Pfiffner, L. J., Calzada, E. and McBurnett, K. (2000). Interventions to enhance social competence. *Child and Adolescent Psychiatric Clinics of North America, 9,* 689–709.

Philips, E. L. (1978). *The social skills basis of psychopathology.* New York: Grune and Stratton.

Phillips, M. L., Drevets, W. C., Rausch, S. L. and Lane, R. D. (2003). Neurobiology of emotion perception I: The neural basis of normal emotion perception. *Biological Psychiatry, 54,* 504–14.

Piasecki, T. M., Hufford, M. R., Solhan, M. and Trull, T. J. (2007). Assessing clients in their natural environments with electronic diaries: Rationale, benefits, limitations, and barriers. *Psychological Assessment, 19,* 25–43.

Pichot, P. (1994). Nosological models in psychiatry. *British Journal of Psychiatry, 164,* 232–40.

Pierce, G. R., Lakey, B., Sarason, I. G., Sarason, B. R., and Joseph, H.J. (1997). Personality and social support processes: A conceptual overview. In G.R. Pierce, B. Lakey, I.G. Sarason, & B.R. Sarason (Eds.), Sourcebook of social support and personality (pp. 3–18). New York: Plenum.

Pies, R. (2009). Should DSM-V designate "internet addiction" a mental disorder. *Psychiatry, 6,* 31–7.

Pike, A. and Atzaba-Poria, N. (2003). Do sibling and friend relationships share the same temperamental origins? A twin study. *Journal of Child Psychology and Psychiatry and Allied Disciplines, 44,* 598–611.

Pilecki, M. and Jozefik, B. (2008). Self-image of girls with different subtypes of eating disorders. *Archives of Psychiatry and Psychotherapy, 10,* 17–22.

Pina, A. A. and Silverman, W. K. (2004). Clinical phenomenology, somatic symptoms, and distress in Hispanic/Latino and European American youths with anxiety disorders. *Journal of Clinical Child and Adolescent Psychology, 33,* 227–36.

Pinault, J. R. (1992). *Hippocratic Lives and Legends.* Leiden: Brill Academic Publishers.

Pine, D. S., Cohen, P., Gurley, D., Brook, J. and Ma, Y. (1998). The risk for early-adulthood anxiety and depressive disorders in adolescents with anxiety and depressive disorders. *Archives of General Psychiatry, 55,* 56–64.

Pine, D. S. and Cohen, J. A. (2002). Trauma in children and adolescents: Risk and treatment of psychiatric sequelae. *Society of Biological Psychiatry, 51,* 519–31.

Pine, D. S., Guyer, A. E. and Leibenluft, E. (2008). Functional magnetic resonance imaging and pediatric anxiety. *Journal of the American Academy of Child and Adolescent Psychiatry, 47,* 1217–21.

Pine, D. S. and Klein, R. G. (2010). Anxiety disorders. In M. Rutter, D. Bishop, D. Pine, S. Scott, J. Stevenson, E. Taylor and A. Thapar (Eds.), *Rutter's child and adolescent psychiatry* (pp. 628–47). Oxford: Blackwell.

Pine, D. S., Costello, E. J., Dahl, R., James, R., Leckman, J., Leibenluft, E.,...Zeanah, C. (2010). Increasing the developmental focus in DSM-V: Broad issues and specific potential applications in anxiety. Retrieved from American Psychiatric Association DSM-5 Development website: www.dsm5.org/ProposedRevisions/Documents/APA%20Developmental%20Focus%20in%20DSM-5%20Pine%20et%20al.pdf

Pinhas, L., Heinmaa, M., Bryden, P., Bradley, S. and Toner, B. (2008). Disordered eating in Jewish adolescent girls. *Canadian Journal of Psychiatry, 53,* 601–8.

Pinker, S. (2002). *The blank slate: The modern denial of human nature.* New York: Viking.

Pitzer, M. and Schmidt, M. H. (2000). Reference tables for representation of ICD-10 diagnoses in DSM-IV. *Zeitschrift fur Kinder- und Jugendpsychiatrie und Psychotherapie, 28,* 119–28.

Plant, R. W., Panzarella, P. (2009). Residential treatment of adolescents with substance use disorders: Evidence-based approaches and best practice recommendations. In C. Leukefeld, T. P. Gullotta and M. Staton-Tindall (Eds.), *Adolescent substance abuse: Evidence-based approaches to prevention and treatment* (Vol. IX, pp. 135–54). New York: Springer.

Pleck, J. (1997). Parental involvement: Levels, sources, and consequences. In M. Lamb (Ed.), *The role of the father in child development* (3rd edn., pp. 66–103). New York: Wiley.

Pleck, J. H. (2007). Why could father involvement benefit children? Theoretical perspectives. *Applied Developmental Science, 11,* 196–202.

Pliszka, S. R., Glahn, D. C., Semrud-Clikeman, M., Franklin, C., Perez, R., 3rd, Xiong, J. et al. (2006). Neuroimaging of inhibitory control areas in children with attention deficit hyperactivity disorder who were treatment naive or in long-term treatment. *American Journal of Psychiatry, 163*(6), 1052–60.

Plomin, R., DeFries, J. C. and Loehlin, J. C. (1977). Genotype–environment interaction and correlation in the analysis of human behavior. *Psychological Bulletin, 84,* 309–22.

Plomin, R. and Walker, S. O. (2003). Genetics and educational psychology. *British Journal of Educational Psychology, 73,* 3–14.

Plomin, R. and Davis, O. S. P. (2009). The future of genetics in psychology and psychiatry: Microarrays, genome-wide association, and non-coding RNA. *Journal of Child Psychology and Psychiatry, 50,* 63–71.

Plomin, R., Kovas, Y. and Haworth, C. M. A. (2007). Generalist genes: Genetic links between brain, mind, and education. *Mind, Brain, and Education, 1,* 11–19.

Polak, M. A. and Nijman, H. (2005). Pharmacological treatment of sexually aggressive forensic psychiatric patients. *Psychology, Crime and Law, 11,* 457–65.

Polanczyk, G., de Lima, M. S., Horta, B. L., Biederman, J. and Rohde, L. A. (2007). The worldwide prevalence of ADHD: A systematic review and metaregression analysis. *The American Journal of Psychiatry, 164,* 942–8.

Polivy, J. and Herman, C. P. (1987). Diagnosis and treatment of normal eating. *Journal of Consulting and Clinical Psychology, 55,* 635–44.

Polivy, J. and Herman, C. P. (2002). Causes of eating disorders. *Annual Review of Psychology, 53,* 187–213.

Pollak, S., Cicchetti, D. and Klorman, R. (1998). Stress, memory, and emotion: Developmental considerations from the study of child maltreatment. *Development and Psychopathology, 10,* 811–28.

Pollak, Y., Shomaly, H. B., Weiss, P. L., Rizzo, A. A. and Gross-Tsur, V. (2010). Methylphenidate effect in children with ADHD can be measured by an ecologically valid continuous performance test embedded in virtual reality. *CNS Spectrums, 15,* 125–30.

Pomery, E. A. et al. (2005). Families and risk: Prospective analyses of familial and social influences on adolescent substance use. *Journal of Family Psychology, 19*(4), 560–70.

Popma, A., Jansen, L. M., Vermeiren, R., Steiner, H., Raine, A., van Goozen, S. H. et al. (2006). Hypothalamus pituitary adrenal axis and autonomic activity during stress in delinquent male adolescents and controls. *Psychoneuroendocrinology, 31,* 948–57.

Popma, A., Vermeiren, R., Geluk, C. A., Rinne, T., van den Brink, W., Knol, D. L. et al. (2007). Cortisol moderates the relationship between testosterone and aggression in delinquent male adolescents. *Biological Psychiatry, 61,* 405–11.

Porges, S. W. (2011). *The polyvagal theory: Neurophysiological foundations of emotions, attachment, communication, and self-regulation.* New York: W. W. Norton and Co.

Portes, A. (1971). On the emergence of behavior therapy in modern society. *Journal of Counseling Psychology, 36,* 303–13.

Post, R. M. (1992). Transduction of psychosocial stress into the neurobiology of recurrent affective disorder. *American Journal of Psychiatry, 149,* 999–1010.

Post, R. M., and Leverich, G. S. (2006). The role of psychosocial stress in the onset and progression of bipolar disorder and its comorbidities: The need for earlier and alternative modes of therapeutic intervention. *Development and Psychopathology, 18,* 1181–211.

Postert, C., Averbeck-Holocher, M., Beyer, T., Muller, J. and Furniss, T. (2009). Five systems of psychiatric classification for preschool children: Do differences in validity, usefulness and reliability make for competitive or complimentary constellations? *Child Psychiatry and Human Development, 40*, 25–41.

Posthumus, J. A., Bocker, K. B., Raaijmakers, M. A., van Engeland, H. and Matthys, W. (2009). Heart rate and skin conductance in four-year-old children with aggressive behavior. *Biological Psychology, 82*, 164–8.

Poston, J. M. and Hanson, W. E. (2010). Meta-analysis of psychological assessment as a therapeutic intervention. *Psychological Assessment, 22*, 203–12.

Poulin, F., Cillessen, A. H. N., Hubbard, J. A., Coie, J. D., Dodge, K. A. and Schwartz, D. (1997). Children's friends and behavioral similarity in two social contexts. *Social Development, 6*, 224–36.

Poulin, F., Dishion, T. J. and Haas, E. (1999). The peer influence paradox: Friendship quality and deviancy training within male adolescent friendships. *Merrill-Palmer Quarterly, 45*, 42–61.

Poulin, F., Cantin, S., Vitaro, F. and Boivin, M. (2009). Amitiés et conduites agressives à l'enfance. In B. H. Schneider, S. Normand, M. Allès-Jardel, M. A. Provost and G. M. Tarabulsy (Eds), *Conduites agressives chez l'enfant: Perspectives développementales et psychosociales* (pp. 175–98). Québec, QC: Presses de l'Université du Québec.

Poulter, M. O., Du, L., Weaver, I. C. G., Palkovits, M., Faludi, G., Merali, Z. et al. (2008). GABAA receptor promoter hypermethylation in suicide brain: Implications for the involvement of epigenetic processes. *Biological Psychiatry, 8*, 645–52.

Power, T. J., Karustis, J. L. and Habboushe, D. F. (2001). *Homework success for children with ADHD: A family-school intervention program*. New York: Guilford Press.

Pratt, V. (1977). Foucault and the history of classification theory. *Studies in History and Philosophy of Science, 8*, 163–71.

Pretorius, N., Arcelus, J., Beecham, J., Dawson, H., Doherty, F., Eisler, I.,…Schmidt, U. (2009). Cognitive-behavioural therapy for adolescents with bulimic symptomatology: The acceptability and effectiveness of internet-based delivery. *Behaviour Research and Therapy, 47*, 729–36.

Preyde, M. and Adams, G. R. (2008). Foundations of addictive problems: Developmental, social and neurobiological problems. In C. A. Esau (Ed.), *Adolescent addiction: Epidemiology, assessment, and treatment* (pp. 3–16). Philadelphia: Elsevier.

Prinstein, M. J., Borelli, J. L., Cheah, C. S. L., Simon, V. A. and Aikins, J. W. (2005). Adolescent girls' interpersonal vulnerability to depressive symptoms: A longitudinal examination of reassurance-seeking and peer relationships. *Journal of Abnormal Psychology, 114*, 676–88.

Prinstein, M. J. and Dodge, K. A. (2008). *Understanding peer influence in children and adolescents*. New York: Guilford Press.

Proner, K. (1998). Learning and teaching the theories of Melanie Klein. *Journal of Child Psychotherapy, 24*, 449–60.

Pruessner, J. C., Kirschbaum, C., Meinlschmid, G., Hellhammer, D. H. (2003). Two formulas for the computation of the area under the curve represent measures of total hormone concentration versus time-dependent change. *Psychoneuroendocrinology, 28*, 916–93.

Purdie, N., Hattie, J. and Carroll, A. (2002). A review of the research on interventions for attention deficit hyperactivity disorder: What works best? *Review of Educational Research, 72*, 61–99.

Puhl, R. M. and Latner, J. D. (2007). Stigma, obesity, and the health of the nation's children. *Psychological Bulletin, 133*, 557–80.

Punamaki, R.-L. and Puhakka, T. (1997). Determinants and effectiveness of children's coping with political violence. *International Journal of Behavioral Development, 21*, 349–70.

Punamaki, R.-L., Qouta, S. and El-Sarraj, E. (2001). Resiliency factors predicting psychological adjustment after political violence among Palestinian children. *International Journal of Behavioral Development, 25*, 256–67.

Purvis, K. B. and Cross, D. R. (2007). Improvements in salivary cortisol, depression, and representations of family relationships in at-risk adopted children utilizing a short-term therapeutic intervention. *Adoption Quarterly, 10*, 25–43.

Putnam, W. J. (2008). *Transformative assessment*. Alexandria, VA: Association for Supervision and Curriculum Development.

Qiu, J. (2006). Epigenetics: Unfinished symphony. *Nature, 441*, 143–5.

Quay, H. C. (1997). Inhibition and attention deficit hyperactivity disorder. *Journal of Abnormal Child Psychology, 25*, 7–13.

Quiggle, N. L., Garber, J., Panak, W. E. and Dodge, K. A. (1992). Social information processing in aggressive and depressed children. *Child Development, 63*, 1305–20.

Quinodoz, J. M. and Alcorn, D. (2005). *Reading Freud: A chronological exploration of Freud's writings* (David Alcorm trans.). Hove, East Sussex: Routledge.

Rabinowitz, F. E. and Cochran, S. V. (2008). Men and therapy: A case of masked male depression. *Clinical Case Studies, 7*, 575–91.

Radden, J. (1996). Lumps and bumps: Kantian faculty psychology, phrenology, and twentieth-century psychiatric classification. *Philosophy, Psychiatry, and Psychology, 3*, 1–14.

Raine, A. (1993). *The psychopathology of crime: Criminal behaviour as a clinical disorder.* San Diego, CA: Academic Press.

Raine, A. (1997). Antisocial behavior and psychophysiology: A biosocial perspective and a prefrontal dysfunction hypothesis. In D. M. Stoff, J. Breiling and J. D. Maser (Eds.), *Handbook of antisocial behavior* (pp. 289–304). New York: Wiley.

Raine, A. (2002). Biosocial studies of antisocial and violent behaviour in children and adults: A review. *Journal of Abnormal Child Psychology, 30*, 311–26.

Raine, A., O'Brien, M., Smiley, N., Scerbo, A. and Chan, C. J. (1990). Reduced lateralization in verbal dichotic-listening in adolescent psychopaths. *Journal of Abnormal Psychology, 99*, 272–7.

Raine, A., Venables, P. H. and Williams, M. (1990). Relationships between central and autonomic measures of arousal at age 15 years and criminality at age 24 years. *Archives of General Psychiatry, 47*, 1003–7.

Raine, A., Venables, P. H. and Mednick, S. (1997). Low resting heart rate at age 3 predisposes to aggression at age 11 years: Evidence from the Mauritius child health project. *Journal of the American Academy of Child and Adolescent Psychiatry, 36*, 1457–64.

Raine, A., Liu, J., Venables, P. H., Mednick, S. A. and Dalais, C. (2010). Cohort profile: The Mauritius child health project. *International Journal of Epidemiology, 39*, 1441–51.

Randazzo, W. T., Dockray, S. and Susman, E. J. (2008). The stress response in adolescents with inattentive type ADHD symptoms. *Child Psychiatry and Human Development, 39*, 27–38.

Rank, B. (1949). Adaptation of the psychoanalytic techniques for the treatment of young children with atypical development. *American Journal of Orthopsychiatry, 19*, 130–9.

Rao, U., Hammen, C., Ortiz, L. R., Chen, L. A., Poland, R. E. (2008). Effects of early and recent adverse experiences on adrenal response to psychosocial stress in depressed adolescents. *Biological Psychiatry, 64*, 521–6.

Rapee, R. M., Kennedy, S., Ingram, M., Edwards, S. and Sweeney, L. (2005). Prevention and early intervention of anxiety disorders in inhibited preschool children. *Journal of Consulting and Clinical Psychology, 73*, 488–97.

Rapee, R. M., Schniering, C. A. and Hudson, J. L. (2009). Anxiety disorders during childhood and adolescence: Origins and treatment. *Annual Review of Clinical Psychology, 5*, 311–41.

Rapee, R. M. and Coplan, R. J. (2010). Conceptual relations between anxiety disorder and fearful temperament. In H. Gazelle and K. H. Rubin (Eds.), *Social anxiety in childhood: Bridging developmental and clinical perspectives* (pp. 17–32). San Francisco, CA: Wiley Subscription Services.

Rapport, M. D., Bolden, J., Kofler, M. J., Sarver, D. E., Raiker, J. S. and Alderson, R. M. (2009). A ubiquitous core symptom or manifestation of working memory deficits? *Journal of Abnormal Child Psychology, 37*, 521–34.

Rascle, O., Coulomb-Cabagno, G. and Delsarte, A. (2005). Perceived motivational climate and observed aggression as a function of competitive level in youth male French handball. *Journal of Sport Behavior, 28*, 51–67.

Rawana, J. S., Morgan, A. S., Nguyen, H. and Craig, S. G. (2010). The relation between eating- and weight-related disturbances and depression in adolescence: A review. *Clinical Child and Family Psychology Review, 13*, 213–30.

Ray, D. C., Stulmaker, H. L., Lee, K. R. and Silverman, W. K. (2013). Child-centered play therapy and impairment: Exploring relationships and constructs. *International Journal of Play Therapy, 22*, 13–27.

Ray, S. L. (2004). Eating disorders in adolescent males. *Professional School Counseling, 8*, 98–101.

Razin, A. and Riggs, A. D. (1980). DNA methylation and gene function. *Science, 210*, 604–10.

Recchia, H. E. and Howe, N. (2009). Associations between social understanding, sibling relationship quality, and siblings' conflict strategies and outcomes. *Child Development, 80*, 1564–78.

Reebye, R. N. and Eble, D. (2009). The role of pharmacotherapy in the management of self-regulation difficulties in young children. *Journal of the Canadian Academy of Child and Adolescent Psychiatry, 18*, 150–9.

Reger, M. A. and Gahm, G. A. (2009). A meta-analysis of the effects of internet- and computer-based cognitive-behavioral treatments for anxiety. *Journal of Clinical Psychology, 65*, 53–75.

Regier, D. A. (2008). Foreword: Dimensional approaches to psychiatric classification. In J. E. Helzer, H. C. Kraemer, R. F. Krueger, H. Wittchen, P. J. Sirovatka and D. A. Regier (Eds.), *Dimensional approaches in diagnostic classification: Refining the research agenda for DSM-V.* Washinton, DC: American Psychiatric Association.

Reid, M. J., Webster-Stratton, C. and Hammond, M. (2003). Follow-up of children who received the Incredible Years Intervention of oppositional-defiant disorder: Maintenance and prediction of 2-year outcome. *Behavior Therapy, 34*, 471–91.

Reinecke, M. A., Ryan, N. E. and DuBois, D. L. (1998). Cognitive-behavioral therapy of depression and depressive symptoms during adolescence: A review and meta-analysis. *Journal of the American Academy of Child and Adolescent Psychiatry, 37*, 26–34.

Reinecke, M. A. and Ginsburg, G. S. (2008). Cognitive-behavioral treatment of depression during childhood and adolescence. In J. R. Z. Abela and B. L. Hankin (Eds.), *Handbook of depression in children and adolescents* (pp. 179–206). New York: Guilford Press.

Rekers, G. A. and Varni, J. W. (1977). Self-monitoring and self-reinforcement processes in a pre-transsexual boy. *Behaviour Research and Therapy, 15*, 177–80.

Rendell, R. (1977). *A judgement in stone*. London: Hutchinson & Co.

Reschly, D. J. and Hosp, J. L. (2004). State SLD identification policies and practices. *Learning Disability Quarterly, 27*, 197–213.

Resnick, R. J. (2005). Attention deficit hyperactivity disorder in teens and adults: They don't all outgrow it. *Journal of Clinical Psychology, 61*, 529–33.

Rettew, D. C., Stanger, C., McKee, L., Doyle, A. and Hudziak, J. J. (2006). Interactions between child and parent temperament and child behavior problems. *Comprehensive Psychiatry, 47*, 412–20.

Reuther, E. T., Davis, T. E., Moree, B. N. and Matson, J. L. (2011). Treating selective mutism using modular CBT for child anxiety: A case study. *Journal of Clinical Child and Adolescent Psychology, 40*, 156–63.

Reyno, S. M. and McGrath, P. J. (2006). Predictors of parent training efficacy for child externalizing behaviour problem – a meta-analytic review. *Journal of Child Psychology and Psychiatry, 47*, 99–111.

Reynolds, C. R. (2010). Measurement and assessment: An editorial view. *Psychological Assessment, 22*, 1–4.

Reynolds, S., Lane, S. J. and Gennings, C. (2010). The moderating role of sensory overresponsivity in HPA activity: A pilot study with children diagnosed with ADHD. *Journal of Attention Disorders, 13*, 46–78.

Rhee, S. H. et al. (2006). Comorbidity between alcohol dependence and illicit drug dependence in adolescents with antisocial behavior and matched controls. *Drug and Alcohol Dependence, 84*(1), 85–92.

Rhule, D. M., McMahon, R. J. and Vando, J. (2009). The acceptability and representativeness of standardized parent–child interaction tasks. *Behavior Therapy, 40*, 393–402.

Rice, F. (2009). The genetics of depression in childhood and adolescence. *Current Psychiatry Reports, 11*, 167–73.

Rice, F., Harold, G. and Thapar, A. (2002). The genetic aetiology of childhood depression: A review. *Journal of Child Psychology and Psychiatry, 43*, 65–79.

Rich, B. A., Vinton, D. T., Roberson-Nay, R., Hommer, R. E., Berghorst, L. H., McClure, E. B.,…Leibenluft, E. (2006). Limbic hyperactivation during processing of neutral facial expressions in children with bipolar disorder. *Proceedings of the National Academy of Sciences, 103*, 8900–5.

Richardson, R. C. (1995). The relationship of individualism to psychopathology. *Dissertation Abstracts International: Section B: The Sciences and Engineering, 55*, 5115.

Richmond, M. E. (1917). *Social diagnosis*. New York: Sage.

Rieger, E., van Buren, D. J., Bishop, M., Tanofsky-Kraff, M., Welch, R. and Wilfley, D. E. (2010). An eating disorder-specific model of interpersonal psychotherapy (IPT-ED): Causal pathways and treatment implications. *Clinical Psychology Review, 30*, 400–10.

Riggins-Caspers, K. M., Cadoret, R. J., Knutson, J. F. and Langbehn, D. (2003). Biology–environment interaction and evocative biology–environment correlation: Contributions of harsh discipline and parental psychopathology to problem adolescent behaviors. *Behavior Genetics, 33*, 205–20.

Riley-Tillman, T. C., Methe, S. A. and Weegar, K. (2009). Examining the use of direct behavior rating on formative assessment of class-wide engagement: A case study. *Assessment for Effective Intervention, 34*, 224–30.

Rilling, J., Gutman, D., Zeh, T., Pagnoni, G., Berns, G. and Kilts, C. (2002). A neural basis for social cooperation. *Neuron, 35*, 395–405.

Rivard, L. M., Missiuna, C., Hanna, S. and Wishart, L. (2007). Understanding teachers' perceptions of the motor difficulties of children with developmental coordination disorder (DCD). *British Journal of Educational Psychology, 77*, 633–48.

Rivera, M. S. and Nangle, D. W. (2008). Peer intervention. In M. Hersen and A. M. Gross (Eds.), *Handbook of clinical psychology*, Vol. II: *Children and adolescents* (pp. 759–85). Hoboken, NJ: John Wiley and Sons.

Rivett, M. (2008). Towards a metamorphosis: Current developments in the theory and practice of family therapy. *Child and Adolescent Mental Health, 13*, 102–6.

Rivett, M. and Street, E. (2009). *Family therapy: 100 key points and techniques*. New York: Routledge.

Rizzo, A. A., Buckwalter, J. G., Bowerly, T., van der Zaag, C., Humphrey, L., Neumann, U.,…Sisemore, D. (2000). The virtual classroom: A virtual reality environment for the assessment and rehabilitation of attention deficits. *Cyber Psychology and Behavior, 3*, 483–99.

Robb, A., Cueva, J., Sporn, J., Yang, R. and Vanderburg, D. (2008). Efficacy of sertraline in childhood posttraumatic stress disorder. In *Scientific proceedings*. Chicago, IL: American Academy of Child and Adolescent Psychiatry.

Roberts, A. L., Rosario, M., Slopen, N., Calzo, J. P. and Austin, S. B. (2013). Childhood gender nonconformity, bullying victimization, and depressive symptoms across adolescence and early adulthood: An 11-year longitudinal study. *Journal of the American Academy of Child and Adolescent Psychiatry, 52*, 143–52.

Roberts, R. E. and Roberts, C. R. (2007). Ethnicity and risk of psychiatric disorder among adolescents. *Research in Human Development, 4*, 89–117.

Robin, A. L., Gilroy, M. and Dennis, A. B. (1998). Treatment of eating disorders in children and adolescents. *Clinical Psychology Review, 18*, 421–46.

Robins, E. and Guze, S. B. (1970). Establishment of diagnostic validity in psychiatric illness: Its application to schizophrenia. *The American Journal of Psychiatry, 126*, 983–6.

Robins, L. N. and Price, R. K. (1991). Adult disorders predicted by childhood conduct problems: Results from the NIMH Epidemiologic Catchment Area Project. *Psychiatry, 54*, 116–32.

Robinson, D. J. (2003). *Reel psychiatry: Movie portrayals of psychiatric conditions*. Port Huron, MI: Rapid Psychler Press.

Robinson, E. S. (1920). The compensatory function of make-believe play. *Psychological Review, 27*, 434–8.

Roeckelein, J. E. (1998). *Dictionary of theories, laws, and concepts in psychology*. Westport, CT: Greenwood.

Rockhill, C. M., Fan, M., Katon, W. J., McCauley, E., Crick, N. R. and Pleck, J. H. (2007). Friendship interactions in children with and without depressive symptoms: Observation of emotion during game-playing interactions and post-game evaluations. *Journal of Abnormal Child Psychology, 35*, 429–41.

Rogers, C. R. (1951). *Client-centered therapy; its current practice, implications, and theory*. Oxford: Houghton Mifflin.

Rogers, S. J. and Vismara, L. A. (2008). Evidence-based comprehensive treatments for early autism. *Journal of Clinical Child and Adolescent Psychology, 37*, 8–38.

Rohde, L. A. (2002). ADHD in Brazil: The DSM-IV criteria in a culturally different population. *Journal of the American Academy of Child and Adolescent Psychiatry, 41*, 1131–3.

Rohde, L. A., Biederman, J., Busnello, E. A., Zimmermann, H., Schmitz, M., Martins, S. and Tramontina, S. (1999). ADHD in a school sample of Brazilian adolescents: A study of prevalence, comorbid conditions, and impairments. *Journal of the American Academy of Child and Adolescent Psychiatry, 38*, 716–22.

Rohde, L. A., Szobot, C., Polanczyk, G., Schmitz, M., Martins, S. and Tramontina, S. (2005). Attention-deficit/ hyperactivity disorder in a diverse culture: Do research and clinical findings support the notion of a cultural construct for the disorder? *Biological Psychiatry, 57*, 1436–41.

Rohde, P., Lewinsohn, P. M., Seely, J. R. and Rohling-Langhinrichsen, J. (1996). The Life Attitudes Schedule short form: An abbreviated measure of life-enhancing and life-threatening behaviors in adolescents. *Suicide and Life-Threatening Behavior, 26*, 272–81.

Rohde, P., Lewinsohn, P. M. and Seeley, J. R. (1996). Psychiatric comorbidity with problematic alcohol use in high school students. *Journal of the American Academy of Child and Adolescent Psychiatry, 35*, 101–9.

Rohleder, N., Wolf, J. M., Maldonado, E. F. and Kirschbaum, C. (2006). The psychosocial stress-induced increase in salivary alpha-amylase is independent of saliva flow rate. *Psychophysiology, 43*, 645–52.

Rohrer, F. (2008, September 22). The path from cinema to playground. *BBC News Magazine*. Retrieved from http://news.bbc.co.uk/2/hi/uk_news/magazine/7629376.stm

Rollett, B. (1997). The Vienna school of developmental psychology. In W. Bringmann, H. Lück, R. Miller and C. Early (Eds.) *A pictorial history of psychology* (pp. 348–51). Chicago: Quintessence.

Romano, E., Tremblay, R. E., Vitaro, F., Zoccolillo, M. and Pagani, L. (2005). Sex and informant effects on diagnostic comorbidity in an adolescent community sample. *The Canadian Journal of Psychiatry, 50*, 479–89.

Rorschach, H. (1927). *Rorschach test – psychodiagnostic plates*. Cambridge, MA: Hogrefe Publishing.

Rosario, V. A. (2002). Science and sexual identity: An essay review. *Journal of the History of Medicine and Allied Science, 57*, 79–85.

Rose, R. J. (2002). How do adolescents select their friends? A behavior-genetic perspective. In L. Pulkkinen and A. Caspi (Eds.), *Paths to successful development: Personality in the life course* (pp. 106–25). New York: Cambridge University Press.

Rosenfeld, D. and Faircloth, C. (Eds.). (2006). *Medicalized masculinities*. Philadelphia, PA: Temple University Press.

Rosenhan, D. L. (1973). On being sane in insane places. *Science, 179*, 250–8.

Rosenthal, R. (1991). *Meta-analytic procedures for social research*. Newbury Park, CA: Sage.

Ross, H. and Howe, N. (2009). Family influences on children's peer relationships. In K. H. Rubin, W. M. Bukowski and B. Laursen (Eds.), *Handbook of peer interactions, relationships, and groups* (pp. 508–27). New York: Guilford Press.

Rossman, B. B. R. and Ho, J. (2000). Posttraumatic response and children exposed to parental violence.

Journal of Aggression, Maltreatment and Trauma, 3, 85–106.

Rotenberg, V. (2012). Religious education as a prevention of learned helplessness and depression: Theoretical consideration. *Activitas Nervosa Superiro, 54,* 1–9.

Rothbart, M. K. and Posner, M. I. (2006). Temperament, attention, and developmental psychopathology. In D. Cicchetti (Ed.), *Developmental Psychopathology* (Vol. II; pp. 465–501), *Developmental Neuroscience* (2nd edn.). New York: Wilcy.

Rottenberg, J., Clift, A., Bolden, S. and Salomon, K. (2007). RSA fluctuation in major depressive disorder. *Psychophysiology, 44,* 450–8.

Rotter, J. B., Lah, M. I. and Rafferty, J. E. (1992). *Rotter incomplete sentences blanks, second edition (RISB-2).* San Antonio, TX: Harcourt Brace.

Rourke, B. P. (1989). *Nonverbal learning disabilities: The syndrome and the model.* New York: Guilford Press.

Rourke, B. P. (1995). Introduction: The NLD syndrome and the white matter model. In B. P. Rourke (Ed.), *Syndrome of non-verbal learning disabilities: Neurodevelopmental manifestations* (pp. 1–26). New York: Guilford Press.

Rourke, B. P., Del Dotto, J. E., Bourke, S. B. and Casey, J. E. (1990). Nonverbal learning disabilities: The syndrome and a case study. *Journal of School Psychology, 28,* 361–85.

Rowe, R., Maughan, B., Pickles, A., Costello, E. J. and Angold, A. (2002). The relationship between DSM-IV oppositional defiant disorder and conduct disorder: Findings from the Great Smoky Mountains Study. *Journal of Child Psychology and Psychiatry, 43,* 365–73.

Rowe, R., Maughan, B., Costello, E. J. and Angold, A. (2005). Defining oppositional defiant disorder. *Journal of Child Psychology and Psychiatry, 46,* 1309–16.

Rubia, K., Overmeyer, S., Taylor, E., Brammer, M., Williams, S. C., Simmons, A. et al. (1999). Hypofrontality in attention deficit hyperactivity disorder during higher-order motor control: A study with functional MRI. *American Journal of Psychiatry, 156*(6), 891–6.

Rubia, K., Smith, A. B., Brammer, M. J. and Taylor, E. (2007). Temporal lobe dysfunction in medication-naive boys with attention-deficit/hyperactivity disorder during attention allocation and its relation to response variability. *Biological Psychiatry, 62,* 999–1006.

Rubin, K. H. and Krasnor, L. R. (1986). Social-cognitive and social behavioural perspectives on problem solving. In M. Perlmutter (Ed.), *Cognitive perspectives on children's social and behavioural development. The Minnesota Symposia on Child Psychology* (Vol. XVIII, pp. 1–68). Hillsdale, NJ: Erlbaum.

Rubin, K. H., and Mills, R. S. (1991). Conceptualizing developmental pathways to internalizing disorders in childhood. *Canadian Journal of Behavioural Science, 23,* 300–317.

Rubin, K. H. and Burgess, K. B. (2001). Social withdrawal and anxiety. In M. W. Vasey and M. R. Dadds (Eds.), *The developmental psychopathology of anxiety* (pp. 407–34). New York: Oxford University Press.

Rubin, K. H., Burgess, K. B. and Hastings, P. D. (2002). Stability and social-behavioral consequences of toddlers' inhibited temperament and parenting behaviors. *Child Development, 73,* 483–95.

Rubin, K. H., Burgess, K. B., Dwyer, K. M. and Hastings, P. D. (2003). Predicting preschoolers' externalizing behaviours from toddler temperament, conflict, and maternal negativity. *Developmental Psychology, 39,* 164–76.

Rubin, K. H., Wojslawowicz, J. C., Rose-Krasnor, L., Booth-LaForce, C. and Burgess, K. B. (2006). The best friendships of shy/withdrawn children: Prevalence, stability, and relationship quality. *Journal of Abnormal Child Psychology, 34,* 143–57.

Rubin, K. H., Bukowski, W. and Parker, J. (2006). Peer interactions, relationships, and groups. In W. Damon, R. M. Lerner and N. Eisenberg (Eds.), *Handbook of child psychology: Social, emotional, and personality development* (6th edn., pp. 571–645). New York: Wiley.

Rubin, K. H., Coplan, R. J. and Bowker, J. C. (2009). Social withdrawal in childhood. *Annual Review of Psychology, 60,* 141–71.

Ruble, D. N., Taylor, L. J., Cyphers, L., Greulich, F. K., Lurye, L. E. and Shrout, P. E. (2007). The role of gender constancy in early gender development. *Child Development, 78,* 1121–136.

Ruchkin, V., Sukhodolsky, D. G., Vermeiren, R., Koposov, R., Schwab-Stone and M. (2006). Depressive symptoms and associated psychopathology in urban adolescents: A cross-cultural study of three countries. *Journal of Nervous and Mental Disease, 94,* 106–13.

Rucklidge, J. J. (2006). Gender differences in neuropsychological functioning of New Zealand adolescents with and without attention deficit hyperactivity disorder. *International Journal of Disability, Development and Education, 53,* 47–66.

Rucklidge, J. J. and Tannock, R. (2001). Psychiatric, psychosocial, and cognitive functioning of female adolescents with ADHD. *Journal of the American Academy of Child and Adolescent Psychiatry, 40,* 530–40.

Rudolph, K. D. and Clark, A. G. (2001). Conceptions of relationships in children with aggressive and depressive symptoms: Social-cognitive distortion or reality? *Journal of Abnormal Child Psychology, 29,* 41–56.

Rudolph, K. D., Hammen, C. and Burge, D. (1994). Interpersonal functioning and depressive symptoms in childhood: Addressing the issues of specificity and comorbidity. *Journal of Abnormal Child Psychology, 22*, 355–71.

Rudolph, K. D., Ladd, G. and Dinella, L. (2007). Gender differences in the interpersonal consequences of early-onset depressive symptoms. *Merrill-Palmer Quarterly, 53*, 461–88.

Rudolph, K. D., Flynn, M. and Abaied, J. L. (2008). A developmental perspective on interpersonal theories. In J. R. Z. Abela and B. L. Hankin (Eds.) *Handbook of depression in children and adolescents* (pp. 79–101). New York: Guilford Press.

Ruggiero, G. M. (2003). *Eating disorders in the Mediterranean area*. Hauppauge, NY: Nova Science Publishers.

Ruiz, S. Y., Pepper, A. and Wilfley, D. (2004). Obesity and body image among ethnically diverse children and adolescents. In J. K. Thompson (Ed.), *Handbook of eating disorders and obesity* (pp. 656–78). Hoboken, NJ: John Wiley and Sons, Inc.

Ruiz-Lazaro, P. M., Alonso, J. P., Comet, P., Lobo, A. and Velillia, M. (2005). Prevalence of eating disorders in Spain: A survey on a representative sample of adolescents. In P. I. Swain (Ed.), *Trends in eating disorders research* (pp. 85–108). Hauppauge, NY: Nova Biomedical Books.

Runyon, R. S. (1984). Freud and Adler: A conceptual analysis of their differences. *Psychoanalytic Review, 71*, 413–21.

Rushton, J. P. (1990). Sir Francis Galton, epigenetic rules, genetic similarity theory, and human life-history analysis. *Journal of Personality, 58*, 117–40.

Ruskin, M. (2007). John Bowlby at the Tavistock. *Attachment and Psychopathology, 9*, 355–9.

Rutgers, A. H., Bakermans-Kranenburg, M. J., van IJzendoorn, M. H. and van Berckelaer-Onnes, I. A. (2004). Autism and attachment: A meta-analytic review. *Journal of Child Psychology and Psychiatry, 45*, 1123–34.

Rutten, T. (2008). Rufus' legacy in the psychopathological literature of the (early) modern period. In P. E. Pormann (Ed.), *Rufus of Ephesus: On Melancholy* (pp. 245–62). Tubingen, Germany: Mohr Siebeck.

Rutter, M. (2001). Autism: Two-way interplay between research and clinical work. In J. Green and W. Yule (Eds.), *Research and innovation on the road to modern child psychiatry*, Vol. I: *Festschrift for Professor Sir Michael Rutter* (pp. 54–80). London: Gaskell and the Association for Child Psychology and Psychiatry.

Rutter, M. (2005). Incidence of autism spectrum disorders: Changes over time and their meaning. *Acta Paediatrica, 94*, 2–15.

Rutter, M. (2011). Progress in understanding autism: 2007–2010. *Journal of Autism and Developmental Disorders, 41*, 395–404.

Rutter, M. and Yule, W. (1975). The concept of specific reading retardation. *Journal of Child Psychology and Psychiatry, 16*, 181–97.

Rutter, M., Graham, P., Chadwick, O. F. and Yule, W. (1976). Adolescent turmoil: Fact or fiction? *Journal of Child Psychology and Psychiatry, 17*, 35–56.

Rutter, M. and Sroufe, L. A. (2000). Developmental psychopathology: Concepts and challenges. *Development and Psychopathology, 12*, 265–96.

Rutter, M. and Silberg, J. (2002). Gene–environment interplay in relation to emotional and behavioral disturbance. *Annual Review of Psychology, 53*, 463–90.

Rutter, M., Le Couteur, A. and Lord, C. (2003). *ADI-R: The Autism Diagnostic Interview-Revised*. Los Angeles, CA: Western Psychological Services.

Rutter, M. and Maughan, B. (2005). Dyslexia: 1965–2005. *Behavioural and Cognitive Psychotherapy, 33*, 389–402.

Rutter, M., Moffitt, T. E. and Caspi, A. (2006). Gene-environment interplay and psychopathology: Multiple varieties but real effects. *Journal of Child Psychology and Psychiatry, 47*, 226–61.

Rutter, M., Bishop, D., Pine, S., Scott, J., Stevenson, Taylor, E. and Thapar, A. (2008) (Eds.), *Rutter's child and adolescent psychiatry* (5th edn., pp. 820–40). Oxford: Blackwell.

Rutter, M., Caspi, A. and Moffitt, T. E. (2003). Using sex differences in psychopathology to study causal mechanisms: Unifying issues and research strategies. *Journal of Child Psychology and Psychiatry, 8*, 1092–115.

Rutter, M. and Plomin, R. (2009). Pathways from science findings to health benefits. *Psychological Medicine, 39*, 529–42.

Rutter, M. and Stevenson, J. (2010). Developments in child and adolescent psychiatry over the last 50 years. In M. Rutter, D. Bishop, D. Pine, S. Scott, J. Stevenson, E. Taylor and A. Thapar. (Eds.) *Rutter's child and adolescent psychiatry* (pp. 1–17). Oxford: Blackwell.

Ryan, N. D. (1998). Psychoneuroendocrinology of children and adolescents. *Psychiatric Clinics of North America, 21*, 435–41.

Ryckman, R. (2004). *Theories of Personality*. Belmont, CA: Thomson/Wadsworth.

Rynn, M., Puliafico, A., Heleniak, C., Rikhi, P., Ghalib, K. and Vidair, H. (2011). Advances in pharmacotherapy for pediatric anxiety disorders. *Depression and Anxiety, 28,* 76–87.

Saarni, C., Mumme, D. L. and Campos, J. J. (1998). Emotional development: Action, communication, and understanding. In W. Damon and N. Eisenberg (Eds.), *Handbook of child psychology* (5th edn., Vol. III, pp. 237–309). Hoboken, NJ: John Wiley and Sons Inc.

Sabatier, C. (2003). Assessment and culture: Psychology tests with minority populations. *Journal of Cross-Cultural Psychology, 34,* 484–5.

Sabshin, M. (1990). Turning points in twentieth-century American psychiatry. *The American Journal of Psychiatry, 147,* 1267–74.

Sadler, J. Z., Wiggins, O. P. and Schwartz, M. A. (1994). *Philosophical perspectives on psychiatric diagnostic classification.* Baltimore, MD: Johns Hopkins University Press.

Safren, S. A. and Pantalone, D. W. (2006). Social anxiety and barriers to resilience among lesbian, gay, and bisexual adolescents. In A. M. Omoto and H. S. Kurtzman (Eds.), *Sexual orientation and mental health: Examining identity and development in lesbian, gay, and bisexual people* (pp. 55–71). Washington, DC: American Psychological Association.

Salisbury, C. L. and Palombaro, M. M. (1998). Friends and acquaintances: Evolving relationships in an inclusive elementary school. In L. H. Meyer, H.-S. Park, M. Grenot-Scheyer, I. S. Schwartz and B. Harry (Eds.), *Making friends: The influences of culture and development* (pp. 81–104). Baltimore, MD: Paul H. Brookes.

Salloum, A., Carter, P., Burch, B., Garfinkel, A. and Overstreet, S. (2011). Impact of exposure to community violence, Hurricane Katrina, and Hurricane Gustav on posttraumatic stress and depressive symptoms among school age children. *Anxiety, Stress and Coping, 24,* 27–42.

Salmivalli, C. (2001). Peer-led intervention campaign against school bullying: Who considered it useful, who benefited? *Educational Research, 43,* 263–78.

Salmivalli, C., Lagerspetz, K., Bjorkqvist, K., Osterman, K. and Kaukiainen, A. (1996). Bullying as a group process: Participant roles and their relations to social status within the group. *Aggressive Behavior, 22,* 1–15.

Salmivalli, C., Kärnä, A. and Poskiparta, E. (2011) Counteracting bullying in Finland: The KiVa program and its effects on different forms of being bullied. *International Journal of Behavioral Development, 35,* 405–11.

Salmon, K. and Bryant, R. A. (2002). Posttraumatic stress disorder in children: The influence of

developmental factors. *Clinical Psychology Review, 22,* 163–88.

Saltzman, K. M., Weems, C. F. and Carrion, V. G. (2006). IQ and posttraumatic stress symptoms in children exposed to interpersonal violence. *Child Psychiatry and Human Development, 36,* 261–72.

Sameroff, A. (2010). A unified theory of development: A dialectic integration of nature and nurture. *Child Development, 81,* 6–22.

Santor, D. and Bagnell, A. (2008). Enhancing the effectiveness and sustainability of school based mental health programs: Maximizing program participation, knowledge uptake and ongoing evaluation using internet based resources. *Advances in School Mental Health Promotion, 1,* 17–28.

Santrock, J. W. (2007). *Essentials of life-span development.* Boston: McGraw-Hill.

Satterfield, J. H., Faller, K. J., Crinella, F. M., Schell, A. M., Swanson, J. M. and Homer, L. D. (2007). A 30-year prospective follow-up study of hyperactive boys with conduct problems: adult criminality. *Journal of the American Academy of Child and Adolescent Psychiatry, 46,* 601–10.

Satterfield, J. H., Schell, A. M., Backs, R. W. and Hidaka, K. C. (1984). A cross-sectional and longitudinal study of age effects of electrophysiological measures in hyperactive and normal children. *Biological Psychiatry, 19,* 973–90.

Sattler, J. M. and Hoge, R. D. (2006). *Assessment of children: Behavioral, social, and clinical foundations.* La Mesa, CA: Jerome M. Sattler.

Saunders, B. E., Berliner, L. and Hanson, R. F. (Eds.) (2004). *Child physical and sexual abuse: Guidelines for treatment (Revised report: April 26, 2004).* Charleston, SC: National Crime Victims Research and Treatment Center.

Sauter, F. M., Heyne, D. and Westenberg, P. M. (2009). Cognitive behaviour therapy for anxious adolescents: Developmental influences on treatment design and delivery. *Clinical Child and Family Psychology Review, 12,* 310–35.

Saxena, K., Nakonezny, P. A., Simmons, A., Mayes, T., Walley, A. and Emslie, G. (2009). Outpatient diagnosis and clinical presentation of bipolar youth. *Journal of the Canadian Academy of Child and Adolescent Psychiatry, 18,* 215–20.

Scahill, L. and Schwab-Stone, M. (2000). Epidemiology of ADHD in school-age children. *Child and Adolescent Psychiatric Clinics of North America, 9,* 541–55.

Scarr, S. and McCartney, K. (1983). How people make their own environments: A theory of genotype environment effects. *Child Development, 54,* 424–35.

Scerri, T. S. and Schulte-Körne, G. (2010). Genetics of developmental dyslexia. *European Child and Adolescent Psychiatry, 19*, 179–97.

Schachar, R., Taylor, E., Wieselberg, M., Thorley, G. and Rutter, M. (1987). Changes in family function and relationships in children who respond to methylphenidate. *Journal of the American Academy of Child and Adolescent Psychiatry, 26*, 728–32.

Schalock, R. L., Luckasson, R. A., Shogren, K. A., Borthwick-Duffy, S., Bradley, V., Buntinx, W. H. E., ... Yeager, M. H. (2007). The renaming of mental retardation: Understanding the change to the term intellectual disability. *Intellectual and Developmental Disabilities, 45*, 116–24.

Schendel, E. and Kourany, R. F. (1980). Cacodemonomania and exorcism in children. *Journal of Clinical Psychiatry, 41*, 119–23.

Scherrer, J. F., True, W. R., Xian, H., Lyons, M. J., Eisen, S. A., Goldberg, J., Lin, N. and Tsuang, M. T. (2000). Evidence for genetic influences common and specific to symptoms of generalized anxiety and panic. *Journal of Affective Disorders, 57*, 25–35.

Schiefelbein, V. L. and Susman, E. J. (2006). Cortisol levels and longitudinal cortisol change as predictors of anxiety in adolescents. *Journal of Early Adolescence, 26*, 397–413.

Schlachter, S. (2008). Diagnosis, treatment, and educational implications for students with attention-deficit/hyperactivity disorder in the United States, Australia, and the United Kingdom. *Peabody Journal of Education, 83*, 154–69.

Schmidt, L. A., Fox, N. A., Rubin, K. H., Sternberg, E. M., Gold, P. W., Smith, C. C. et al. (1997). Behavioral and neuroendocrine responses in shy children. *Developmental Psychobiology, 164*, 127–40.

Schmidt, U., Lee, S., Beecham, J., Perkins, S., Treasure, J., Yi, I., ... Eisler, I. (2007). A randomized controlled trial of family therapy and cognitive behavior therapy guided self-care for adolescents with bulimia and related disorders. *The American Journal of Psychiatry, 164*, 591–8.

Schneider, B. H. (1992). Didactic methods for enhancing children's peer relations: A quantitative review. *Clinical Psychology Review, 12*, 363–82.

Schneider, B. H. (1993a). *Children's social competence in context*. Oxford: Pergamon.

Schneider, B. H. (1993b). Social skills training and the aggressive child: On the value of small, paradoxical gain. *Exceptionality Education Canada, 3*, 195–203.

Schneider, B. H. (1999). A multi-method exploration of the friendships of children considered socially withdrawn by their school peers. *Journal of Abnormal Child Psychology, 27*, 115–23.

Schneider, B. H. (2000). *Friends and enemies: Peer relations in childhood*. London: Arnold.

Schneider, B. H. (2006). How much stability in attachment styles does Bowlby's theory imply?: Commentary on Lopez. *Infancia y Aprendizaje/Journal for the Study of Education and Development, 29*, 25–30.

Schneider, B. H. (2009). An observational study of the interactions of socially withdrawn/anxious early adolescents and their friends. *Journal of Child Psychology and Psychiatry, 50*, 799–806.

Schneider, B. H. and Amichai-Hamburger, Y. (2010). Electronic communication: Escape mechanism or relationship-building tool for shy, withdrawn children and adolescents? In K. H. Rubin and R. J. Coplan (Eds.), *The development of shyness and social withdrawal* (pp. 236–61). New York: Guilford Press.

Schneider, B. H. and Byrne, B. M. (1987). Individualizing social skills training for behaviour-disordered children. *Journal of Consulting and Clinical Psychology, 55*, 444–5.

Schneider, B. H., Wiener, J. and Murphy, K. (1994). Children's friendships: The giant step beyond peer acceptance. *Journal of Social and Personal Relationships, 11*, 323–40.

Schneider, B. H., Karcher, M. J. and Schlapkohl, W. (1999). Relationship counselling across cultures: Cultural sensitivity and beyond. In P. Pedersen (Ed.), *Multiculturalism: A fourth force in psychological interventions?* (pp. 167–90). Washington, DC: Taylor & Francis.

Schneider, B. H., Atkinson, L. and Tardif, C. (2001). Child–parent attachment and children's peer relations: A quantitative review. *Developmental Psychology, 37*, 86–100.

Schneider, B. H., Normand, S., Soteras-de Toro, M. d. P., Santana-Gonzalez, Y., Guilarte Tellez, J. A., Naranjo, M. C., Musle, M., Diaz-Socarras, F. and Robaey, P. (2011). Distinguishing features of Cuban children referred for professional help because of ADHD: Looking beyond the symptoms. *Journal of Attention Disorders, 15*, 328–7.

Schneider, B. H. and Tessier, N. (2007). Close friendship as understood by socially withdrawn, anxious early adolescents. *Child Psychiatry and Human Development, 38*, 339–51.

Schneider, B. H., Tomada, G., Normand, S., Tonci, E. and de Domini, P. (2008). Social support as a predictor of school bonding and academic motivation following the transition to Italian middle school. *Journal of Social and Personal Relationships, 25*, 287–310.

Schneider, B. H., Normand, S., Allès-Jardel, M., Provost, M. A. and Tarabulsy, G. M. (2009). *Conduites agressives chez les enfants: Perspectives développementales et psychosociales*. Québec: Presses de l'Université du Québec.

Schneider, B. H., Lee, M. D. and Alvarez-Valdivia, I. (2012). Adolescent friendship bonds in cultures of connectedness. In Laursen, B. and Collins, W. A. (Eds.), *Relationship pathways: From adolescence to young adulthood* (pp. 114–34). Thousand Oaks, CA: Sage.

Schneider, B. H., Normand, S., del Pilar Soteras de Toro, M., Santana Gonzalez, Y., GuilarteTellez, J. A., Carbonell Naranjo, M., Musle, M. et al. (in press). Distinguishing features of Cuban children referred for professional help because of ADHD: Looking beyond the symptoms. *Journal of Attention Disorders*.

Scholte, R. H. J., van Lieshout, C. F. M. and van Aken, M. A. G. (2001). Perceived relational support in adolescence: Dimensions, configurations, and adolescent adjustment. *Journal of Research on Adolescence, 11*, 71–94.

Schope, R. D. and Eliason, M. J. (2004). Sissies and tomboys: Gender role behaviors and homophobia. *Journal of Gay and Lesbian Social Services: Issues in Practice, Policy and Research, 16*, 73–97.

Schrag, P. and Divoky, D. (1975). *The myth of the hyperactive child*. New York: Pantheon.

Schreier, S.-S., Heinrichs, N., Alden, L., Rapee, R. M., Hofmann, S. G., Chen, J., Oh, K. J. and Bögels, S. (2010). Social anxiety and social norms in individualistic and collectivistic countries. *Depression and Anxiety, 27*, 1128–34.

Schulte-Markwort, M., Marutt, K. and Riedesser, P. (2003). *Cross-walks: ICD-10 – DSM-IV-TR*. Gottingen, Germany: Hogrefe and Huber Publishers.

Schultz, W. (2006). Behavioral theories and the neurophysiology of reward. *Annual Review of Psychology, 26*, 87–115.

Schumann, C. M. and Amaral, D. G. (2006). Stereological analysis of amygdala neuron number in autism. *The Journal of Neuroscience, 26*, 7674–9.

Schumann, C. M., Hamstra, J., Goodlin-Jones, B. I., Lotspeich, L. J., Kwon, H., Buonocore, M. H.,…Amaral, D. G. (2004). The amygdala is enlarged in children but not adolescents with autism; the hippocampus is enlarged at all ages. *Journal of Neuroscience, 24*, 6392–401.

Schwartz, C. E., Snidman, N. and Kagan, J. (1999). Adolescent social anxiety as an outcome of inhibited temperament in childhood. *Journal of the American Academy of Child and Adolescent Psychiatry, 38*, 1008–15.

Schwartz, C. E., Wright, C. I., Shin, L. M., Kagan, J. and Rausch, S. L. (2003). Inhibited and uninhibited infants "grown up": Adult amygdalar response to novelty. *Science, 300*, 1952–3.

Schwartz, D., Dodge, K. A., Pettit, G. S. and Bates, J. E. (2000). Friendship as a moderating factor in the pathway between early harsh home environment and later victimization in the peer group. *Developmental Psychology, 36*, 646–62.

Schwartz, D., Gorman, A. H., Duong, M. T. and Nakamoto, J. (2008). Peer relationships and academic achievement as interacting predictors of depressive symptoms during middle childhood. *Journal of Abnormal Psychology, 117*, 289–99.

Schwartz, S. H. and Ros, M. (1995). Value priorities in West European nations: A cross-cultural perspective. In G. Ben-Shakhar and A. Lieblich (Eds.), *Studies in psychology in honor of Solomon Kugelmass* (pp. 322–47). Jerusalem, Israel: Magnes Press.

Schwartzberg, S. (2000). *Casebook of psychological disorders: The human face of emotional distress*. Boston: Allyn & Bacon.

Schweitzer, J. B., Lee, D. O., Hanford, R. B., Zink, C. F., Ely, T. D., Tagamets, M. A. et al. (2004). Effect of methylphenidate on executive functioning in adults with attention-deficit/hyperactivity disorder: Normalization of behavior but not related brain activity. *Biological Psychiatry, 56*(8), 597–606.

Schweitzer, J. B., Faber, T. L., Grafton, S. T., Tune, L. E., Hoffman, J. M. and Kilts, C. D. (2000). Alterations in the functional anatomy of working memory in adult attention deficit hyperactivity disorder. *Am J Psychiatry, 157*(2), 278–80.

Schweinhart, L. J. and Weikart, D. P. (1989). The High/Scope Perry Preschool study: Implications for early childhood care and education, *Prevention in Human Services, 7*, 109–32.

Seelinger, G. and Mannel, M. (2007). Drug treatment in juvenile depression – is St. John's Wort a safe and effective alternative? *Child and Adolescent Mental Health, 12*, 143–9.

Seginer, R. (1992). Sibling relationships in early adolescence: A study of Israeli Arab sisters. *The Journal of Early Adolescence, 12*, 96–110.

Segman, R. H., Meltzer, A., Gross-Tsur, V., Kosov, A., Frisch, A., Inbar, E.,…Galili-Weisstub, E. (2002). Preferential transmission of interleukin-1 receptor antagonist alleles in attention deficit hyperactivity disorder. *Molecular Psychiatry, 7*, 72–4.

Segrave, J. O. and Hastad, D. N. (1982). Delinquent behaviour and interscholastic athletic participation. *Journal of Sport Behavior, 5*, 96–111.

Seidman, L. J., Biederman, J., Monuteaux, M. C., Valera, E., Doyle, A. E. and Farone, S. V. (2005). Impact of gender and age on executive functioning: Do girls and boys with and without attention deficit hyperactivity disorder differ neuropsychologically in preteen and teenage years? *Developmental Neuropsychology, 27*, 79–105.

Seifer R., et al. (2000). *Handbook of developmental psychopathology* (2nd edn.). Dordrecht, Netherlands: Kluwer Academic Publishers.

Seligman, L. D. and Ollendick, T. H. (1998). Comorbidity of anxiety and depression in children and adolescents: An integrative review. *Clinical Child and Family Psychology Review, 1*, 125–44.

Seligman, M. E. P. and Csikszentmihalyi, M. (2000). Positive psychology: An introduction. *American Psychologist, 55*, 5–14.

Selman, R. L. (1980). *The growth of interpersonal understanding.* Orlando, FL: Academic Press.

Selvini Palazzoli, M. (1978). *Self-starvation: From individual to family therapy in the treatment of anorexia nervosa.* New York: Aronson.

Semrud-Clikeman, M., Steingard, R. J., Filipek, P., Biederman, J., Bekken, K. and Renshaw, P. F. (2000). Using MRI to examine brain–behavior relationships in males with attention deficit disorder with hyperactivity. *Journal of the American Academy of Child and Adolescent Psychiatry, 39*, 477–84.

Serbin, L. A. and Karp, J. (2004). The intergenerational transfer of psychosocial risk: Mediators of vulnerability and resilience. *Annual Review of Psychology, 55*, 333–63.

Serketich, W. J. and Dumas, J. E. (1996). The effectiveness of behavioural parent training to modify antisocial behaviour in children: A meta-analysis. *Behavior Therapy, 27*, 171–86.

Serna, L. A., Nielsen, E., Mattern, N. and Forness, S. (2003). Primary prevention in mental health for Head Start classrooms: Partial replication with teachers as intervenors. *Behavioural Disorders, 28*, 124–9.

Seymour, B., O'Doherty, J. P., Dayan, P., Koltzenburg, M., Jones, A. K., Dolan, R. J. et al. (2004). Temporal difference models describe higher-order learning in humans. *Nature, 429*, 664–7.

Shackman, J. E., Shackman, A. J. and Pollak, S. D. (2007). Physical abuse amplifies attention to threat and increases anxiety in children. *Emotion, 7*, 838–52.

Shaffer, D., Fisher, P., Lucas, C. P., Dulcan, M. K. and Schwab-Stone, M. E. (2000). NIMH diagnostic interview schedule for children version IV (NIMH DISC-IV): Description, differences from previous version, and reliability of some common diagnoses. *Journal of the American Academy of Child and Adolescent Psychiatry, 39*, 28–38.

Shahar, G., Cohen, G., Grogan, K. E., Barile, J. P. and Henrich, C. C. (2009). Terrorism-related perceived stress, adolescent depression, and social support from friends. *Pediatrics, 124*, 235–40.

Shanahan, M. and Hofer, S. (2005). Social context in gene-environment interactions: Retrospect and prospect. *Journal of Gerontology: Series B, 60B*, 65–76.

Shannon, K. E., Beauchaine, T. P., Brenner, S. L., Neuhaus, E. and Gatzke-Kopp, L. (2007). Familial and temperamental predictors of resilience in children at risk for conduct disorder and depression. *Development and Psychopathology, 19*, 701–27.

Shapiro, A. K. (1960). A contribution to the history of the placebo effect. *Behavioral Sciences, 5*, 398–430.

Shapiro, J. R., Berkman, N. D., Brownley, K. A., Sedway, J. A., Lohr, K. N. and Bulik, C. M. (2007). Bulimia nervosa treatment: A systematic review of randomized controlled trials. *International Journal of Eating Disorders, 40*, 321–36.

Sharabany, R. (2006). The cultural context of children and adolescents: Peer relationships and intimate friendships among Arab and Jewish children in Israel. In X. Chen, D. C. French and B. H. Schneider (Eds.), *Peer relationships in cultural context* (pp. 452–78). New York: Cambridge University Press.

Shaw, D. S., Beck, J., Criss, M. and Schonberg, M. (2004). The development of family hierarchies and their relation to children's conduct problems. *Development and Psychopathology, 16*, 483–500.

Shaw, P., Eckstrand, K., Sharp, W., Blumenthal, J., Lerch, J. P., Greenstein, D. et al. (2007). Attention-deficit/hyperactivity disorder is characterized by a delay in cortical maturation. *PNAS, 104*(49), 19649–4.

Shaw, P., Lerch, J., Greenstein, D., Sharp, W., Clasen, L., Evans, A. et al. (2006). Longitudinal mapping of cortical thickness and clinical outcome in children and adolescents with attention-deficit/hyperactivity disorder. *Archives of General Psychiatry, 63*(5), 540–9.

Shaywitz, B. A., Shaywitz, S. E., Pugh, K. R., Mencl, W. E., Fulbright, R. K., Skudlarksi, P.,…Gore, J. C. (2002). Disruption of posterior brain systems for reading in children with developmental dyslexia. *Biological Psychiatry, 52*, 101–10.

Shaywitz, S. E. (1996). *Dyslexia. Scientific American, 275*, 98–104.

Shaywitz, S. E. (2003). *Overcoming dyslexia: A new and complete science-based program for reading problems at any level.* New York: Knopf.

Shaywitz, S. E., Morris, R. and Shaywitz, B. A. (2008). The education of dyslexic children from childhood to young adulthood. *Annual Review of Psychology, 59,* 451–75.

Shelton, T. L., Barkley, R. A., Crosswait, C., Moorehouse, M., Fletcher, K., Barrett, S.,...Metevia, L. (1998). Psychiatric and psychological morbidity as a function of adaptive disability in preschool children with aggressive and hyperactive-impulsive-inattentive behavior. *Journal of Abnormal Child Psychology, 26,* 475–94.

Shen, A. C. (2009). Long-term effects of interparental violence and child physical maltreatment experiences on PTSD and behavior problems: A national survey of Taiwanese college students. *Child Abuse and Neglect, 33,* 148–60.

Sheppard, A. (2011). The non-sense of raising school attendance. *Emotional and Behavioural Difficulties, 16*(3), 239–47.

Shibagaki, M. and Furuya, T. (1997). Baseline respiratory sinus arrhythmia and heart-rate responses during auditory stimulation of children with attention-deficit hyperactivity disorder. *Perceptual and Motor Skills, 84,* 967–75.

Shih, J., Chen, K. and Ridd, M. (1999). Monoamine oxidase: From genes to behavior. *Annual Review of Neuroscience, 22,* 197–217.

Shirk, S. R. and Russell, R. L. (1992). A reevaluation of estimates of child therapy effectiveness. *Journal of the American Academy of Child and Adolescent Psychiatry, 31,* 703–9.

Shochet, I. M., Homel, R., Cockshaw, W. D. and Montgomery, D. T. (2008). How do school connectedness and attachment to parents interrelate in predicting adolescent depressive symptoms?*Journal of Clinical Child and Adolescent Psychology, 37,* 676–81.

Shoham-Solomon, V. and Rosenthal, R. (1987). Paradoxical interventions: A meta-analysis. *Journal of Consulting and Clinical Psychology, 55,* 22–8.

Shomaker, L. B. and Furman, W. (2009). Interpersonal influences on late adolescent girls' and boys' disordered eating. *Eating Behaviors, 10,* 97–106.

Shorter, E. (2005). The history of the biopsychosocial approach in psychiatry: Before and after Engel. In P. White (Ed.), *Biopsychosocial medicine: An integrated approach to understanding illness* (pp. 1–19). Oxford: Oxford University Press.

Sideridis, G. D. (2007a). International approaches to learning disabilities: More alike or more different? *Learning Disabilities Research and Practice, 22,* 210–15.

Sideridis, G. D. (2007b). Why are students with LD depressed? A goal orientation model of depression vulnerability. *Journal of Learning Disabilities, 40,* 526–39.

Siegel, L. S. (1999). Issues in the definition and diagnosis of learning disabilities: A perspective on Guckenberger v. Boston University. *Journal of Learning Disabilities, 32,* 304–19.

Siegel, R. S., La Greca, A. M. and Harrison, H. M. (2009). Peer victimization and social anxiety in adolescents: Prospective and reciprocal relationships. *Journal of Youth and Adolescence, 38,* 1096–109.

Siegler, R. S. (1992). The other Binet. *Developmental Psychology, 28,* 179–90.

Siever, M. D. (1994). Sexual orientation and gender as factors in socioculturally acquired vulnerability to body dissatisfaction and eating disorders. *Journal of Consulting and Clinical Psychology, 62,* 252–60.

Sijtsema, J. J., Veenstra, R., Lindenberg, S., van Roon, A. M., Verhulst, F. C., Ormel, J. et al. (2010). Mediation of sensation seeking and behavioral inhibition on the relationship between heart rate and antisocial behavior: The TRAILS study. *Journal of the American Academy of Child and Adolescent Psychiatry, 49,* 493–502.

Silk, J. S., Nath, S. R., Siegel, L. R. and Kendall, P. C. (2000). Conceptualizing mental disorders in children: Where have we been and where are we going? *Development and Psychopathology, 12,* 713–35.

Silver, M. and Oakes, P. (2001). Evaluation of a new computer intervention to teach people with autism or Asperger syndrome to recognize and predict emotions in others. *Autism, 5,* 299–316.

Silverman, W. K. and Albano, A. M. (1996). *The anxiety disorders interview schedule for DSM-IV child and parent versions.* London: Oxford University Press.

Silverman, W. K. and Albano, A. M. (2004). *Anxiety Disorders Interview Schedule (ADIS-IV) child and parent interview schedules.* London: Oxford University Press.

Silverman, W. K., Pina, A. A. and Viswesvaran, C. (2008). Evidence-based psychosocial treatments for phobic and anxiety disorders in children and adolescents. *Journal of Clinical Child and Adolescent Psychology, 37,* 105–30.

Silverman, W. K. and Hinshaw, S. P. (2008). The second special issue on evidence-based psychosocial treatments for children and adolescents: A 10-year update. *Journal of Clinical Child and Adolescent Psychology, 37,* 1–7.

Silverthorn, P. and Frick, P. J. (1999). Developmental pathways to antisocial behavior: The delayed-onset pathway in girls. In D. Cicchetti (Ed.), *Development and psychopathology* (pp. 101–26). New York: Cambridge University Press.

Simon, B. (1992). Shame, stigma, and mental illness in ancient Greece. In P. J. Fink and A. Tasman (Eds.), *Stigma and mental illness* (pp. 29–39). Washington, DC: American Psychiatric Association.

Simonoff, E., Pickles, A., Charman, T., Chandler, S., Loucas, T. and Baird, G. (2008). Psychiatric disorders in children with autism spectrum disorders: Prevalence, comorbidity, and associated factors in a population-derived sample. *Journal of the American Academy of Child and Adolescent Psychiatry, 47*, 921–9.

Simonsen, J. (2011). Knowledge and power: The relevance of scientific doctrine and psychiatric evaluation to the American eugenics movement (Doctoral dissertation). Retrieved from Dissertation Abstracts International Section A: Humanities and Social Sciences (3311).

Simpkins, S. D., Eccles, J. S. and Becnel, J. N. (2008). The mediational role of adolescents' friends in relations between activity breadth and adjustment. *Developmental Psychology, 44*, 1081–94.

Simpson, J. A. and Weiner, E. S. C. (Eds.) (1989). *The Oxford English dictionary.* Oxford: Clarendon Press.

Sinclair, E., Salmon, K. and Bryant, R. A. (2007). The role of panic attacks in acute stress disorder in children. *Journal of Traumatic Stress, 20*, 1069–73.

Siperstein, G. N. and Leffert, J. S. (1997). Comparison of socially accepted and rejected children with mental retardation. *American Journal on Mental Retardation, 101*, 339–51.

Siperstein, G. N., Norins, J. and Mohler, A. (2006). Social acceptance and attitude change: Fifty years of research. In J. W. Jacobson, J. A. Mulick and J. Rojahn (Eds.), *Handbook of intellectual and developmental disabilities* (pp. 133–54). New York: Springer Publishing.

Siperstein, G. N. and Parker, R. C. (2008). Toward an understanding of social integration: A special issue. *Exceptionality, 16*, 119–24.

Siperstein, G. N., Glick, G. C. and Parker, R. C. (2009). Social inclusion of children with intellectual disabilities in a recreational setting. *Intellectual and Developmental Disabilities, 47*, 97–107.

Siperstein, G. N., Pociask, S. E. and Collins, M. A. (2010). Sticks, stones, and stigma: A study of students' use of the derogatory term "retard."*Intellectual and Developmental Disabilities, 48*, 126–34.

Skinner, B. F. (1948). *Walden two.* Indianapolis: Hackett.

Skounti, M., Philalithis, A. and Galanakis, E. (2007). Variations in prevalence of attention deficit hyperactivity disorder worldwide. *European Journal of Pediatrics, 166*, 117–23.

Slater, A. and Tiggemann, M. (2010). Body image and disordered eating in adolescent girls and boys: A test of objectification theory. *Sex Roles, 63*, 42–9.

Slesnick, N., Kaminer, Y. and Kelly, J. (2008). Psychosocial interventions for adolescent substance use disorders. In O. Bukstein and Y. Kaminer (Eds.), *Adolescent substance abuse: Psychiatric comorbidity and high risk behaviors.* New York: Haworth Press.

Slopen, N., Fitzmaurice, G., Williams, D. R. and Gilman, S. E. (2010). Poverty, food insecurity, and the behavior for childhood internalizing and externalizing disorders. *Journal of the American Academy of Child and Adolescent Psychiatry, 49*, 444–52.

Small, D. M., Simons, A. D., Yovanoff, P., Silva, S. G., Lewis, C. C., Murakami, J. L. and March, J. (2008). Depressed adolescents and comorbid psychiatric disorders: Are there differences in the presentation of depression? *Journal of Abnormal Child Psychology, 36*, 1015–28.

Smider, N. A., Essex, M. J., Kalin, N. H., Buss, K. A., Klein, M. H., Davidson, R. J. et al. (2002). Salivary cortisol as a predictor of socioemotional adjustment during kindergarten: A prospective study. *Child Development, 73*, 75–92.

Smidts, D. and Oosterlaan, J. (2007). How common are symptoms of ADHD in typically developing preschoolers? A study on prevalence rates and prenatal/demographic risk factors. *Cortex: A Journal Devoted to the Study of the Nervous System and Behavior, 43*, 710–17.

Smiley, E. and Cooper, S. (2003). Intellectual disabilities, depressive episode, diagnostic criteria and diagnostic criteria for psychiatric disorders for use with adults with learning disabilities/mental retardation (DC-LD). *Journal of Intellectual Disability Research, 47*, 62–71.

Smith, M. L., Glass, G. V. and Miller, T. I. (1980). *The benefits of psychotherapy.* Baltimore, MD: Johns Hopkins University Press.

Smolak, L. (2009). Risk factors in the development of body image, eating problems, and obesity. In L. Smolak and J. K. Thompson (Eds.), *Body image, eating disorders, and obesity in youth: Assessment, prevention, and treatment* (2nd edn., pp. 135–55). Washington, DC: American Psychological Association.

Smolak, L., Levine, M. P. and Striegel-Moore, R. (1996). *The developmental psychopathology of eating disorders: Implications for research, prevention, and treatment.* Mahwah, NJ: Lawrence Erlbaum Associates Inc.

Smoller, J. W. and Finn, C. T. (2003). Family, twin, and adoption studies of bipolar disorder. *American Journal of Medical Genetics, 123C*, 48–58.

Smoller, J. W., Gardner-Schuster, E. and Misiaszek, M. (2008). Genetics of anxiety: Would the genome recognize the DSM? *Depression and Anxiety, 25*, 368–77.

Smoller, J. W., Block, S. R. and Young, M. M. (2009). Genetics of anxiety disorders: The complex road from DSM to DNA. *Depression and Anxiety, 26*, 965–75.

Smythe, I., Everatt, J., Al-Menaye, N., He, X., Capellini, S., Gyarmathy, E. and Siegel, L. S. (2008). Predictors of word-level literacy amongst grade 3 children in five diverse languages. *Dyslexia: An International Journal of Research and Practice, 14*, 170–87.

Snoek, H., van Goozen, S. H., Matthys, W., Buitelaar, J. K. and van Engeland, H. (2004). Stress responsivity in children with externalizing behavior disorders. *Development and Psychopathology, 16*, 389–406.

Snyder, J., Horsch, E. and Childs, J. (1997). Peer relationships of young children: Affiliative choices and the shaping of aggressive behaviour. *Journal of Clinical Child Psychology, 26*, 145–56.

Socolar, R. R. S. (1997). A classification scheme for discipline: Type, mode of administration, context. *Aggression and Violent Behavior, 2*, 355–64.

Sokoloff, N. J. and Pratt, C. (2005). *Domestic violence at the margins: Readings on race, class, gender, and culture*. Piscataway, NJ: Rutgers University Press.

Solanto, M. V., Arnsten, A. F. T. and Castellanos, F. X. (2001). *Stimulant drugs and ADHD: Basic and clinical neuroscience*. New York: Oxford University Press.

Solish, A., Minnes, P. and Kupferschmidt, A. (2003). Integration of children with developmental disabilities in social activities. *Journal on Developmental Disabilities, 10*, 115–21.

Solish, A., Perry, A. and Minnes, P. (2010). Participation of children with and without disabilities in social, recreational and leisure activities. *Journal of Applied Research in Intellectual Disabilities, 23*, 226–36.

Solomon, M., Goodlin-Jones, B. L. and Anders, T. F. (2004). A social adjustment enhancement intervention for high functioning autism, Asperger's syndrome, and pervasive developmental disorder NOS. *Journal of Autism and Developmental Disorders, 34*, 649–68.

Solomon, M., Bauminger, N. and Rogers, S. J. (2011). Abstract reasoning and friendship in high functioning preadolescents with autism spectrum disorders. *Journal of Autism and Developmental Disorders, 41*, 32–43.

Sommers, C. H. and Satel, S. (2005). *One nation under therapy*. New York: St. Martin's Press.

Sommers, C. H. (2000). *The war against boys: How misguided feminism is harming our young men*. New York: Simon & Schuster.

Sondeijker, F. E., Ferdinand, R. F., Oldehinkel, A. J., Veenstra, R., Tiemeier, H., Ormel, J. et al. (2007). Disruptive behaviors and HPA-axis activity in young adolescent boys and girls from the general population. *Journal of Psychiatric Research, 41*, 570–8.

Sonuga-Barke, E. J., Dalen, L. and Remington, B. (2003). Do executive deficits and delay aversion make independent contributions to preschool attention-deficit/hyperactivity disorder symptoms? *Journal of the American Academy of Child and Adolescent Psychiatry, 42*, 1335–42.

Sonuga-Barke, E. J. S. (1998). Categorical models of childhood disorder: A conceptual and empirical analysis. *Journal of Child Psychology and Psychiatry, 39*, 115–33.

Sonuga-Barke, E. J. S. and Halperin, J. M. (2010). Developmental phenotypes and causal pathways in attention deficit hyperactivity disorder: Potential targets for early intervention? *Journal of Child Psychology and Psychiatry, 51*, 368–89.

Soomro, G. M., Crisp, A. H., Lynch, D., Tran, D. and Joughin, N. (1995). Anorexia nervosa in non-white populations. *British Journal of Psychiatry, 167*, 380–4.

Soomor, M., Crisp, A. H., Lynch, D., Tran, D. and Joughin, N. (1995). Anorexia nervosa in "non-white" populations. *British Journal of Psychiatry, 167*, 385–9.

Sooraksa, N. (2009). Influences of family and peers on amphetamine use behaviors in Thailand and implication for counseling. *International Journal of Child Health and Human Development, 2*, 2009, 449–60.

Sorensen, M. J., Mors, O. and Thomsen, P. H. (2005). DSM-IV or ICD-10-DCR diagnoses in child and adolescent psychiatry: Does it matter? *European Child and Adolescent Psychiatry, 14*, 335–40.

Southam-Gerow, M. A. and Kendall, P. C. (2002). Emotion regulation and understanding: Implications for child psychopathology and therapy. *Clinical Psychology Review, 22*, 189–222.

Souza, I., Pinheiro, M. A., Denardin, D., Mattos, P. and Rohde, L. A. (2004). Attention-deficit/hyperactivity disorder and comorbidity in Brazil: Comparisons between two referred samples. *European Child and Adolescent Psychiatry, 13*, 243–8.

Sowell, E. R., Thompson, P. M., Welcome, S. E., Henkenius, A. L., Toga, A. W. and Peterson, B. S. (2003). Cortical abnormalities in children and adolescents with attention-deficit hyperactivity disorder. The *Lancet, 362*, 1699–707.

Sowell, E. R., Peterson, B. S., Thompson, P. M., Welcome, S. E., Henkenius, A. L. and Toga, A. W. (2003). Mapping cortical change across the human life span. *Nature Neuroscience, 6*, 309–15.

Spaulding, J. and Balch, P. (1983). A brief history of primary prevention in the twentieth century: 1908–1980. *American Journal of Community Psychology, 11*, 59–80.

Speltz, M. L., McClellan, J., DeKlyen, M. and Jones, K. (1999). Preschool boys with oppositional defiant disorder: Clinical presentation and diagnostic change. *Journal of the American Academy of Child and Adolescent Psychiatry, 38*, 838–45.

Spence, S. H., Donovan, C. and Brechman-Toussaint, M. (1999). Social skills, social outcomes, and cognitive features of childhood social phobia. *Journal of Abnormal Psychology, 108*, 211–21.

Spencer, T. J., Biederman, J. and Mick, E. (2007). Attention-deficit/hyperactivity disorder: Diagnosis, lifespan, comorbidities, and neurobiology. *Journal of Pediatric Psychology, 32*, 631–42.

Spielmans, G. I., Pasek, L. F. and McFall, J. P. (2007). What are the active ingredients in cognitive and behavioral psychotherapy for anxious and depressed children? A meta-analytic review. *Clinical Psychology Review, 27*, 642–54.

Spielmans, G. I., Gatlin, E. T. and McFall, J. P. (2010). The efficacy of evidence-based psychotherapies versus usual care for youths: Controlling confounds in a meta-reanalysis. *Psychotherapy Research, 20*, 234–46.

Spika, B., Hood, R. W. and Gorsuch, R. J. (1985). *The psychology of religion*. Englewood Cliffs, NJ: Prentice Hall.

Spinrad, T. L., Eisenberg, N., Granger, D. A., Eggum, N. D., Sallquist, J., Haugen, R. G. et al. (2009). Individual differences in preschoolers' salivary cortisol and alpha-amylase reactivity: Relations to temperament and maladjustment. *Hormones and Behavior, 56*, 133–9.

Spock. B. and Needlman, R. (2004). *Dr. Spock's baby and child care: a handbook for parents of the developing child from birth through adolescence*. New York: Pocket Books.

Spoth, R., Redmond, C. and Shin, C. (1998). Direct and indirect latent-variable parenting outcomes of two universal family-focused preventive interventions: Extending a public health-oriented research base. *Journal of Consulting and Clinical Psychology, 66*, 385–99.

Sroufe, L. A. (1997). Psychopathology as an outcome of development. *Development and Psychopathology, 9*, 251–68.

Sroufe, L. A., Sonies, B. C., West, W. D. and Wright, F. S. (1973). Anticipatory heart-rate deceleration and reaction-time in children with and without referral for learning disability. *Child Development, 44*, 267–73.

Sroufe, L. A. and Rutter, M. (1984). The domain of developmental psychopathology. *Child Development, 55*, 17–29.

Sroufe, L. A., Carlson, E. A., Levy, A. K. and Egeland, B. (1999). Implications of attachment theory for developmental psychopathology. *Development and Psychopathology, 11*, 1–13.

Sroufe, L. A., Duggal, S., Weinfield, N. and Carlson, E. (2000). Relationships, development, and psychopathology. In A. J. Sameroff, M. Lewis and S. M. Miller (Eds.), *Handbook of developmental psychopathology* (pp. 75–92). New York: Springer Science and Business Media.

Stage, S. A. and Quiroz, D. R. (1997). A meta-analysis of interventions to decrease disruptive classroom behavior in public education settings. *School Psychology Review, 26*, 333–68.

Stahl, S. (2000). *Essential psychopharmacology of depression and bipolar disorder*. New York: Cambridge University Press.

Stallard, P., Richardson, T. and Velleman, S. (2010). Clinicians' attitudes towards the use of computerized cognitive behaviour therapy (cCBT) with children and adolescents. *Behavioural and Cognitive Psychotherapy, 38*, 545–60.

Stanton, M. D. (1981). Strategic approaches to family therapy. In A. S. Gurman and D. P. Kniskern (Eds.), *Handbook of family therapy* (pp. 361–402). New York: Brunner/Mazel.

Stark, W. (1992). Empowerment and social change: Health promotion within the Healthy Cities Project of WHO: Steps toward a participative prevention program. In G. W. Albee, L. A. Bond and T. V. C. Monsey (Eds.) *Improving children's lives: Global perspectives on prevention* (pp. 167–76). Newbury Park, CA: Sage Publications.

Statham, H., Ponder, M., Richards, M., Hallowell, N. and Raymond, F. L. (2011). A family perspective of the value of a diagnosis for intellectual disability: Experiences from a genetic research study. *British Journal of Learning Disabilities, 39*, 46–56.

Statt, D. A. (2003). *A student's dictionary of psychology*. New York: Psychology Press.

Stavrakaki, C., Vargo, B., Boodoosingh, L. and Roberts, N. (1987). The relationship between anxiety and depression in children: Rating scales and clinical variables. *The Canadian Journal of Psychiatry, 32*, 433–9.

Steele, R. G., Forehand, R. and Armisted, I. (1997). The role of family processes and coping strategies in the relationship between parental chronic illness and childhood internalizing problems. *American Journal of Community Psychology, 18*, 407–21.

Stefan, C. A. and Miclea, M. (2013). Effects of a multifocused prevention program on preschool children's competencies and behavior problems. *Psychology in the Schools, 50*, 382–402.

Stein, D., Latzer, Y. and Merick, J. (2009). Eating disorders: From etiology to treatment. *International Journal of Child and Adolescent Health, 2*, 139–51.

Stein, M. T., Blum, N. J. and Lukasik, M. K. (2005). Self-injury and mental retardation in a 7-year-old boy. *Developmental and Behavioral Pediatrics, 26*, 241–5.

Steinberg, L. and Silverberg, S. B. (1986). The vicissitudes of autonomy in early adolescence. *Child Development, 57*, 841–51.

Steinberg, L., Graham, S., O'Brien, L., Woolard, J., Cauffman, E. and Banich, M. (2009). Age differences in future orientation and delay discounting. *Child Development, 80*, 28–44.

Sternberg, R. G. and Kaufman, S. B. (2011). *Cambridge handbook of intelligence.* Cambridge: Cambridge University Press.

Steingard, R. J., Renshaw, P. F., Yurgelun-Todd, D., Appelmans, K. E. et al. (1996). Structural abnormalities in brain magnetic resonance images of depressed children. *Journal of the American Academy of Child and Adolescent Psychiatry, 35*, 307–11.

Steinhausen, H.-C. (2002). The outcome of anorexia nervosa in the 20th century. *The American Journal of Psychiatry, 159*, 1284–93.

Steinhausen, H.-C. (2009). Outcome of eating disorders. *Child and Adolescent Psychiatric Clinics of North America, 18*, 225–42.

Sterba, S. K. Prinstein, M. J. and Cox, M. J. (2007). Trajectories of internalizing problems across childhood: Heterogeneity, external validity, and gender differences. *Development and Psychopathology. 19*, 345–66.

Sternberg, R. J. (1990). Intellectual styles: Theory and classroom implications. In B. Z. Presseisen, R. J. Sternberg, K. W. Fischer, C. C. Knight and R. Feuerstein (Eds.), *Learning and thinking styles: Classroom interaction.* Washington, DC: National Education Association.

Sterns, P. N. (2008). *Oxford encyclopedia of the modern world.* Oxford: Oxford University Press.

Sterzer, P., Stadler, C., Krebs, A., Kleinschmidt, A. and Poustka, F. (2005). Abnormal neural responses to emotional visual stimuli in adolescents with conduct disorder. *Biological Psychiatry, 57*, 7–15.

Stevens, E. A. and Prinstein, M. J. (2005). Peer contagion of depressogenic attributional styles among adolescents: A longitudinal study. *Journal of Abnormal Child Psychology, 33*, 25–37.

Stevens, E. P. (1973). Marianismo: The other face of machismo in Latin America. In A. Pescatelo (Ed.), *Female and male in Latin America* (pp. 89–102). Pittsburgh, PA: University of Pittsburgh Press.

Stevens, N. R., Gerhart, J., Goldsmith, R. E., Heath, N. M., Chesney, S. A. and Hobfoll, S. E. (2013). Emotion regulation difficulties, low social support, and interpersonal violence mediate the link between childhood abuse and posttraumatic stress symptoms. *Behavior Therapy, 44*, 152–61.

Stevenson, A. (2010). *Oxford dictionary of English* (3rd cdn.). Oxford: Oxford University Press.

Stevenson, A, and Lindberg, C. A. (Eds.) (2010). *New Oxford American dictionary* (3rd edn.). Oxford: Oxford University Press.

Stewart, R. B., Beilfuss, M. L. and Verbrugge, K. M. (1995). That was then, this is now: An empirical typology of adult sibling relationships. Paper presented at the biennial meeting of the Society for Research on Child Development, Indianapolis.

Stewart, S., Kennard, B., Lee, P., Hughes, C., Mayes, T., Emslie, G. and Lewinsohn, P. (2004). A cross-cultural investigation of cognitions and depressive symptoms in adolescents. *Journal of Abnormal Psychology, 113*, 248–57.

Stice, E. (1998). Modeling of eating pathology and social reinforcement of the thin-ideal predict onset of bulimic symptoms. *Behaviour Research and Therapy, 36*, 931–44.

Stice, E. and Agras, W. S. (1999). Subtyping bulimic women along dietary restraint and negative affect dimensions. *Journal of Consulting and Clinical Psychology, 67*, 460–9.

Stice, E. and Shaw, H. (2004). Eating disorder prevention programs: A meta-analytic review. *Psychological Bulletin, 130*, 206–27.

Stice, E., Ragan, J. and Randall, P. (2004). Prospective relations between social support and depression: Differential direction of effects for parent and peer support? *Journal of Abnormal Psychology, 113*, 155–9.

Stice, E., Shaw, H. and Marti, C. N. (2007). A meta-analytic review of eating disorder prevention programs: Encouraging findings. *Annual Review of Clinical Psychology, 3*, 207–31.

Stice, E., Shaw, H., Becker, C. B. and Rohde, P. (2008). Dissonance-based interventions for the prevention of eating disorders: Using persuasion principles to promote health. *Prevention Science, 9*, 114–28.

Stice, E., Shaw, H., Bohon, C., Marti, C. N. and Rohde, P. (2009). A meta-analytic review of depression prevention programs for children and adolescents: Factors that predict magnitude of intervention effects. *Journal of Consulting and Clinical Psychology, 77*, 486–503.

Still, G. F. (1931). *The history of paediatrics: The progress of the study of the diseases of children up to the end of the 18th century.* Oxford: Oxford University Press.

Stith, S. M., Rosen, K. H. and McCollum, E. (2002). Developing a manualized couples' treatment for domestic violence: Overcoming challenges, *Journal of Marital and Family Therapy, 28,* 21–5.

Stockdill, J. W. (2005). National mental health policy and the community mental health centers, 1963–1981. In W. E. Pickren and S. F. Schneider (Eds.), *Psychology and the National Institute of Mental Health: A historical analysis of science, practice, and policy* (pp. 261–93). Washington, DC: American Psychological Association.

Stormshak, E. A. and Dishion, T. J. (2009). A school-based, family-centered intervention to prevent substance use: The Family Check-Up. *The American Journal of Drug and Alcohol Abuse, 35*(4), 227–32.

Storch, E. A., Masia-Warner, C., Crisp, H. and Klein, R. G. (2005). Peer victimization and social anxiety in adolescence: A prospective study. *Aggressive Behavior, 31,* 437–52.

Strain, P. S. (1985). Programmatic research on peer-mediated interventions. In B. H. Schneider, J. E. Ledingham and K. H. Rubin (Eds.), *Research strategies in children's social skill training.* Baltimore, MD: Paul Brookes.

Strang, N. M., Hanson, J. L. and Pollak, S. D. (2012). The importance of biological methods in linking social experience with social and emotional development. *Monographs of the Society for Research in Child Development, 77,* 61–6.

Strang, N. M., Hanson, J. L. and Pollak, S. D. (2012). The importance of biological methods in linking social experience with social and emotional development. In T. A. Dennis, K. A. Dennis and P. D. Hastings (Eds.), *Physiological measures of emotion from a developmental perspective: State of the science.* Monographs of the Society for Research in Child Development.

Straus, M. A., Hamby, S. L., Boney-McCoy, S. and Sugarman, D. B. (1996). The revised Conflict Tactics Scales (CTS2): Development and preliminary psychometric data. *Journal of Family Issues, 17,* 283–316.

Strauss, A. A. and Werner, H. (1942). Disorders of conceptual thinking in the brain-injured child. *Journal of Nervous and Mental Disease, 96,* 153–72.

Strauss, J., Muday, T., McNall, K. and Wong, M. (1997). Response style theory revisited: Gender differences and stereotypes in rumination and distraction. *Sex Roles, 36,* 771–92.

Strauss, K., Dapp, U., Anders, J., von Renteln-Kruse, W. and Schmidt, S. (2011). Range and specificity of war-related trauma to posttraumatic stress; depression and general health perception: Displaced former World War II children in late life. *Journal of Affective Disorders, 128,* 267–76.

Streiner, D. L. (2003). Diagnosing tests: Using and misusing diagnostic and screening tests. *Journal of Personality Assessment, 81,* 209–19.

Strelau, J. and Zawadzki, B. (2008). Temperament from a psychometric perspective: Theory and measurement. In G. J. Boyle, G. Matthews and D. H. Saklofske (Eds.), *The SAGE handbook of personality theory and assessment* (pp. 352–73). Thousand Oaks, CA: Sage Publications.

Striegel-Moore, R. H., Dohm, F. A., Kraemer, H. C., Taylor, C. B., Daniels, S., Crawford, P. B. and Schreiber, G. B. (2003). *The American Journal of Psychiatry, 160,* 1326–31.

Strober, M., Green, J. and Carlson, G. A. (1981). Phenomenology and subtypes of major depressive disorder in adolescence. *Journal of Affective Disorders, 3,* 281–90.

Strober, M., Freeman, R. and Morrell, W. (1997). The long-term course of severe anorexia nervosa in adolescents: Survival analysis of recovery, relapse, and outcome predictors over 10–15 years in a prospective study. *International Journal of Eating Disorders, 22,* 339–60.

Strober, M., Freeman, R., Lampert, C., Diamond, J. and Kaye, W. (2000). Controlled family study of anorexia nervosa and bulimia nervosa: Evidence of shared liability and transmission of partial syndromes. *The American Journal of Psychiatry, 157,* 393–401.

Stuebing, K. K., Fletcher, J. M., LeDoux, J. M., Lyon, G. R., Shaywitz, S. E. and Shaywitz, B. A. (2002). Validity of IQ-discrepancy classifications of reading disabilities: A meta-analysis. *American Educational Research Journal, 39,* 469–518.

Sturge-Apple, M. L., Davies, P. T. and Cummings, E. M. (2010). Typologies of family functioning and children's adjustment during the early school years. *Child Development, 81,* 1320–35.

Sukhodolsky, D. G. and Butter, E. M. (2007). Social skills training for children with intellectual disabilities. In J. W. Jacobson, J. A. Mulick and J. Rojahn (Eds.), *Handbook of intellectual and developmental disabilities* (pp. 601–18). New York: Springer Publishing.

Suliman, S., Mkabile, S. G., Fincham, D. S., Ahmed, R., Stein, D. J. and Seedat, S. (2009). Cumulative effect of multiple trauama on symptoms of posttraumatic stress disorder, anxiety, and depression in adolescents. *Comprehensive Psychiatry, 50,* 121–7.

Sullivan, H. S. (1953). *The interpersonal theory of psychiatry.* New York: Norton.

Sullivan, H. S. (1972). *Personality pathology.* New York: Norton.

Sullivan, P. F., Neale, M. and Kendler, R. S. (2000). Genetic epidemiology of major depression: Review and meta-analysis. *American Journal of Psychiatry, 157,* 1552–62.

Suzuki, K., Takei, N., Kawai, M., Minabe, Y. and Mori, N. (2003). Is Taijin Kyofusho a culture-bound syndrome? *The American Journal of Psychiatry, 160,* 1358.

Swanson, H. L., Carson, C. and Saches-Lee, C. M. (1996). A selective synthesis of intervention research for students with learning disabilities. *School Psychology Review, 25,* 370–91.

Swanson, H. L., Zheng, X. and Jerman, O. (2009). Working memory, short-term memory, and reading disabilities: A selective meta-analysis of the literature. *Journal of Learning Disabilities, 42,* 260–87.

Swanson, J., Posner, M. I., Cantwell, D., Wigal, S., Crinella, F., Filipek, P., Emerson, J., Tucker, D. and Nalcioglu, O. (1998). Attention-deficit/hyperactivity disorder: Symptom domains, cognitive processes, and neural networks. In R. Parasuraman (Ed.), *The attentive brain* (pp. 445–460). Cambridge, MA: The MIT Press.

Swanson, J. M., Flodman, P., Kennedy, J., Spence, M. A., Moyzis, R., Schuck, S.,...Posner, M. (2000). Dopamine genes and ADHD. *Neuroscience and Biobehavioral Reviews, 24,* 21–5.

Swanson, J. M., Greenhill, L., Wigal, T., Kollins, S., Stehli, A., Davies, M.,...Wigal, S. (2006). Stimulant-related reductions of growth rates in the PATS. *Journal of the American Academy of Child and Adolescent Psychiatry, 45,* 1304–13.

Swanson, J. M., Elliott, G. R., Greenhill, L. L., Wigal, T., Arnold, L. E., Vitiello, B.,...Volkow, N. D. (2007). Effects of stimulant medication on growth rates across 3 years in the MTA. *Journal of the American Academy of Child and Adolescent Psychiatry, 46,* 1015–27.

Swanson, J. M. and Volkow, N. D. (2009). Psychopharmacology: Concepts and opinions about the use of stimulant medications. *Journal of Child Psychology and Psychiatry, 50,* 180–93.

Swedo, S. (2009). *Report of the DSM-5 neurodevelopmental disorders work group.* Retrieved from American Psychiatric Association DSM5 development website: www.dsm5.org/progressreports/pages/0904reportofthedsm-vneurodevelopmentaldisordersworkgroup.aspx

Switzky, H. N. and Greenspan, S. (2006). *What is mental retardation: Ideas for an evolving disability in the 21st century.* Washington, DC: American Association on Mental Retardation.

Szasz, T. (1974). *The myth of mental illness: Foundations of a theory of personal conduct.* New York: Harper & Row.

Szasz, T. (2007). *The medicalization of everyday life: Selected essays.* Syracuse, NY: Syracuse University Press.

Szyf, M., McGowan, P. and Meaney, M. J. (2008). The social environment and the epigenome. *Environmental and Molecular Mutagenesis, 49,* 46–60.

Tager-Flusberg, H., Paul, R. and Lord, C. E. (2005). Language and communication in autism. In F. Volkmar, R. Paul, A. Klin and D. J. Cohen (Eds.), *Handbook of autism and pervasive developmental disorder* (3rd edn) (Vol. I, pp. 335–64). New York: Wiley.

Taghavi, M. R., Neshat-Doost, H. T., Moradi, A. R., Yule, W. and Dalgleish, T. (1999). Biases in visual attention in children and adolescents with clinical anxiety and mixed anxiety-depression. *Journal of Abnormal Child Psychology, 27,* 215–23.

Tamm, L., Menon, V. and Reiss, A. L. (2002). Maturation of brain function associated with response inhibition. *Journal of the American Academy of Child and Adolescent Psychiatry, 41,* 1231–8.

Tarter, R. E., Vanyukov, M. and Kirisci, L. (2008). Etiology of substance use disorder: Developmental perspective. In Y. Kaminer and O. G. Bukstein (Eds.), *Adolescent substance abuse: Psychiatric comorbidity and high-risk behaviors* (pp. 5–27). New York: Routledge/Taylor & Francis Group.

Taylor, C. B. (2010). Depression, heart rate, related variables and cardiovascular disease. *International Journal of Pyschophysiology, 78,* 80–8.

Taylor, E. (2009). Developing ADHD. *Journal of Child Psychology and Psychiatry, 50,* 126–32.

Taylor, E. and Rutter, M. (2010). Classification. In M. Rutter, D. Bishop, D. Pine, S. Scott, J. Stevenson, E. Taylor and A. Thapar (Eds.), *Rutter's child and adolescent psychiatry* (pp. 18–31). Oxford: Blackwell.

Taylor, S., Klein, L., Lewis, B., Gruenewald, T., Gurung, R. and Updegraff, J. (2000). Biobehavioral responses to stress in females: Tend-and-befriend, not fight or flight. *Psychological Review, 107,* 411–29.

Taylor, S., Klein, L., Lewis, B., Gruenwald, T., Gurung, R. and Updegraff, J. (2002). Sex differences in biobehavioral responses to threat: Reply to Geary and Flinn (2002). *Psychological Review, 109,* 751–3.

Taylor, S. E., Sherman, D. K., Kim, H. S., Jarcho, J., Takagi, K. and Dunagan, M. S. (2004). Culture and social support: Who seeks it and why? *Journal of Personality and Social Psychology, 87,* 354–62.

Tebes, J. K., Kauffman, J. S. and Connell, C. M. (2003). The evaluation of prevention and health promotion programs. In T. P. Gullotta and M. Bloom (Eds.), *Encyclopedia of primary prevention* (pp. 43–69). New York: Kluwer.

Teicher, M. H., Anderson, C. M., Polcari, A., Glod, C. A., Maas, L. C. and Renshaw, P. F. (2000). Functional deficits in basal ganglia of children with attention-deficit/hyperactivity disorder shown with functional magnetic resonance imaging relaxometry. *Nature Medicine, 6*, 470–3.

Tennant, A. (2007). Goal attainment scaling: Current methodological challenges. *Disability and Rehabilitation, 29*, 1583–8.

Teo, A. R. and Gaw, A. C. (2010). Hikikomori, a Japanese culture-bound syndrome of social withdrawal? A proposal for DSM-5. *Journal of Nervous and Mental Disease, 198*, 444–9.

Terr, L. C. (1979). Children of Chowchilla: A study of psychic trauma. *The Psychoanalytic Study of the Child, 34*, 547–623.

Terr, L. C. (1981). Psychic trauma in children: Observations following the Chowchilla school-bus kidnapping. *The American Journal of Psychiatry, 138*, 14–19.

Terr, L. C. and Watson, A. S. (1968). The battered child rebrutalized: 10 cases of medical-legal confusion. *The American Journal of Psychiatry, 124*, 1432–9.

Thalbitzer, S. (2008). *Emotion and insanity.* London: Routledge. (Original edition published in 1926.)

Thambirajah, M. S., Grandison, K. J. and De-Hayes, L. (2008). *Understanding school refusal.* London: Kingsley.

Thapar, A., Langley, K., Owen, M. J. and O'Donovan, M. C. (2007). Advances in genetic findings on attention deficit hyperactivity disorder. *Psychological Medicine, 37*, 1681–92.

Thapar, A., Harold, G., Rice, F., Langley, K. and O'Donovan, M. (2007). The contribution of gene–environment interaction to psychopathology. *Development and Psychopathology, 19*, 989–1004.

Thayer, J. F. and Lane, R. D. (2000). A model of neurovisceral integration in emotion regulation and dysregulation. *Journal of Affective Disorders, 61*, 201–16.

Thiemann, K. S. and Goldstein, H. (2004). Effects of peer training and written text cueing on social communication of school-age children with pervasive developmental disorder. *Journal of Speech, Language, and Hearing Research, 47*, 126–44.

Thienkrua, W., Cardozo, B. L., Chakkraband, M. L. S., Guadamuz, T. E., Pengjuntr, W., Tantipiwatanaskul, P.,...van Griensven, F. (2006). Symptoms of posttraumatic stress disorder and depression among children in tsunami-affected areas in southern Thailand. *Journal of the American Medical Association, 296*, 549–59.

Thome, J. and Jacobs, K. A. (2004). Attention deficit hyperactivity disorder (ADHD) in a 19th century children's book. *European Psychiatry, 19*, 303–6.

Thomas, A., Chess, S. and Birch, H. G. (1970). The origin of personality. *Scientific American, 223*, 102–9.

Thomas, C. R. and Penn, J. V. (2002). Juvenile justice mental health services. *Child and Adolescent Psychiatric Clinics of North America, 11*, 731–48.

Thomas, K. M., Drevets, W. C., Dahl, R. E., Ryan, N. D., Birmaher, B., Eccard, C. H. et al. (2001). Amygdala response to fearful faces in anxious and depressed children. *Archives of General Psychiatry, 58*, 1057–63.

Thompson, L. J. (1950). The contributions of mental hygiene and the future. In M. J. Shore (Ed.), *Twentieth century mental hygiene: New directions in mental health.* New York: Social Science Publishers.

Thompson, R. A. (1994). Emotion regulation: A theme in search of definition. In N. A. Fox (Ed.), *The development of emotion regulation: Biological and behavioral considerations* (Vol. LIX, pp. 25–52). Chicago: The University of Chicago Press.

Thompson, R. A. (2006). The development of the person: Social understanding, relationships, conscience, self. In N. Eisenberg, W. Damon and R. M. Lerner (Eds.), *Handbook of child psychology*: Vol. III, *Social, emotional, and personality development* (6th edn.) (pp. 24–98). Hoboken, NJ: John Wiley and Sons.

Thompson-Brenner, H., Eddy, K. T., Satir, D. A., Boisseau, C. L. and Westen, D. W. (2009). Personality subtypes in adolescents with eating disorders: Validation of a classification approach. *Infanzia e Adolescenza, 8*, 85–97.

Thornton, L. C., Frick, P. J., Crapanzano, A. M. and Terranova, A. M. (2013). The incremental utility of callous-unemotional traits and conduct problems in predicting aggression and bullying in a community sample of boys and girls. *Psychological Assessment, 25*, 366–78.

Thorpe, K. and Gardner, K. (2006). Twins and their friendships: Differences between monozygotic, dizygotic same-sex and dizygotic mixed-sex pairs. *Twin Research and Human Genetics, 9*, 155–64.

Tiedemann, M. (2008, October 20). *Health care at the Supreme Court of Canada.* Ottawa, ON: Parliament of Canada. Retrieved from www.parl.gc.ca/Content/LOP/ ResearchPublications/prb0519-e.htm

Timimi, S. (2002). *Pathological child psychiatry and the medicalization of childhood.* Hove: Brunner-Routledge.

Timimi, S. (2002). *Pathological child psychiatry and the medicalization of childhood.* New York: Brunner-Routledge.

Timimi, S. (2004). A critique of the International Consensus Statement on ADHD. *Clinical Child and Family Psychology Review, 7*, 59–63.

Timimi, S. (2005). *Naughty boys: Anti-social behavior, ADHD and the role of culture.* New York: Palgrave Macmillan.

Timimi, S. and Taylor, E. (2004). ADHD is best understood as a cultural construct. *The British Journal of Psychiatry, 184*, 8–9.

Timmons-Mitchell, J., Chandler-Holtz, D. and Semple, W. E. (1997). Post-traumatic stress disorder symptoms in child sexual abuse victims and their mothers. *Journal of Child Sexual Abuse: Research, Treatment, and Program Innovations for Victims, Survivors, and Offenders, 6,* 1–14.

Tobler, N. S., Roona, M. R., Ochshorn, P., Marshall, D. G., Streke, A. V. and Stackpole, K. M., School-based adolescent drug prevention programs: 1998 meta-analysis. *Journal of Primary Prevention, 20,* 275–336.

Tolin, D. F. and Foa, E. B. (2008). Sex differences in trauma and posttraumatic stress disorder: A quantitative review of 25 years of research. *Psychological Trauma: Theory, Research, Practice, and Policy, S,* 37–85.

Tonhajzerova, I., Ondrejka, I., Javorka, K., Turianikova, Z., Farsky, I. and Javorka, M. (2010) Cardiac autonomic regulation is impaired in girls with major depression. *Progress in Neuro-Psychopharmacology and Biological Psychiatry, 34,* 613–18.

Toplak, M. E., Connors, L., Shuster, J., Knezevic, B. and Parks, S. (2008). Review of cognitive, cognitive-behavioral, and neural-based interventions for attention-deficit/hyperactivity disorder. *Clinical Psychology Review, 28,* 801–23.

Toth, S. L., Rogosch, F. A., Sturge-Apple, M. and Cicchetti, D. (2009). Maternal depression, children's attachment security and representational development: An organizational perspective. *Child Development, 80,* 192–208.

Tremblay, R. E. (2000). The development of aggressive behavior during childhood: What have we learned in the past century?*International Journal of Behavioral Development, 24,* 129–41.

Tremblay, R. E., Nagin, D. S., Seguin, J. R., Zoccolillo, M., Zelazo, P. D., Boivin, M. et al. (2004). Physical aggression during early childhood: Trajectories and predictors. *Pediatrics, 114,* 43–50.

Trent, J. (2001). "Who shall say who is a useful person?" Abraham Myerson's opposition to the eugenics movement. *History of Psychiatry, 12,* 33–57.

Triandis, H. C., Marin, G., Lisansky, J. and Betancourt, H. (1984). Simpatia as a cultural script of Hispanics. *Journal of Personality and Social Psychology, 47,* 1363–75.

Trickett, E. J. (2007). George Albee and the nurturing spirit of primary prevention. *The Journal of Primary Prevention, 28,* 61–4.

Trowell, J., Kolvin, I., Weeramanthri, T., Sadowski, H., Berelowitz, M., Glasser, D. and Leitch, I. (2002). Psychotherapy for sexually abused girls: Psychopathological outcome findings and patterns of change. *British Journal of Psychiatry, 180,* 234–47.

Trull, T. J. (2007). Expanding the aperture of psychological assessment: Introduction to the special section on innovative clinical assessment technologies and methods. *Psychological Assessment, 19,* 1–3.

Trzesniewski, K. H., Moffitt, T. E., Caspi, A., Taylor, A. and Maughan, B. (2006). Revisiting the association between reading achievement and antisocial behaviour: New evidence of an environmental explanation from a twin study. *Child Development, 77,* 72–88.

Turner, S. M., Beidel, D. C. and Epstein, L. H. (1991). Vulnerability and risk for anxiety disorders. *Journal of Anxiety Disorders, 5,* 151–66.

Turner, S. M., Beidel, D. C. and Roberson-Nay, R. (2005). Offspring of anxious parents: Reactivity, habituation, and anxiety-proneness. *Behaviour Research and Therapy, 43,* 1263–79.

Tuvblad, C., Grann, M. and Lichtenstein, P. (2006). Heritability for adolescent antisocial behavior differs with socioeconomic status: Gene–environment interaction. *Journal of Child Psychology and Psychiatry, 47,* 734–43.

Tuvblad, C., Zheng, M., Raine, A. and Baker, L. A. (2009). A common genetic factor explains the covariation among ADHD ODD and CD symptoms in 9–10 year old boys and girls. *Journal of Abnormal Child Psychology, 37,* 153–67.

Twemlow, S. W. and Harvey, E. (2010). Power issues and power struggles in mental illness and everyday life. *International Journal of Applied Psychoanalytic Studies, 7,* 307–28.

Twohig, M. P., Field, C. E., Armstrong, A. B. and Dahl, A. L. (2010). Acceptance and mindfulness as mechanisms of change in mindfulness-based interventions for children and adolescents. In R. A. Baer (Ed.), *Assessing mindfulness and acceptance processes in clients: Illuminating the theory and practice of change* (pp. 226–49). Oakland, CA: Context Press/New Harbinger Publications.

Tzourio-Mazoyer, N., de Schonen, S., Crivello, F., Reutter, B., Aujard, Y. and Mazoyer, B. (2002). Neural correlates of woman face processing by 2-month-old infants. *Neuroimage, 15,* 454–61.

United States Office of Technology Assessment (1980). The efficacy and cost-effectiveness of psychotherapy. Background Paper No. 3. The implications of cost-effectiveness analysis of medical technology. Washington, DC: US Government Printing Office.

Unruh, S. and McKellar, N. A. (2013). Evolution, not revolution: School psychologists' changing practices in determining specific learning disabilities. *Psychology in the Schools, 50,* 353–65.

Urban, J. B., Lewin-Bizan, S. and Lerner, R. M. (2009). The role of neighbourhood ecological assets and activity involvement in youth developmental outcomes: Differential impacts of asset poor and asset rich neighborhoods. *Journal of Applied Developmental Psychology, 30*, 601–14.

US Department of Education (2007). *Twenty-five years of progress in educating children with disabilities through IDEA.* Retrieved from www2.ed.gov/policy/speced/leg/idea/history.html

US Department of Education (2010). *29th Annual report to congress on the implementation of the individuals with disabilities education act, 2007*, Vol. 1. Washington, DC: US Department of Education, Office of Special Education and Rehabilitative Services, Office of Special Education Programs.

US Department of Health and Human Services, Administration for Children and Families, Administration on Children, Youth and Families, Children's Bureau. (2010). *Child maltreatment 2009.* Retrieved from www.acf.hhs.gov/programs/cb/stats_research/index.htm%23;can

Useem, J., Useem, R. and Donoghue, J. (1963). Men in the middle of the Third Culture: The roles of American and non-Western people in cross-cultural administration. *Human Organization, 22*, 169–79.

Utendale, W. T. (2005). Cardiovascular reactivity during stress induction differentiates ADHD subtypes. Unpublished Masters. Concordia University, Montreal.

Vaidya, C. J., Austin, G., Kirkorian, G., Ridlehuber, H. W., Desmond, J. E., Glover, G. H. et al. (1998). Selective effects of methylphenidate in attention deficit hyperactivity disorder: A functional magnetic resonance study. *Proc Natl Acad Sci USA, 95*(24), 14494–9.

Vakili, N. and Gorji, A. (2006). Psychiatry and psychology in medieval Persia. *Journal of Clinical Psychiatry, 67*, 1862–9.

Valdivia, I. A., Schneider, B. H., Chavez, K. L. and Chen, X. (2005). Social withdrawal and maladjustment in a very group-oriented society. *International Journal of Behavioral Development, 29*, 219–28.

Valera, E. M., Faraone, S. V., Murray, K. E. and Seidman, L. J. (2006). Meta-analysis of structural imaging findings in attention-deficit/hyperactivity disorder. *Biological Psychiatry, 16*, 1361–9.

Valera, E. M., Faraone, S. V., Murray, K. E. and Seidman, L. J. (2007). Meta-analysis of structural imaging findings in attention-deficit/hyperactivity disorder. *Biological Psychiatry, 61*(12), 1361–9.

Vallbo, A. B., Hagbarth, K. E. and Wallin, B. G. (2004). Microneurography: How the technique developed and its role in the investigation of the sympathetic nervous system. *Journal of Applied Physiology, 96*, 1262–9.

van Beijsterveldt, C. E. M., Hudziak, J. J. and Boomsma, D. I. (2006). Genetic and environmental influences on cross-gender behavior and relation to behavior problems: A study of Dutch twins at ages 7 and 10 years. *Archives of Sexual Behavior, 35*, 647–58.

van Bokhoven, I., Matthys, W., van Goozen, S. H. M. and van Engeland, H. (2005). Prediction of adolescent outcome in children with disruptive behaviour disorders: A study of neurobiological, psychological and family factors. *European Child and Adolescent Psychiatry, 14*, 153–63.

van de Vijver, F. J. R. and Leung, K. (1997). *Methods and data analysis for cross-cultural research.* Thousand Oaks, CA: Sage Publications.

van de Vijver, F. J. R. and Poortinga, Y. H. (1997). Towards and integrated analysis of bias in cross-cultural assessment. *European Journal of Psychological Assessment, 13*, 29–37.

van de Wiel, N. M. H., van Goozen, S. H. M., Matthys, W., Snoek, H. and van Engeland, H. (2004). Cortisol and treatment effect in children with disruptive behaviour disorders: A preliminary study. *Journal of the American Academy of Child and Adolescent Psychiatry, 43*, 1011–18.

van den Berg, P., Thompson, J. K., Obremski-Brandon, K. and Coovert, M. (2002). The tripartite influence model of body image and eating disturbance: A covariance structure modeling investigation testing the meditational role of appearance comparison. *Journal of Psychosomatic Research, 53*, 1007–20.

van den Bergh, B. R. H., van Calster, B., Puissant, S. P. and van Huffel, S. (2008). Self-reported symptoms of depressed mood, trait anxiety and aggressive behavior in post-pubertal adolescents: Associations with diurnal cortisol profiles. *Hormones and Behavior, 54*, 253–7.

van der Bruggen, C. O., Stams, G. J. J. M. and Bögels, S. M. (2008). Research review: The relation between child and parent anxiety and parental control: A meta-analytic review. *Journal of Child Psychology and Psychiatry, 49*, 1257–69.

van der Bruggen, C. O., Bögels, S. M. and van Zeilst, N. (2010). What influences parental controlling behaviour? The role of parent and child trait anxiety. *Cognition and Emotion, 24*, 141–9.

van der Eijnden, R. J. J. M., Meerkerk, G. J., Vermulst, A. A., Spijkerman, R and Engels, R. C. M. E. (2008). Online communication, compulsive internet use, and psychosocial well-being among adolescents: A longitudinal study. *Developmental Psychology, 44*, 655–65.

van der KolkBA. and van der HartO. (1989). Pierre Janet and the breakdown of adaptation in psychological trauma. *American Journal of Psychiatry. 146*, 1530–40.

van der Oord, S., Prins, P. J. M., Oosterlaan, J. and Emmelkamp, P. M. G. (2008). Efficacy of methylphenidate, psychosocial treatments and their combination in school-aged children with ADHD: A meta-analysis. *Clinical Psychology Review, 28*, 783–800.

van der Veer, R. and Valsiner, J. (1988). Lev Vygotsky and Pierre Janet: On the social origin of the concept of sociogenesis. *Developmental Review, 8*, 52–65.

van Goozen, S. H. M., Matthys, W., Cohen-Kettenis, P. T., Gispen-de Wied, C., Wiegant, V. M. and van Engeland, H. (1998). Salivary cortisol and cardiovascular activity during stress in oppositional-defiant disorder boys and normal controls. *Biological Psychiatry, 43*, 531–9.

van Goozen, S. H. M., Fairchild, G., Snoek, H. and Harold, G. T. (2007). The evidence for a neurobiological model of childhood antisocial behaviour. *Psychological Bulletin, 133*, 149–82.

van Goozen, S. H. M., Fairchild, G. and Harold, G. T. (2008). The role of neurobiological deficits in childhood antisocial behavior. *Current Directions in Psychological Science, 17*, 224–8.

van Hoof, A., Raaijmakers, Q.A.W., van Beek, Y., Hale, W.W. and Aleva, L. (2008). A multi-mediation model on the relations of bullying, victimization, identity, and family with adolescent depressive symptoms. *Journal of Youth and Adolescence, 37*, 772–82.

van Kraayenoord, C. (2002). Celebrity and disability. *International Journal of Disability, Development and Education, 49*, 333–6.

van IJzendoorn, M. H., Schuengel, C. and Bakermans-Kranenburg, M. J. (1999). Disorganized attachment in early childhood: Meta-analysis of precursors, concomitants, and sequelae. *Development and Psychopathology, 11*, 225–49.

van IJzendoorn, M. H., Bakermans-Kranenburg, M. J. and Juffer, F. (2008). Video-feedback intervention to promote positive parenting: Evidence-based intervention for enhancing sensitivity and security. In F. Juffer, M. J. Bakermans-Kranenburg and M. H. van IJzendoorn (Eds.), *Promoting positive parenting: An attachment-based intervention* (pp. 193–202). New York: Taylor & Francis Group.

van Lier, P. A. and Koot, H. M. (2010). Developmental cascades of peer relations and symptoms of externalizing and internalizing problems from kindergarten to fourth-grade elementary school. *Development and Psychopathology, 22*, 569–82.

Varela, R. E., Vernberg, E. M., Sanchez-Sosa, J. J., Riveros, A., Mitchell, M. and Mashunkashey, J. (2004). Anxiety reporting and culturally associated interpretation biases and cognitive schemas: A comparison of Mexican, Mexican American, and European American Families.

Journal of Clinical Child and Adolescent Psychology, 33, 237–47.

Varela, R. E., Sanchez-Sosa, J. J., Biggs, B. K. and Luis, T. M. (2008). Anxiety symptoms and fears in Hispanic and European American children: Cross-cultural measurement equivalence. *Journal of Psychopathology and Behavioral Assessment, 30*, 132–45.

Varela, R. E. and Hensley-Maloney, L. (2009). The influence of culture on anxiety in Latino youth: A review. *Clinical Child and Family Psychology Review, 12*, 217–33.

Vasey, P. L. and Bartlett, N. H. (2007). What can the Samoan "fa'afafine" teach us about the western concept of gender identity disorder in childhood? *Perspectives in Biology and Medicine, 50*, 481–90.

Vaughn, S., Kim, A., Sloan, C. V. M., Hughes, M. T., Elbaum, B. and Sridhar, D. (2003). Social skills interventions for young children with disabilities: A synthesis of group design studies. *Remedial and Special Education, 24*, 2–15.

Vazsonyi, A. T. and Belliston, L. M. (2006). The cultural and developmental significance of parenting processes in adolescent anxiety and depression symptoms. *Journal of Youth and Adolescence, 35*, 491–505.

Vazsonyi, A. T. and Chen, P. (2010). Entry risk into the juvenile justice system: African American, American Indian, Asian American, European American, and Hispanic children and adolescents. *Journal of Child Psychology and Psychiatry, 51*, 668–78.

Verduin, T. L. and Kendall, P. C. (2008). Peer perceptions and liking of children with anxiety disorders. *Journal of Abnormal Child Psychology, 36*, 459–69.

Vernberg, E. M., Abwender, D. A., Ewell, K. K. and Beery, S. H. (1992). Social anxiety and peer relationships in early adolescence: A prospective analysis. *Journal of Clinical Child Psychology, 21*, 189–96.

Villarreal, G., Hamilton, D. A., Graham, D. P., Driscoll, I., Qualls, C., Petropoulos, H. and Brooks, W. M. (2004). Reduced area of the corpus callosum in posttraumatic stress disorder. *Psychiatry Research, 131*, 227–35.

Virués-Ortega, J. (2010). Applied behavior analytic intervention for autism in early childhood: Meta-analysis, meta-regression and dose-response meta-analysis of multiple outcomes. *Clinical Psychology Review, 30*, 387–99.

Vitaro, F., Tremblay, R. E., Kerr, M., Pagani, L. and Bukowski, W. M. (1997). Disruptiveness, friends' characteristics, and delinquency in early adolescence: A test of two competing models of development. *Child Development, 68*, 676–89.

Vitaro, F., Boivin, M. and Tremblay, R. E. (2007). Peers and violence: A two-sided developmental perspective. In D. J. Flannery, A. T. Vazsonyi and I. D. Waldman

(Eds.), *The Cambridge handbook of violent behaviour and aggression* (pp. 361–87). New York: Cambridge University Press.

Vitiello, B., Silva, S. G., Rohde, P., Kratochvil, C. J., Kennard, B. D., Reinecke, M. A., Mayes, T. L. et al. (2009). Suicidal events in the Treatment for Adolescents with Depression Study (TADS). *Journal of Clinical Psychiatry, 70,* 741–7.

Vitoroulis, I. et al. (2012) Social support and academic intrinsic motivation in three cultural settings: The roles of parents and peers. *Journal of Cross-Cultural Psychology, 43,* 704–22.

Vivanti, G., McCormick, C., Young, G. S., Abucayan, F., Hatt, N., Nadig, A., Ozonoff, S. and Rogers, S. J. (2011). Intact and impaired mechanisms of action understanding in autism. *Developmental Psychology, 47,* 841–56.

Volker, M. A. and Lopata, C. (2008). Autism: A review of biological bases, assessment, and intervention. *School Psychology Quarterly, 23,* 258–70.

Volkmar, F. R. (1998). Categorical approaches to the diagnosis of autism: An overview of DSM-IV ad ICD-10. *Autism, 2,* 45–59.

Volkow, N. D. and Swanson, J. M. (2003). Variables that affect the clinical use and abuse of methylphenidate in the treatment of ADHD. *The American Journal of Psychiatry, 160,* 1909–18.

von Stauffenberg, C. and Campbell, S. B. (2007). Predicting the early developmental course of symptoms of attention deficit hyperactivity disorder. *Journal of Applied Developmental Psychology, 28,* 536–52.

Vrabel, K. R., Hoffart, A., Ro, O., Martinsen, E. W. and Rosenvinge, J. H. (2010). Co-occurrence of avoidant personality disorder and child sexual abuse predicts poor outcome in long-standing eating disorder. *Journal of Abnormal Psychology, 119,* 623–9.

Vreeburg, S. A., Hoogendijk, W. J. G., van Pelt, J., DeRijk, R. H., Verhagen, J. C. M., van Dyck, R. et al. (2009). Major depressive disorder and hypothalamic-pituitary-adrenal axis activity results from a large cohort study. *Archives of General Psychiatry, 66,* 617–26.

Vuijk, P., van Lier, P., Crijnen, A. A. M. and Huizink, A. C. (2007). Testing sex-specific pathways from peer victimization to anxiety and depression in early adolescents through a randomized intervention trial. *Journal of Affective Disorders, 100,* 221–6.

Waas, G. A. and Graczyk, P. A. (1999). Child behaviors leading to peer rejection: A view from the peer group. *Child Study Journal, 29,* 291–306.

Wachtel, P. L. (2010). Beyond "ESTs": Problematic assumptions in the pursuit of evidence-based practice. *Psychoanalytic Psychology, 27,* 251–72.

Wainright, J. L., Russell, S. T. and Patterson, C. J. (2004). Psychosocial adjustment, school outcomes, and romantic relationships of adolescents with same-sex parents. *Child Development, 75,* 1886–98.

Wagner, R. K. and Sternberg, R. J. (1986). *Practical intelligence: Nature and origins of competence in the everyday world.* Cambridge: Cambridge University Press.

Wakabayashi, A., Baron-Cohen, S., Uchiyama, T., Yoshida, Y., Kuroda, M. and Wheelwright, S. (2007). Empathizing and systemizing in adults with and without autism spectrum conditions: Cross-cultural stability. *Journal of Autism and Developmental Disorders, 37,* 1823–32.

Wake, N. (2008). On our memory of gay Sullivan: A hidden trajectory. *Journal of Homosexuality, 55,* 150–65.

Wakefield, A. J., Murch, S. H., Anthony, A., Linnell, J., Casson, D. M., Malik, M.,…Walker-Smith, J. A. (1998). Ileal-lymphoid-nodular hyperplasia, non-specific colitis, and pervasive developmental disorder in children. *Lancet, 351,* 637–41.

Wakefield, J. C. (2007). Attachment and sibling rivalry revisited: The fantasy of the two giraffes revisited. *Psychoanalytic Study of the Child, 62,* 61–91.

Wakefield, J. C. (2008). New myths and harsh realities: Reply to Paul on the implications of Paul and Lentz (1977) for generalization from token economies to uncontrolled environments. *Behavior and Social Issues, 17,* 86–110.

Wakefield, J. C., Pottick, K. J. and Kirk, S. A. (2002). Should the DSM-IV diagnostic criteria for conduct disorder consider social context? *The American Journal of Psychiatry, 159,* 380–6.

Wakefield, J. C., Horwitz, A. V. and Schmitz, M. F. (2005). Are we overpathologizing the socially anxious? Social phobia from a harmful dysfunction perspective. *The Canadian Journal of Psychiatry, 50,* 317–19.

Waldron, H. B. et al. (2001). Treatment outcomes for adolescent substance abuse at 4- and 7-month assessments. *Journal of Consulting and Clinical Psychology, 69,* 802–13.

Walker, A., Flatley, J., Kershaw, C. and Moon, D. (2009). *Crime in England and Wales 2008/09: Findings from the British Crime Survey and police recorded crime,* Vol. I. Home Office Statistical Bulletin, No. 11/09. London, UK: Home Office.

Walker, J. S., Coleman, D., Lee, J., Squire, P. N. and Friesen, B. J. (2008). Children's stigmatization of childhood depression and ADHD: Magnitude and demographic variation in a national sample. *Journal of the American Academy of Child and Adolescent Psychiatry, 47,* 912–20.

Wallander, J. L., Dekker, M. C. and Koot, H. M. (2003). Psychopathology in children and adolescents with intellectual disability: Measurement, prevalence, course, and risk. In L. M. Glidden (Ed.), *International review of research in mental retardation* (Vol. XXVI, pp. 93–134). San Diego, CA: Academic Press.

Wallien, M. S. C., Swaab, H. and Cohen-Kettenis, P. T. (2007). Psychiatric comorbidity among children with gender identity disorder. *Journal of the American Academy of Child and Adolescent Psychiatry, 46*, 1307–14.

Wallien, M. S. C. and Cohen-Kettenis, P. T. (2008). Psychosexual outcome of gender-dysphoric children. *Journal of the American Academy of Child and Adolescent Psychiatry, 47*, 1413–23.

Wallien, M. S. C., Veenstra, R., Kreukels, B. P. C. and Cohen-Kettenis, P. T. (2010). Peer group status of gender dysphoric children: A sociometric study. *Archives of Sexual Behavior, 39*, 553–60.

Wallis, D., Russell, H. F. and Muenke, M. (2008). Review: Genetics of attention deficit/hyperactivity disorder. *Journal of Pediatric Psychology, 33*, 1085–99.

Walsh, B. T. and Garner, D. M. (1997). Diagnostic issues. In D. M. Garner and P. E. Garfinkel (Eds.), *Handbook of treatment for eating disorders* (2nd edn., pp. 25–33). New York: Guilford Press.

Walters, G. D. (2002). The heritability of alcohol abuse and dependence: A meta-analysis of behavior genetic research. *The American Journal of Drug and Alcohol Abuse, 28*, 557–84.

Wang, J., Simons-Morton, B. G., Farhardt, T. and Luk, J. W. (2009). Socio-demographic variability in adolescent substance use: Mediation by parents and peers. *Prevention Science, 10*, 387–96.

Wang, P. and Spillane, A. (2009). Evidence-based social skills interventions for children with autism: A meta-analysis. *Education and Training in Developmental Disabilities, 44*, 318–42.

Warren, C. S. and Messer, S. B. (1999). Brief psychodynamic therapy with anxious children. In S. W. Russ and T. H. Ollendick (Eds.), *Handbook of psychotherapies with children and families* (pp. 219–37). Dordrecht, Netherlands: Kluwer Academic Publishers.

Waschbusch, D. A., Pelham, W. E., Waxmonsky, J. and Johnston, C. (2009). Are there placebo effects in the medication treatment of children with attention-deficit hyperactivity disorder? *Journal of Developmental and Behavioral Pediatrics, 30*, 158–68.

Watamura, S. E., Donzella, B., Alwin, J. and Gunnar, M. R. (2003). Morning-to-afternoon increases in cortisol concentrations for infants and toddlers at child care: Age differences and behavioral correlates. *Child Development, 74*, 1006–20.

Waters, E. and Cummings, E. M. (2000). A secure base from which to explore close relationships. *Child Development, 71*, 164–72.

Watkins, B. and Lask, B. (2009). Defining eating disorders in children. In L. Smolak and J. K. Thompson (Eds.), *Body image, eating disorders, and obesity in youth: Assessment, prevention, and treatment* (2nd edn.) (pp. 35–46). Washington, DC: American Psychological Association.

Watson, D. (2005). Rethinking the mood and anxiety disorders: A quantitative hierarchical model for DSM-V. *Journal of Abnormal Psychology, 114*, 522–36.

Watson, J. B. and Raynor, R. (1920). Conditioned emotional reactions. *Journal of Experimental Psychology, 3*, 1–14.

Watters, E. (2010). *Crazy like use: The globalization of the American psyche.* New York: Free Press.

Watts, C. L., Nakkula, M. J. and Barr, D. J. (1997). Person-in-pairs, pairs-in-programs: Pairs in different institutional contexts. In R. L. Selman, C. L. Watts, and L. H. Schultz (Eds.), *Fostering friendship: Pair therapy for treatment and prevention.* Hawthorne, NY: Aldine Transaction.

Watzlawick, P., Weakland, J. H. and Fisch, R. (1974). *Change: Principles of problem formation and problem resolution.* Oxford: W. W. Norton.

Way, N. (2004). Intimacy, desire, and distrust in the friendships of adolescent boys. In N. Way and J. Y. Chu (Eds.), *Adolescent boys: Exploring diverse cultures of boyhood* (pp. 167–96). New York: New York University Press.

Wazana, A., Bresnahan, M. and Kline, J. (2007). The autism epidemic: Fact or artifact? *Journal of the American Academy of Child and Adolescent Psychiatry, 46*, 721–30.

Weaver, I. C., Cervoni, N., Champagne, F. A., D'Alessio, A. C., Sharma, S., Seckl, J. R. et al. (2004). Epigenetic programming by maternal behavior. *Nature Neuroscience, 7*, 847–54.

Webb, B. J., Miller, S. P., Pierce, T. B., Strawser, S. and Jones, W. P. (2004). Effects of social skill instruction for high-functioning adolescents with autism spectrum disorders. *Focus on Autism and Other Developmental Disabilities, 19*, 53–62.

Webster, A. A. and Carter, M. (2007). Social relationships and friendships of children with developmental disabilities: Implications for inclusive settings. A systematic review. *Journal of Intellectual and Developmental Disability, 32*, 200–13.

Webster-Stratton, C. H. and Reid, M. J. (2003). Treating conduct problems and strengthening social and emotional competence in young children: The Dina Dinosaur treatment program. *Journal of Emotional and Behavioral Disorder, 11*, 130–43.

Webster-Stratton, C. H. and Reid, J. M. (2011). The Incredible Years program for children from infancy to pre-adolescence: Prevention and treatment of behavior problems. In R. C. Murrihy, A. D. Kidman and T. H. Ollendick (Eds.), *Clinical handbook of assessing and treating conduct problems in youth*. New York: Springer Publishing.

Wechsler, D. (2003). *Wechsler Intelligence Scale for Children – Fourth Edition*. San Antonio, TX: Psychological Corporation.

Wedding, D., Boyd, M. A. and Niemiec, R. M. (2005). *Movies and mental illness: Using films to understand psychopathology*. Cambridge, MA: Hogrefe and Huber.

Weems, C. F., Zakem, A. H., Costa, N. M., Cannon, M. F. and Watts, S. E. (2005). Physiological response and childhood anxiety: Association with symptoms of anxiety disorders and cognitive bias. *Journal of Clinical Child and Adolescent Psychology, 34*, 712–23.

Weikart, D. (1983). Intervention programming for preschool children. In M. Perlmutter (Ed.), *Minnesota symposium in child psychology, 16*. New Jersey: Lawrence Erlbaum Associates.

Wehmeyer, M. L. (2003). Eugenics and sterilization in the heartland. *Mental Retardation, 41*, 57–60.

Weinberg, N. Z. (2001). Risk factors for adolescent substance abuse. *Journal of Learning Disabilities, 34*, 343–51.

Weinberg, R. A. (1989). Intelligence and IQ: Landmark issues and great debates. *American Psychologist, 44*, 98–104.

Weiss, B. and Weisz, J. R. (1990). The impact of methodological factors on child psychotherapy outcome research: A meta-analysis for researchers. *Journal of Abnormal Child Psychology, 18*, 639–70.

Weiss, B. and Garber, J. (2005). Developmental differences in the phenomenology of depression. *Development and Psychopathology*, 403–30.

Weissberg, R. P., Kumpfer, K. L. and Seligman, M. E. P. (2003). Prevention that works for children and youth: An introduction. *American Psychologist, 58*, 425–32.

Weissman, M. M., Paykel, E. and Klerman, G. (1972). *The depressed woman as a mother. Social Psychiatry, 7*, 98–108.

Weisz, J. and Bearman, S. K. (2010). Psychological treatments: Overview and critical issues for the field. In M. Rutter, D. Bishop, D. Pine, S. Scott, J. Stevenson, E. Taylor and A. Thapar (Eds.), *Rutter's child and adolescent psychiatry* (pp. 251–68). Oxford: Blackwell.

Weisz, J. R., Weiss, B., Alicke, M. D. and Klotz, M. L. (1987). Effectiveness of psychotherapy with children and adolescents: A meta-analysis for clinicians. *Journal of Consulting and Clinical Psychology, 55*, 542–9.

Weisz, J. R., Suwanlert, S., Chaiyasit, W., Weiss, B., Walter, B. R. and Anderson, W. W. (1988). Thai and American perspectives on over- and undercontrolled child behaviour problems: Exploring the threshold model among parents, teachers, and psychologists. *Journal of Consulting and Clinical Psychology, 56*, 601–9.

Weisz, J. R. and Eastman, K. R. (1995). Cross-national research in child and adolescent psychopathology. In F.C. Verhulst and H. M. Koot (Ed.), *The epidemiology of child and adolescent psychopathology*. (pp. 42–65). New York: Oxford University Press.

Weisz, J. R., Chaiyasit, W., Weiss, B., Eastman, K. L. and Jackson, E. W. (1995). A multimethod study of problem behaviour among Thai and American children in school: Teacher reports versus direct observations. *Child Development, 66*, 402–15.

Weisz, J. R., McCarty, C. A., Eastman, K. L., Suwanlert, S. and Chaiyasit, W. (1997). Developmental psychopathology and culture: Ten lessons from Thailand. In S. S. Luthar, J. A. Burack, D. Cicchetti and J. R. Weisz (Eds.), *Developmental psychopathology* (pp. 568–92). Cambridge: Cambridge University Press.

Weisz, J. R., Weiss, B., Suwanlert, S. and Chaiyasit, W. (2006). Culture and youth psychopathology: Testing the syndromal sensitivity model in Thai and American adolescents. *Journal of Consulting and Clinical Psychology, 74*, 1098–107.

Weisz, J. R., McCarty, C. A. and Valeri, S. M. (2006). Effects of psychotherapy for depression in children and adolescents: A meta-analysis. *Psychological Bulletin, 132*, 132–49.

Weisz, J. R., Jensen-Doss, A. and Hawley, K. M. (2006). Evidence-based youth psychotherapies versus usual clinical care: A meta-analysis of direct comparisons. *American Psychologist, 61*, 671–89.

Weisz, J. R. and Kazdin, A. E. (2010). *Evidence-based psychotherapies for children and adolescents* (2nd edn.). London: Guilford Press.

Wells, K. C., Pelham, W. E., Kotkin, R. A., Hoza, B., Abikoff, H. B., Abramowitz, A.,...Schiller, E. (2000). Psychosocial treatment strategies in the MTA study: Rationale, methods, and critical issues in design and implementation. *Journal of Abnormal Child Psychology, 28*, 483–505.

Werner, E. E. (1989). High-risk children in young adulthood: A longitudinal study from birth to 32 years. *American Journal of Orthopsychiatry, 59,* 72–81.

Werning, R., Loser, J. M. and Urban, M. (2008). Cultural and social diversity: An analysis of minority groups in German schools. *The Journal of Special Education, 42,* 47–54.

Wertsch, J. V. (1985). *Vygotsky and the social formation of the mind.* Cambridge, MA: Harvard University Press.

West, A. E., Jacobs, R. H., Westerholm, R., Lee, A., Carbray, J., Heidenreich, J. and Pavuluri, M. N. (2009). Child and family-focused cognitive-behavioral therapy for pediatric bipolar disorder: Pilot study of group treatment format. *Journal of the Canadian Academy of Child and Adolescent Psychiatry, 18,* 239–46.

Weyandt, L. L. (2005). Executive function in children, adolescents, and adults with attention deficit hyperactivity disorder: Introduction to the special issue. *Developmental Neuropsychology, 27,* 1–10.

Whalen, P. J., Rausch, S. L., Etcoff, N. L., McInerney, S. C., Lee, M. B. and Jenike, M. A. (1998a). Masked presentations of emotional facial expressions modulate amygdala activity without explicit knowledge. *Journal of Neuroscience, 18,* 411–18.

Whalen, P. J., Shin, L. M., McInerney, S. C., Fischer, H., Wright, C. I. and Rauch, S. L. (2001). A functional MRI study of human amygdala responses to facial expressions of fear versus anger. *Emotion, 1,* 70–83.

Wheeler, J. and Carlson, C. L. (1994). The social functioning of children with ADD and hyperactivity and ADD without hyperactivity: A comparison of their peer relations and social deficits. *Emotional and Behavioral Disorders, 2,* 2–12.

White, B. P. and Mulligan, S. E. (2005). Behavioral and physiologic response measures of occupational task performance: A preliminary comparison between typical children and children with attention disorder. *American Journal of Occupational Therapy, 59,* 426–36.

Winters, K. C., Leitten, W., Wagner, E. and O'Leary-Tevyaw, T. (2007). Use of brief interventions for drug abusing teenagers within a middle and high school setting. *Journal of School Health, 77,* 196–206.

Winters, K. C., Stinchfield, R. and Bukstein, O. G. (2008). Assessing Adolescent Substance Abuse. In Y. Kaminer and O. G. Bukstein (Eds.), *Adolescent substance abuse: Psychiatric comorbidity and high risk behaviors* (pp. 53–85). Binghamton, NY: Haworth Press.

White, J. and Halliwell, E. (2010). Examination of a sociocultural model of excessive exercise among male and female adolescents. *Body Image, 7,* 227–33.

White, S. H. (1992). Stanley Hall: From philosophy to developmental psychology. *Developmental Psychology, 28,* 25–34.

Wiener, J. and Schneider, B. H. (2002). A multisource exploration of the friendship patterns of children with and without learning disabilities. *Journal of Abnormal Child Psychology, 30,* 127–41.

Wiesner, M. and Capaldi, D. M. (2003). Relations of childhood and adolescent factors to offending trajectories of young men. *Journal of Research in Crime and Delinquency, 40,* 231–62.

Wilens, T. E. (2003). Does the medicating ADHD increase or decrease the risk for later substance abuse? *Revista Brasileira de Psiquiatria, 25,* 127–8.

Wilfley, D. E., Welch, R. R., Stein, R. I., Spurrell, E. B., Cohen, L. R., Saelens, B. E., . . . Matt, G. E. (2002). A randomized comparison of group cognitive-behavioral therapy and group interpersonal psychotherapy for the treatment of overweight individuals with binge-eating disorder. *Archives of General Psychiatry, 59,* 713–21.

Wilksch, S. M. (2010). Universal school-based eating disorder prevention: Benefits to both high- and low-risk participants on the core cognitive feature of eating disorders. *Clinical Psychologist, 14,* 62–9.

Willcutt, E. G., Betjemann, R. S., Pennington, B. F., Olson, R. K., DeFries, J. C. and Wadsworth, S. J. (2007). Longitudinal study of reading disability and attention-deficit/hyperactivity disorder: Implications for education. *Mind, Brain, and Education, 1,* 181–92.

Willcutt, E. G., Doyle, A. E., Nigg, J. T., Faraone, S. V. and Pennington, B. F. (2005). Validity of the executive function theory of ADHD: A meta-analytic review. *Biological Psychiatry, 57,* 1336–46.

Willem, L., Bijttebier, P., Claes, L. and Raes, F. (2011). Rumination subtypes in relation to problematic substance use in adolescence. *Personality and Individual Differences, 57,* 1–21.

Willemen, A. M., Schuengel, C. and Koot, H. M. (2009). Physiological regulation of stress in referred adolescents: The role of the parent–adolescent relationship. *Journal of Child Psychology and Psychiatry, 50,* 482–90.

Williams, K. D. (2007). Ostracism. *Annual Review of Psychology, 58,* 425–52.

Williams, L. R. et al. (2010). Early temperament, propensity for risk-taking and adolescent substance-related problems: A prospective multi-method investigation. *Addictive Behaviors. 35*(12), 1148–51.

Williams, R. J. and Chang, S. Y. (2000). A comprehensive and comparative review of adolescent substance abuse treatment outcome. *Clinical Psychology: Science and Practice, 7,* 138–66.

Williams, L. R., Fox, N. A., Lejuez, C. W., Reynolds, E. K., Henderson, H. A., Perez-Edgar, K. E., Steinberg, L. and Pine, D. S. (2010). Early temperament, propensity for risk-taking and adolescent substance-related problems: A prospective multi-method investigation. *Addictive Behaviors, 35*, 1148–51.

Williams, S. K. and Kelly, F. D. (2005). Relationships among involvement, attachment, and behavioral problems in adolescence: Examining father's influence. *The Journal of Early Adolescence, 25*, 168–96.

Willoughby, M. T., Angold, A. and Egger, H. L. (2008). Parent-reported attention-deficit/hyperactivity disorder symptomatology and sleep problems in a preschool-age pediatric clinic sample. *Journal of the American Academy of Child and Adolescent Psychiatry, 47*, 1086–94.

Wilson, A. M., Armstrong, C. D., Furrie, A. and Walcot, E. (2009). The mental health of Canadians with self-reported learning disabilities. *Journal of Learning Disabilities, 42*, 24–40.

Wilson, D. (2010, September, 1). Child's ordeal shows risks of psychosis drugs for young. The *New York Times.* Retrieved from www.nytimes.com

Wilson, D. (2010, October, 2). Side effects may include lawsuits. The *New York Times.* Retrieved from www. nytimes.com

Wilson, S. J. and Lipsey, M. W. (2000). Wilderness challenge programs for delinquent youth: A meta-analysis of outcome evaluations. *Evaluation and Program Planning, 23*, 1–12.

Wing, L. (1997). The history of ideas on autism: Legends, myths and reality. *Autism, 1*, 13–23.

Wing, L., Yeates, S. R., Brierley, L. M. and Gould, J. (1976). The prevalence of early childhood autism: Comparison of administrative and epidemiological studies. *Psychological Medicine, 6*, 89–100.

Winston, J. S., Strange, B. A., O'Doherty, J. and Dolan, R. J. (2002). Automatic and intentional brain responses during evaluation of trustworthiness of faces. *Nature Neuroscience, 5*, 277–83.

Winters, K. (2006). Gender dissonance: Diagnostic reform of gender identity disorder for adults. *Journal of Psychology and Human Sexuality, 17*, 71–89.

Winters, K. C., Botzet, A. M., Fahnhorst, T., Stinchfield, R. and Koskey, R. (2009). Adolescent substance abuse treatment: A review of evidence-based research. *Adolescent Substance Abuse, 9*, 73–96.

Wise, R. A. (2004). Dopamine, learning and motivation. *Nat Rev Neurosci, 5*, 483–94.

Wiseman, M. C. and Moradi, B. (2010). Body image and eating disorder symptoms in sexual minority men: A test and extension of objectification theory. *Journal of Counseling Psychology, 57*, 154–66.

Wolf, E. M. and Collier, C. S. (2005). Assessment and treatment of child and adolescent eating disorders. In L. VandeCreek and J. B. Allen (Eds.), *Innovations in clinical practice: Focus on health and wellness* (pp. 105–30). Sarasota, FL: Professional Resource Press.

Wolfe, D. A., Crooks, C. V., Lee, V., McIntyre-Smith, A. and Jaffe, P. G. (2003). The effects of children's exposure to domestic violence: A meta-analysis and critique. *Clinical Child and Family Psychology Review, 6*, 171–87.

Wolfe, V. V., Gentile, C. and Wolfe, D. A. (1989). The impact of sexual abuse on children: The PTSD formulation. *Behavior Therapy, 20*, 215–28.

Wolfensberger, W. and Tullman, S. (1982). A brief outline of the principle of normalization. *Rehabilitation Psychology, 27*, 131–45.

Wolff, S. (2004). The history of autism. *European Child and Adolescent Psychiatry, 13*, 201–8.

Wolraich, M. L., Hannah, J. N., Pinnock, T. Y., Baumgaertel, A. and Brown, J. (1996). Comparison of diagnostic criteria for attention-deficit hyperactivity disorder in a country-wide sample. *Journal of the American Academy of Child and Adolescent Psychiatry, 35*, 319–24.

Wong, B. Y. L. (2003). General and specific issues for researchers' consideration in applying the risk and resilience framework to the social domain of learning disabilities. *Learning Disabilities Research and Practice, 18*, 68–76.

Wood, J. (2006). Effect of anxiety reduction on children's school performance and social adjustment. *Developmental Psychology, 42*, 345–9.

Wood, J. J. (2012). School attendance problems and youth psychopathology: Structural cross-lagged regression models in three longitudinal data sets. *Child Development, 83*, 351–66.

Wood, J. J., McLeod, B. D., Sigman, M., Hwang, W. and Chu, B. C. (2003). Parenting and childhood anxiety: Theory, empirical findings, and future directions. *Journal of Child Psychology and Psychiatry, 44*, 134–51.

Wood, J. J., Piacentini, J. C., Southam-Gerow, M., Chu, B. C. and Sigman, M. (2006). Family cognitive behavioral therapy for child anxiety disorders. *Journal of the American Academy of Child and Adolescent Psychiatry, 45*, 314–21.

Wood, W. and Eagly, A. (2002). A cross-cultural analysis of the behaviour of women and men: Implications for the origins of sex differences. *Psychological Bulletin, 128*, 699–727.

Woodward, L. J. and Fergusson, D. M. (2001). Life course outcomes of young people with anxiety disorders in adolescence. *Journal of the American*

Academy of Child and Adolescent Psychiatry, 40, 1086–93.

World Health Organization. (n.d.). *History of the development of the ICD.* Retrieved March 3, 2014 from www.who.int/classifications/icd/en/HistoryOfICD.pdf

World Health Organization (1992). *The ICD-10 classification of mental and behavioural disorders; Clinical descriptions and diagnostic guidelines.* Geneva, Switzerland: World Health Organization.

World Health Organization (1996). *ICD-10 guide for mental retardation.* Geneva, Switzerland: World Health Organization of Mental Health and Prevention of Substance Abuse. Retrieved from www.who.int/mental_health/media/en/69.pdf

World Health Organization (n.d). *Mental health and substance abuse: Facts and figures: Mental retardation: From knowledge to action.* Retrieved from http://209.61.208.233/en/Section1174/Section1199/Section1567/Section1825_8086.htm, retrieved March 3, 2014.

Wozniak, J., Biederman, J., Kwon, A., Mick, E., Faraone, S., Orlovsky, J.,...van Grondelle, A. (2005). How cardinal are cardinal symptoms in pediatric bipolar disorder? An examination of clinical correlates. *Biological Psychiatry, 58,* 583–8.

Wright, R., John, L., Livingstone, A., Shepherd, N. and Duku, E. (2007). Effects of school-based interventions on secondary school students with high and low risks for antisocial behaviour. *Canadian Journal of School Psychology, 22,* 32–49.

Wu, G. H., Chong, M. Y., Cheng, A. T. and Chen, T. H. (2007). Correlates of family, school, and peer variables with adolescent substance use in Taiwan. *Social Science and Medicine, 64*(12), 2594–600.

Wuang, Y.-P., Chiang, C.-S., Su, C.-Y. and Wang, C.-C. (2011). Effectiveness of virtual reality using Wii gaming technology in children with Down syndrome. *Research in Developmental Disabilities, 32,* 312–21.

Wykes, T. and Callard, F. (2010). Diagnosis, diagnosis, diagnosis: Towards DSM-5. *Journal of Mental Health, 19,* 301–4.

Yang, T. T., Menon, V., Eliez, S., Blasey, C., White, C. D., Reid, A. J. et al. (2002). Amygdalar activation associated with positive and negative facial expressions. *Neuroreport, 13,* 1737–41.

Yates, A. (1989). Current perspectives on the eating disorders: I. History, psychological and biological aspects. *Journal of the American Academy of Child and Adolescent Psychiatry, 28,* 813–28.

Yeh, H.-C. and Lempers, J. D. (2004). Perceived sibling relationships and adolescent development. *Journal of Youth and Adolescence, 33,* 133–47.

Yeh, K. H. (2006). The impact of filial piety on the problem behaviours of culturally Chinese adolescents. *Journal of Psychology in Chinese Societies, 7,* 237–57.

Yeh, M. and Weisz, J. R. (2001). Why are we here at the clinic? Parent–child (dis)agreement on referral problems at outpatient treatment entry. *Journal of Consulting and Clinical Psychology, 69,* 1018–25.

Yen, J., Ko, C., Yen, C., Wu, H. and Yang, M. (2007). The comorbid psychiatric symptoms of internet addiction: Attention deficit and hyperactivity disorder (ADHD), depression, social phobia, and hostility. *Journal of Adolescent Health, 41,* 93–8.

Yabiku, S. T., Flavio, F., Kulis, S. and Parsai, M. B., Becerra, D. and Del-Colle, M. (2010). Parental monitoring and changes in substance use among Latino/a and non-Latino/a pre-adolescents in the Southwest. *Substance Use and Misuse, 45,* 2524–50.

Yirmiya, N. and Charman, T. (2010). The prodome of autism: Early behavioral and biological signs, regression, peri- and post-natal development and genetics. *Journal of Child Psychology and Psychiatry, 51,* 432–58.

Yoshikawa, H., Weisner, T. S., Kalil, A. and Way, N. (2008). Mixing qualitative and quantitative research in developmental science: Uses and methodological choices. *Developmental Psychology, 44,* 344–54.

Young, J. F., Mufson, L. and Davies, M. (2006). Efficacy of interpersonal psychotherapy-adolescent skills training: an indicated preventive intervention for depression. *Journal of Child Psychology and Psychiatry, 47,* 1254–62.

Young, S. and Amarasinghe, J. M. (2010). Practitioner review: Non-pharmacological treatments for ADHD: A lifespan approach. *Journal of Child Psychology and Psychiatry, 51,* 116–33.

Young, S. E., Smolen, A., Hewitt, J. K., Haberstick, B. C., Stallings, M. C., Corley, R. P. and Crowley, T. J. (2006). Interaction between MAO-A genotype and maltreatment in the risk for conduct disorder: Failure to confirm in adolescent patients. *The American Journal of Psychiatry, 163,* 1019–25.

Young, S. E. et al. (2006). Genetic and environmental vulnerabilities underlying adolescent substance use and problem use: General or specific?*Behavior Genetics. 36*(4), 603–15.

Young-Bruehl, E. (2004). Anna Freud and Dorothy Burlingham at Hempstead: The origins of psychoanalytic parent–infant observation, *The Annual of Psychoanalysis, 32,* 185–97.

Youssef, H. A, Youssef, F. A. and Dening, T. R (1996). Evidence for the existence of schizophrenia in medieval Islamic society. *History of Psychiatry, 7,* 55–62.

Yu, D. and Atkinson, L. (1993). Intellectual disability with and without psychiatric involvement: Prevalence estimates for Ontario. *Journal on Intellectual Disabilities, 2*, 92–9.

Yu, D. L. and Seligman, M. E. P. (2002). Preventing depressive symptoms in Chinese children. *Prevention and Treatment, 5*.

Yu, X. (2011). Three professors face sanctions following Harvard Medical School inquiry. *The Crimson*, July 2. Retrieved from http://www.thecrimson.com/article/2011/7/2/school-medical-harvard-investigation/

Yule, W., Perrin, S. and Smith, P. (1999). Post-traumatic stress disorders in children and adolescents. In W. Yule (Ed.), *Post-traumatic stress disorders: Concepts and therapy* (pp. 25–50). New York: John Wiley and Sons.

Zachar, P. (2009). Psychiatric comorbidity: More than a Kuhnian anomaly. *Philosophy, Psychiatry, and Psychology, 16*, 13–22.

Zagrina, N. A. (2009). Ivan Petrovich Pavlov and the authorities. *Neuroscience and Behavioral Physiology, 39*, 383–5.

Zahn, T. P., Schooler, C. and Murphy, D. L. (1986). Autonomic correlates of sensation seeking and monoamine-oxidase activity – Using confirmatory factor-analysis on psychophysiological data. *Psychophysiology, 23*, 521–31.

Zahn, T. P., Rapoport, J. L. and Thompson, C. L. (1980). Autonomic and behavioral effects of dextroamphetamine and placebo in normal and hyperactive prepubertal boys. *Journal of Abnormal Child Psychology, 8*, 145–60.

Zahn, T. P., Little, B. C. and Wender, P. H. (1978). Pupillary and heart-rate reactivity in children with minimal brain-dysfunction. *Journal of Abnormal Child Psychology, 6*, 135–47.

Zahn-Waxler, C., Shirtcliff, E. A. and Marceau, K. (2008). Disorders of childhood and adolescence: Gender and psychopathology. *Annual Review of Clinical Psychology, 4*, 275–303.

Zaider, T. I., Johnson, J. G. and Cockell, S. J. (2000). Psychiatric comorbidity associated with eating disorder symptomatology among adolescents in the community. *International Journal of Eating Disorders, 28*, 58–67.

Zalot, A., Jones, D. J., Kincaid, C. and Smith, T. (2009). Hyperactivity, impulsivity, inattention (HIA) and conduct problems among African American youth: The roles of neighbourhood and gender. *Journal of Abnormal Child Psychology, 27*, 535–49.

Zebracki, K. and Stancin, T. (2007). Cultural considerations in facilitating coping to a father's illness and bereavement in a Latino child. *Clinical Case Studies, 6*, 3–16.

Zehe, J. M., Colder, C. R., Read, J. P., Wieczorek, W. F. and Lengua, L. J. (2013). Social and generalized anxiety symptoms and alcohol and cigarette use in early adolescence: The moderating role of perceived peer norms. *Addictive Behaviors, 38*, 1931–9.

Zelli, A., Dodge, K. A., Lochman, J. E., Laird, R. D. and Conduct Problems Prevention Research Group (1999). The distinction between beliefs legitimizing aggression and deviant processing of social cues: Testing measurement validity and the hypothesis that biased processing mediates the effects of beliefs on aggression. *Journal of Personality and Social Psychology, 77*, 150–66.

Zetlin, A. G. and Murtaugh, M. (1988). Friendship patterns of mildly learning handicapped and nonhandicapped high school students. *American Journal on Mental Retardation, 92*, 447–54.

Zhou, J., Hofman, M. A., Gooren, L. J. G. and Swaab, D. F. (1995). A sex difference in the human brain and its relation to transsexuality. *Nature, 378*, 68–70.

Ziegler, J. C. and Goswami, U. (2005). Reading acquisition, developmental dyslexia, and skilled reading across languages: A psycholinguistic grain size theory. *Psychological Bulletin, 131*, 3–29.

Zoccolillo, M. (1992). Co-occurrence of conduct disorder and its adult outcomes with depressive and anxiety disorders: A review. *Journal of the American Academy of Child and Adolescent Psychiatry, 31*, 547–56.

Zoellner, L. A., Foa, E. B., Brigidi, B. D. and Przeworski, A. (2000). Are trauma victims susceptible to "false memories?" *Journal of Abnormal Psychology, 109*, 517–24.

Zubin, J. and Spring, B. (1977). Vulnerability: A new view on schizophrenia. *Journal of Abnormal Psychology, 86*, 103–26.

Zucker, K. J. (1985). Cross-gender-identified children. In B. W. Steiner (Ed.), *Gender dysphoria: Development, research, management* (pp. 75–174). New York: Plenum Press.

Zucker, K. J. (2006). Commentary on Langer and Martin's (2004) "How dresses can make you mentally ill: Examining gender identity disorder in children."*Child and Adolescent Social Work Journal, 23*, 533–55.

Zucker, K. J. (2007). Gender identity disorder in children, adolescents, and adults. In G. O. Gabard (Ed.), *Gabbard's treatments of psychiatric disorders* (4th edn., pp. 683–701). Washington, DC: American Psychiatric Press.

Zucker, K. J. and Bradley, S. J. (1995). *Gender identity disorder and psychosexual problems in children and adolescents*. New York: Guilford Press.

Zucker, K. J., Bradley, S. J. and Sanikhani, M. (1997). Sex differences in referral rates of children with gender identity disorder: Some hypotheses. *Journal of Abnormal Child Psychology*, *25*, 217–27.

Zucker, K. J. and Bradley, S. J. (2004). Gender identity and psychosexual disorders. In J. M. Wiener and M. K. Dulcan (Eds.), *The American Psychiatric Publishing textbook of child and adolescent psychiatry* (3rd edn., pp. 813–35). Arlington, VA: American Psychiatric Publishing.

Zucker, K. J. and Spitzer, R. L. (2005). Was the gender identity disorder of childhood diagnosis introduced into DSM-III as a backdoor maneuver to replace homosexuality? A historical note. *Journal of Sex and Marital Therapy*, *31*, 31–42.

Zucker, K. J. and Seto, M. C. (2010). Gender identity and sexual disorders. In M. Rutter, D. Bishop, D. Pine, S. Scott, J. Stevenson, E. Taylor and A. Thapar (Eds.), *Rutter's child and adolescent psychiatry* (5th edn., pp. 864–81). Oxford: Blackwell.

Zuroff, D. C., Mongrain, M. and Santor, D. A. (2004). Conceptualizing and measuring personality vulnerability to depression: Comment on Coyne and Whiffen. *Psychological Bulletin*, *130*, 489–511.

Zuvekas, S. H., Vitiello, B. and Norquist, G. S. (2006). Recent trends in stimulant medication use among US children. *The American Journal of Psychiatry*, *163*, 579–85.

INDEX

NOTE: Page numbers in **bold type** refer to glossary entries.